Principles and Practice of Surgery

Edited by

O. James Garden BSc MB ChB MD FRCS(Glasg) FRCS(Ed) FRACS(Hon)

Regius Professor of Clinical Surgery, Clinical and Surgical Sciences (Surgery), University of Edinburgh; Honorary Consultant Surgeon, Royal Infirmary of Edinburgh, UK

Andrew W. Bradbury BSc MB ChB MD MBA FRCS(Ed)

Head of Surgery and Professor of Vascular Surgery, University of Birmingham; Consultant Vascular Surgeon and Director of Research and Development, Heart of England NHS Foundation Trust Office, Birmingham, UK

John L.R. Forsythe MD FRCS(Ed) FRCS(Eng)

Consultant Transplant Surgeon, Transplant Unit, Royal Infirmary of Edinburgh; Reader in Clinical and Surgical Sciences (Surgery), University of Edinburgh, UK

Rowan W. Parks MD FRCSI FRCS(Ed)

Reader in Clinical and Surgical Sciences (Surgery), University of Edinburgh; Honorary Consultant Surgeon, Royal Infirmary of Edinburgh, UK

Surgery

CHURCHILL LIVINGSTONE

ELSEVIER

Fifth Edition

Edinburgh London New York Oxford Philadelphia St Louis Sydney Toronto 2007

CHURCHILL
LIVINGSTONE
ELSEVIER

An imprint of Elsevier Limited

© Longman Group Limited 1985
© Harcourt Brace and Company Limited 1998
© Harcourt Publishers Limited 2002
© 2007, Elsevier Limited. All rights reserved.

First edition 1985
Second edition 1991
Third edition 1995
Fourth edition 2002
Fifth edition 2007

ISBN: 978-0-443-10157-1

International edition ISBN: 978-0-443-10158-8

British Library Cataloguing in Publication Data
A catalogue record for this book is available from the British Library

Library of Congress Cataloging in Publication Data
A catalog record for this book is available from the Library of Congress

Note
Neither the Publisher nor the Editors assume any responsibility for any loss or injury and/or damage to persons or property arising out of or related to any use of the material contained in this book. It is the responsibility of the treating practitioner, relying on independent expertise and knowledge of the patient, to determine the best treatment and method of application for the patient.

The Publisher

Working together to grow
libraries in developing countries

www.elsevier.com | www.bookaid.org | www.sabre.org

ELSEVIER   BOOK AID
International   Sabre Foundation

The publisher's policy is to use **paper manufactured from sustainable forests**

ELSEVIER   your source for books, journals and multimedia in the health sciences
www.elsevierhealth.com

Commissioning Editor:
Laurence Hunter
Development Editor:
Barbara Simmons
Project Manager:
Andrew Palfreyman
Designer:
Stewart Larking
Illustration Manager:
Gillian Richards
Illustrators:
Gillian Lee and Barking Dog Illustrators

Printed in Spain

Contents

Section 3 **UPPER GASTROINTESTINAL SURGERY**

Section 4 **LOWER GASTROINTESTINAL SURGERY**

Section 5 **SURGICAL SPECIALTIES**

Preface

The production of this fifth edition of *Principles and Practice of Surgery* builds on the popularity of its predecessors and its companion volume *Davidson's Principles and Practice of Medicine.* Despite the ongoing changes to undergraduate curricula, the continuing success of these texts does suggest that there remains a need for an undergraduate textbook which provides a readable account of those facts that are relevant to current surgical practice. While the tendency to develop teaching modules across disciplines has a sound educational basis, there is still a place for a text which provides a ready source of information to the undergraduate and for the recently qualified doctor on the surgical ward. It is also apparent that a text such as this should not be focused on the preparation for final examinations alone but rather guide the student through the key core surgical topics which will be encountered within an integrated undergraduate curriculum and in subsequent clinical practice.

The editors welcome to the editorial team Mr Rowan Parks, Reader in Surgery at the University of Edinburgh. He has had the remit of ensuring a consistent style between chapters and sought to highlight relevant areas of evidence-based surgical practice. This edition sees the introduction of colour and considerable effort has been put into improving further the quality of radiographs and illustrations.

We remain indebted to the founders of this book, Professors Sir Patrick Forrest, Sir David Carter and Mr Ian Macleod who established the reputation of the textbook with students and doctors around the world. We are grateful to Laurence Hunter of Elsevier for his encouragement and enthusiasm and thank Barbara Simmons and Wendy Lee for keeping our contributors and ourselves in line during all stages of publication.

We very much hope that this edition continues the tradition and high standards set by our predecessors and that the revised content and presentation of the fifth edition satisfies the needs of tomorrow's doctors.

Edinburgh
2007

OJG, AWB, JLRF, RWP

Contributors

Andrew C. de Beaux MD FRCS MBChB
Consultant General and Oesophago-gastric Surgeon;
Honorary Senior Lecturer, University of Edinburgh, UK

Andrew W. Bradbury BSc MB ChB MD MBA FRCS(Ed)
Head of Surgery and Professor of Vascular Surgery,
University of Birmingham; Consultant Vascular
Surgeon and Director of Research and Development,
Heart of England NHS Foundation Trust Office,
Birmingham, UK

Roderick T. A. Chalmers MB ChB FRCS(Ed) MD FRCS(Gen)
Consultant Vascular Surgeon and Honorary Senior
Lecturer in Surgery, Royal Infirmary of Edinburgh, UK

Trevor J. Cleveland BMedSci BM BS FRCS FRCR
Consultant Vascular Radiologist, Sheffield Vascular
Institute, Sheffield Teaching Hospitals, Sheffield, UK

Fiona J Cutler MBChB MRCP MRCPath
Consultant, Scottish National Blood Transfusion
Service, Edinburgh, UK
Consultant Haemotologist, Ayr and Crosshouse
Hospitals, Ayrshire, UK

J. Michael Dixon BSc(Hons) MBChB MD FRCS FRCS(Ed)
FRCP
Consultant Surgeon and Senior Lecturer in Surgery,
Edinburgh Breast Unit, Western General Hospital,
Edinburgh, UK

Malcolm G. Dunlop MB ChB FRCS MD FMedSci
Professor of Coloproctology, University of Edinburgh;
Honorary Consultant Surgeon, Coloproctology Unit,
Western General Hospital, Edinburgh, UK

Kenneth C. H. Fearon MD FRCS(Gen)
Professor of Surgical Oncology, University of
Edinburgh; Honorary Consultant Surgeon, Western
General Hospital, Edinburgh

John L.R. Forsythe MD FRCS (Edin) FRCS(Eng)
Consultant Transplant Surgeon, Transplant Unit, Royal
Infirmary of Edinburgh, UK

O. James Garden BSc FRCS(Glasg) FRCS(Ed)
Regius Professor of Clinical Surgery, Clinical and
Surgical Sciences (Surgery), University of Edinburgh;
Honorary Consultant Surgeon, Royal Infirmary of
Edinburgh, UK

Marcus A. Green MB ChB FRCS(Ortho) Dip IMC RCS(Ed)
Consultant Orthopaedic Surgeon, Royal Orthopaedic
Hospital, Birmingham, UK

Rachel H. A. Green MBChB BMed Biol FRCP FRCPath
Clinical Director, West of Scotland Blood
Transfusion Centre at Gartnavel General Hospital,
Glasgow, UK

Ian F. Laurenson MA MD FRCP(Ed) FRCPath
Consultant Microbiologist, Royal Infirmary of
Edinburgh; Honorary Clinical Senior Lecturer,
University of Edinburgh, UK

T.W.J. Lennard MBBS (Hons) MD FRCS
Head of School of Surgical and Reproductive
Sciences, The Medical School, University of Newcastle
upon Tyne, UK

Paramananthan Mariappan MBBS FRCS(Urol) FEBU
FRCSEd, Board of Urology Cert (Mal)
Consultant Urological Surgeon,
Department of Urology, Western General Hospital,
Edinburgh, UK

Lorna P. Marson MB BS FRCS MD
Senior Lecturer in Transplant Surgery, University of
Edinburgh; Honorary Consultant Transplant Surgeon,
Royal Infirmary of Edinburgh, UK

D. Brian L. McClelland MBChB BSc(Hons) MD(London)
FRCP(Ed) FRCPath
Consultant, Scottish National Blood Transfusion
Service, Edinburgh, UK

Dermot W. McKeown MBChB FRCA FRCS(Ed) FCEM
Consultant in Anaesthesia and Intensive Care, Royal
Infirmary of Edinburgh, UK

Robert P. Mills MBBS FRCS(Eng) FRCS(Ed) MS MPhil
Consultant Otolaryngologist, Lothian Health University
Hospitals Division; Senior Lecturer, University of
Edinburgh, Edinburgh, UK

Lynn Myles MB ChB BSc(Hons) MD FRCP(Ed) SN
Consultant Neurosurgeon, Western General Hospital,
Edinburgh, and Royal Hospital for Sick Children,
Edinburgh, UK

Rowan W. Parks MD FRCSI FRCS(Ed)
Senior Lecturer in Clinical and Surgery Sciences
(Surgery), University of Edinburgh; Royal Infirmary of
Edinburgh

Simon Paterson-Brown MBBS MPhil MS FRCS
Honorary Senior Lecturer, Clinical and Surgical
Sciences (Surgery), University of Edinburgh; Consultant
General and Upper Gastrointestinal Surgeon, Royal
Infirmary of Edinburgh, UK

Anthony J. Pollok BSC MB ChB FRCA
Consultant Anaesthetist, Intensive Care Unit, Royal
Infirmary of Edinburgh, UK

Mark A. Potter BSc MBChB MD FRCS
Consultant Colorectal Surgeon, Western General
Hospital, Edinburgh, UK

Colin E. Robertson BA(Hons) MBChB MRCP(UK) FRCP(Ed)
FRCS(Ed) FFAEM
Honorary Professor of Accident and Emergency
Medicine and Surgery, University of Edinburgh;
Consultant, Accident and Emergency Department,
Royal Infirmary of Edinburgh

Laurence H. Stewart MBChB MD FRCS(Ed) FRCS(Urol)
Consultant Urological Surgeon, Western General
Hospital, Edinburgh, UK

William S. Walker MA MB BChir FRCS(Eng), FRCS(Ed)
Consultant Cardiothoracic Surgeon, Royal Infirmary of
Edinburgh, UK

Timothy S. Walsh MB ChB(Hons) BSc(Hons) MRCP FRCA
MD
Consultant in Anaesthetics and Intensive Care, The
Royal Infirmary of Edinburgh, UK

James D. Watson MB ChB FRCSEd FRCSG(Plast)
Consultant Plastic Surgeon, St John's Hospital,
Livingston; Honorary (Clinical) Senior Lecturer in
Surgery, University of Edinburgh, Edinburgh, UK

Stephen J. Wigmore BSc MBBS MD FRCS(Ed)
Professor of Transplantation Surgery, University of
Birmingham, UK

John A. Wilson MB ChB MRCP(UK) FRCA
Consultant in Anaesthesia and Pain Medicine, The
Royal Infirmary of Edinburgh, UK

Section 1
PRINCIPLES OF SURGICAL CARE

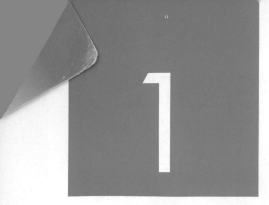

1

T.S. WALSH

The metabolic response to injury

INTRODUCTION

Following accidental or deliberate injury, a characteristic series of changes occurs, both locally at the site of injury and within the body generally; these changes are intended to restore the body to its pre-injury condition. They are mediated via many different systems, which interact in a complex manner and may be modified by external factors, such as drugs and other treatments administered to the patient. The magnitude of the metabolic response is generally proportional to the severity of tissue injury, but can be modified by additional factors such as infection. The response to injury has probably evolved to aid recovery, by mobilizing substrates and mechanisms of preventing infection, and by activating repair processes. However, many of these physiological changes can now be modified or corrected by treatments. Although the metabolic response aims to return an individual to health, it can sometimes have harmful effects. For example, a major response can damage organs distant to the injured site itself. In modern surgery, a major goal is to minimize the metabolic response to surgery in order to shorten recovery times. This has been achieved through surgical techniques that minimize tissue damage. When a major metabolic response does occur, the emphasis is on managing the patient in a way that minimizes further tissue damage either at the original site of injury or in other organs. This chapter describes the principal physiological systems involved in the metabolic response to injury, how they function and are controlled, and at what stage they are important.

FEATURES OF THE METABOLIC RESPONSE WHEN NOT MODIFIED BY MEDICAL INTERVENTIONS

Early observations of the metabolic response to injury were made in patients before the advent of medical treatments such as intravenous fluids. This unmodified response was divided into two phases: the 'ebb' and the 'flow'. During the ebb phase, which usually comprised the first few hours after injury, the individual was cold and hypotensive. In current medical practice this corresponds to the period of traumatic shock before or during resuscitation. When fluid therapies and blood transfusions were introduced into medical practice, the shock that occurred in this phase was sometimes found to be reversible ('reversible shock') and in other cases irreversible ('irreversible shock'). Irreversible shock probably occurs when the metabolic response has initiated inflammatory processes that cause a downward spiral of further injury in other organs.

The flow phase followed if the individual survived, and was also described in two parts. The initial catabolic phase was characterized by a high metabolic rate, breakdown of proteins and fats, a net loss of body nitrogen (negative nitrogen balance) and weight loss. This phase usually lasted about a week and was followed by an anabolic phase, during which protein and fat stores were restored and weight gain

Table 1.1	SOME CYTOKINES INVOLVED IN THE ACUTE INFLAMMATORY RESPONSE
Cytokine	**Relevant actions**
TNF-α	Pro-inflammatory; release of leucocytes by bone marrow; activation of leucocytes and endothelial cells
IL-1	Fever; T-cell and macrophage activation
IL-6	Growth and differentiation of lymphocytes; activation of the acute-phase protein response
IL-8	Chemotactic for neutrophils and T cells
IL-10	Inhibits immune function
(TNF = tumour necrosis factor; IL = interleukin)	

occurred (positive nitrogen balance). The recovery phase usually lasted 2–4 weeks.

This characteristic pattern probably occurs after all types of injury, but the degree depends on the magnitude of tissue injury and how the response is modified by interventions.

FACTORS MEDIATING THE METABOLIC RESPONSE TO INJURY

The metabolic response is a complex interaction between many body systems.

THE ACUTE INFLAMMATORY RESPONSE

Inflammatory cells (macrophages and neutrophils) and cytokines (molecules with the capacity to act on a wide range of cell types, both at the site of injury and at distant sites in the body) are mediators of the acute inflammatory response. Physical damage to tissues results in local activation of cells such as tissue macrophages. These cells release a variety of cytokines (Table 1.1). Some of these, such as interleukin-8 (IL-8), attract large numbers of circulating macrophages and neutrophils to the site of injury. Other cytokines, such as tumour necrosis factor alpha (TNF-α), IL-1 and IL-6, activate these inflammatory cells, enabling them to clear dead tissue and kill bacteria. Although these cytokines are produced locally, their release into the circulation initiates some of the systemic features of the metabolic response, such as fever (IL-1) and the acute-phase protein response (IL-6, see below). An important determinant of the effects of the inflammatory response is whether the effects of mediators remain localized (paracrine effect) or become generalized in the body (endocrine effect). This cascade of events results in rapid amplification of the initial injurious stimulus so that, within a few hours, large numbers of inflammatory cells are present at the injured site, controlling and mediating the inflammatory response via cytokines (Fig. 1.1).

Other pro-inflammatory substances are released in association with tissue injury, leucocyte activation and

1

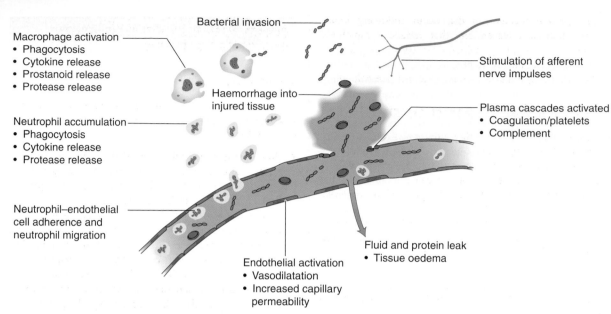

Bacterial invasion

Macrophage activation
• Phagocytosis
• Cytokine release
• Prostanoid release
• Protease release

Haemorrhage into injured tissue

Stimulation of afferent nerve impulses

Plasma cascades activated
• Coagulation/platelets
• Complement

Neutrophil accumulation
• Phagocytosis
• Cytokine release
• Protease release

Neutrophil–endothelial cell adherence and neutrophil migration

Endothelial activation
• Vasodilatation
• Increased capillary permeability

Fluid and protein leak
• Tissue oedema

Fig. 1.1   Key events occurring at the site of tissue injury.

cytokine production. These include prostaglandins, kinins, complement, various proteases (such as elastase and cathepsin) and free radicals. Anti-inflammatory substances and mechanisms also exist, such as antioxidants (for example, glutathione, vitamin A and vitamin C), protease enzyme inhibitors (for example, α_2-macroglobulin) and IL-10. The balance between pro- and anti-inflammatory processes is extremely important but is not yet fully understood.

THE ENDOTHELIUM AND BLOOD VESSELS

Leucocyte accumulation in injured tissues relies on a stepwise process whereby cells initially adhere 'lightly' to the endothelium, subsequently adhere 'tightly', and then migrate between endothelial cells into tissues (Fig. 1.1). These processes are controlled via specific molecules released by endothelial cells and inflammatory cells following cell activation. 'Light' adhesion is mediated via the selectins, and 'tight' adhesion via integrins and the intercellular adhesion molecule (ICAM) family.

When tissues are injured, the local blood flow increases because of vasodilatation. This steps up the local delivery of inflammatory cells, oxygen and nutrient substrates that are important in the healing process. Vasodilatation is caused by substances such as kinins, prostaglandins and nitric oxide, which are generated in response to injury and inflammation. Nitric oxide, which is synthesized in endothelial cells, is particularly important in controlling blood flow to tissues, both in health and following injury. In addition to vasodilatation, capillaries in injured tissues become more permeable to plasma because endothelial activation increases the size of intercellular pores. As a result, fluid and colloid particles (principally albumin) leak into injured tissues, resulting in oedema formation. If

tissue injury is severe and widespread (for example, following severe burns), fluid loss into tissues can amount to many litres.

At sites of injury, tissue factor is exposed which promotes coagulation to decrease haemorrhage. This involves a complex interaction between endothelial cells, platelets, and circulating coagulation and inflammatory factors. A situation of excess pro-coagulant activity can cause impaired blood flow by occluding capillaries. This can occur when inflammatory processes become generalized in the circulation, commonly as a result of infection, and cause disseminated intravascular coagulation.

AFFERENT NERVE IMPULSES AND SYMPATHETIC NERVOUS SYSTEM ACTIVATION

Impulses generated in afferent nerve endings at the site of tissue injury have a role in mediating the metabolic response to injury. The most important nerves are probably pain fibres which comprise both unmyelinated C fibres and myelinated A fibres. These are stimulated via direct trauma or the release of nerve stimulants such as prostaglandins. Nerve impulses reach the thalamus via the dorsal horn of the spinal cord and the lateral spinothalamic tract. Afferent impulses reaching the thalamus mediate the metabolic response via several mechanisms:

1. *Stimulation of the sympathetic nervous system.* Increased discharge of sympathetic nerves results in tachycardia and increased cardiac output. Noradrenaline (norepinephrine) release from sympathetic nerve endings and adrenaline (epinephrine) release from the adrenal gland increase circulating catecholamine concentrations. This contributes to the changes in carbohydrate, fat

and protein metabolism that occur following injury (see below). Interventions that reduce sympathetic stimulation, such as epidural or spinal anaesthesia, may attenuate these changes.

2. *Stimulation of pituitary hormone release* (see below).

THE ENDOCRINE RESPONSE TO SURGERY

Changes occur to circulating concentrations of many hormones following injury (Table 1.2). These take place as a result of direct stimulation of the various glands that produce the hormones, and also because normal negative feedback mechanisms are altered as part of the response to injury. Hormonal changes are mainly involved in maintaining the body's fluid balance and in the changes to substrate metabolism that occur following injury (see below).

BOX 1.1 FACTORS MEDIATING THE METABOLIC RESPONSE TO INJURY

The acute inflammatory response
Inflammatory cells (macrophages, monocytes, neutrophils)
Pro-inflammatory cytokines and other inflammatory mediators

Endothelial cell activation
Adhesion of inflammatory cells
Vasodilatation
Increased permeability

Nervous system
Afferent nerve stimulation

Endocrine response
Increased secretion of stress hormones
Decreased secretion of anabolic hormones

Bacterial infection

CONSEQUENCES OF THE METABOLIC RESPONSE TO INJURY

HYPOVOLAEMIA

A reduced circulating volume is characteristic following moderate to severe injury, and can occur for various reasons (Table 1.3):

- *Fluid loss* may be in the form of blood (haemorrhage), electrolyte-containing fluid (for example, nasogastric suction, vomiting or sweating) or water (evaporation from exposed organs during surgery).
- *Fluid sequestration* of plasma-like fluid in injured tissues (sometimes termed third-space losses) occurs in proportion to the severity and extent of injury. It results from the increased 'leakiness' of the endothelium described above, usually lasts 24–48 hours, and after major surgery can amount to several litres. The extent and duration of this leakiness may be prolonged if the acute inflammatory response is exaggerated: for example, by infection or the ischaemia–reperfusion syndrome.

Decreased circulating volume is important because it may reduce oxygen delivery to organs and tissues, lowering rates of healing or even causing further damage. The neuroendocrine response to hypovolaemia and a reduced circulating volume attempts to restore normal fluid status and maintain perfusion to vital organs. These interrelated processes can be considered as fluid-conserving measures and blood flow-conserving measures. With modern management of patients, this response is less crucial to survival because fluids and blood products can be administered to correct hypovolaemia.

Table 1.2 HORMONAL CHANGES IN RESPONSE TO SURGERY AND TRAUMA

Hormonal change	Pituitary	Adrenal	Pancreatic	Others
Increased secretion	Growth hormone (GH) Adrenocorticotrophic hormone (ACTH) Prolactin Antidiuretic hormone/arginine vasopressin (ADH/AVP)	Adrenaline Cortisol Aldosterone	Glucagon	Renin Angiotensin
Unchanged secretion	Thyroid-stimulating hormone (TSH) Luteinizing hormone (LH) Follicle-stimulating hormone (FSH)	–	–	–
Decreased secretion	–	–	Insulin	Testosterone Oestrogen Thyroid hormones

1

Table 1.3   CAUSES OF FLUID LOSS FOLLOWING SURGERY AND TRAUMA

Nature of fluid	Mechanism	Contributing factors
Blood	Haemorrhage	Site and magnitude of tissue injury
		Poor surgical haemostasis
		Abnormal coagulation
Electrolyte-containing fluids	Vomiting	Anaesthesia/analgesia (e.g. opiates)
		Ileus
	Nasogastric drainage	Ileus
		Gastric surgery
	Diarrhoea	Antibiotic-related infection
		Enteral feeding
	Sweating	Pyrexia
Water	Evaporation	Prolonged exposure of viscera during surgery
Plasma-like fluid (third-space losses)	Capillary leak/sequestration in tissues	Acute inflammatory response
		Infection
		Ischaemia–reperfusion syndrome

Fluid-conserving measures

Oliguria, together with sodium and water retention, is very common after major surgery or injury. It may occur because of decreased renal perfusion as a result of hypovolaemia, but frequently arises even after normal circulating volume is restored. Characteristic changes affect urine after major surgery, which result from neuroendocrine responses.

Antidiuretic hormone (ADH)

Synthesis and secretion of ADH (sometimes called arginine vasopressin or AVP) by the posterior pituitary are increased in response to the following stimuli:

- direct afferent nerve impulses from the site of injury
- increased plasma osmolality (principally sodium ions) detected by hypothalamic osmoreceptors
- afferent nerve impulses from atrial stretch receptors (responding to reduced volume) and the aortic and carotid baroreceptors (responding to reduced pressure)
- input from higher centres in the brain (pain, emotion and anxiety).

ADH promotes the retention of free water (without electrolytes) by cells of the distal renal tubule and collecting duct. If excess water is administered during the period of increased ADH secretion, plasma hypotonicity and hyponatraemia may occur.

Aldosterone

Aldosterone secretion from the adrenal cortex is increased by the following mechanisms (Fig. 1.2):

- Secretion is raised via the renin–angiotensin system at the juxtaglomerular apparatus within nephrons. Renin is released from afferent arteriolar cells in response to stimuli activated during hypovolaemia and reduced renal blood flow. These include reduced afferent arteriolar pressure, tubuloglomerular feedback (signalling via the macula densa of the distal tubule according to electrolyte concentration) and activation of the renal sympathetic nerves. Renin, a proteolytic enzyme, converts circulating angiotensinogen to angiotensin I. Angiotensin I is converted to angiotensin II by angiotensin-converting enzyme (ACE), which is found in plasma and in various tissues, particularly the lung. Angiotensin II has several actions, which include potent vasoconstriction of arterioles and stimulation of aldosterone secretion by the adrenal cortex.

- ACTH secretion by the anterior pituitary is increased in response to hypovolaemia and hypotension via afferent nerve impulses from stretch receptors in the atria, aorta and carotid arteries. It is also raised by ADH.

- Hyponatraemia or hyperkalaemia directly stimulates adrenal cortex cells to increase secretion.

Aldosterone acts mainly via receptors on distal renal tubular cells. The net effect is reabsorption of sodium ions and simultaneous excretion of hydrogen and potassium ions into urine. Aldosterone also effects ion transfer across some other cell types: for example, cardiac muscle.

The duration of increased ADH and aldosterone secretion is usually 48–72 hours. Urine volume is often reduced during this period (about 0.5 ml/kg/hr), and urine is concentrated as a result of water retention. Urinary sodium excretion decreases, typically to 10–20 mmol/24 hrs (normal 50–80 mmol/24 hrs). Urinary potassium excretion increases, typically to > 100 mmol/24 hrs (normal 50–80 mmol/24 hrs), but hypokalaemia is relatively rare in the 24–48 hours following injury because a net efflux of

BOX 1.2   URINARY CHANGES DURING THE METABOLIC RESPONSE TO INJURY

Reduced urine volume in response to hypovolaemia and ADH release
Low urinary sodium and increased urinary potassium excretion due to aldosterone release
Increased urinary nitrogen excretion due to the catabolic response to injury

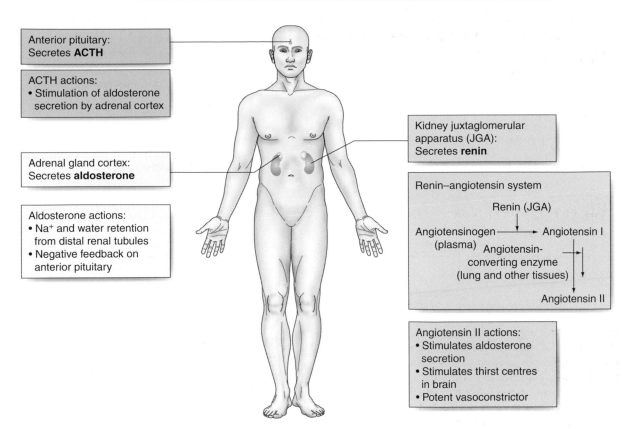

Fig. 1.2   The renin–angiotensin–aldosterone system.
(ACTH = adrenocorticotrophic hormone)

potassium from cells occurs. This typical pattern may be modified by fluid and electrolyte administration.

Blood flow-conserving measures

An important potential consequence of hypovolaemia is reduced cardiac output, resulting in decreased blood flow to organs. Cardiac output is determined by the cardiac preload (the amount of blood returning to the heart), the heart rate, the contractility of cardiac muscle (the rate at which each contraction occurs) and the afterload (a measure of the resistance against which the heart pumps). Blood pressure is determined by the cardiac output and the peripheral resistance of blood vessels (mainly arterioles). Following injury, several mechanisms act to maintain or increase cardiac output and blood pressure despite hypovolaemia (Fig. 1.3).

INCREASED ENERGY METABOLISM AND SUBSTRATE CYCLING

Metabolic rate (the energy expenditure of the body) can be considered in three parts: energy required for physical work, energy associated with heat production (thermogenesis) and basal metabolic rate (BMR, comprising the energy needed for enzyme reactions and ion pumps).

Physical work

Following injury physical work is usually decreased because of inactivity, although heart and respiratory muscle work may increase. Resting energy expenditure (the sum of BMR and thermogenesis) is increased by up to 50% following severe injury as a result of metabolic changes (Fig. 1.4).

Thermogenesis

Patients are frequently mildly pyrexial for 24–48 hours following injury. This occurs because cytokines, principally IL-1, reset temperature-regulating centres in the hypothalamus. Pyrexia may also complicate infection occurring after injury. Metabolic rate increases by 6–10% for each 1°C change in body temperature.

Basal metabolic rate

Following injury, there is increased activity of protein, carbohydrate and fat-related metabolic pathways (see below) and of many ion pumps. The activity of some cycles is apparently 'futile'; for example, glucose–lactate cycling and triglyceride turnover involve simultaneous synthesis and degradation. This general increase in substrate cycling is energy-dependent, but probably evolved to increase the ability of the body to respond to altering demands.

CATABOLISM AND STARVATION

Catabolism is the breakdown of complex substances, such as muscle proteins, to form simpler molecules (glucose, amino acids and fatty acids) that are basic substrates for metabolic pathways. Starvation is the inadequate intake

1

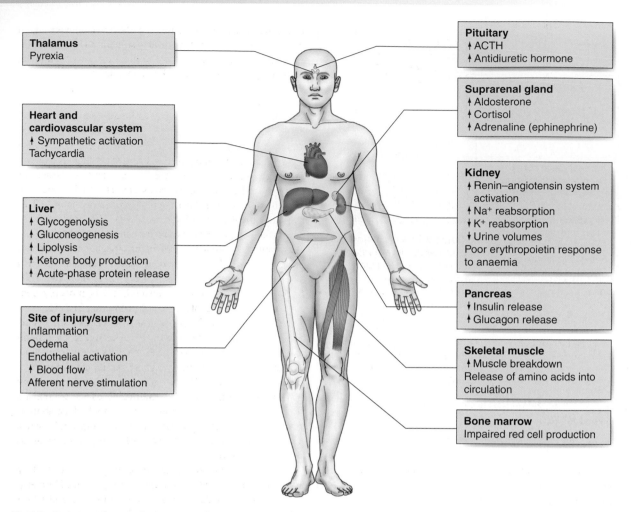

Thalamus
Pyrexia

Heart and cardiovascular system
↑ Sympathetic activation
Tachycardia

Liver
↑ Glycogenolysis
↑ Gluconeogenesis
↑ Lipolysis
↑ Ketone body production
↑ Acute-phase protein release

Site of injury/surgery
Inflammation
Oedema
Endothelial activation
↑ Blood flow
Afferent nerve stimulation

Pituitary
↑ ACTH
↑ Antidiuretic hormone

Suprarenal gland
↑ Aldosterone
↑ Cortisol
↑ Adrenaline (ephinephrine)

Kidney
↑ Renin–angiotensin system activation
↑ Na⁺ reabsorption
↓ K⁺ reabsorption
↓ Urine volumes
Poor erythropoietin response to anaemia

Pancreas
↓ Insulin release
↑ Glucagon release

Skeletal muscle
↑ Muscle breakdown
Release of amino acids into circulation

Bone marrow
Impaired red cell production

Fig. 1.3 Summary of metabolic responses to surgery and trauma.

BOX 1.3 PHYSIOLOGICAL CHANGES OCCURRING DURING CATABOLISM

Carbohydrate metabolism

- ↑ Glycogenolysis (stores last about 10 hours)
- ↑ Hepatic gluconeogenesis
- Insulin resistance of tissues
- Hyperglycaemia

Fat metabolism

- ↑ Lipolysis
- Free fatty acids used as energy substrate by tissues (except brain)
- Some conversion of free fatty acids to ketones in liver (used by brain)
- Glycerol converted to glucose in the liver

Protein metabolism

- ↑ Skeletal muscle breakdown
- Amino acids converted to glucose in liver and used as substrate for acute-phase protein production
- Negative nitrogen balance

Total energy expenditure increased in proportion to injury severity and other modifying factors.
Progressive reduction in fat and muscle mass until stimulus for catabolism ends.

---

of food to meet metabolic demand. Following severe injury or major surgery, these two processes generally occur simultaneously. The metabolic changes associated with each process are different, and so the changes occurring in any individual patient depend on which process predominates. Generally, uncomplicated surgery or moderate trauma is followed by a period of starvation but little catabolism. Major trauma or surgery complicated by sepsis may result in marked catabolism, which outweighs any effect of simultaneous starvation.

Catabolism

Catabolism is mediated by catecholamines, cytokines and other substances generated in response to injury and released into the circulation. These bring about changes in carbohydrate, protein and fat metabolism.

Carbohydrate metabolism

Glycogenolysis in the liver results in rapid depletion of glycogen stores, which last for only 8–12 hours. Gluconeogenesis is increased, particularly in the liver, which converts substrates released from other tissues, such as amino acids, into glucose. Insulin secretion is decreased as a result of inhibition of pancreatic β-cells by cate-

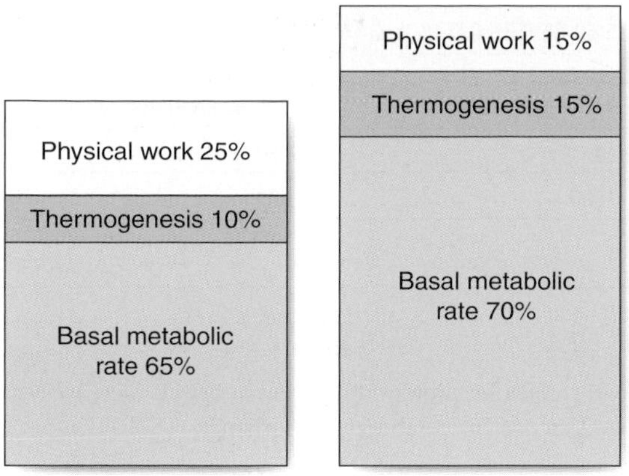

Physical work 15%

Thermogenesis 15%

Basal metabolic
rate 70%

Physical work 25%

Thermogenesis 10%

Basal metabolic
rate 65%

**Healthy sedentary
70 kg man**
• Total energy expenditure
  about 1800 kcal/day
• Basal metabolic rate
  comprises enzymes and
  ion pumps (85%) and the
  mechanical work of the
  heart and respiratory
  system (15%)

**24 hours following major
surgery or moderate injury**
• Total energy expenditure
  increased 10–30%
• Relative reduction in physical
  work due to inactivity
• Thermogenesis/heat energy
  increased by mild pyrexia
• Basal metabolic rate increased
  by raised enzyme and ion
  pump activity and increased
  cardiac work

**Fig. 1.4 Components of body energy expenditure in health and
following injury.**

cholamines. In addition, a state of insulin resistance occurs, meaning that cells become less sensitive to the effects of insulin. This is caused by changes to the insulin receptor/intracellular signal pathway. Together, these factors result in hyperglycaemia, which provides glucose substrate for the inflammatory and repair processes that follow injury. However, the degree of control of glucose in the perioperative setting and during critical illness may have an effect on recovery (see below).

Catecholamines and glucagon also increase gluconeogenesis. There is a correlation between the degree of hyperglycaemia that occurs and the severity of surgery or injury.

Fat metabolism
Adipose tissue is a large triglyceride store that constitutes the principal source of energy following trauma. The stress hormones released as part of the metabolic response to injury (catecholamines, glucagon, cortisol and growth hormone) are all capable of activating the enzyme, triglyceride lipase, within fat cells. This process is exacerbated by the state of insulin resistance. Cortisol is a potent stimulus for lipolysis, and circulating cortisol concentrations increase from normal baseline levels of ≅ 400 nmol/l to levels of > 1500 nmol/l within hours of major surgery. Triglycerides are broken down into glycerol and free fatty acids. Glycerol is a substrate for gluconeogenesis, and free fatty acids can be directly metabolized by most tissues to generate energy. The brain is unable to use free fatty acids for energy production, and in health relies on glucose supply. Animals are unable to convert

free fatty acids into glucose, but the liver converts them into ketone bodies that are water-soluble and can support cerebral energy metabolism. Following severe trauma, 200–500 g of fat may be broken down daily.

Protein metabolism
Skeletal muscle is the major labile protein store in the body. Following major injury, skeletal muscle is broken down, releasing amino acids into the circulation. These are metabolized principally in the liver, which converts a major proportion into glucose for re-export to tissues for energy metabolism. Amino acids are also used in the liver as substrate for the 'acute-phase protein response'. This response involves the liver increasing the production of one group of proteins (positive acute-phase proteins) and decreasing the production of others (negative acute-phase proteins) (Table 1.4). The acute-phase response is mediated in the liver by cytokines, especially IL-1, IL-6 and TNF. Its function is not fully understood, but is probably concerned with fighting infection and promoting healing.

The mechanism by which muscle catabolism occurs is also incompletely understood. It is mediated by inflammatory mediators and hormones, such as cortisol, released as part of the metabolic response to injury. Trauma or surgery associated with a minimal metabolic response is usually accompanied by minimal muscle catabolism. In patients with major tissue injury, marked catabolism and loss of skeletal muscle can occur, especially when factors that enhance the metabolic response, such as sepsis, are present.

In health, 80–120 g/day dietary protein (12–20 g nitrogen) is ingested (1 g nitrogen = 6 g protein). Normally, approximately 2 g/day nitrogen is lost in faeces and 10–18 g/day in urine (mainly in the form of urea). During catabolism, nitrogen intake is often reduced but urinary losses can increase markedly, reaching 20–30 g/day in patients with severe trauma, sepsis or burns. Following uncomplicated surgery, this negative nitrogen balance usually lasts only 5–8 days, but in patients with prolonged sepsis, burns or conditions associated with prolonged inflammation (for example, acute pancreatitis) it may persist for many weeks. Severe catabolism and negative nitrogen balance cannot be reversed by feeding, but the provision of protein and calories can attenuate the processes. Even patients undergoing uncomplicated abdominal surgery

**Table 1.4 PROTEINS SYNTHESIZED BY THE LIVER WHICH ALTER
AS PART OF THE ACUTE-PHASE PROTEIN RESPONSE**

Positive acute-phase proteins (↑ after injury)
• C-reactive protein
• Haptoglobins
• Ferritin
• Fibrinogen
• α_1-Antitrypsin
• α_2-Macroglobulin
• Plasminogen

Negative acute-phase proteins (↑ after injury)
• Albumin
• Transferrin

Table 1.5   A COMPARISON OF NITROGEN AND ENERGY LOSSES IN A MODERATE TO SEVERE CATABOLIC STATE AND DURING THE DIFFERENT PHASES OF STARVATION*

	Catabolic state	Acute starvation	Compensated starvation
Nitrogen loss (g/day)	20–25	14	3
Energy expenditure (kcal/day)	2200–2500	1800	1500

* Values are approximate and relate to a 70 kg man.

can lose about 600 g muscle protein (1 g protein = 5 g wet muscle mass), amounting to 6% of total body protein. This is usually regained within 3 months.

Starvation

Starvation occurs in relation to trauma and surgery for several reasons:

- the illness requiring treatment (for example, gastric carcinoma), which may have reduced nutritional intake for weeks/months prior to surgery
- fasting prior to surgery
- fasting after surgery, especially to the gastrointestinal tract
- loss of appetite associated with illness.

The response of the body to starvation can be described in two phases (Table 1.5).

Acute starvation

This is accompanied by metabolic changes that preserve the glucose supply to the brain. Glycogenolysis and gluconeogenesis occur in the liver, releasing glucose for cerebral energy metabolism. Lipolysis in fat stores releases free fatty acids for use by other tissues, and glycerol which is converted to glucose in the liver. These processes can sustain the normal energy requirements of the body (about 1800 kcal/day for a 70 kg adult) for approximately 10 hours.

Chronic starvation

This is initially accompanied by muscle breakdown to release amino acids, which are converted to glucose by hepatic gluconeogenesis. In addition, fatty acids released from adipose tissue are converted by the liver to ketones. Tissue energy supply is in the form of glucose, fatty acids and ketones. The brain is unable to utilize free fatty acids and uses about 70% of the glucose generated by hepatic gluconeogenesis. With prolonged starvation, the brain adapts to utilize ketones as the primary energy substrate, rather than glucose. This adaptation reduces muscle protein loss and switches metabolism to increase fat consumption, so that net body nitrogen loss is reduced. Hepatic gluconeogenesis from amino acids decreases to about 25% of its previous rate, and overall metabolic rate and energy requirements fall, the latter from 1800 kcal/day to about 1500 kcal/ day (Table 1.5). This state is termed compensated starvation, which continues until body fat stores are depleted. At this stage, when an individual is often close to death, muscle protein breakdown again increases to provide glucose for cerebral metabolism.

CHANGES IN RED BLOOD CELL SYNTHESIS AND BLOOD COAGULATION

Anaemia is common after major surgery or trauma because of bleeding and the haemodilution that occurs when blood losses are replaced with crystalloid or colloid fluids (Ch. 2). In addition, the bone marrow production of new red cells is impaired. The reasons for this are unclear, but include an inappropriately low release of erythropoietin by the kidney and impaired maturation of red blood cell precursors. In addition, changes to iron metabolism occur that increase storage iron (bound to ferritin) and decrease the available iron (bound to transferrin). These changes are probably due to the effects of inflammation, but how this may be of benefit is unclear. Recent evidence suggests that actively correcting anaemia in patients after surgery or during critical illness when they are not bleeding is not beneficial (Ch. 4).

Following tissue injury, the blood may become hypercoagulable. This is usually a transient feature lasting 1–2 days, but it increases the risk of thromboembolism after surgery or trauma. Contributing factors include:

- endothelial injury and activation, which in turn activates the coagulation pathways
- increased activation of platelets in response to circulating mediators such as adrenaline (epinephrine) and cytokines
- dehydration and/or reduced venous blood flow due to immobility
- an increase in circulating concentrations of procoagulant factors, such as fibrinogen, and a decrease in circulating natural anticoagulants, such as protein C.

Rarely, patients develop hypocoagulable states. These are usually found in association with shock, massive blood transfusion or sepsis. The most extreme form of coagulopathy is disseminated intravascular coagulation.

FACTORS MODIFYING THE METABOLIC RESPONSE TO INJURY

The magnitude and duration of the metabolic response to injury are influenced by many factors. Some of these are summarized in Table 1.6. There has been considerable research into ways of decreasing the metabolic response and

Table 1.6   FACTORS ASSOCIATED WITH THE MAGNITUDE OF THE METABOLIC RESPONSE TO INJURY

Factor	Comment
PATIENT-RELATED FACTORS	
Genetic predisposition	Recent evidence shows that gene subtype for inflammatory mediators is associated with how an individual responds to injury and infection
Coexisting disease	The presence of disease, such as cancer and chronic inflammatory disease, may influence the metabolic response
Drug treatments	Pre-existing anti-inflammatory or immunosuppressive therapy, such as steroids, may alter responses
Nutritional status	Malnourished patients may have decreased immune function or deficiency in important substrates. Malnutrition prior to surgery or trauma is associated with poor outcomes
ACUTE SURGICAL/TRAUMA-RELATED FACTORS	
Severity of injury	Greater tissue damage is associated with a greater metabolic response
Nature of injury	Some types of tissue injury cause a proportionate metabolic response. An example is major burn injury, which is associated with a major response
Ischaemia–reperfusion injury	If resuscitation is not quick and/or effective, the reperfusion of previously ischaemic tissues can set off a cascade of inflammation that further injures organs. This is called ischaemia–reperfusion injury
Temperature	Extreme hypothermia and hyperthermia are both detrimental to the metabolic response
Infection	The occurrence of infection is often associated with an exaggerated response to injury. If infection spreads to the systemic circulation, it can result in sepsis or septic shock, which are associated with a massive inflammatory response
Anaesthetic techniques	The use of certain drugs, such as opioids, can reduce the release of stress hormones. Regional anaesthetic techniques for major surgery can reduce the release of cortisol, adrenaline (epinephrine) and other hormones, but has little effect on cytokine responses

how this might affect patient outcome. In surgical practice, the major advances have been in reducing the extent of tissue injury through improvements in surgical techniques. In situations of exaggerated metabolic response, where the patient either has undergone major surgery or is critically ill, several recent trials have suggested that interventions to alter aspects of the metabolic response can improve patient survival.

CONTROL OF BLOOD GLUCOSE

Hyperglycaemia is a major component of the stress response, and is usually more severe following major trauma or surgery. Recent evidence suggests that, after major (particularly cardiac) surgery and during critical illness, tighter control of blood glucose using insulin is associated with lower mortality and complication rates (EBM 1.1).

MANIPULATION OF INFLAMMATION AND COAGULATION IN SEVERE INFECTION

When severe infection complicates an illness, the metabolic response becomes exaggerated and is thought to contribute to further tissue injury and organ failure. This is called sepsis syndrome and is a major cause of morbidity and mortality in hospitals. The concentrations of many cytokines and other inflammatory factors in the circulation are markedly increased. Many large RCTs have tested whether using therapeutic interventions such as monoclonal antibodies to neutralize certain factors (for example, TNF-α, IL-6 or endotoxin) could improve survival of patients in these situations. The majority of these studies have shown no benefit from such interventions and indeed sometimes show harm. However, a recent large RCT in which activated human protein C was administered to patients with severe sepsis demonstrated a clear improvement in survival (EBM 1.2). This factor, which has anti-inflammatory and anticoagulant actions, is normally present in the circulation but is deficient in patients with severe sepsis. The drug is recommended for use in many countries under the guidance of intensive care specialists.

EBM 1.1   BLOOD GLUCOSE CONTROL

'A large single-centre RCT in patients who had had major surgery or with critical illness (most of whom had undergone cardiac surgery) found that tight blood glucose control in the post-operative period using insulin infusions decreased operative mortality and complication rates.'

Van den Berghe G, et al. New Engl J Med 2001; 345:1359–1367.

EBM 1.2   MANAGEMENT OF SEVERE SEPSIS

'Recombinant human activated protein C reduces 28-day mortality in severe sepsis, even if multiple organ failure has already developed.'

Taylor FB, et al. J Clin Invest 1987; 79:918–925.
Bernard GR, et al. N Engl J Med 2001; 344:699–709.

ANABOLISM

Anabolism is the process of regaining weight, restoring skeletal muscle mass and strength, and replenishing fat stores. It is unlikely to occur until the processes associated with catabolism, such as the release of inflammatory mediators, have subsided. This point is often associated with an obvious clinical improvement in the patient, who feels better and regains his or her appetite. Hormones contributing to the process of anabolism include insulin, growth hormone, insulin-like growth factors, androgens and the 17-ketosteroids. The factors controlling the rate of anabolism are complex, but nutritional support and the activity level of the patient are important contributing factors.

2

T.S. WALSH
A.J. POLLOK

Principles of fluid and electrolyte balance in surgical patients

INTRODUCTION

Many patients undergoing surgery do not ingest oral fluids, either in preparation for surgery or as a result of the surgery itself. If fluid ingestion is restricted for a prolonged period, fluid requirements need to be met by intravenous administration. In addition to reduced intake from fasting, surgery can alter fluid and electrolyte status by:

- stimulating the secretion of stress hormones (antidiuretic hormone (ADH), aldosterone, cortisol) that alter the body's handling of water and electrolytes (Ch. 1)

- causing fluid and electrolyte loss from the gastrointestinal tract, including the pre-operative use of laxatives for bowel preparation
- increasing insensible fluid losses: for example, sweating secondary to fever
- sequestration of fluids and electrolytes at the site of surgery ('third-space' losses)
- fluid loss from surgical drains or fistulae.

Fluid and electrolyte status may also be altered during the perioperative period by the patient's normal medical treatments, such as diuretic and antihypertensive drugs. Careful monitoring of fluid balance (input and output) is therefore important in the perioperative period. An adequate

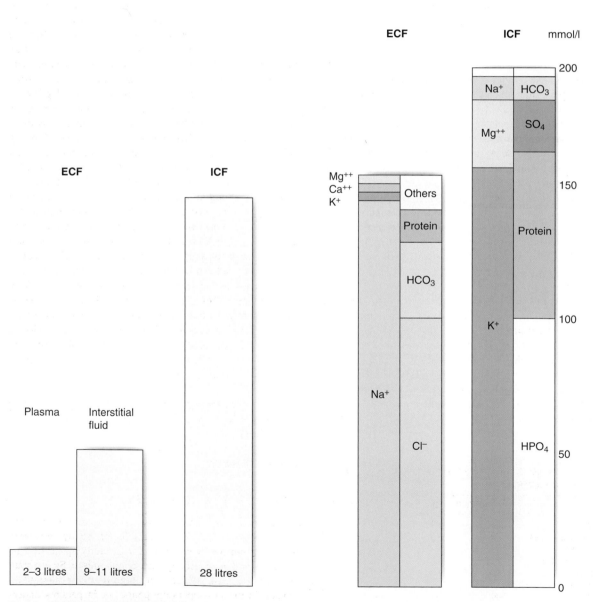

Fig. 2.1 Distribution of fluid and electrolytes between the intracellular and extracellular fluid compartments.
A Approximate values for water in a 70 kg man. B Cations and anions.

volume of water, together with an appropriate amount of sodium and potassium, needs to be given. In surgical conditions associated with excessive and prolonged fluid loss (such as prolonged gastrointestinal loss or fistulae), consideration should be given to other electrolytes, such as calcium, magnesium and phosphate. This chapter describes the important aspects of fluid and electrolyte balance relevant to the surgical patient.

NORMAL WATER AND ELECTROLYTE BALANCE

The body of a healthy 70 kg male contains about 42 litres of water, which is distributed into the compartments shown in Figure 2.1A. Electrolytes are dissolved in body water, but distributed differently between the various compartments (Fig. 2.1B). This distribution is maintained by membrane ion pumps, is essential for normal cellular function, and is an energy-dependent process that uses a significant proportion of basal energy requirements. The osmolality of extracellular fluid is determined primarily by sodium and chloride concentrations, whereas the major intracellular ions are potassium, magnesium, phosphate and sulphate. The distribution of fluid between the intra- and extravascular compartments is dependent on the oncotic pressure of plasma and the permeability of the endothelium. The plasma oncotic pressure is determined by the presence of colloid particles, of which albumin is the most important. Both the colloid oncotic pressure and the endothelial permeability may alter following surgery (Ch. 1). The control of total body electrolytes and water is primarily a function of the kidneys in conjunction with hormonal regulation by factors such as aldosterone, ADH and atrial natriuretic peptide. It follows that patients with abnormal renal function are more likely to develop fluid and electrolyte abnormalities in the perioperative period.

A healthy individual loses fluid and electrolytes by three routes: via the kidneys, via the gastrointestinal tract, and by evaporation from the skin and respiratory tract (Table 2.1). A rise in core temperature (pyrexia) and/or sweating increases insensible fluid and electrolyte losses significantly. In health, water is taken in as fluids and in solid foods, and an additional 200–300 ml per 24 hours is provided endogenously by oxidation of carbohydrate and fat (i.e. metabolic water).

Table 2.1 NORMAL DAILY LOSSES AND REQUIREMENTS FOR FLUIDS AND ELECTROLYTES

	Volume (ml)	Na+ (mmol)	K+ (mmol)
Urine	2000	80	60
Insensible losses (skin and respiratory tract)	700	–	–
Faeces	300	–	10
Minus endogenous water	300	–	–
Total	2700	80	70

In the absence of sweating, almost all sodium loss is via the urine. Under the influence of aldosterone, the kidney can reduce sodium loss to a minimum of approximately 10–20 mmol/24 hrs. Potassium is also excreted mainly via the kidney (60–100 mmol/24 hrs) and about 10 mmol/day is lost via the gastrointestinal tract. In severe potassium deficiency, losses can be reduced to about 20 mmol/day, but increased aldosterone secretion, high urine flow rates and metabolic alkalosis all limit the ability of the kidneys to conserve potassium.

The percentage water content of newborn babies and children is higher than in adults. As a consequence, the maintenance fluid requirements of the paediatric surgical patient are higher than the adult counterpart. In the first few days of life, the newborn is relatively waterlogged and the kidneys are relatively immature. The maintenance fluid requirement at birth is about 75 ml/kg body weight (BW)/day. This increases during the first week of life to 150 ml/kg BW/day. Premature infants can require as much as 200 ml/kg BW/day of maintenance fluids. After the first month of life, fluid requirements decrease. The '4/2/1 formula' is widely used to calculate the fluid requirements of the average paediatric patient after the neonatal period. The first 10 kg BW requires approximately 4 ml/kg BW/hr (equates to 100 ml/kg/day); the next 10 kg BW requires approximately 2 ml/kg BW/hr (equates to 50 ml/kg BW/day); every kg BW thereafter requires approximately 1 ml/kg BW/hr (equates to 25 ml/kg BW/day). Using this formula, a 35 kg child would require $(10 \times 4\ ml) + (10 \times 2\ ml) + (15 \times 1\ ml) = 40 + 20 + 15 = 75$ ml/hr of maintenance fluids.

Electrolyte and mineral requirements are also calculated by body weight. For example, the daily requirement for sodium and potassium in children is approximately 2–3 mmol/kg BW/day. It will be clear that the sodium content of normal saline (150 mmol/l) would result in serious sodium overload if this were used as the maintenance fluid for neonates and children. A 3 kg neonate whose daily fluid requirement is 450 ml/day (150 ml/kg BW/day) needs approximately 9 mol of sodium per day. A 450 ml quantity of normal saline contains 67.5 mmol of sodium; 450 ml of fifth strength (0.18%) contains 13.5 mmol of sodium. It is for this reason that the normal maintenance intravenous fluid used in children is not normal saline.

ASSESSING LOSSES IN THE SURGICAL PATIENT

(See also Table 2.2.)

INSENSIBLE FLUID LOSSES

Hyperventilation increases insensible water loss via the respiratory tract, but this increase is not usually very large unless the normal mechanisms for humidifying inhaled air (the nasal and upper airways) are compromised. Such a state can occur in patients receiving high-flow non-humidified oxygen in the post-operative period, or in patients undergoing mechanical ventilation without humidification of gases. In these situations gas humidifiers should be used.

2

Table 2.2	SOURCES OF FLUID LOSS IN SURGICAL PATIENTS	
	Typical losses per 24 hrs	Factors modifying volume
Insensible losses	700–2000 ml	Pyrexia, sweating, use of non-humidified oxygen (increase loss)
Urine	1000–2500 ml	Aldosterone and ADH secretion (stress response to surgery) (decrease) Diuretic therapy (increase)
Gut	300 ml normal Diarrhoea, obstruction, fistulae > 1000 ml	Obstruction, fistulae, diarrhoea (may increase substantially)
Third-space losses	0–1000 ml	Extent of surgery and tissue trauma (increase)

Pyrexia increases water loss from the skin by approximately 200 ml/day for each 1°C rise in temperature. Sweating increases fluid loss considerably, by up to 1 litre per hour, but is difficult to quantify. Sweat contains significant amounts of sodium (20–70 mmol/l) and potassium (10 mmol/l), which should be considered when assessing losses.

EFFECT OF SURGERY

The stress response

This was considered in Chapter 1. ADH release conserves water and typically reduces urine volume to 1000–1500 ml for 2–3 days following major surgery. Excess water administration during this period is therefore likely to result in excess total body water, which may cause hyponatraemia (see below). Aldosterone secretion conserves sodium and further contributes to oliguria. In the first 2 days after operation, urinary excretion of sodium typically falls to approximately 30 mmol/24 hrs. Potassium excretion is increased during this period to approximately 120 mmol/day, as a result of the action of aldosterone and

the release of intracellular potassium from damaged tissues. Hypokalaemia is the most common electrolyte disorder in the perioperative period, typically occurring 2–3 days after major surgery. The endocrine response to surgery, which promotes water and sodium retention, means that accumulation of excess water and sodium in the body can occur easily if excessive fluid replacement therapy is administered during the perioperative period. This emphasizes the importance of providing appropriate replacement.

'Third-space' losses

Sequestration of extracellular fluid (ECF) at the site of operation produces local oedema. This fluid contains water, electrolytes and colloid particles because it results from local tissue injury, inflammation and capillary leak. As a result, third-space losses can significantly decrease the circulating fluid volume in the immediate post-operative period. Sequestration typically persists for approximately 48 hours and may involve up to 4 litres of fluid, depending on the severity of the operation or injury. Third-space losses are higher after major surgery, particularly to abdominal organs. Minimally invasive techniques reduce tissue injury and third-space losses. These losses are an important consideration in the post-operative period because they significantly reduce ECF status and circulating volume.

Loss from the gastrointestinal tract

The magnitude and content of gastrointestinal fluid losses depend mainly on the site of loss. The approximate electrolyte content and volumes of various gastrointestinal fluids are shown in Table 2.3. Gastrointestinal losses may result from various factors:

- *Intestinal obstruction.* In general, the higher an obstruction occurs in the intestine, the greater the fluid loss. This is because fluids secreted by the upper gastrointestinal tract fail to reach the absorptive areas of the distal jejunum and ileum. Thus a patient with a high small-bowel obstruction loses fluid more rapidly than one with a low small-bowel obstruction.
- *Adynamic ileus.* This condition, in which propulsion in the small intestine ceases, has various possible causes (Box 2.1). The most common is probably handling of

Table 2.3	THE APPROXIMATE DAILY VOLUMES AND ELECTROLYTE CONCENTRATIONS OF VARIOUS GASTROINTESTINAL FLUIDS (ML)*				
	Volume	Na$^+$	K$^+$	Cl$^-$	HCO$_3$
Plasma	–	140	5	100	25
Gastric juice	2500	50	10	80	40
Intestinal fluid (upper)	3000	140	10	100	25
Bile and pancreatic juice	1500	140	5	80	60
Mature ileostomy	500	50	5	20	25
Diarrhoea (inflammatory)	–	110	40	100	40

* If gastrointestinal loss continues for more than 2–3 days, samples of fluid and urine should be collected regularly and sent to the laboratory for measurement of electrolyte content.

<hr>

BOX 2.1 CONDITIONS ASSOCIATED WITH INCREASED RISK OF ADYNAMIC ILEUS

- Trauma to the GI tract (including operative handling)
- Infection
- Systemic inflammatory conditions (e.g. severe pancreatitis)
- Electrolyte imbalance (particularly potassium, calcium and magnesium deficiency)
- Poorly controlled diabetes (especially with evidence of ketoacidosis)
- Hypoproteinaemia
- Retroperitoneal trauma or haemorrhage
- Hypoxaemia
- Head injury or neurosurgical operations
- Shock

<hr>

and trauma to the bowel during surgery, which usually resolves within 1–2 days of the operation. Occasionally, adynamic ileus persists for longer, and in this case the less common causes should be sought and corrected if possible. During adynamic ileus the stomach should be decompressed using nasogastric tube drainage, and fluid losses monitored by measuring nasogastric aspirates. Adynamic ileus can sometimes be distinguished from obstruction by the presence or absence of bowel sounds.

- *Intestinal fistula.* Losses of fluid and electrolytes from an intestinal fistula can be considerable. As with obstruction, fistulae occurring high in the gut are usually associated with the greatest fluid losses. The electrolyte content of fistula losses can be high and the composition can vary depending on the site of the fistula. It may be useful to measure the electrolyte content of fistula fluid in order to determine the type of fluid replacement required to maintain balance.

- *Diarrhoea.* Patients may present with diarrhoea or develop it during the perioperative period: for example, as a result of antibiotic use. Fluid and electrolyte loss from diarrhoea may be considerable.

INTRAVENOUS FLUID ADMINISTRATION

The composition of commonly administered intravenous fluids is shown in Table 2.4. When choosing and administering intravenous fluids it is important to decide:

- from what deficiencies the patient suffers
- the compartments that require replacement
- which fluid is most appropriate.

TYPES OF INTRAVENOUS FLUID

Dextrose solution 5%

Dextrose solution 5% (5 g of dextrose/100 ml water) does not contain any electrolytes. The dextrose is rapidly metabolized in the body, such that dextrose solution is equivalent to administering water, which distributes rapidly and evenly throughout the entire body fluid compartments. It follows that 1 litre of intravenous dextrose solution expands the ECF compartment by 330 ml and the intravas-

Table 2.4 COMPOSITION OF COMMONLY ADMINISTERED INTRAVENOUS FLUIDS

	Na^+ (mmol/l)	K^+ (mmol/l)	Cl^- (mmol/l)	HCO_3^- (mmol/l)	Misc. (mmol/l)	Oncotic pressure (mmH_2O)	Typical plasma half-life	pH
5% dextrose	–	–	–	–	–	0	–	4.0
0.9% NaCl	154	0	154	0	0	0	–	5.0
Ringer's lactate (Hartmann's solution)	131	5	112	29*	Ca^{2+} 1 Mg^{2+} 1	0	–	6.5
Haemaccel (succinylated gelatin)	145	5.1	145	0	Ca^{2+} 6.25	370	5 hours	7.4
Gelofusine (polygeline gelatin)	154	0.4	125	0	Ca^{2+} 0.4 Mg^{2+} 0.4	465	4 hours	7.4
Hetastarch	154	0	154	0	0	310	17 days	5.5
Human albumin solution 4.5% (HAS)	150	0	120	0	0	275	–	7.4

* The lactate present in Ringer's lactate solution is rapidly metabolized in the liver. This generates bicarbonate ions. Bicarbonate cannot be directly added to the solutions because it is unstable (tends to precipitate).

2

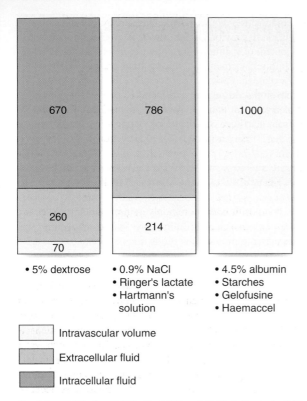

- 5% dextrose

- 0.9% NaCl
- Ringer's lactate
- Hartmann's solution

- 4.5% albumin
- Starches
- Gelofusine
- Haemaccel

☐ Intravascular volume

▨ Extracellular fluid

▨ Intracellular fluid

Fig. 2.2 Distribution (1000 ml) of different fluids in the body fluid compartments 30–60 minutes after rapid intravenous infusion.

cular compartment by only about 70 ml (Fig. 2.2); 5% dextrose is therefore of value for replacing water losses but has no use as a resuscitation fluid to expand the intravascular volume. More concentrated dextrose solutions (10%, 20% and 50%) are available, but their use is limited to the management of diabetic patients or patients with hypoglycaemia. These solutions are irritant to veins.

Sodium chloride 0.9% ('normal saline') and Ringer's lactate

These fluids are isotonic to ECF. After intravenous administration they distribute rapidly into the ECF compartment, and are appropriate when the main fluid deficiency derives from this source: for example, gastrointestinal losses or intra-operative losses other than bleeding. It follows that 1 litre of these fluids administered intravenously will increase the intravascular volume by about 220 ml after equilibration (Fig. 2.2). These fluids are therefore useful for resuscitation of the circulating volume, but it must be remembered that only about one-quarter remains in the circulating volume after redistribution. Under normal conditions, redistribution is complete within 30–60 minutes, but this time may be considerably shorter in conditions such as sepsis and burns that cause capillary leakiness.

Colloid solutions

Colloid solutions are those containing particles that exert an oncotic pressure. These particles may occur naturally or be synthetic (Table 2.4). When a colloid solution is administered, the solution remains in the circulation until the colloid particles are removed (predominantly by the reticulo-endothelial system), after which it distributes into the ECF volume because it also contains electrolytes. Most solutions remain in the circulation for between 6 and 24 hours, but this time can be shorter in conditions associated with leaky capillaries. Colloid solutions are good resuscitation fluids because all the volume administered stays in the circulation. Some starch solutions have a greater oncotic pressure than normal plasma, so fluid is drawn into blood vessels and the circulating volume is increased by more than the volume administered. Various starch solutions are available; their properties (amount of volume expansion achieved and duration of action) depend on the structure of the starch molecules used.

Hypertonic saline solutions

These are not true colloids, although some formulations contain additional colloid particles. Their use is limited to resuscitation, but there is little evidence at present that they have any benefit over more traditional solutions.

MAINTENANCE FLUID REQUIREMENTS

In the prescription of the normal daily fluid and electrolyte requirements (Table 2.5), sodium and chloride are usually provided as a 0.9% sodium chloride solution. Under normal conditions, daily sodium and chloride requirements are contained in 1 litre of 0.9% saline. Potassium requirements are usually met by adding potassium chloride according to plasma potassium concentrations (typically 60 mmol in 24 hours). Potassium should not be administered at a rate greater than 10–20 mmol/hr, except in severe potassium deficiency. (Continuous electrocardiogram (ECG) monitoring is then essential.) It must never be given as an intravenous bolus, as cardiac arrest can occur. The remaining water requirement to maintain hydration is typically provided as 5% dextrose solution. An example of how short-term requirements may be provided for a patient with ileus is shown in Table 2.6.

In patients requiring replacement for more than 3–4 days, correction of 'trace' ions may be needed, particularly if intestinal fluid loss is significant. Magnesium, calcium and phosphate are most commonly required (see below), and are best guided by direct measurement of plasma concentrations. In this situation, the provision of parenteral nutrition also requires consideration (Ch. 5).

Table 2.5 PROVISION OF NORMAL 24-HOUR FLUID AND ELECTROLYTE REQUIREMENTS BY INTRAVENOUS INFUSION

Intravenous fluid	Additive	Duration (hrs)
500 ml 0.9% NaCl	20 mmol KCl	4
500 ml 5% dextrose	–	4
500 ml 5% dextrose	20 mmol KCl	4
500 ml 0.9% NaCl	–	4
500 ml 5% dextrose	20 mmol KCl	4
500 ml 5% dextrose	–	4

Table 2.6 HOW TO ESTIMATE FLUID AND ELECTROLYTE REQUIREMENTS (ML) IN A PATIENT WITH ILEUS*			
	Volume	Na⁺	K⁺
Urine	1500	80	60
Nasogastric aspirate	2000	240	20
Insensible loss	800	–	–
Minus endogenous water	−300	–	–
Net losses/requirements	4000	320	80

2 litres of normal saline would supply 300 mmol of Na^+.
2 litres of 5% dextrose would supply water.
The required 60–80 mmol of K^+ can be added as 20 mmol to alternate 500 ml bags.

* Assuming that the patient is in electrolyte balance and is losing 2 litres/day as nasogastric aspirate and 1.5 litres/day as urine, 24-hour losses can be calculated as shown.

TREATING HYPOVOLAEMIA AND/OR HYPOTENSION

Hypotension and hypovolaemia are common in the early post-operative period because of the fluid losses described. The use of regional analgesia (especially epidural block) may make hypotension more likely when intravascular hypovolaemia occurs. In hypotensive patients, other potential causes of shock, such as poor cardiac function or sepsis, should be considered before assuming the cause is simple hypovolaemia (Ch. 3). Boluses of 200–400 ml of fluid should be given over 10–30 minutes, followed by reassessment. The amount of fluid needed can be judged by the patient's blood pressure, pulse rate, urine output and peripheral skin temperature (a good indicator of peripheral blood flow). If a central venous catheter is in place, central venous pressure is very useful.

There is controversy as to whether crystalloid or colloid solutions should be the first choice for treating intravascular hypovolaemia (EBM 2.1). Recent evidence in intensive care patients shows that crystalloids and albumin are equally safe. The most important principle is to provide the correct volume of the fluid chosen to restore perfusion of organs.

EBM 2.1   CRYSTALLOIDS VERSUS ALBUMIN TO TREAT INTRAVASCULAR HYPOVOLAEMIA

'A very large multicentre study in patients in intensive care units (the SAFE study) showed that mortality was the same for patients treated with albumin and with crystalloids as first-choice fluids for management of hypovolaemia.'

Finfer S, et al. New Engl J Med 2004; 350:2247–2256.

SPECIFIC WATER AND ELECTROLYTE ABNORMALITIES

WATER AND SODIUM IMBALANCE

Water depletion

A decrease in total body water of 1–2% (350–700 ml) causes an increase in blood osmolarity sufficient to stimulate brain osmoreceptors and produce the sensation of thirst. Clinically obvious dehydration, with thirst, a dry tongue and loss of skin turgor, indicates at least 4–5% deficiency of total body water (1.5–2 litres). Pure water depletion is rare in surgical practice, and is usually combined with sodium loss. The most frequent causes are inadequate intake or the excessive loss of gastrointestinal secretions.

Water excess

Water excess is common in surgical patients, particularly in post-operative patients who receive large volumes of intravenous 5% dextrose during the period of increased ADH secretion (Ch. 1). In this situation the patient is commonly hyponatraemic (see below). Patients with water excess usually remain well, but may develop dependent oedema. In patients with poor cardiac function or renal failure, water accumulation can result in pulmonary oedema.

Sodium balance

Sodium is the principal extracellular cation. Changes in the concentration of sodium in ECF therefore result in changes in the tonicity of this fluid compartment. Sodium concentration is closely related to the relative amount of water in the ECF space. The presence of hypo- or hypernatraemia therefore reflects the balance between sodium and water content.

Hypernatraemia

Hypernatraemia is most commonly a result of water depletion or pure dehydration (Box 2.2). In the surgical patient, the common causes are reduced water intake due to anorexia, nausea or fasting in relation to the surgical procedure. Increased water loss can result from fever, sweating and hyperventilation. The treatment is usually to increase the patient's water intake. This can be achieved via the oral route, by encouraging the patient to drink or adding additional water to nasogastric feeds, or by administering additional intravenous water as 5% dextrose solution.

Hyponatraemia

Hyponatraemia is a more complex disorder because it can occur in the presence of decreased, normal or increased extracellular volume (Box 2.2). In the surgical patient, the common causes of hyponatraemia are volume depletion, excessive administration of water as 5% dextrose (particularly during the post-operative period of increased ADH secretion) and diuretic use. Comorbidity, such as cirrhosis, cardiac failure and renal impairment, is a potential contributing factor. The treatment of hyponatraemia depends on identifying its cause correctly. The most important assessment is to judge whether plasma and/or extracellular volume is increased, normal or decreased. If

2

2

BOX 2.2   THE AETIOLOGY OF HYPER- AND HYPONATRAEMIA

Hypernatraemia

Reduced intake

- Fasting*
- Nausea and vomiting*
- Ileus*
- Reduced conscious level

Increased loss

- Sweating (pyrexia, hot environment)*
- Respiratory tract loss (increased ventilation, administration of dry gases)
- Burns*

Inappropriate urinary water loss

- Diabetes insipidus (pituitary or nephrogenic)
- Diabetes mellitus
- Excessive sodium load (hypertonic fluids, parenteral nutrition)

Hyponatraemia

Low extracellular fluid volume

- Volume depletion (vomiting, diarrhoea, burns, decreased fluid intake)*
- Salt-losing renal disease
- Hypoadrenalism
- Diuretic use*

Normal extracellular fluid volume

- Hypothyroidism
- Syndromes of inappropriate ADH secretion (SIADH)

Increased extracellular fluid volume

- Excessive water administration*
- Excessive mannitol use
- Cardiac failure
- Cirrhosis
- Nephrotic syndrome
- Renal failure

* Causes commonly encountered in the surgical patient are denoted with an asterisk.

BOX 2.3   CONSEQUENCES OF HYPER- AND HYPOKALAEMIA

Hyperkalaemia

- Arrhythmias (broad-complex rhythms, bradycardia, heart block, ventricular fibrillation)
- Muscle weakness
- Ileus

Hypokalaemia

- ECG changes (flattened T-waves, U-waves)
- Ectopic beats
- Muscle weakness

POTASSIUM IMBALANCE

Potassium is the principal intracellular cation. Only 60 mmol of the normal total body potassium (typically about 3500 mmol) is extracellular. Plasma potassium concentration (typically 4 mmol/l) is therefore a poor indicator of the total body potassium. Changes in the distribution of potassium between plasma and intracellular fluid can have a dramatic effect on the plasma K^+ concentration. Potassium distribution is tightly controlled by Na^+/K^+ ATPase and other ion pumps present in cell membranes. The Na^+/K^+ ATPase is pH-sensitive, and during acidosis reduced activity results in a net efflux of potassium from cells and thence hyperkalaemia. Conversely, during alkalosis increased activity results in hypokalaemia. These abnormalities are exacerbated by renal compensatory mechanisms that correct acid–base balance at the expense of potassium homeostasis. The consequences of hyper- and hypokalaemia are listed in Box 2.3.

Hyperkalaemia

This has several causes (Box 2.4). Most are characterized by an increased efflux of potassium from cells as a result of tissue damage or altered membrane pump function. Hyperkalaemia is often asymptomatic until dangerous arrhythmias develop, or is diagnosed incidentally as a

---

BOX 2.4   CAUSES OF HYPERKALAEMIA

Excess intravenous or oral intake

Efflux of potassium from cells

- Haemolysis
- Rhabdomyolysis (e.g. crush syndromes, compartment syndromes)*
- Massive tissue damage (e.g. ischaemic bowel or liver)*

Acidosis

Impaired excretion

- Acute renal failure*
- Chronic renal failure
- Drugs (ACE inhibitors, spironolactone)

Abnormalities of the renin–angiotensin system (e.g. Addison's disease)

* Frequent causes in surgical patients are denoted with an asterisk.

ECF volume is normal or increased in the surgical patient who does not have comorbidity such as cardiac failure or liver disease, the most likely cause of hyponatraemia is excessive intravenous water administration. This will correct spontaneously if water intake is reduced. In patients with decreased ECF volume, hyponatraemia usually indicates combined water and sodium deficiency, which will correct if adequate 0.9% sodium chloride is administered. Severe hyponatraemia (plasma sodium < 120 mmol/l) is usually a result of coexisting cardiac, liver or renal disease or, if these are not present, the syndromes of inappropriate ADH secretion (SIADH). Severe hyponatraemia requires careful management with water restriction, cautious 0.9% sodium chloride therapy, and occasionally diuretic use. Hypertonic saline solutions are rarely indicated and can be dangerous. The condition can be complicated by confusion, cerebral oedema, seizures and coma. Plasma sodium requires slow correction (at about 1 mmol/hr) with regular monitoring, because rapid increases in sodium concentration can cause permanent neurological damage.

BOX 2.5   MANAGEMENT OF SEVERE ACUTE HYPERKALAEMIA (K^+ > 7 MMOL/L)

1. Identify and treat cause
2. 10–20 ml intravenous 10% calcium gluconate over 10 mins in patients with ECG abnormalities (reduces risk of ventricular fibrillation)
3. 50 ml 50% dextrose plus 10 units short-acting insulin over 2–3 mins Monitor plasma glucose and K^+ over next 30–60 mins Start infusion of 10 or 20% dextrose solution 50–100 ml/hr
4. Regular salbutamol nebulizers
5. Consider oral or rectal calcium resonium (ion exchange resin), although this is more effective for non-acute hyperkalaemia
6. Haemodialysis for persistent hyperkalaemia

---

result of ECG changes or measurement of plasma concentration. Severe hyperkalaemia (K^+ > 7 mmol/l) requires immediate treatment and identification of the likely cause (Box 2.5).

Hypokalaemia

This is a common disorder in surgical patients. Dietary intake of potassium is normally 60–80 mmol/day, and > 85% is excreted via the kidneys. Maintenance of potassium balance depends on normal renal tubular regulation. Potassium excretion is increased by alkalosis, increased urine flow rates and increased aldosterone release, which all occur frequently in the surgical patient. The causes of hypokalaemia are listed in Box 2.6. Hypokalaemia is treated by administering additional potassium orally as a potassium salt, or intravenously. The oral or nasogastric route is preferable and safer whenever possible.

OTHER ELECTROLYTE DISTURBANCES

Abnormalities in calcium and magnesium balance are rarely of major significance in the surgical patient, except in specific conditions such as acute pancreatitis (hypocalcaemia) or in relation to endocrine surgery (such as parathyroid surgery). These are described in the relevant chapters of this book. Hypophosphataemia is a frequent and important disorder in the surgical patient that merits specific consideration. About 80% of total body phosphate is in the skeleton, and the remaining 20% is a major intracellular anion. Phosphate molecules are critical in many biochemical processes, notably in storing energy as adenosine triphosphate (ATP), in signalling messengers, and in synthesizing nucleic acids during cell division and healing. Severe hypophosphataemia (< 0.4 mmol/l; normal range 0.8–1.4 mmol/l) causes widespread cellular dysfunction and, notably, muscle weakness. Hypophosphataemia commonly occurs in patients recovering from major illness and surgery, particularly after nutrition is reintroduced, either naturally or artificially. Like hypokalaemia, hypophosphataemia is also precipitated by alkalosis. Plasma phosphate concentration should therefore be measured regularly following major surgery and in patients receiving artificial nutrition. Phosphate can be replaced via oral supplements or by slow intravenous infusion.

ACID–BASE BALANCE

There are four main types of acid–base disturbance: acidosis or alkalosis can occur, and each may be respiratory or metabolic in origin. These disturbances can occur in isolation or as mixed disorders. The diagnosis of acid–base disturbance relies on the measurement of arterial blood gases, and occasionally on blood lactate concentration (Ch. 10). Arterial blood gas analysis is a straightforward technique. Samples can be analysed rapidly by ward- or laboratory-based machines (Fig. 2.3). The common conditions encountered in the surgical patient are discussed below.

BOX 2.6   CAUSES OF HYPOKALAEMIA

Reduced/inadequate intake*

Gastrointestinal tract losses

- Vomiting*
- Gastric aspiration/drainage*
- Fistulae*
- Diarrhoea*
- Ileus*
- Intestinal obstruction*
- Potassium-secreting villous adenomas*

Urinary losses

- Metabolic alkalosis*
- Hyperaldosteronism*
- Diuretic use*
- Renal tubular disorders (e.g. Bartter's syndrome, renal tubular acidosis, amphotericin-induced tubular damage)

* Common causes in the surgical patient are denoted by an asterisk.

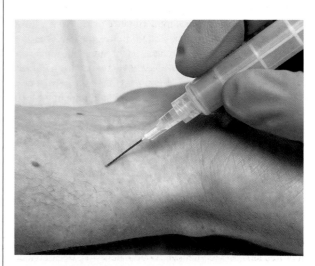

Fig. 2.3   A blood gas sample being taken from the radial artery under local anaesthesia.

2

BOX 2.7 ACID–BASE FINDINGS AND COMMON CAUSES OF METABOLIC ACIDOSIS IN THE SURGICAL PATIENT

Common surgical causes of metabolic acidosis

Lactic acidosis
- Shock (any cause)
- Severe hypoxaemia
- Severe haemorrhage/anaemia
- Liver failure

Accumulation of other acids
- Diabetic ketoacidosis
- Acute or chronic renal failure
- Poisoning (ethylene glycol, methanol, salicylates)

Increased bicarbonate loss
- Diarrhoea
- Intestinal fistulae

Acid–base findings

Acute uncompensated
- H^+ ions ↑
- $PaCO_2$ →
- Actual HCO_3^- ↓
- Standard HCO_3^- ↓

With respiratory compensation (hyperventilation)
- H^+ ions → (full compensation), ≠(partial compensation)
- $PaCO_2$ ↓
- Actual HCO_3^- ↓
- Standard HCO_3^- ↓

BOX 2.8 ACID–BASE FINDINGS AND COMMON CAUSES OF METABOLIC ALKALOSIS IN THE SURGICAL PATIENT

Common surgical causes of metabolic alkalosis

Loss of sodium, chloride and water
- Vomiting
- Aspiration of gastric secretions (e.g. nasogastric suction)
- Diuretic administration

Hypokalaemia
- Box 2.6

Acid–base findings

Acute uncompensated
- H^+ ions ↓
- $PaCO_2$ →
- Actual HCO_3^- ↑
- Standard HCO_3^- ↑

With respiratory compensation (hypoventilation)
- H^+ ions → (full compensation), ↓ (partial compensation)
- $PaCO_2$ ↑
- Actual HCO_3^- ↑
- Standard HCO_3^- ↑

METABOLIC ACIDOSIS

Metabolic acidosis is characterized by an increase in plasma hydrogen ions in conjunction with a decrease in bicarbonate concentration (Box 2.7). Respiratory compensation decreases the $PaCO_2$ to levels lower than normal secondary to hyperventilation. Metabolic acidosis can occur as a result of increased production of lactic acid, the accumulation of acids other than lactic acid, or increased loss of bicarbonate.

The most common cause in surgical practice is lactic acidosis, which stems from impaired tissue perfusion due to shock (Ch. 3). A low total CO_2 estimation on routine blood urea and electrolytes should alert the physician to the possibility of the presence of a metabolic acidosis, particularly if there are clinical signs of tissue hypoperfusion, such as oliguria, hypotension or cold peripheries. Therapy is directed towards restoring the circulating blood volume and tissue perfusion. With normal cardiorespiratory and renal function, the metabolic acidosis will correct spontaneously after adequate resuscitation.

METABOLIC ALKALOSIS

Metabolic alkalosis is characterized by a decrease in plasma hydrogen ion concentration and an increase in bicarbonate concentration (Box 2.8). A compensatory respiratory acidosis may occur, resulting in an increase in $PaCO_2$. Metabolic alkalosis is commonly associated with hypokalaemia and hypochloraemia. The body has an enormous capacity to generate bicarbonate ions, and this is stimulated particularly by chloride losses that can only be reversed by exogenous administration. This is a major factor causing metabolic alkalosis following chloride losses from the gastrointestinal tract, especially when combined with loss of acid from conditions such as gastric outlet obstruction. Hypokalaemia is often associated with metabolic alkalosis because hydrogen ions shift into cells, and because distal renal tubular cells retain potassium in preference to hydrogen ions. Treatment of most forms of metabolic alkalosis involves the administration of adequate 0.9% NaCl together with sufficient potassium to correct hypokalaemia.

RESPIRATORY ACIDOSIS

Respiratory acidosis is characterized by increased $PaCO_2$, hydrogen ions and plasma bicarbonate concentration, and is a common post-operative problem (Box 2.9). It usually results from excessive opiate administration because of a shift in the response of chemoreceptors to CO_2. This form of respiratory acidosis is harmless in most patients, requires no specific treatment, and will resolve as opiate requirements for pain decrease. Occasionally, respiratory acidosis occurs because of pulmonary complications such as pneumonia, but usually only in very sick patients or those with pre-existing respiratory disease. Patients with this cause of respiratory acidosis may require respiratory support with artificial ventilation, because the problem is inadequate respiratory muscle strength, often in association with respiratory complications that increase the work of breathing.

RESPIRATORY ALKALOSIS

Respiratory alkalosis is caused by excessive loss of CO_2 owing to hyperventilation of the lungs. $PaCO_2$ and hydrogen

BOX 2.9 ACID–BASE FINDINGS AND COMMON CAUSES OF RESPIRATORY ACIDOSIS ENCOUNTERED IN SURGICAL PRACTICE

Common surgical causes of respiratory acidosis

Central respiratory depression

- Opioid drugs
- Head injury or intracranial pathology

Pulmonary disease

- Severe asthma
- COPD
- Severe chest infection

Acid–base findings

Acute uncompensated

- H^+ ions ↑
- $PaCO_2$ ↑
- Actual HCO_3^- → or ↑
- Standard HCO_3^- →

With metabolic compensation (renal bicarbonate retention)

- H^+ ions → (full compensation), ↑ (partial compensation)
- $PaCO_2$ ↑
- Actual HCO_3^- ↑
- Standard HCO_3^- ↑↑

BOX 2.10 ACID–BASE FINDINGS AND CAUSES OF RESPIRATORY ALKALOSIS

Causes of respiratory alkalosis

- Pain
- Apprehension/hysterical hyperventilation
- Pneumonia
- Central nervous system disorders (meningitis, encephalopathy)
- Pulmonary embolism
- Septicaemia
- Salicylate poisoning
- Liver failure

Acid–base findings

Acute uncompensated

- H^+ ions ↓
- $PaCO_2$ ↓
- Actual HCO_3^- → or ↓
- Standard HCO_3^- →

With metabolic compensation (renal bicarbonate excretion)

- H^+ ions → (full compensation), ↑ (partial compensation)
- $PaCO_2$ ↓
- Actual HCO_3^- ↓
- Standard HCO_3^- ↓

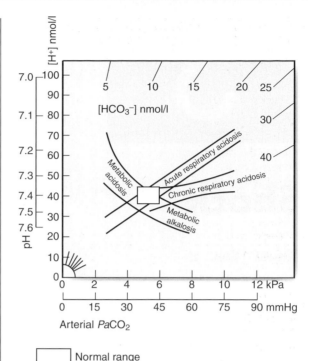

Normal range

95% Confidence limits

Fig. 2.4 Changes in blood [H^+].
The rectangle indicates limits of normal reference ranges for [H^+] and $PaCO_2$. The bands represent 95% confidence limits of single disturbances in human blood in vivo. When the point obtained by plotting [H^+] against P does not fall within one of the labelled bands, compensation is incomplete or a mixed disorder is present.

MIXED PATTERNS OF ACID–BASE IMBALANCE

Mixed patterns of acid–base disturbance are common, particularly in very sick patients. In this situation acid–base nomograms can be very useful in clarifying the contributing factors (Fig. 2.4).

ion concentration decrease (Box 2.10). Respiratory alkalosis is rarely chronic and usually does not need specific treatment. It usually corrects spontaneously when the precipitating condition resolves.

23

3

A.J. POLLOK

Shock

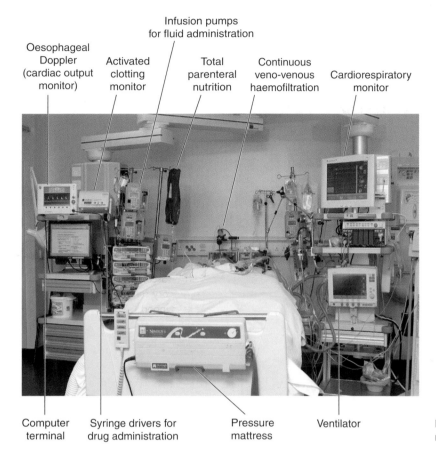

Oesophageal Doppler (cardiac output monitor)

Activated clotting monitor

Infusion pumps for fluid administration

Total parenteral nutrition

Continuous veno-venous haemofiltration

Cardiorespiratory monitor

Computer terminal

Syringe drivers for drug administration

Pressure mattress

Ventilator

Fig. 3.1   ICU bed pictured with invasive monitoring and life-support devices.

3

BOX 3.1   DEFINITION OF SHOCK

- Shock is an imbalance between oxygen delivery and demand, resulting in cellular dysfunction and death, which is reflected in organ failure

DEFINITION OF SHOCK

Shock exists when, despite a normal oxygen content of arterial blood, oxygen delivery fails to meet the metabolic requirements of tissues. Shock is sometimes considered to be synonymous with hypotension. However, it is very important to realize that hypotension is often a late sign of shock; cardiac output and oxygen delivery may be critically low, even though the blood pressure remains normal. It is important to identify this state and intervene, if at all possible.

CAUSES OF SHOCK

A broad classification is as follows.

Hypovolaemia

A reduction in circulating blood volume may result from many conditions, including haemorrhage, severe burns, dehydration (e.g. diabetic ketoacidosis) or severe gastrointestinal losses due to vomiting and diarrhoea.

Cardiogenic shock

Here there is an adequate circulating blood volume but the heart fails to act as a satisfactory pump. Examples include myocardial infarction, severe valvular incompetence or situations in which the heart is obstructed (such as massive pulmonary embolism, cardiac tamponade or tension pneumothorax).

Neurogenic shock

This is caused by major brain or spinal injury and may be associated with neurogenic pulmonary oedema.

Anaphylaxis

This can occur following the administration of any drug or may be triggered by other allergens, e.g. bee sting. Inappropriate vasodilatation is triggered, producing flushing and oedema.

Sepsis

This can be brought about either by infection or by other causes of a systemic inflammatory response that produce widespread endothelial damage. There is vasodilatation, arteriovenous shunting and microvascular occlusion. These result in decreased oxygen delivery to the capillary beds of vital organs. Septic shock and the systemic inflammatory response syndrome are defined in Tables 3.1 and 3.2.

The clinical features and possible diagnosis in different types of shock are illustrated in Figure 3.2.

3

Table 3.1 SEPTIC SHOCK

- Commonly due to infections with Gram-negative bacteria but can be due to Gram-positive bacteria or fungi
- Endotoxin from bacterial cell walls triggers a localized inflammatory cascade within the vascular compartment, which in susceptible individuals becomes systemic
- The haemodynamic response is vasodilatation due to a reduction in the systemic vascular resistance
- A reflex increase in cardiac output may maintain the blood pressure, and the hyperdynamic circulation results in a patient who appears deceptively well, with pink warm peripheries
- Significant organ hypoperfusion (splanchnic circulation) may be occurring, with arteriovenous shunting within the capillary beds of many organs, resulting in cellular hypoxia and organ dysfunction

---

Table 3.2 SYSTEMIC INFLAMMATORY RESPONSE SYNDROME (SIRS)

Systemic response to either an infective or a non-infective insult (trauma, pancreatitis, vasculitis etc.). Two or more features must be present for the diagnosis:
- Temperature > 38C° or < 36°C
- Heart rate > 90 beats per minute
- Respiratory rate > 20 per minute
- Mean arterial pressure < 65 mmHg or evidence of organ dysfunction
- White cell count > $12 \times 10^9/l$ or < $4 \times 10^9/l$

Severe sepsis is diagnosed when two of the above are present with evidence of infection

---

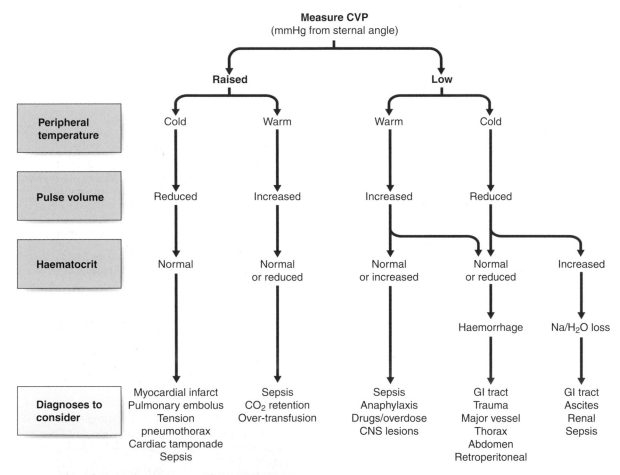

Fig. 3.2 Clinical features and possible diagnosis in different types of shock. (CVP = central venous pressure)

PATHOPHYSIOLOGY OF SHOCK

Irrespective of the aetiology underlying a low-output state (either hypovolaemia or pump failure), the sympathetic stimulation and catecholamine release that occur result in a similar clinical picture. Whereas slight differences can be detected at the level of the macrocirculation, alterations in the microcirculation are indistinguishable. Prolonged sym-

pathetic overactivity and catecholamine release, due either to unrecognized shock or to an inability to correct the precipitating cause, will lead to organ and tissue hyperperfusion. In turn, this will produce generalized hypoxia and a deterioration in acid–base status. Without intervention, cell dysfunction and organ failure will occur. In septic shock, elevated levels of circulating vasoactive substances are responsible for the physiological abnormalities observed. At the level of the macrocirculation there is a reduction in whole-body systemic vascular resistance. This picture masks serious inequalities in blood flow between various organs and therefore there is still hypoxia at tissue level.

MACROCIRCULATION

The classic signs associated with a low-output state are cold, pale, clammy skin and collapsed peripheral veins. These signs occur because low blood pressure causes catecholamine release from the adrenal medulla. The resultant increase in heart rate, myocardial contractility and systemic vascular resistance helps to maintain cardiac output. However, it also causes clinically obvious peripheral vasoconstriction and less obvious splanchnic hypoperfusion. It is this reduced blood supply to the gut which is implicated in many of the complications associated with prolonged or untreated shock. There is also a reduction in renal cortical blood flow, which stimulates the renin–angiotensin system. The resultant elevated levels of circulating angiotensin II further contribute to systemic vasoconstriction.

In a patient with septic shock, elevated levels of circulating vasoactive substances result in vasodilatation and a fall in systemic vascular resistance. The cardiovascular response is a reflex tachycardia and increased cardiac output, so that patients demonstrate a hyperdynamic circulation with warm pink peripheries and venodilatation. Fit young patients may compensate for these changes relatively well, although oxygen delivery and utilization at a capillary level are compromised. Therefore the fit young patient with normal blood pressure and heart rate within normal limits, but who has an unexplained metabolic acidosis, should alert the physician to the possibility of serious sepsis.

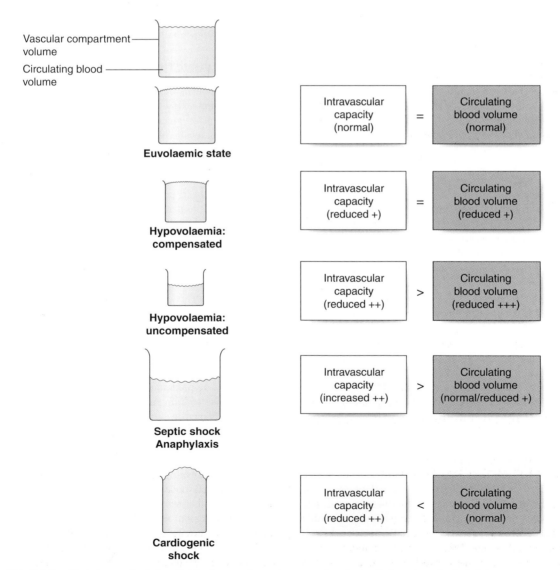

Fig. 3.3 Relationship between circulating blood volume and vascular compartment capacity in various shocked states.

3

As cardiogenic shock is also a low-output state, the physiological changes are similar to those seen with severe hypovolaemia but on a background of normovolaemia. If there is associated left ventricular failure, then there may be increased pressure in the pulmonary veins, resulting in pulmonary oedema that may manifest itself as tachypnoea and shortness of breath. Right-sided heart failure may be present in isolation or as a consequence of left-sided failure leading to an elevation in central venous pressure (CVP, Fig. 3.3).

MICROCIRCULATION

Irrespective of the aetiology, the microcirculatory abnormality is an imbalance between the supply of and demand for oxygen at a cellular level. Vasoconstriction, seen in early hypovolaemic and cardiogenic shock, results in constriction of capillary beds, helping to maintain a satisfactory mean arterial pressure. This mechanism also produces a fall in the capillary hydrostatic pressure, encouraging a net transfer of fluid from the interstitial space into the vascular compartment in an attempt to augment the decreased circulating blood volume. This results in a high vascular resistance in non-vital organs: specifically, skin, muscle and gut. Reduced skin blood flow can be identified by an increase in the difference between core and peripheral temperature. Falls in muscle and splanchnic blood flow are not so easily detected. A 10% reduction in circulating blood volume produces an alteration to heart rate or systolic blood pressure but masks a significant reduction in splanchnic blood flow and oxygen delivery. In the case of septic shock, the characteristic fall in systemic vascular resistance reflects a pathological increase in arteriovenous shunts in tissue capillary beds. This diversion of oxygenated blood away from capillary beds, together with an increase in capillary permeability, contributes to tissue hypoxia, which is reflected by an elevated lactate and associated metabolic acidosis. These microcirculatory responses to shock will be modified by underlying cardiovascular disease, such as hypertension or atherosclerosis, and this explains why elderly patients frequently do not demonstrate the classic signs mentioned above and may decompensate at an earlier stage in the process.

If shock remains uncorrected, the local accumulation of the products of anaerobic metabolism, such as lactic acid and carbon dioxide, together with the release of vasoactive substances from the endothelium, reverses the sympathetic effects and leads to pre-capillary vasodilatation. However, if there is persistent post-capillary venoconstriction, then the result is pooling of blood within the capillary bed and endothelial cell damage secondary to the presence of stimulants, such as microemboli, vasoactive substances, activated leucocytes and complement. Vessel permeability increases with the loss of fluid from the capillary into the interstitium, resulting in oedema. Haemoconcentration means increased viscosity and this adds to the already increased viscosity associated with low-flow states. These conditions predispose to reduced red blood cell deformability and a tendency for red blood cell and platelet aggregation. A combination of microemboli and increased local levels of noradrenaline (norepinephrine), prostaglandins and thrombin, together with capillary endothelial damage on a background of low flow and increased viscosity, sets the scene for platelet aggregation and clot formation within the capillary beds. This will further exacerbate existing tissue ischaemia and oedema, contributing to ongoing damage to organs.

At the capillary level, the activation of coagulation that is occurring in many tissue beds results in consumption of both platelets and coagulation factors, leading to abnormal clotting with thrombocytopenia and prolonged prothrombin and activated partial thromboplastin times. A parallel activation of the fibrinolytic pathway via plasminogen results in a breakdown of these intracapillary clots and an elevation in the circulating levels of fibrin and fibrinogen (D-dimers). The somewhat paradoxical finding of increased capillary coagulation and systemic anti-coagulation on a background of thrombocytopenia and elevated levels of D-dimers is referred to as disseminated intravascular coagulation (DIC). This serious abnormality of coagulation is uncommon and tends to be associated with more severe cases of shock, especially if there is underlying sepsis.

CELLULAR FUNCTION

Aerobic metabolism requires a continuous supply of oxygen for the efficient extraction of energy from carbohydrate substrates such as glucose. This occurs within the mitochondria and results in the production of high-energy adenosine triphosphate (ATP). ATP is the energy source for the majority of active processes within the cell. The free hydrogen associated with ATP generation is temporarily scavenged by NAD^+ prior to its ultimate combination with oxygen and disposal as water. Early in shock the oxygen debt results in a saturation of NAD^+ and other scavengers and an accumulation of the intermediate metabolite, pyruvic acid, which is prevented from entering the citric acid cycle. In the absence of oxygen, pyruvic acid itself can facilitate the oxidation of NADH to NAD^+ by converting to lactic acid. This allows limited ATP production to continue. Lactic acid accumulates in the systemic circulation and can be monitored biochemically. In the absence of significant renal or liver disease, serum lactate concentration is a useful marker of cellular hypoxia and systemic oxygen debt.

Sodium is a predominantly extracellular ion and the cell membrane 'sodium pump' is central to the maintenance of cellular homeostasis. The movement of the sodium ion against a concentration gradient is an active process requiring ATP. Any reduction in the ATP supply will lead to intracellular accumulation of sodium. This in turn results in an osmotic gradient across the cell membrane, encouraging cell oedema. When this is combined with the failure of other vital cell functions and the breakdown of lysosomal membranes, leading to the release of enzymes, cell death becomes the inevitable consequence. If the pathophysiological changes responsible for these cellular alterations are widespread and remain uncorrected, multiple organ failure (MOF) supervenes and recovery is unlikely.

BOX 3.2 METABOLIC MONITORING IN SHOCK

- Regular arterial blood gas sampling, with measurement of acid–base status and serum lactate concentration, will assist the physician in assessing the effectiveness of resuscitation

---

EFFECTS ON INDIVIDUAL ORGAN SYSTEMS

Intrinsic organ autoregulation, combined with an increase in sympathetic activity and circulating catecholamines, is the major compensatory mechanism responsible for the maintenance of an adequate perfusion and oxygen supply to vital organs. This occurs at the expense of both the periphery and non-essential organs. However, these 'sparing' mechanisms have limits and, in the case of severe, prolonged and uncorrected shock, the clinical effects of vital organ hypoperfusion become apparent.

NERVOUS SYSTEM

In early shock the effects of pain and increased sympathetic activity may predominate, with the patient appearing inappropriately anxious. As compensatory mechanisms reach their limit and cerebral hypoperfusion and hypoxia supervene, there is increasing restlessness, progressing to confusion, stupor and coma. Unless hypoxia has been prolonged, effective resuscitation will quickly correct the depressed conscious level. In septic shock, the clinical picture may be complicated by the presence of an underlying encephalopathy caused by other factors. This should be considered if, after the shocked state has been reversed, the patient remains confused with altered cognitive function. Unlike the effects of hypoperfusion, the encephalopathy may take significantly longer to recover.

KIDNEYS

The clinical effects of shock on the kidneys reflect the combined effects of increased sympathetic activity, circulating catecholamines, antidiuretic hormone (ADH) and aldosterone. Reduced renal blood flow, with diversion of blood from the cortex to the medulla, together with sodium and water conservation, results in a low urine output, or oliguria (< 0.5 ml/kg/hr). This pre-renal abnormality is characterized by urine that has a normal to high specific gravity and low sodium concentration. If the shocked state is not reversed, prolonged hypoxia of the tubular cells will result in damage and ultimately cell death. Acute tubular necrosis (ATN) results in renal failure and is associated with a very low volume of urine, which has a low specific gravity, high sodium concentration and osmolality close to that of plasma. Over the subsequent days, a rising blood urea and creatinine in the presence of normovolaemia and an adequate blood pressure will confirm the clinical impression of ATN.

Temporary renal replacement therapy may be required while the return of renal function is awaited. Recovery of the tubular function may be signalled by the development of a marked diuresis on a background of high urea and creatinine (diuretic phase of acute renal failure).

Patients in septic shock may present with an inappropriately high urine output in the presence of hypotension. However, an increasing blood urea and creatinine will confirm the presence of acute renal failure (high-output renal failure).

RESPIRATORY SYSTEM

In the initial phase of shock, the patient is frequently tachypnoeic. The reasons for this include the central effects of pain, anxiety and increased sympathetic drive, together with peripheral chemoreceptor stimulation. Early arterial blood gas estimation may reveal a predominantly uncompensated respiratory alkalosis. With the onset of a metabolic acidosis, respiratory compensation involves an increase in depth (tidal volume) and rate of breathing in order to raise the minute ventilation and increase CO_2 excretion. In hypovolaemic states, the reduction in systemic blood flow is mirrored by an identical reduction in pulmonary blood flow. This decrease in pulmonary perfusion pressure increases the mismatching between lung ventilation and perfusion, so that increased areas of the lung are ventilated but not perfused.

In contrast, during cardiogenic shock, left ventricular failure and pulmonary oedema are frequently present. There are areas of lung where the presence of pulmonary oedema fluid compromises alveolar ventilation and gas transfer across the alveolar–capillary membrane. This results in alveoli being perfused but not adequately ventilated (increasing the shunt fraction, Qs/Qt). This pathological process will contribute to a low arterial oxygen saturation, which may not be reversed by simply increasing the inspired oxygen concentration.

Direct thoracic trauma may lead to pulmonary contusion, fractured ribs, pneumothorax or haemothorax, which can all result in a deterioration in pulmonary gas exchange. Additional insults, such as aspiration of gastric contents, fluid overload following resuscitation, smoke inhalation or central respiratory depression, may contribute to pulmonary insufficiency or precipitate acute respiratory failure. Any severe insult, such as multiple trauma, shock or sepsis, can trigger the systemic cascade of inflammatory mediators mentioned above, resulting in increased capillary permeability. The pulmonary manifestation of this systemic process is pulmonary oedema. This pathophysiological process is thought to be responsible for the delayed (24–48 hours) failure of ventilation and oxygenation that is often seen. This is the non-specific but well-defined syndrome of adult respiratory distress (ARDS). The diagnosis of ARDS can only be considered after other causes of pulmonary oedema, such as pneumonia, left ventricular failure and pulmonary contusion, have been excluded. Irrespective of the cause, hypoxia will have profound consequences in patients in whom oxygen delivery to tissues is already compromised by haemodynamic factors.

3

HEART

In cardiogenic shock, the primary abnormality is one of sudden pump failure, commonly due to extensive muscle damage from myocardial infarction. Myocardial function may also be compromised indirectly by a variety of factors associated with other causes of shock. Despite the presence of coronary autoregulation, severe hypotension will eventually result in an imbalance between myocardial oxygen supply and demand. This global decrease in oxygen supply causes ischaemia in the watershed area of the endocardial layer and will impair myocardial contractility. Hypoxia and acidosis deplete myocardial stores of noradrenaline (norepinephrine) and diminish the cardiac response to endogenous and exogenous catecholamines. Acid–base and electrolyte abnormalities, when combined with local hypoxia, create conditions that are ideal for increasing myocardial excitability and generating dysrhythmias. Myocardial contractility and ventricular function may be further depressed by the direct action of a variety of circulating humoral factors and activated inflammatory mediators implicated in sepsis and the systemic inflammatory response (SIRS; see above).

GUT

To the body undergoing the process of shock, the gut is considered a non-vital organ and a marked reduction in splanchnic blood flow occurs early in the genesis of shock. However, prolonged mucosal hypoperfusion and hypoxia predispose the gastric mucosa to acid damage, stress ulceration and haemorrhage, and, in addition, subtle mucosal barrier damage to the remainder of the gastrointestinal tract will occur. This process has been implicated in the movement (translocation) of toxic substances, gut bacterial endotoxins as well as the bacteria themselves, from the intestinal lumen to the portal blood stream. Their presence in the systemic circulation has been closely linked to the mechanisms underlying both SIRS and MOF.

LIVER

The liver is somewhat protected from ischaemic damage by its dual blood supply from the portal vein and hepatic artery. A significant elevation in serum transaminase levels indicates a major hepatocellular ischaemic–hypoxic injury, and is more commonly observed in severe cardiogenic shock and hepatic venous congestion. Irrespective of the aetiology of the shock state, the presence of biochemical (elevated transaminases) and haematological (prolonged prothrombin time) markers of severe liver damage suggests a very significant insult that carries a very poor prognosis.

NEUROHUMORAL RESPONSE

Many of the clinical signs of shock reflect the central nervous system's attempt to preserve oxygen delivery to vital tissues by maintaining an adequate circulating blood volume, cardiac output and perfusion pressure. Multiple afferent inputs (arterial and venous pressures, vascular

---

BOX 3.3 EFFECTS OF SHOCK ON VARIOUS ORGANS

CNS
- Progressive hypoperfusion: anxiety, restlessness, confusion, stupor, coma
- Sepsis: encephalopathy—prolonged alteration in conscious level

Kidneys
- Oliguria: < 0.5 ml/kg/hr
- Acute renal failure
    Increasing blood urea, creatinine and acidosis
    Anuria: acute tubular necrosis (ATN)
    High-output renal failure

Lungs
- Hypovolaemia
    Alveolar ventilation/perfusion ($\dot{V}/\dot{Q}$) mismatch, leading to hypoxia; reversed by increasing F_{IO_2}
- Cardiogenic
    Pulmonary oedema: increased proportion of cardiac output through alveoli that are not ventilated, leading to an increase in shunt (Qs/Qt), increasing hypoxia which may not respond to increasing F_{IO_2}

Heart
- Decrease in diastolic pressure → fall in coronary perfusion pressure
- Increase in heart rate → decrease in period of diastole → decreased coronary blood flow
- Reduced oxygen delivery → ischaemia → increased excitability
- Depressed contractility
- Acidosis, electrolyte disturbances, hypoxia → dysrhythmias

Gut
- Hypoperfusion ⇓ breakdown of gut mucosal barrier
- Translocation of bacteria/bacterial wall contents into blood stream

---

volume, osmolality, acidosis, pain, anxiety and tissue damage) trigger an increase in sympathetic outflow activity, leading to peripheral sympathetic stimulation and increased circulating catecholamines from the adrenal glands. This increase in sympathetic activity results in a diversion of blood from the renal cortex to the medulla and stimulates the juxtaglomerular cells to release renin. This in turn activates the renin–angiotensin cascade, leading to elevated circulating levels of the potent vasoconstrictor angiotensin II. In the attempt to maintain the circulating blood volume, angiotensin II stimulates the adrenocortical release of aldosterone, resulting in increased sodium and water retention. This early endocrine response is followed by elevations in the concentrations of a number of other stress hormones. Antidiuretic hormone (ADH) acts on the distal tubules of the kidney to conserve water. Adrenocorticotrophic hormone (ACTH) stimulates the adrenal cortex to release cortisol, which plays a major role in the initial protection from the effects of hypovolaemia. Elevated levels of growth hormone and glucagons can also be detected. The combined effect of this complex neurohumoral response is to activate mechanisms that will help to maintain an adequate circulating blood volume and, by mobilizing energy reserves in the form of increased blood glucose, prepare the body for stress.

PRINCIPLES OF MANAGEMENT

Resuscitation should not be delayed because of lack of a diagnosis; however, ultimate treatment success will depend largely on the detection and management of the cause of shock.

HYPOVOLAEMIC SHOCK

Clinical features and examination

Although obtaining a history from either the patient or witnesses can be helpful, it may often prove impossible when the patient's consciousness is impaired from head injury, alcohol or drugs, or as a direct result of cerebral hypoperfusion.

In many cases, such as major trauma or burns, the presence of volume loss is obvious. In other situations (diabetic ketoacidosis, diarrhoea and vomiting, dehydration), both assessment and diagnosis become more problematical.

Cardiovascular assessment begins with observing the patient's colour, a pale skin suggesting a reduction of oxygenated blood through the skin capillaries. Palpation of a peripheral pulse will give valuable information on rate and volume and whether the skin feels warm and dry or cold and clammy. Capillary refill following nailbed pressure can be assessed. With this information alone, the physician can make a quick and often accurate assessment of the patient's volume status. Clearly, if the patient is pale, with a rapid low-volume pulse, skin that is cold and moist,

> **BOX 3.4 CLINICAL FEATURES OF HYPOVOLAEMIC SHOCK**
>
> - Patient often anxious, restless and confused
> - Skin pale, cool and clammy, with collapsed veins
> - Pulse fast and thready; may be difficult to palpate limb pulses
> - JVP not seen

delayed capillary refill and collapsed veins, the clinical picture is one of reduced cardiac output on a background of hypovolaemia and excess sympathetic activity. In contrast, a lucid patient with warm, dry, pink skin and rapid capillary refill is unlikely to have significant hypovolaemia. The volume status may be further assessed by observing the height of the JVP as an estimate of CVP.

The successful management of shock depends on early and frequent clinical monitoring of the patient's volume status and perfusion, as described above. In addition, there are a number of simple measurements of cardiovascular function and organ perfusion that can be made to help in the clinical assessment.

Blood pressure

Blood pressure will depend on the patient's volume status (relative in the case of septic shock and absolute in hypovolaemic shock), myocardial function and the efficiency of the compensatory mechanisms initiated by the sympathetic nervous system. These in turn will be influenced by the patient's pre-morbid cardiovascular state, age (which influences 'normal' blood pressure), ongoing

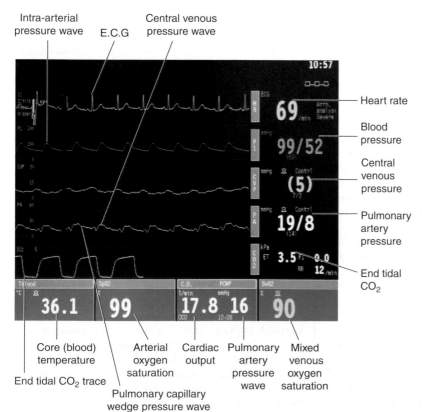

Fig. 3.4 Monitoring screen for a patient in ICU showing multiple physiological measurements.

3

resuscitation measures and additional comorbidities. Taken in isolation, a satisfactory blood pressure does not exclude the presence of a shocked state and is only of use when placed in the context of a full clinical assessment.

Electrocardiogram (ECG) monitoring

The ECG (Fig. 3.4) is a measure of myocardial electrical activity and not of the heart's ability to act as a mechanical pump. It will detect dysrhythmias and severe myocardial ischaemia, and is more useful in cardiogenic shock, myocardial dysfunction secondary to ischaemia, or contusion as a result of severe thoracic injury. Severe hypoxia, electrolyte abnormality or acid–base disturbance can aggravate or precipitate abnormalities in electrical activity and myocardial contractility.

Pulse oximetry

When attached peripherally to a finger or earlobe, the pulse oximeter will give information on pulse volume, which may serve as an estimate of peripheral perfusion. It measures the oxygen saturation of the haemoglobin on the arterial side of the capillary. The screen will display a pulse waveform and a value for the percentage oxygen saturation of haemoglobin. As a simple non-invasive monitor, it gives valuable information on the adequacy of arterial oxygenation and peripheral tissue perfusion. In the poorly perfused state, it will provide a visual and audible warning of a poor signal and confirm the clinical impression.

Core to periphery temperature gradient

Peripheral and core (axillary, nasopharyngeal) temperature measurement can be made and the gradient calculated (ΔT, Fig. 3.5). This is a useful measure of peripheral perfusion, as the gradient can be significant in the presence of severe vasoconstriction (> 10° C). With volume replacement, improved cardiac output and reduced sympathetic activity, there will be an increase in the flow of warm blood through the skin, a rise in peripheral temperature and a decrease in the gradient. The gradient can be used as a simple but accurate index of adequacy of resuscitation

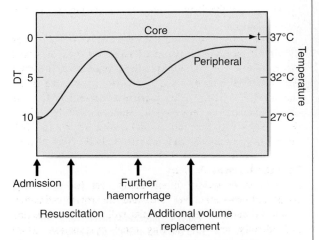

Fig. 3.5 Response of temperature gradient to resuscitation.

and an early indicator of ongoing blood loss. A lower than normal core temperature (hypothermia) is frequently found in trauma patients who have lain in a cold environment, but may also be seen in those who have received large volumes of unwarmed intravenous fluids. Measurement of the core to peripheral temperature gradient is particularly useful in small children and neonates.

Urine output

Unless there is a contraindication (such as the possibility of urethral injury from severe pelvic fractures), the transurethral insertion of a bladder catheter connected to a graduated collecting device will allow an hourly measurement of urine output. This can be used as an indirect measurement of vital organ perfusion: namely, that of the kidney. An adequate urine output (> 0.5 ml/kg/hr) would suggest satisfactory renal perfusion. An increase in the urine output is frequently used as indicator of successful resuscitation.

Central venous catheterization

With the increasing availability of multilumen catheter packs, a catheter can be inserted percutaneously over a wire into a large central vein and the tip positioned in the superior vena cava (SVC). These catheters give the clinician secure vascular access for the rapid administration of large volumes of fluid, at the same time as continuously monitoring the filling pressures on the right side of the heart (CVP). They are not essential in the early stages of the resuscitation process, as fluid can be administered by the insertion of one or two peripheral large-bore intravenous cannulae and volume status assessed by clinical examination. However, following the initial resuscitation, CVP estimation can help in deciding the requirement for further measures. It can also aid the identification of patients who may appear to be clinically normovolaemic but remain volume-deplete (subclinical hypovolaemia).

At the extremes of measurement, the CVP gives an accurate indication of volume status (Fig. 3.6), negative values being associated with significant hypovolaemia and high values (> 20 mmHg) indicating volume overload, as seen in cardiac failure or cardiogenic shock. Between these extremes, however, isolated measurements become unreliable as an indicator of volume status. With minor to moderate hypovolaemia, patients may not exhibit any classic signs of shock and have a CVP value within the normal range. These patients can be identified by observing the response of their CVP to a fluid challenge (i.e. 200 ml colloid over 10 minutes).

Fluid administration

The first step in the resuscitation process is to obtain reliable venous access. This can be done by siting one or two large-bore intravenous cannulae (16 G or larger) in a peripheral vein. If vasoconstriction is intense, access may be difficult and central vein cannulation or a formal cut-down should be considered. This is performed in the antecubital fossa or on to the long saphenous vein in front of the medial malleolus. In hypovolaemic children under the age of 6, placement of an intra-osseous needle into the anterior aspect of the

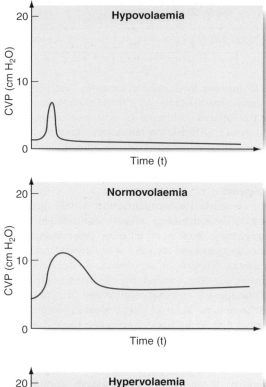

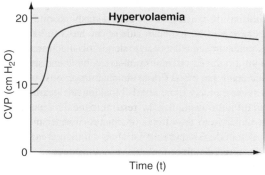

Fig. 3.6 Response of central venous pressure (CVP) to fluid challenge.

blood will result in the dilution of clotting factors and platelets which, when combined with their consumption in major bleeding, may result in a generalized coagulopathy, contributing to further blood loss. By the time the volume transfused equates to the patient's calculated blood volume (approximately 5 litres), consideration should be given to requesting a coagulation screen and administering replacement in the form of fresh frozen plasma and platelet concentrate.

Unless active measures are taken to warm all fluids to 37° C, the administration of large volumes of stored blood at 4° C or colloid/crystalloid at room temperature will result in hypothermia, with effects on coagulation and oxygen delivery being particularly relevant. The use of blood-warming equipment, such as the 'Level 1' (Fig. 3.7), will allow the administration of up to 1000 ml/min of intravenous fluids warmed to body temperature.

Metabolic monitoring

In addition to venous blood being sent for full blood count and cross-matching, urea and electrolyte estimation should be undertaken. The results will provide a baseline and identify any pre-existing renal dysfunction. More importantly, arterial blood gas samples taken both early

upper tibia (taking care to avoid damaging the epiphyseal growth plate) is an excellent alternative route for fluid administration.

Successful resuscitation depends on quick and adequate volume replacement in order to restore a satisfactory cardiac output and peripheral perfusion. The type of fluid lost has no influence on the initial choice of intravenous fluid replacement, both colloid and/or crystalloid being utilized in the first instance (EBMs 3.1 and 3.2). In the case of continued haemorrhage and shock, red cell concentrates or whole blood will be required early in the resuscitation in order to maintain tissue oxygen delivery. Ideally, suitably cross-matched blood should be administered, but in the emergency situation most accident and emergency departments hold a 'shock pack', which will include a quantity of group O Rhesus-negative blood. This can be used until such time as cross-matched blood becomes available. Infusion of large volumes of crystalloid, colloid or stored

3

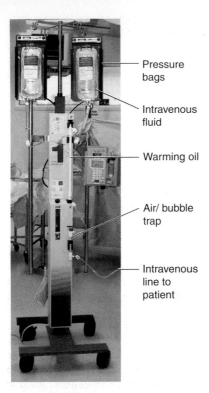

Fig. 3.7 'Level 1' blood warmer.

Pressure bags

Intravenous fluid

Warming oil

Air/ bubble trap

Intravenous line to patient

BOX 3.5 AIDS TO THE CLINICAL ASSESSMENT OF SHOCK

- Blood pressure measurement
- ECG monitoring
- Pulse oximetry
- Core to periphery temperature gradient
- Urine output
- CVP measurement

In isolation, single measurements are not helpful. They become useful when used in combination with the findings of the clinical examination to confirm the clinical impression. Repeated measurements over time, trends and patterns, together with the changes associated with therapeutic interventions, increase their usefulness

---

and frequently will aid in the early identification of respiratory failure, as indicated by the presence of hypoxia and/or hypercarbia. A low PaO_2 may simply require an increase in inspired oxygen concentration (40–60% via face mask), but should this prove to be inadequate, thought should be given as to potential causes and assisted ventilation should be considered. An elevated $PaCO_2$ indicates respiratory insufficiency which, if confirmed on clinical examination, requires assisted ventilation, together with identification of the underlying cause. Metabolic acidosis with increased base deficit, reduced level of bicarbonate (HCO_3) and an elevated blood lactate are the most frequently encountered abnormalities. They will correct rapidly when the circulating blood volume and cardiac output are restored. In severe cases (pH < 7.2 and base excess > 10) not responding to volume replacement, a small volume of intravenous 8.5% sodium bicarbonate (50–100 ml) may

---

BOX 3.6 USE OF OPIATES IN SHOCK

- Shocked patients are more sensitive to the effects of opiates

---

help to improve myocardial contractility and correct any associated hyperkalaemia. As with the clinical examination, it is the frequent estimation of acid–base status, arterial blood gases and lactate concentrations over time that will give the most information on the effectiveness of the resuscitation process.

Analgesia

In the conscious patient with severe trauma there is no indication for withholding effective analgesia. In addition to its primary purpose of relieving pain, analgesia also reduces the associated sequelae of anxiety and sympathetic overactivity that may be contributing to the pathophysiological derangements underlying the shocked state. Short-acting analgesics are inappropriate and in hypovolaemic shock there is no place for subcutaneous or intramuscular administration, as the reduced peripheral blood flow results in unreliable and unpredictable absorption. A long-acting agent such as morphine, given in 1–2 mg increments and titrated against effect, is appropriate. With constant monitoring of conscious level and respiratory function, it should be possible to obtain satisfactory pain control without any significant sequelae of parenteral opiate administration.

With a reduced circulating blood volume and decreased hepatic and renal blood flows, the pharmacokinetics of drugs such as morphine will be altered, making analgesic requirements difficult to predict. In general, patients appear to be more sensitive to the effects of opiates, with a subsequent reduction in dose requirements. Their duration of action will also be unpredictable, making recommendations difficult, but additional doses may be required every 30–60 minutes.

Although the use of local anaesthetic techniques, such as local infiltration and regional nerve blockade, should be considered, they are frequently impractical in the presence of multiple injuries and are contraindicated in coagulopathy. With unilateral rib fractures, multiple intercostal nerve blocks will produce superior analgesia while reducing the requirements for parenteral opiates.

SEPTIC SHOCK

The principles of resuscitation in septic shock are:

1. volume replacement in order to maintain the cardiac preload or CVP
2. the administration of oxygen to optimize total body oxygen delivery
3. maintaining a blood pressure that would be considered appropriate for the individual patient, in the hope that it might ensure adequate organ perfusion
4. investigating the cause of sepsis (Table 3.3).

Against the background of a high cardiac output, an intravenous infusion of a vasoconstrictor, such as noradrenaline (norepinephrine), may be considered. In the most

---

Table 3.3 SURVIVING SEPSIS

1. Recognize severe sepsis/septic shock (see definitions, Ch. 6)
2. Measure serum lactate (arterial)
3. Resuscitation:

    A: airway—if patient obtunded, consider intubation for protection

    B: breathing—high-flow oxygen (minimum 40%)

    C: circulation—central venous pressure (CVP) 8–12 mmHg
    See EBM 3.3.

    > Mean arterial pressure (MAP) > 65 mmHg
    > Urine output > 0.5 ml/kg/hr

4. Microbiology: specimens—blood, sputum, urine, wound, pus
5. Antibiotic: early, empirical
6. Source: identification and control (surgical and/or radiological)
7. Consider adjuvants:

    Steroids—if patient requiring high-dose inotropes

    Activated protein C: endogenous anticoagulant with anti-inflammatory properties (EBM 3.4)

EBM 3.3 EARLY GOAL-DIRECTED THERAPY IN SEVERE SEPSIS

'In patients with severe sepsis or septic shock managed initially in A&E, early goal-directed therapy (EGT) reduced 60-day mortality from 57% to 44%. Both groups were resuscitated with similar targets for central venous pressure, arterial blood pressure and urine output, but in the EGT group additional goals were central venous oxygen saturation > 70% and haematocrit > 30%, resulting in more rapid fluid resuscitation and higher red blood cell transfusion rates in the first 6 hours.'

Rivers E, et al. N Engl J Med 2001; 345:1368–1377.

EBM 3.4 ACTIVATED PROTEIN C IN SEVERE SEPSIS

'Recombinant human activated protein C reduces 28-day mortality in severe sepsis, even if multiple organ failure has already developed.'

Taylor FB, et al. J Clin Invest 1987; 79:918–925.
Bernard GR, et al. N Engl J Med 2001; 344:699–709.

---

severe cases, where there is evidence of organ dysfunction despite aggressive resuscitation and cardiovascular monitoring, admission to an intensive care unit (ICU) for additional monitoring and/or organ support may be indicated. Although an infective agent is frequently implicated, this is not always the case and SIRS can be associated with non-infective conditions such as severe pancreatitis, trauma or vasculitis. Where an infective organism is being considered, common sites are the chest, abdomen and urinary tract. Blood cultures, together with appropriate samples (urine, sputum, discharges), should be sent for urgent Gram staining, culture and sensitivities. Where the source is not obvious, repeated blood cultures should be obtained, and consideration should also be given to atypical organisms and, in certain groups of patients (the immunocompromised), infections with fungi. Multiresistant organisms may be responsible in patients who have received broad-spectrum antibiotics or those who have had a long hospital stay. In the case of many intra-abdominal conditions, antibiotic therapy should only be considered as a supplement to surgical intervention. Initial therapy is usually empirical, with a broad-spectrum antibiotic to cover the most likely organisms. Following bacteriological culture and sensitivity, the antibiotic may have to be changed or the spectrum narrowed.

CARDIOGENIC SHOCK

The clinical diagnosis of pump failure is made on the basis of a low-output state similar to that seen with hypovolaemia on a background of an adequate circulating blood volume (high jugular venous pulse, or JVP). Following the diagnosis, the patient should be moved to a high-dependency area for continuous monitoring of blood pressure, ECG, SaO_2, CVP and urine output. Immediate therapy may include the administration of high-flow oxygen (minimum 40%), together with intravenous opiates (morphine in 1–2 mg increments) to control pain, reduce anxiety and produce vasodilatation. The presence of a severe metabolic acidosis will contribute to poor myocardial function, which will not improve until there is an increase in cardiac output. The administration of small volumes of 8.5% sodium bicarbonate (50–100 ml), together with the regular monitoring of acid–base status and serum sodium, will allow for temporary pharmacological correction in the hope that this will result in an improvement in myocardial contractility, reflected in an increase in cardiac output. Should these simple measures fail to improve the patient's clinical condition, transfer to a coronary or intensive care area should be considered, as additional invasive monitoring in the form of a pulmonary artery flotation catheter, together with the intravenous administration of vasodilators and/or inotropes, may be required in order to optimize myocardial function.

Along with cardiovascular monitoring and support, the clinical diagnosis should be confirmed. This will require serial 12-lead ECGs and cardiac enzyme estimations to confirm myocardial damage. A transthoracic echocardiogram will give useful information on the state of left ventricular contractility, as well as excluding other cardiac causes of cardiogenic shock, such as pericardial tamponade, acute valve rupture and massive pulmonary embolus.

ANAPHYLAXIS

See Table 3.4.

ADVANCED MONITORING AND ORGAN SUPPORT

CARDIOVASCULAR SUPPORT

Intra-arterial measurement of blood pressure

By use of the Seldinger technique, a 20 G cannula can be inserted percutaneously into the radial artery. If the patient

3

Table 3.4 ANAPHYLAXIS

1. Stop administration of causative agent (drug/fluid)
2. Call for help
3. Lie patient flat, feet elevated
4. Maintain airway: give 100% O_2
5. Adrenaline (epinephrine)
   - 0.5–1.0 mg (0.5–1.0 ml of 1:10 000) i.v.
   - 50–100 μg (0.5–1.0 ml of 1:10 000) i.v.
   - Repeated doses titrated against response
6. Intravascular volume expansion with crystalloid or colloid
7. Second-line therapy
   - Antihistamine: Chlorphenamine
     - 10–20 mg slow i.v.
   - Corticosteroid: Hydrocortisone
     - 100–300 mg i.v.
   - Consider catecholamine infusion

---

is vasoconstricted, the femoral artery is often used. Via a saline-filled line, the mechanical pressure wave can be electrically transduced at a point distal to the artery and a continuous pressure wave displayed on a monitor. These lines allow access for the multiple arterial blood gas sampling that is an integral part of patient monitoring.

Pulmonary artery flotation catheter (PAFC)

In those patients who do not respond to the normal resuscitation measure of fluid replacement and remain shocked despite CVP evidence of normovolaemia, the PAFC gives the physician the opportunity to measure and monitor additional variables of cardiac function. The PAFC is a 100 cm long catheter with multiple lumina, one of which opens at the tip. An additional channel is connected to a small balloon at the tip, which can be inflated by means of a 2 ml syringe. The catheter is inserted percutaneously through a large-bore cannula sited in a central vein. Once the catheter is within the blood vessel, the balloon is inflated. The catheter will then float with the blood flow through the right side of the heart, lodging itself in a branch

of the pulmonary artery. If the pressure within the catheter lumen that is in continuity with the tip is transduced, the passage of the catheter can be monitored by observing the characteristic changes in the pressure waveform as it passes down the SVC and through the right atrium and ventricle, before coming to rest in the pulmonary artery. The balloon is deflated and the pulmonary artery pressure monitored continuously. If the balloon is inflated in the pulmonary artery, it will move forward and become wedged in a more distal arterial branch. A pressure measurement taken at this point is called a pulmonary capillary wedge pressure (PCWP). Because there is now a solid uninterrupted column of blood between the end of the catheter and the left atrium, the measurement taken will in most instances provide an accurate estimate of left atrial filling pressure.

Modern catheters now have the additional facility of continuously and automatically measuring cardiac output. Thus a PAFC can directly measure CVP, right atrial pressure, right ventricular pressure, pulmonary artery pressure, PCWP (estimate of left atrial filling pressure) and cardiac output. By sampling blood from the distal lumen of the catheter, oxygen saturation of the mixed venous blood from the pulmonary artery can be measured. From these values, together with heart rate and arterial blood pressure, it is possible to calculate a large number of derived values, such as systemic vascular resistance, oxygen delivery (DO_2) and oxygen consumption (VO_2), which help in monitoring of shocked patients and assessing the effectiveness of any therapeutic manoeuvres undertaken.

Gastric tonometry

It is now recognized that the splanchnic circulation is one of the earliest vascular beds to be compromised in shock. By monitoring the CO_2 gap between an air-filled intragastric tonometry balloon and an arterial blood sample, one can identify splanchnic hypoperfusion and cellular hypoxia resulting in anaerobic metabolism and increasing acidosis.

Vasoactive drug administration

Many drugs can be used in a critical care setting to overcome the pathophysiology of shock, as shown in Table 3.5.

Table 3.5 CIRCULATORY EFFECTS OF COMMONLY USED VASOACTIVE DRUG INFUSIONS

Drug	Cardiac contractility	Heart rate	Blood pressure	Cardiac output	Splanchnic blood flow	Systemic vascular resistance
Dopamine						
(< 5 mg/kg/min)	↑	→/↑	→/↑	↑	→/↑	→/↑
(> 5 mg/kg/min)	↑↑	↑	↑	↑↑	→	↑
Adrenaline (epinephrine)	↑↑	↑	↑↑	↑↑↑	↓	↑
Noradrenaline (norepinephrine)	→/↑	→/↓	↑↑	→/↓	→/↓	↑↑
Isoprenaline	↑	↑↑	→/↓	↑	→/↑	→/↓
Dobutamine	↑	↑	→/↓	↑↑	→	↓
Dopexamine	↑	↑↑	→/↓	↑	↑	↓
Glyceryl trinitrate	→	↑	↑	↑	↑	↓
Nitroprusside	→	↑	↑	↑	↑	↓

Note These effects are guidelines only. The exact response will depend on the circulatory state of the patient and the dose of the drug.

EBM 3.5   OXYGEN DELIVERY IN CRITICALLY ILL PATIENTS

'Two RCTs have shown that, for patients already on the ICU with established organ failure, treatment with aggressive volume-loading and inotropes in an attempt to achieve high levels of oxygen delivery ('goal-directed therapy') not only often fails to achieve these goals but also does not improve survival and may be harmful. However, a subsequent single-centre RCT applying goal-directed therapy early to patients with severe sepsis and septic shock in the A & E department before ICU admission and before they had developed established organ failure did reduce 28- and 60-day mortality.'

Hayes MA, et al. Chest 1993; 103:886–895.
Gattinoni L, et al. N Engl J Med 1995; 333:1025–1032.
Rivers E, et al. N Engl J Med 2001; 345:1368–1377.

For further information: 🖥 www.nejm.org

Table 3.6   INDICATIONS FOR RENAL REPLACEMENT THERAPY

These reflect the lost functions of the kidney and include:
- Control of fluid balance to prevent fluid overload and pulmonary oedema
- Reduction of blood urea to avoid the systemic effects of severe uraemia
- Control of hyperkalaemia
- Normalization of acid–base status

BOX 3.7   INDICATIONS FOR INTUBATION/VENTILATION

- Inability to maintain oxygen saturations whilst breathing spontaneously
- Inability to maintain carbon dioxide excretion and physical exhaustion
- Depressed conscious level
    Cerebral hypoperfusion
    Septic encephalopathy
- Severe cardiovascular instability

RESPIRATORY SUPPORT

As a result of the pathophysiological derangements in shock, there is frequently an increase in the mismatch between perfusion and ventilation in the lungs. This abnormality results in an increase in the venous blood mixing with the fully oxygenated blood entering the left atrium (increasing shunt), reducing the overall oxygen content of the blood entering the arterial circulation. This is reflected in a fall in the oxygen saturation, as measured with the pulse oximeter. The defect can usually be corrected by increasing the fraction of inspired oxygen from room air (21%) by administering supplemental oxygen (40–60%).

In a small number of patients in whom the process is so severe that increasing the inspired oxygen concentration is not sufficient to correct the hypoxia, exhaustion will set in owing to the increased effort of breathing (identified on clinical examination and arterial blood gas evidence of an inability to excrete CO_2). In these patients, additional measures must be taken to protect the airway and assist ventilation (EBM 3.5). This is also the case with patients in whom cerebral hypoperfusion or septic encephalopathy has resulted in a reduced level of consciousness, putting their airway at risk from obstruction or aspiration. Induction of anaesthesia is necessary to aid endotracheal intubation and artificial ventilation until the underlying cause is reversed.

RENAL SUPPORT

In more severe cases of shock there is renal vasoconstriction and hypoperfusion. Acute tubular necrosis (ATN) may occur if resuscitation is not adequate. ATN is irreversible in the very short term, but if the pre-morbid renal function was normal and the underlying precipitating insult is treated, renal function will usually return within 3–6 weeks. In the interim, replacement is required (Table 3.6).

CONTINUOUS VENO-VENOUS HAEMOFILTRATION (CVVH)

This is the replacement therapy of choice in the early stage of the patient's ICU stay, when there may be ongoing cardiovascular instability. Via a double-lumen large-bore catheter introduced into a large central vein, blood can be mechanically withdrawn and pumped through a haemofil-

tration circuit at 200–300 ml/min. This is sufficient to produce a filtrate volume in excess of 1000 ml/hr, which can be replaced with an equal volume of an appropriate electrolyte solution. The technique is continuous and requires a minimal amount of anticoagulation to prevent clotting with the filter. As only a relatively small volume of blood passes through the extracorporeal circuit, it confers a degree of cardiovascular stability not obtainable with other methods.

Intermittent haemodialysis

Although this technique is more effective than CVVH at solute removal, it is rarely the initial choice for replacement therapy. It results in a greater degree of cardiovascular instability and disequilibrium (acute changes in osmolality), which would not be tolerated by the unstable patient. Haemodialysis is frequently started in the convalescent phase, when the patient is recovering and waiting for the return of native renal function. It can be undertaken over short periods (4 hours), often on alternate days, and should not delay the patient's mobilization or further recovery.

NUTRITION

Consideration should always be given to the patient's nutritional state. The shocked state is an intensively catabolic condition in which there is rapid protein break-down. This can have significant effects on both wound healing and immune status. In an attempt to attenuate these effects, artificial nutrition should be considered early on in the disease process. If the gastrointestinal tract is intact and there is no contraindication, then enteral nutrition is the method of choice.

Failure to institute enteral nutrition will mean the insertion of a dedicated line into a central vein and the administration of total parenteral nutrition in an attempt to attenuate the stress response to shock, thereby reducing complications and speeding up recovery.

F.J. CUTLER
R.H.A. GREEN
D.B.L. MCCLELLAND

Transfusion of blood and blood products

INTRODUCTION

Blood transfusion can be life-saving and many areas of surgery could not be undertaken without reliable transfusion support. However, as with any treatment, transfusion of blood and its components carries potential risks, which must be outweighed by the patient's need. The magnitude of risk depends on factors such as the prevalence of infectious disease in the donor population, the resources and dedication of the organization collecting, processing and issuing the blood and blood products, and the care with which the clinical team administers these products.

BLOOD DONATION

In the UK, whole blood is donated by healthy adult volunteers aged 17–65 years with normal haemoglobin levels. The standard 480 ml donation contains approximately 200 mg of iron, the loss of which is easily tolerated by healthy donors. Blood components (platelets and plasma) can be separated from the donated blood or obtained from the donor as separate products by the use of a cell separator, in a process called apheresis.

Strict donor selection and the testing of all donations are essential to exclude blood that may be hazardous to the recipient, as well as ensuring the welfare of the donor.

4

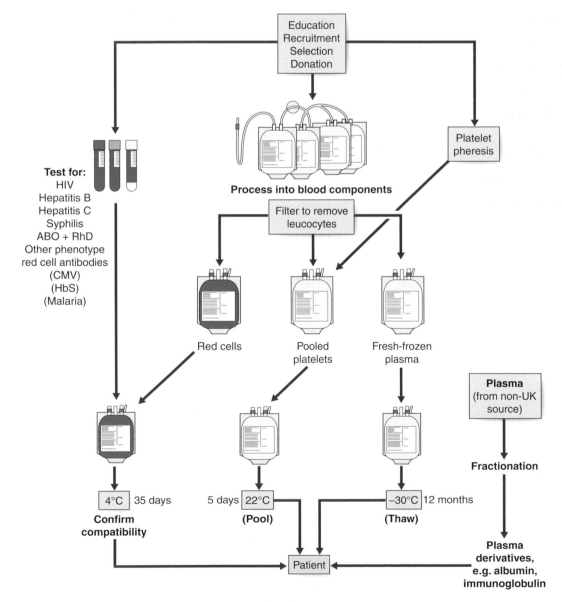

Fig. 4.1   Products that can be obtained from 1 unit of donated whole blood.

All donations are ABO-grouped, Rhesus (Rh) D-typed, antibody-screened, and tested for evidence of hepatitis B, hepatitis C, human immunodeficiency virus (HIV) I and II, human T-cell leukaemia virus (HTLV) I and II and syphilis, using tests for antibody to the virus, viral antigen or nucleic acid. Some donations are also tested for antibody to cytomegalovirus (CMV), so that CMV-negative blood can be provided for patients such as transplant recipients and premature infants. Dependent on epidemiology, other testing may be required, e.g. Chagas disease.

Due to concerns regarding transmission of variant Creutzfeldt–Jakob disease (vCJD) by transfusion, a number of precautions have been introduced. Since 1999 all blood donated in the UK has been filtered to remove white blood cells (leucodepletion), UK plasma has been excluded from fractionation, and from April 2004 people who have received a blood or blood product transfusion in the UK after 1980 are excluded from donating blood. Some countries currently exclude donations from individuals who resided in the UK during the time of the bovine spongiform encephalitis (BSE) epidemic.

BLOOD COMPONENTS

The components that can be prepared from donated blood are shown in Figure 4.1 and their descriptions follow.

FRESH BLOOD COMPONENTS

Red blood cells in additive solution

Donated whole blood is collected into an anticoagulant (citrate), nutrient (phosphate, dextrose and adenine) solution. Centrifugation removes virtually all of the associated plasma, and a saline, adenine and glucose solution is then added. The final product has a haematocrit of 55–65% and a volume of approximately 300 ml. The blood is not sterilized, so that blood transfusion can transmit organisms not detected by donor screening.

Transfused blood must be ABO- and Rh(D)-compatible with the recipient and transfused through a sterile blood administration set with an appropriate filter, designed for the procedure. The set should be primed with saline and no other solutions transfused simultaneously. This product is indicated for most forms of anaemia and is the most widely available form of red cells for transfusion.

Platelets

Platelet concentrates can be made either from centrifugation of whole blood or from an individual donor using apheresis. An adult dose is manufactured from four separate donations pooled together or one apheresis collection. Platelet concentrates carry a greater risk of bacterial contamination as they cannot be refrigerated. Platelets are infused through a standard blood-giving set over less than 30 minutes. As the concentrate contains some red cells and plasma, it should ideally be ABO- and Rh(D)-compatible with the recipient. RhD-negative females of child-bearing age

must receive Rh(D)-compatible platelets, or prophylactic Rh(D) immunoglobulin should be given. An adult dose should raise an adult platelet count by $20–40 \times 10^9/l$.

Platelet concentrates are indicated in thrombocytopenia, when platelet function is defective, and in patients receiving massive blood transfusions when there is microvascular bleeding (oozing from mucous membranes, needle puncture sites and wounds).

Fresh frozen plasma (FFP)

Some 200–300 ml of plasma can be removed from a unit of whole blood and stored frozen at $-30°C$. FFP contains albumin, immunoglobulins and, most importantly, all of the coagulation factors. FFP can be stored at $-30°C$ for a year and is thawed to $37°C$ before issue. FFP must be ABO-compatible with the recipient and should be transfused within 4 hours of thawing. The average adult dose is 3–4 units. Virally inactivated plasma (treated with methylene blue or solvent detergent) is available for use in recipients who will require repeated exposures to FFP, and in the UK for children born after 1 January 1996.

FFP is used when there are multiple coagulation factor deficiencies (e.g. disseminated intravascular coagulation, DIC) associated with severe bleeding and in inherited clotting factor deficiencies for which no virus-safe fractionated product is available. It may be indicated in selected patients who are over-anticoagulated with warfarin, but there are now, however, heat-treated products that should usually be used in preference. In the case of massive blood loss arising during or after surgery, the decision whether to use FFP and, if so, how much to use, should be guided by timely tests of coagulation. FFP should not be used to correct prolonged clotting times in patients who are not bleeding or who are not about to undergo immediate surgery, e.g. in the ICU; in these circumstances, vitamin K should be given.

Cryoprecipitate

A single unit of cryoprecipitate can be removed from 1 unit of FFP after controlled thawing. After resuspension in 10–20 ml plasma, the cryoprecipitate is frozen once more to $-30°C$, in which condition it can be stored for up to a year. It contains fibrinogen, factor VIII, von Willebrand factor, factor XIII and fibronectin. A normal adult dose is 10 units. ABO-compatible units should be given, and the product infused as soon as possible after thawing. Cryoprecipitate is used when fibrinogen levels are low, as in DIC and in bleeding associated with uraemia.

PLASMA FRACTIONS

Fractionated products are manufactured from large pools (several thousand donations) of donor plasma that undergo some form of viral inactivation stage through the manufacturing process. Virus inactivation processes now mean that these products should not transmit HIV I and II or hepatitis B and C, but this may not apply to heat-resistant viruses that have no lipid envelope (e.g. hepatitis A) or to prions.

Table 4.1   INDICATIONS AND DOSES FOR HUMAN IMMUNOGLOBULINS

Problem	Patients eligible for IgG	Preparation	Dose
Hepatitis B	Needle-stick or mucosal exposure victims. Should also be immunized	Hepatitis B IgG	1000 U for adults and 500 U for children < 5 years
Varicella zoster	Immunosuppressed contacts Infants exposed to case Pregnant contacts	Human normal IgG	0.5 ml/kg 0.25 ml/kg 0.2 ml/kg
Tetanus-prone wounds	Non-immune patients with heavily contaminated wounds Toxoid should be administered with IgG	Tetanus IgG	250 U routine prophylaxis 500 U if > 24 hrs since injury or heavily contaminated wound
Accidental transfusions of Rh(D)-positive blood	Women of child-bearing age	Anti-D IgG	125 U/ml of transfused blood

4

Human albumin

Albumin is prepared by fractionation of large pools of plasma that, at the end of processing, is pasteurized at 60°C for 10 hours. There are no compatibility requirements.

Solutions of 4.5 or 5% are used to maintain plasma albumin levels in conditions where there is increased vascular permeability, e.g. burns, and are sometimes used in acute blood volume replacement, although crystalloid or non-plasma colloid solution would be the recommended first-line volume expander until > 20% of the blood volume has been replaced. Randomized controlled trials on the use of albumin (notably the SAFE study and the Cochrane Database systematic review) suggest that there is no clear advantage from the use of albumin solutions in the treatment of hypovolaemia over judicious use of saline. Resuscitation with crystalloid requires volumes of fluid three times greater than with colloid.

Twenty per cent solutions can be used when hypoproteinaemia is associated with oedema that is resistant to diuretics (e.g. liver disease, nephrotic syndrome). Twenty per cent albumin is hyperoncotic, so that there is a risk of acutely expanding the intravascular space and precipitating pulmonary oedema.

Prothrombin complex concentrates

These products contain factors II, IX and X, and may also contain factor VII (vitamin K-dependent clotting factors). Their use is indicated in the prophylaxis and treatment of bleeding in patients with single or multiple deficiencies of these factors, whether congenital or acquired. They are used to reverse the anticoagulant effect of warfarin when there is major bleeding. Care must be taken in patients with liver disease, as this therapy may be thrombogenic.

Immunoglobulin preparations (90% IgG)

These are prepared from fractionation of large pools of plasma from unselected donors or from individuals known to have high levels of specific antibodies. The product may be given intramuscularly or intravenously. The indications for some of the more commonly used immunoglobulins are shown in Table 4.1. Intravenous IgG was originally developed as replacement therapy for inherited immunodeficiency states. It is also used to treat immune thrombocytopenia and other rare diseases such as Guillain–Barré syndrome.

RED CELL SEROLOGY

The red cell membrane is a bilipid layer with which a variety of blood group antigen systems are associated. Over 400 red cell antigens have been described, and although their precise role is uncertain, they play a part in the recognition of self and non-self.

ABO ANTIGENS

Nearly all deaths from transfusion error are due to ABO-incompatible transfusion. ABO antigens are present on many cells of the body, and their presence depends on the inheritance of allelic genes on chromosome 9. Only individuals who lack A or B antigens produce anti-A and anti-B antibodies, respectively. These are usually IgM antibodies (naturally occurring) and are present from the age of 3–6 months. ABO antibodies can react at body temperature and activate complement, and are of major clinical significance as a cause of rapid intravascular haemolysis. For example, transfusion of group A blood to a group B patient results in haemolysis of the transfused red cells because of the anti-A antibodies present in the recipient. Similarly, group O individuals have both anti-A and anti-B antibodies in their plasma that will react with any red cells apart from group O (Table 4.2). Group O blood can be used in all recipients because of the processing that removes the plasma and hence the antibodies contained within.

RHESUS ANTIGENS (RH)

Allelic genes at three closely linked loci on chromosome 1 code for this complex blood group system. Phenotypes

Table 4.2   THE ANTIGENS AND ANTIBODIES OF THE ABO BLOOD GROUP SYSTEM

Blood group	Frequency (UK) %	Red cell antigen	Plasma antibody	Compatible donor blood
A	42	A	Anti-B	A or O
B	8	B	Anti-A	B or O
AB	3	AB	–	AB, A, B or O
O	47	–	Anti-A,B	O only

4

termed Rhesus(D) or no D (termed d), Cc and Ee exist. Individuals with Rh(D) are termed Rhesus-positive and those without Rh(D) are termed Rhesus-negative. Rh(D) is by far the most immunogenic of the Rhesus antigens and is the only one currently cross-matched to ensure compatibility in blood transfusion. Individuals who are Rh(D)-negative do not normally have anti-Rh(D) in their plasma unless they have been immunized by previous transfusion or pregnancy. Antibodies to Rh(D) are IgG antibodies and do not activate complement, although they do cause extravascular haemolysis. Rhesus antibodies can cause transfusion reactions and haemolytic disease of the newborn (HDN). It is essential that Rh(D)-negative women of child-bearing age are not transfused with Rh(D)-positive blood to avoid the stimulation of antibodies to Rh(D), which could cross the placenta in pregnancy and cause haemolysis of Rh(D)-positive cells in the fetus (HDN).

OTHER RED CELL ANTIGENS

Many different types of blood group system exist and the antibodies formed against the antigens are of varying clinical significance, depending on their propensity to cause intra- or extravascular haemolysis and HDN. The most important of these are Kell, Kidd and Duffy.

INDICATIONS FOR TRANSFUSION

The decision to transfuse is a complex one. Clinical judgement plays a vital role, as there is no consensus on the precise indications for red cell transfusion. The clinician prescribing any blood component should consider the risks and benefits of transfusion for each individual patient. Tolerance of anaemia is dependent on a number of factors, including the speed of onset, age, level of activity and coexisting disease. In chronic anaemia, fatigue and shortness of breath, although subjective, are still useful in determining the need for transfusion. In acute anaemia (usually secondary to blood loss), the effects of hypovolaemia need to be differentiated from those of anaemia. Healthy adults can tolerate significant blood loss (30–40% of circulating volume) without adverse effects and would not normally require transfusion. This is largely due to adaptive mechanisms such as a compensatory rise in cardiac output and peripheral vasodilatation, which act to maintain tissue oxygen delivery. The actual haemoglobin

concentration does not in itself indicate a definite need for transfusion; however, it can act as a prompt for the clinician to seek other features that suggest transfusion is required. Red cell transfusion is usually not required with a haemoglobin concentration of ≥ 100 g/l. Generally, in healthy individuals, a transfusion threshold of 70–80 g/l is appropriate, as this leaves a margin of safety over the critical level of 40–50 g/l, at which point oxygen consumption becomes limited by the amount that the circulation can supply. Many patients who have a haemoglobin level of 70–100 g/l will receive a transfusion, yet this is often unnecessary and should therefore not be routine practice. For elderly patients or those with cardiovascular or respiratory disease, who may tolerate anaemia poorly, transfusion should be considered at a haemoglobin concentration of ≤ 80 g/l to maintain a haemoglobin level of around 100 g/l. In the intensive care setting, some studies have shown that maintaining a lower haemoglobin threshold may be associated with better patient outcomes, at least in some patient groups. The best available evidence for this is the randomized, controlled TRICC trial (EBM 4.1), which compared a liberal transfusion strategy (Hb 100–120 g/l) to a restrictive strategy (Hb 70–90 g/l). Overall in-hospital mortality was significantly lower in the restrictive group, although the 30-day mortality rate was not significantly different. However, the 30-day mortality rate was significantly lower in the restrictive transfusion group for those patients who were less ill (APACHE < 20) or younger (< 55 years of age). This shows that a restrictive strategy is at least equivalent, and in some patient groups is superior, to a more liberal transfusion strategy.

EBM 4.1   RED CELL TRANSFUSION IN THE CORRECTION OF A LOW HAEMOGLOBIN IN CRITICALLY ILL PATIENTS

'A single large RCT of red cell transfusion in patients in intensive care showed that patients who were maintained with an Hb in the range of 70–90 g/l had a lower mortality and morbidity compared to those with an Hb maintained in the range of 100–120 g/l. The former groups received approximately half the number of red cell units.'

Hebert PC, et al. with the Canadian Transfusion Requirements in Critical Care Group. N Engl J Med 1999; 340:409–417.
For further information: 🖥 www.transfusionguidelines.org.uk
🖥 www.sign.ac.uk

BOX 4.1   TRANSFUSION TRIGGERS

- Transfusion is likely to be required at haemoglobin levels < 70 g/l
- Transfusion is unjustified at levels > 100 g/l
- Patients with cardiovascular disease, or those expected to have a high incidence of covert cardiovascular disease (the elderly or those with peripheral vascular disease) are likely to benefit from transfusion at haemoglobin levels of < 80 g/l
- Each unit should prepare a set of simple transfusion guidelines for the haemoglobin values/trigger they have demonstrated to have benefited clinical outcome

---

PRE-TRANSFUSION TESTING

Two major forms of pre-transfusion testing are available:

1. *Type and screen/group and save* involves determining the patient's ABO and Rh(D) type and screening a sample of patient serum for the presence of clinically significant antibodies. The sample is then retained for up to 7 days, and if blood is required it can be provided within 10–15 minutes after rapidly excluding ABO incompatibility.
2. *Cross-matching* normally takes about an hour and involves not only typing and screening, but also direct testing of the patient's serum for compatibility with red cells taken from the units of blood to be transfused. If the patient has an antibody, its specificity is determined and donor blood negative for the offending antigen(s) can be issued. This process may take several hours, depending on the population incidence of the antigen(s) in question. Cross-matched units are then allocated to the individual patient and held in reserve for 48 hours.

Emergency requirements for blood make the use of compatibility tests redundant. The laboratory must be told of the urgency and quantity of blood needed immediately, and asked what they can provide in the time available. Group O Rh(D)-negative blood is available in all hospitals for such emergencies. Patient samples can be rapidly ABO- and Rh(D)-typed, and compatible blood released after a rapid test of ABO compatibility while the antibody screen is ongoing and group O Rh(D)-negative blood is being transfused.

BOX 4.2   ORDERING BLOOD IN AN EMERGENCY

- Immediately take samples for cross-matching, ensuring that the sample and the request form are clearly and correctly labelled and are the same on subsequent requests. If the patient is unidentified, then some form of emergency admission number is the best identifier
- Inform the blood bank of the emergency, the volume of blood required, and where blood is to be delivered
- One individual should take responsibility for all communications with the blood bank, and should ensure that it is clear who will be responsible for blood delivery
- In cases of exsanguination, use emergency group O Rh(D)-negative blood
- Do not ask for cross-matched blood in an emergency

Computer cross-matching/issue

Direct compatibility testing may be bypassed in situations where there is accurate patient identification, a historic blood group and antibody screen, patients with no serum antibodies and a secure blood bank computer system that can reliably select and issue blood of compatible type. These systems are currently being implemented in the UK and will allow blood to be selected from remote blood fridges when the patient requires it. Concerns still arise regarding patient identification, as the system is critically dependent on it.

Maximal Surgical Blood Ordering Schedule (MSBOS)

MSBOS lists the number of units of blood routinely cross-matched pre-operatively for elective surgical procedures. This surgical tariff is based on retrospective analysis of actual blood use. The aim is to correlate as closely as possible the number of units cross-matched to the numbers of units transfused. It does not account for individual differences in blood transfusion requirements of different patients undergoing the same procedure, nor does it identify over-transfusion.

BLOOD ADMINISTRATION

Avoidable errors in the requesting, supply and administration of blood lead to significant risks to patients. Multiple errors contribute to more than 50% of 'wrong blood' incidents reported to the UK Serious Hazards of Transfusion (SHOT) scheme. Of these, 70% occur in clinical areas and 30% occur in laboratories. Acute haemolytic transfusion reactions due to ABO incompatibility can be fatal and are most often caused by errors in identification of the patient at the time of blood sampling or administration (EBM 4.2).

The British Committee for Standards in Haematology has produced a guideline for the administration of blood and blood components and the management of transfused patients. This contains a number of recommendations that should be adhered to in order to minimize transfusion error. These include the following:

1. It is crucial that the identity of the patient is established verbally (if possible) *and* by checking the patient identification wristband before blood is taken. The sample must be labelled fully (in handwriting) before leaving the bedside. (Sample tubes must never be pre-labelled.)

EBM 4.2   RISKS OF FATAL TRANSFUSION REACTIONS—CASES REPORTED TO NATIONAL REPORTING SYSTEMS

'In the UK between 1996 and 2000 there were 33 reports of death attributed to transfusion. During this period approximately 10 million units of blood components were supplied. The largest cause of major morbidity remains transfusion of the incorrect unit of blood, leading to an incompatible red cell transfusion reaction.'

Love EM, Soldan K. Serious hazards of transfusion, Annual report 1999–2000. Manchester: SHOT; 2001.

For further information: 🖥 www.shotuk.org
🖥 www.transfusionguidelines.org.uk

---

2. The blood request form should be completed and should provide, as a minimum, the patient's full name, date of birth and hospital number. (Each patient must have a unique identification number.) The location of the patient, number and type of blood or blood components and time when required, the patient's diagnosis and the reason for the request are also essential.

3. Before transfusion is commenced, the following details must be checked by two individuals, at least one of whom must be a State Registered Nurse (SRN) or medical officer:

   a. Full patient identity on the patient wristband, compatibility label on the unit of blood and, where issued, the accompanying report form

   b. ABO and Rh(D) type on the pack, compatibility label and, where issued, the report form

   c. Donation number on the pack, compatibility label and, where issued, the accompanying report form

   d. Expiry date of the pack

   e. Examination of the pack to ensure that there are no leaks or evidence of haemolysis.

If there are any discrepancies, the blood must not be transfused and the laboratory must be informed immediately.

BOX 4.3   SAFETY CHECKS FOR BLOOD ADMINISTRATION

Before administering blood, two staff members (one of whom must be a doctor or trained staff nurse) must check:

- the patient's full identity (wristband, and verbally if possible)
- the blood pack, compatibility label and report form (noting donation number and expiry date)
- the blood pack for signs of haemolysis or leakage from the pack

Any discrepancies mean that the blood must not be transfused and that the laboratory must be informed immediately

---

4. As a minimum, the patient's pulse rate, blood pressure and temperature should be recorded prior to commencing the transfusion, 15 minutes after commencement of each unit (as this is when transfusion reactions are most likely), and on completion of the transfusion. The vital signs should be rechecked if the patient feels unwell during the transfusion.

5. A permanent record of the transfusion of blood and blood components and the administration of blood products must be kept in the medical notes. This should include the sheets used for the prescription of blood or blood components and those used for nursing observations during the transfusion. An entry should also be made in the case notes, documenting the date, the indication for transfusion, the number and type of units used, whether or not the desired effect was achieved, and the occurrence and management of any adverse effects.

ADVERSE EFFECTS OF TRANSFUSION

A voluntary anonymized reporting scheme for serious hazards of transfusion (SHOT) has been in place in the UK since 1996, and the incidence of reported hazards is shown in Figure 4.2. The greatest concern for most patients is the risk of transfusion-transmitted infection, but by far the most common risk is the transfusion of an incorrect blood component.

Transfusion reactions can be divided into those that occur early (acute transfusion reactions, or ATRs, occurring within 24 hours of commencing but usually during the transfusion) and those that occur late (delayed transfusion reactions, or DTRs, occurring more than 24 hours after commencing the transfusion and often once the patient has been discharged). Acute adverse reactions to blood transfusion require urgent investigation and management, as they may be life-

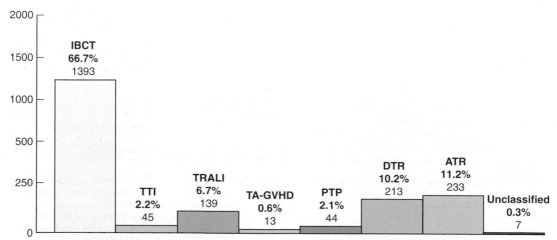

Fig. 4.2   SHOT report for 1996/7–2003 showing the rate (%) of serious hazards of transfusion reported in the UK.
(ATR = acute transfusion reaction; DTR = delayed transfusion reaction; IBCT = incorrect blood component transfused; LVF = left ventricular failure; PTP = post-transfusion purpura; TA-GVHD = transfusion-associated graft-versus-host disease; TRALI = transfusion-related acute lung injury; TTI = transfusion-transmitted infection)

BOX 4.4   TRANSFUSION ERRORS

- Almost all deaths from transfusion reaction are due to ABO incompatibility
- Errors in patient identification at the time of blood sampling or administration are the major cause (occurring in at least 1:1000–1:2000 transfusions)
- When taking the initial blood sample:
    Check the patient's identity verbally and on the wrist identification band
    Label the sample fully before leaving the bedside
    Make sure that the blood request form is clearly and accurately completed

---

threatening. The major acute causes frequently have similar symptoms and signs, and blind treatment may initially be necessary until the exact cause becomes apparent. Acute and delayed adverse effects of transfusion are shown in Tables 4.3 and 4.4 respectively. The risks of infection from blood transfusion are listed in Table 4.5. Management of acute transfusion reactions is illustrated in Figure 4.3.

AUTOLOGOUS TRANSFUSION

As immunological and infective complications can result from donated blood, the use of the patient's own blood may be considered in certain situations to try to reduce the need for allogeneic blood.

PRE-OPERATIVE DONATION

Blood can be withdrawn from otherwise fit patients (in the same way as from a regular blood donor) with a definite date for elective surgery, and stored for up to 35–42 days. Assuming that the haemoglobin concentration is adequate before withdrawal of each unit and that iron therapy is used, up to 5 units of the patient's own blood can be made available, with the last unit being collected 48–72 hours before surgery to allow for re-equilibration of the blood volume. Sepsis and severe myocardial disease are absolute contraindications to autologous transfusion. Autologous units undergo the same testing as allogeneic donations, including the pre-transfusion compatibility test, and their use is restricted to the donor. Autologous pre-deposit virtually eliminates the risks of viral transmission and immunologically mediated side-effects; however, bacterial contamination, volume overload and ABO haemolytic reactions due to administrative or clerical errors (leading to the wrong blood being transfused) are still risks. Autologous blood should only be collected from patients who are likely to require blood during surgery. Recent studies have shown that autologous pre-deposit may reduce allogeneic blood transfusion exposure but it does not reduce the frequency of transfusion, i.e. the autologous units are given whether or not they are required and thus the many other risks of transfusion are not reduced.

Table 4.3   ACUTE TRANSFUSION REACTIONS

	Cause	Implicated components	Clinical features
IMMUNOLOGICAL **Acute haemolytic** **transfusion reaction**	ABO-incompatible transfusion resulting in acute intravascular haemolysis	RCC Platelets FFP Cryo	Develop within mins. Chills, fevers, rigors, chest tightness, infusion site pain, hypotension, shock, DIC and acute renal failure. May be fatal
Transfusion-associated acute lung injury	HLA or neutrophil Abs in donor plasma react with recipient leucocytes	Any plasma-containing component (RCC, FFP, cryo, platelets)	Develop within 4 hrs of transfusion. Dyspnoea, cough, fever, hypoxia, pulmonary infiltrates (ARDS). With supportive care, improvement over 2–4 days in 80% of patients
Febrile non-haemolytic transfusion reaction	Neutrophil Ab in recipient plasma reacts with donor leucocytes	RCC Platelets FFP Cryo	Develops late in course of transfusion. Usually mild. Full recovery expected
Allergic reactions	Reaction to plasma proteins	Any plasma-containing component	Urticaria/itch within minutes of start of transfusion. Occasionally severe with anaphylaxis. Usually full recovery with appropriate management
NON- IMMUNOLOGICAL **Bacterial contamination**	Contamination during collection or storage. Rarely, bacteraemic donor	Platelets most commonly RCC	Symptoms/signs of sepsis develop early in course of transfusion. May be fatal
Cardiac failure	Circulatory overload	Any	Symptoms/signs of acute left ventricular failure. Resolves with appropriate management

(Ab = antibody; Ag = antigen; ARDS = acute respiratory distress syndrome; Cryo = cryoprecipitate; DIC = disseminated intravascular coagulation; FFP = fresh frozen plasma; HLA = human leucocyte antigen; RCC = red cell concentrate)

Table 4.4   DELAYED TRANSFUSION REACTIONS

	Cause	Implicated components	Clinical features
IMMUNOLOGICAL **Delayed haemolytic transfusion reaction**	Patient has red cell Ab at undetectable level. Re-exposure to Ag results in secondary immune response and extravascular haemolysis	Red cells Platelets	May be asymptomatic or develop jaundice, fever and haemoglobinuria with a fall in haemoglobin. Seldom fatal but can result in significant morbidity if the patient is already unwell
Alloimmunization	Recipient forms Ab in response to donor Ag	Red cells	Usually not detected until subsequently grouped and saved or cross-matched
Post-transfusion purpura	Recipient has a platelet-specific Ab and develops secondary immune response on re-exposure, resulting in destruction of donor platelets and, through an unknown mechanism, recipient platelets	Platelets Red cells	Sudden development of severe thrombocytopenia associated with bleeding 5–12 days following transfusion. Complications are related to bleeding. Platelet count usually recovers with appropriate management, which includes i.v. immunoglobulin
Transfusion-associated graft-versus-host disease	Viable T lymphocytes transfused into immunocompromised recipient	Any cellular product	Fever, desquamating rash, abnormal LFTs and pancytopenia develop 1–4 weeks following transfusion. Mortality rate > 90%. Prevent by irradiation of cellular components in patients at high risk

NON-IMMUNOLOGICAL
Transfusion-transmitted infection: Risks shown in Table 4.3
Iron overload: Chronic red cell transfusion leads to accumulation of iron in tissues, e.g. liver, heart, pancreas

(Ag = antigen; Ab = antibody)

Table 4.5   RISKS OF A SINGLE RED CELL UNIT TRANSMITTING DISEASE IN THE UK

Infection	Estimated risk (per unit transfused)
Hepatitis B	1:50 000–1:200 000
Hepatitis C	1:200 000
HIV	1:2 500 000
vCJD	Unknown, not zero
Bacterial	1:2000–10 000

ISOVOLAEMIC HAEMODILUTION

This technique is usually restricted to patients in whom significant blood loss (> 1000 ml) is anticipated. Following induction of anaesthesia, up to 1.5 litres of blood is withdrawn pre-operatively into a clearly labelled blood pack containing a standard anticoagulant, and replaced by saline to maintain blood volume. The fall in haematocrit reduces the loss of red cells (and haemoglobin) during surgical bleeding while maintaining optimal tissue perfusion. The withdrawn blood can be re-infused, either during surgery or post-operatively, with transfusion complete before the patient leaves the responsibility of the anaesthetist. Blood is maintained at the point of care, minimizing the risk of administrative or clerical errors, although standard pre-transfusion checks should be carried out to ensure the correct pack(s) are re-infused.

CELL SALVAGE

Blood can be collected from the operation site either directly during surgery or by the use of collection devices attached to surgical drains. During surgery, blood can be collected by suction, processed by a cell salvage machine in which it is anticoagulated while the cells are washed to remove clots and debris, and then returned to the patient. The process is contraindicated in patients with malignancy or sepsis, and is only appropriate when there is substantial blood loss. Several litres of blood can be salvaged intra-operatively, far more than with other autologous techniques. Post-operative drainage can be returned to the patient, most commonly not washed. This process does require some positive suction pressure, and in some circumstances this may lead to increased blood loss. The other main disadvantage is that salvaged blood is not haemostatically intact, as there may have been clotting in the wound leading to consumption of clotting factors and platelets. Cell salvage can significantly reduce the exposure of patients to allogeneic blood and is used extensively in cardiac surgery, trauma surgery and liver transplantation.

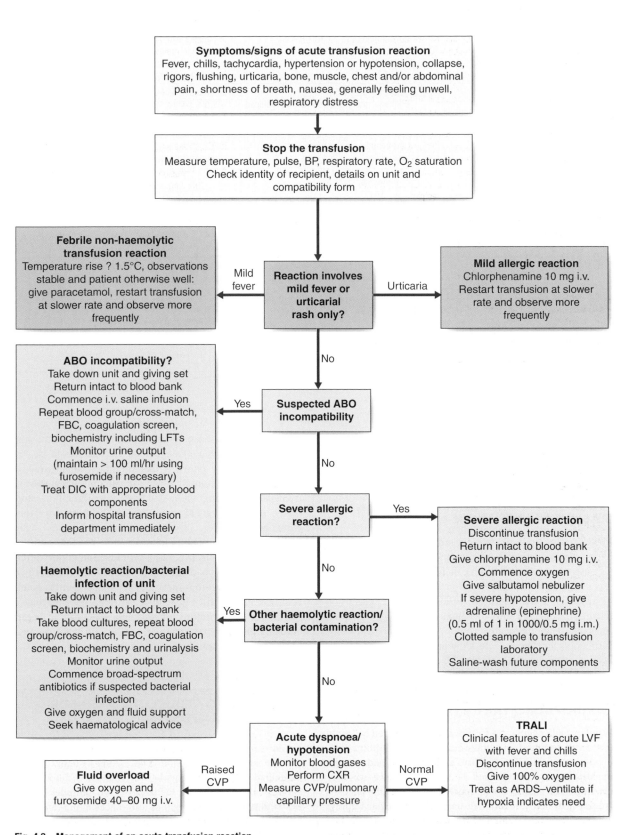

Fig. 4.3 Management of an acute transfusion reaction.
(DIC = disseminated intravascular coagulation; LVF = left ventricular failure; TRALI = transfusion-related acute lung injury)

Table 4.6 COMPLICATIONS OF MASSIVE TRANSFUSION

Complication	Mechanism	Management
Thrombocytopenia	Consumption/DIC Dilutional after 1.5–2.0 blood volumes replaced	In patients with acute bleeding, transfuse platelets to maintain count $> 50 \times 10^9/l$ ($> 100 \times 10^9/l$ if acute trauma or CNS injury)
Coagulopathy	Consumption/DIC Dilutional after 1.0 blood volume replaced	If continued blood loss and PT or APTT ratio $> 1.5 \times$ control levels, give FFP 10–15 ml/kg. If fibrinogen < 1.0 g/l, cryoprecipitate is also indicated
Hypocalcaemia	Citrate anticoagulant binds to ionized Ca, lowering plasma levels (only problematic in neonates and liver disease)	If ECG shows signs of hypocalcaemia, give 5 ml Ca gluconate (or equivalent paediatric dose) over 5 mins. Repeat if ECG remains abnormal
Hyper- or hypokalaemia	Red cell degeneration during storage increases plasma K$^+$ Following transfusion, red cells rapidly normalize Na/K equilibrium, which may lead to $\uparrow$ K$^+$	Careful monitoring of K$^+$ levels in massive transfusion
Hypothermia	Transfusion of blood at 4°C lowers core temperature	Prevent by use of blood warmer when transfusion rate > 50 ml/kg/hr in adults (15 ml/kg/hr in children)
ARDS	Multifactorial	Minimize risk by maintaining tissue perfusion, correct hypotension and avoid over-transfusion

(APTT = activated partial thromboplastin time; ARDS = acute respiratory distress syndrome; DIC = disseminated intravascular coagulation; FFP = fresh frozen plasma; PT = prothrombin time)

TRANSFUSION REQUIREMENTS IN SPECIAL SURGICAL SETTINGS

MASSIVE TRANSFUSION

Massive transfusion denotes the transfusion of the equivalent of the circulating blood volume within a 24-hour period (i.e. 10–12 units in an adult). It is needed most often in severe trauma and in bleeding from the gastrointestinal tract or various obstetric disorders. Although massive transfusion restores circulating blood volume and oxygen-carrying capacity, it is frequently complicated by coagulopathy, particularly in patients with an underlying disorder such as liver disease or DIC. Table 4.6 outlines some of the complications of massive transfusion.

CARDIOPULMONARY BYPASS

Platelets and coagulation factors may be activated or lost in the extracorporeal circulation during cardiopulmonary bypass at open heart surgery, so that FFP and platelet transfusion may be needed to deal with post-operative bleeding. The platelet count may be normal but the platelets are likely to be dysfunctional, having disaggregated during the extracorporeal circuit. Platelet transfusion is indicated if there is microvascular bleeding, or if the bleeding cannot be corrected surgically after the patient is off bypass and once heparin has been reversed with an appropriate dose of protamine sulphate. Coagulation screens should be performed to assess required therapy prior to infusion of coagulation factors in all but life-threatening haemorrhage. Near-patient testing of coagulation, e.g. thromboelastography, may also guide decisions on the need for blood component therapy.

Aspirin is commonly administered to patients awaiting bypass surgery. This drug has a prolonged inhibitory effect on platelet function (5–7 days), and should therefore be stopped 7 days before surgery and commenced immediately post-operatively, when it significantly helps graft patency. It is prudent in the setting of unstable angina or in urgent coronary artery bypass grafting that aspirin is not stopped, and so the use of antifibrinolytics may have a role to play in these patients.

METHODS TO REDUCE THE NEED FOR BLOOD TRANSFUSION

Large variations in transfusion practice are currently seen in the European Union. This is due to many factors, including the patient populations treated, differences in surgical and anaesthetic techniques, and attitudes to and availability of blood, as well as differences in pre- and post-operative care. Such differences in transfusion practice have not been shown to be associated with significant differences in mortality. These findings indicate that transfusion can be avoided or reduced by various interventions and that this does not appear to affect clinical outcomes.

ACUTE VOLUME REPLACEMENT

Non-plasma colloid volume expanders of large molecules, such as dextran, are a relatively inexpensive colloidal alternative to plasma in first-line management of patients who are volume-depleted as a result of bleeding.

In the initial resuscitation of patients with haemorrhagic shock, the adequacy of volume replacement is usually of much greater importance than the choice of fluid. A reasonable guide in adults is 1000 ml of crystalloid (0.9% saline or Ringer's lactate solution), followed by 1000 ml of colloid, and then replacement with red cells. In the elderly and those with cardiac impairment, red cell replacement is started earlier to maintain oxygen-carrying capacity without causing fluid overload.

MECHANISMS FOR REDUCING BLOOD USE IN SURGERY

Pre-operative

When surgery is elective, significant reductions in blood use can be made by ensuring that the patient has a normal haemoglobin and by correcting any pre-existing anaemia, e.g. iron or folic acid deficiency. Drugs that interfere with haemostasis, e.g. non-steroidal anti-inflammatory drugs, aspirin and warfarin, should be stopped where appropriate. An abnormal clotting screen or platelet count should be investigated and corrected prior to surgery. In suitable patients, an autologous pre-deposit programme (see above) may be considered. Recombinant erythropoietin can be used to raise the haemoglobin levels in patients thought likely to need blood, e.g. women with low haemoglobin levels who are undergoing a procedure with a high transfusion requirement. Erythropoietin should be used in conjunction with iron therapy. To ensure optimal management, these issues should be addressed 4–6 weeks prior to surgery at pre-operative assessment clinics.

Intra-operative

The training, experience and competence of the surgeon performing the procedure are the most crucial factors in reducing operative blood loss. The importance of meticulous surgical technique, with attention to bleeding points, cannot be underestimated. Other techniques, such as posture, the use of vasoconstrictors and tourniquets, and avoidance of hypothermia, should always be considered, as these can have a significant impact on perioperative blood loss. Certain pharmacological agents, e.g. antifibrinolytics such as tranexamic acid and aprotinin, can significantly reduce the requirements for blood and are indicated in certain operative procedures.

Fibrin sealant mimics the final stage in the coagulation cascade, in which fibrinogen is converted to fibrin in the presence of thrombin, factor XIII, fibronectin and ionized calcium. Freeze-dried sterilized fibrinogen, fibronectin and factor XIII can be delivered from one barrel of a double-barrelled syringe while thrombin, calcium and aprotinin are delivered from the other. If the two mixtures meet at a surgical bleeding site the solution clots almost immediately, the clot resolving over a period of days. Fibrin sealant has been used in vascular, cardiac and liver surgery and in situations where even small amounts of bleeding can be problematic (e.g. middle ear surgery).

Acute normovolaemic haemodilution and intra-operative blood salvage are two of the autologous methods of blood conservation that can be employed during surgery to reduce exposure to transfusion. They are described in the section on autologous programmes.

Post-operative

Post-operative cell salvage (see above) can reduce the need for allogeneic transfusion.

The decision to transfuse post-operatively should depend on several factors (see 'Indications for transfusion'). Blood transfusion should be limited to the smallest amount of blood required to raise the haemoglobin above the transfusion threshold (even if this is only 1 unit). Appropriate use of antifibrinolytic drugs such as tranexamic acid and the routine prescribing of iron and folic acid also reduce post-operative transfusion. A reduction in transfusion has been shown to result from the introduction of simple protocols that give guidance on when the haemoglobin should be checked and when red cells should be transfused.

BETTER BLOOD TRANSFUSION

In recent times, attention has been focused on blood transfusion practice for a number of reasons. These include concerns about the transmission of vCJD by blood transfusion, increased costs associated with new safety measures such as leucocyte depletion, documented variations in transfusion practice and recommendations arising from the SHOT scheme. The Better Blood Transfusion (BBT) programme has been established to improve transfusion practice and thereby maximize benefits of the supply of blood and blood products. Hospital transfusion committees have been formed and a network of transfusion practitioners has been established. The main purpose is to promote the safe, efficient and appropriate use of blood components and plasma derivatives. The aims of BBT are to establish protocols and guidelines to nationally approved standards, implement an accredited learning programme, generate automated data outputs for transfusion practice to allow comparison of statistics, and achieve a reduction in inappropriate blood use.

FUTURE TRENDS

The demand for blood continued to rise yearly until 2000, when it reached a plateau. Although local shortages occur from time to time, where high demand coincides with low rates of collection, the UK is still self-sufficient in red cells. With ever more stringent donor selection guidelines and an increasingly elderly population, the number of available donors will continue to decrease. This means that blood should be considered a scarce and valuable commodity that should be responsibly prescribed.

Although red cell substitutes are in various stages of clinical trial, no cell-free haemoglobin solution or fluorocarbon oxygen carrier is as yet licensed for clinical use. However, there is every expectation that transfusion therapy will be increasingly supplanted by the use of synthetic or biologically engineered substitutes.

Recombinant growth factors are making an increasing impact on blood requirements. For example, recombinant human erythropoietin raises haemoglobin levels in patients with chronic renal failure and has been used with some success to raise the haemoglobin level pre-operatively with or without autologous pre-deposit.

The objective in managing surgical patients should be to minimize anaemia and bleeding and hence the need for transfusion. Although it is clear that no patient should be transfused unnecessarily, it is equally certain that no patient should be allowed to exsanguinate because of concerns regarding blood safety.

4

5

K.C.H. FEARON

Nutritional support in surgical patients

5

INTRODUCTION

It goes without saying that without food there can be no life, that food is a basic human right, and that it behoves every doctor to pay attention to the nutritional needs of his or her patients. Nevertheless, approximately one-third of all patients admitted to an acute hospital will have evidence of protein–calorie malnutrition and two-thirds will leave hospital either malnourished or having lost weight.

Malnutrition has damaging effects on psychological status, activity levels and appearance. Paradoxically, in the surgical patient a low body fat content may sometimes be viewed as an advantage, making technical aspects of surgery easier. There is, however, clear evidence that patients with severe protein depletion have a significantly greater incidence of post-operative complications, such as pneumonia and wound infection, and a prolonged hospital stay.

Nutritional disorders in surgical practice have two principal components. First, starvation can be initiated by the effects of the disease, by restriction of oral intake, or both. Simple starvation results in progressive loss of the body's energy and protein reserves (i.e. subcutaneous fat and skeletal muscle). Second, there are the metabolic effects of stress/inflammation: namely, increased catabolism and reduced anabolism. These result in a variety of changes, including a low serum albumin concentration, accelerated muscle wasting and water retention. Although malnutrition may be the result of starvation, in most surgical patients it results from a combination of reduced food intake and metabolic change (Fig. 5.1).

ASSESSMENT OF NUTRITIONAL STATUS

The main energy reserves in the body are found in subcutaneous and intra-abdominal fat. Fat reserves are generally in excess and their loss does not greatly impair function. In contrast, there are no true protein reserves in the body. Thus, in the face of starvation or stress, structural tissues such as skeletal muscle and the gut are autocannibalized, resulting in functional impairment that can eventually impede recovery.

The key elements of nutritional assessment include current food intake, levels of energy and protein reserves, and the patient's likely clinical course (Fig. 5.2). Patients who have not eaten for 5 days or more require nutritional support, and those with symptoms such as anorexia, nausea, vomiting or early satiety are at risk of a reduced food intake and hence undernutrition. Levels of energy reserves are most easily assessed by examining for loss of subcutaneous fat (skinfolds), whereas protein depletion is most commonly manifest as skeletal muscle wasting (Fig. 5.3). A history of weight loss of more than 10–15% is highly significant. Patients can also be assessed according to their body mass index (BMI: weight (kg)/height (m^2)). The normal BMI is 18.5–24.9. A value less than 18 is suggestive of severe protein–calorie undernutrition. Finally, it is

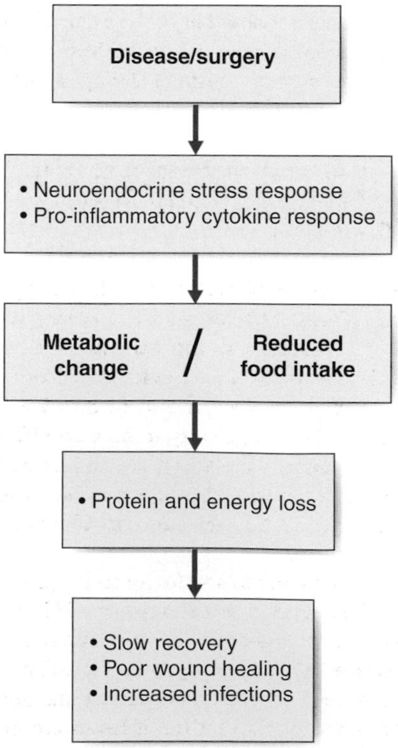

Fig. 5.1 **Mechanisms linking the effects of disease/surgery on patient outcomes.**

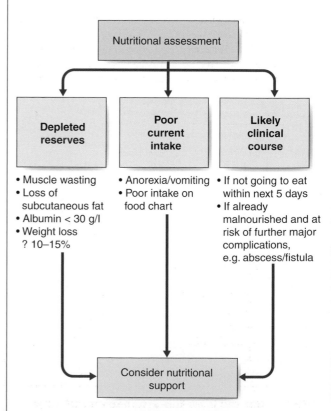

Fig. 5.2 **Nutritional assessment in surgical patients.**

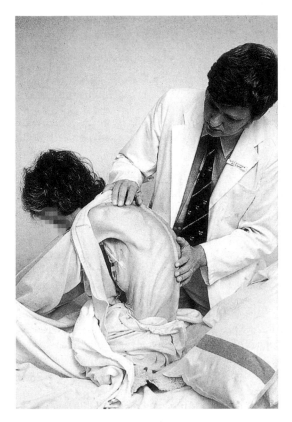

Fig. 5.3 Protein–energy malnutrition in a surgical patient, illustrating depleted muscle and subcutaneous fat stores.

BOX 5.1   BODY MASS INDEX (BMI)

$$BMI = \frac{Weight\ (kg)}{Height\ (m^2)}$$

< 18.4	Underweight for height
18.5–24.9	Ideal weight for height
25–29.9	Over ideal weight for height
30–39.9	Obese
> 40	Very obese

BOX 5.2   NUTRITIONAL STATUS

- Nutritional status in surgical patients may be adversely affected by starvation (effects of disease such as oesophageal cancer, restricted intake), the effects of inflammation (increased catabolism) and the effects of the operation itself (stress/inflammatory response)
- Nutritional status is assessed by current food intake, levels of reserves and likely clinical course

---

important to recognize that in assessing the nutritional status of patients, knowledge of their likely clinical course is vital (Fig. 5.4). For example, if patients are well nourished, they should be able to withstand the brief period of fasting associated with major surgery. However, if

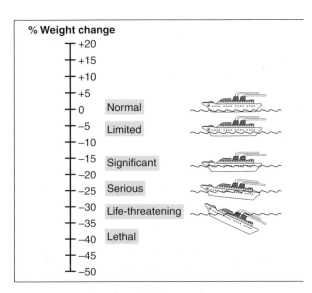

% Weight change

+20	
+15	
+10	
+5	
0	Normal
−5	Limited
−10	
−15	Significant
−20	
−25	Serious
−30	Life-threatening
−35	
−40	Lethal
−45	
−50	

Fig. 5.4   Alterations in nutritional status associated with weight loss.

patients are severely malnourished (e.g. weight loss of 15%, BMI 18), then even a short further period of starvation or catabolism may make them so critically undernourished that this becomes life-threatening in itself. Taken together, a patient's food intake, level of reserve and likely clinical course should alert the astute clinician to the need for nutritional support and should be part of the routine daily appraisal of every patient during a surgical ward round.

ASSESSMENT OF NUTRITIONAL REQUIREMENTS

Energy and protein requirements vary, depending on weight, body composition, clinical status, mobility and dietary intake. For most patients, an approximation based on weight and clinical status is sufficient. Relevant values are given in Table 5.1. Few patients require more than 2500 kcal/day. Additional calories are unlikely to be used effectively and may even constitute a metabolic stress. Particular caution must be exercised when refeeding the chronically starved patient because of the dangers of hypokalaemia and hypophosphataemia.

The most common method for assessing protein requirement is 24-hour urinary urea excretion. This is converted to an estimate of 24-hour urinary nitrogen loss. Most patients require 10–15 g nitrogen per day. (The equivalent amount of protein can be calculated by multiplying by a conversion factor of 6.25.) Even if losses are in excess of this, more than 18 g nitrogen/day (equivalent to 112 g protein) is seldom given because it is unlikely to be used effectively.

Table 5.1   ESTIMATION OF ENERGY AND PROTEIN REQUIREMENTS IN ADULT SURGICAL PATIENTS

	Uncomplicated	Complicated/stressed
Energy (kcal/kg/day)	25	30–35
Protein (g/kg/day)*	1.0	1.3–1.5

* Grams of protein can be converted to the equivalent amount of nitrogen by dividing by 6.25.

CAUSES OF INADEQUATE INTAKE

The ideal way for surgical patients to take in enough nutrients is for them to eat or drink palatable food. Unfortunately, the catering budget is often far too low for the provision of appetizing food, and wastage of unwanted food can account for up to 40% of that served. Other reasons for a poor food intake include the patient being too weak and anorexic, or having a mechanical problem such as obstruction of the gastrointestinal tract. Patients with increased metabolic demands may have some difficulty in taking sufficient food to meet such demands. Patients with a normal functional gut may also have a reduced food intake due simply to the cumulative effects of repeated periods of fasting to undergo investigations such as endoscopy or contrast radiology.

Some patients suffer from what is best described as 'intestinal failure', i.e. a state in which the amount of functioning gut is reduced below a level where enough food can be digested and absorbed for nourishment. The four principal causes of intestinal failure are:

- *short bowel syndrome*, which results from extensive small bowel resection
- *fistula formation*, in which bowel content is lost externally or short-circuited (internal fistula) before it can be adequately digested and absorbed
- *motility disorders*, such as paralytic ileus and chronic intestinal pseudo-obstruction
- extensive *small bowel disease*, such as Crohn's disease.

In these difficult cases, specialized nutritional treatment is required if the patient is to remain normally nourished. The situation of many of these patients, at least in the acute phase, is further complicated by the presence of ongoing inflammation or sepsis. As a general rule, nutritional treatment is not as effective as it might be in the presence of active sepsis. The priority in such patients is to eliminate sepsis at the same time as providing nutritional support.

METHODS OF PROVIDING NUTRITIONAL SUPPORT

Nutrients can be given via the gastrointestinal tract, i.e. enteral nutrition, or intravenously, i.e. parenteral nutrition. Parenteral nutrition is indicated only when enteral feeding is not feasible. Very few patients are not suitable for some form of enteral feeding, which is both safer and cheaper

EBM 5.1   ENTERAL VS PARENTERAL NUTRITION IN SURGICAL PATIENTS

'*Enteral nutrition should be first choice for nutritional support in the critically ill surgical patient.*'

Gramlich L, et al. Nutrition 2004; 20:843–848.

than parenteral nutrition (EBM 5.1). Certainly, all those who have a normal length of functioning gastrointestinal tract, and most of those who have a reduced amount, can be fed by this route. Furthermore, the ingestion of even suboptimal amounts of food may help maintain the integrity of the intestinal mucosa, thereby reducing bacterial and endotoxin translocation, which may compound the metabolic upset in critically ill patients.

ENTERAL NUTRITION

Oral route

As stated previously, it is essential to provide warm, appetizing food on the wards, to make sure there are enough nursing and auxiliary staff available to help elderly/infirm patients take their food, and to encourage nursing staff to be aware of the nutritional needs of all patients. It is against this basic background of nutritional care that the need for artificial nutritional support should be considered.

Many patients suffer from early satiety (feeling full after a meal), and encouraging them to eat small amounts frequently or to sip an oral supplement between meals can help overcome this symptom. Oral supplements come in cartons of about 250 ml and each contains about 250 kcal and 10 g of protein. These should be available to all patients who require them. There is a range of flavours and the texture can be changed if chilled, for example. Most patients manage to take two or three cartons per day if required. However, fatigue with such supplements is commonplace and leads to reduced efficacy in the long run.

Table 5.2   CAUSES OF ANOREXIA IN SURGICAL PATIENTS

- Intestinal obstruction
- Ileus
- Cancer anorexia
- Depression, stress, anxiety
- Drugs, e.g. opiates
- Oral ulceration/infection
- General debility/weakness

5

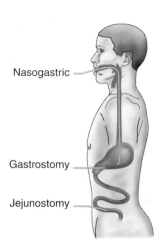

Nasogastric

Gastrostomy

Jejunostomy

Fig. 5.5 Routes of enteral nutrition.

There are numerous reasons why surgical patients may suffer from anorexia (i.e. poor appetite) (Table 5.2). Before embarking on tube enteral feeding, it is important to manage actively any symptoms that can be treated (e.g. oral thrush with nystatin, nausea with anti-emetics) and thus boost spontaneous oral intake. For patients who are unable to swallow, or for those whose anorexia is resistant to other therapy, nasoenteral feeding via a fine-bore tube should be used.

Methods of administration of enteral feeds
(Fig. 5.5)

Nasogastric or nasojejunal tubes
If patients cannot drink or sip a liquid feed for mechanical reasons, or if they are unconscious or on a ventilator, enteral nutrition can be given by a fine-bore nasogastric or nasoenteric tube. The position of the tube tip should be checked radiologically, or by aspirating gastric content and confirming presence of acid by litmus paper, before nutrients are infused. Patients who need prolonged enteral feeding can learn to pass a fine-bore tube each evening and feed themselves overnight. When carried out at home, this is known as home enteral nutrition.

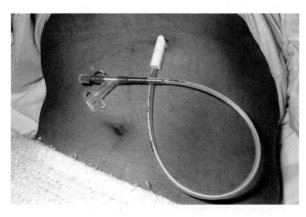

Fig. 5.6 Patient with feeding gastrostomy.

Gastrostomy and jejunostomy
If nasogastric feeding is impossible due to disease or obstruction of the upper alimentary tract, nutrients may be given through a tube placed into the gastrointestinal tract below the lesion (Fig. 5.6). Thus a patient with pseudobulbar palsy or an oesophageal fistula can be fed through a gastrostomy, and a patient with a gastric or duodenal fistula can be fed through a jejunostomy.

Specially designed gastrostomy tubes can now be inserted by a combined percutaneous and endoscopic method, and are particularly valuable for prolonged feeding when there is no impairment of gastric emptying (e.g. stroke patients). Feeding jejunostomy tubes can be inserted at the time of laparotomy when the surgeon anticipates that prolonged nutritional support will be needed post-operatively (e.g. in patients undergoing oesophagectomy and gastrectomy for cancer, or necrosectomy for severe pancreatitis).

Complications of enteral nutrition
Just because enteral feeds are administered directly into the gastrointestinal tract, it cannot be assumed that this technique is free from complications. Diarrhoea may be managed by reducing the rate of infusion and by ensuring the patient is not on broad-spectrum antibiotics. Vomiting can be managed by reducing the rate of feeding and by the use of prokinetic drugs such as metoclopramide or erythromycin. Monitoring of fluid and electrolyte balance is important, at least in the acute phase of a patient's illness (for metabolic complications, see 'Parenteral nutrition').

Complications also occur because of difficulty in placing the tubes. Examples include a fine-bore nasogastric tube inserted wrongly into the respiratory tract, or early accidental removal of a jejunostomy tube, with intraperitoneal leakage. As with other areas of nutrition supplementation, attention to detail is paramount.

BOX 5.3 ENTERAL NUTRITION

- If patients cannot eat adequate amounts of food, they should be reviewed by the ward dietitian
- If oral supplements fail, a fine-bore tube can be used for supplemental or total enteral nutrition
- Most patients tolerate a whole-protein feed (1 kcal/ml), which can be escalated to 100 ml/hr and thus supply about 2400 kcal/day and 14 g nitrogen/day
- If a tube cannot be passed down the oesophagus, gastrostomy and jejunostomy feeding should be considered
- The main complications of enteral feeding relate to patient tolerance (nausea, vomiting and diarrhoea) and to the insertion site (gastrostomy or jejunostomy)

PARENTERAL NUTRITION

Intravenous feeding is indicated when patients cannot be fed adequately by mouth, nasogastric tube or gastrostomy/jejunostomy, or when they have complete or partial intestinal failure. The problem may be permanent, as in most cases of short bowel syndrome, or reversible,

5

5

as in paralytic ileus or fistula. In some cases of short bowel syndrome, the remaining intestine 'adapts' by undergoing mucosal hyperplasia over a period of weeks or months, and normal feeding can then resume.

Parenteral nutrition can provide the patient's total needs for protein, energy, electrolytes, trace metals and vitamins, i.e. total parenteral nutrition (TPN). The need to restrict volume means that concentrated solutions are used. As such solutions are irritant and thrombogenic, they have to be administered through a catheter positioned in a large high-flow vein, such as the superior vena cava.

Indications for TPN

The chief indication for TPN is failure of the gastrointestinal tract. TPN can be both effective and life-saving when post-operative complications develop, especially when these prevent enteral nutrition or are associated with infection. Situations in which TPN is invaluable include prolonged paralytic ileus, gross abdominal sepsis, and in dealing with the increased metabolic demands that follow severe injury.

TPN should continue until intestinal function has recovered sufficiently to allow nutrition to be maintained by the oral or enteral route. In cases of high-output, proximal small bowel fistula, parenteral feeding is continued until the fistula has closed spontaneously or has been closed surgically.

Composition of TPN solutions

Although TPN can be provided by sequential or simultaneous administration of individual glucose, fat or amino acid solutions, it is now standard practice to mix the day's requirements in a 3 litre bag. This is made up in the pharmacy under sterile conditions, and its contents are infused over 18–24 hours using an infusion pump. Many pharmacies now use three or four standard regimens. The solutions contain fixed amounts of energy and nitrogen, and typically provide 1800–2500 kcal (50% glucose, 50% lipid) and 10–14 g nitrogen.

Table 5.3 STANDARD PARENTERAL NUTRITION REGIMEN	
Constituent	Quantity
Non-protein energy	2200 kcal
Nitrogen	13.5 g
Volume	2500 ml
Sodium	115 mmol
Potassium	65 mmol
Calcium	10 mmol
Magnesium	9.5 mmol
Phosphate	20 mmol
Zinc	0.1 mmol
Chloride	113.3 mmol
Acetate	135 mmol
(Adequate vitamins and trace elements)	

Fluid and electrolyte needs are also catered for. Many patients on TPN need additional water, sodium and potassium because of excess loss from, for example, a high-output fistula. Trace elements and vitamins can also be incorporated, and the demands created by infection and excessive loss can be met. An example of a standard TPN regimen is given in Table 5.3.

Administration of TPN

Hypertonic solutions have to be infused into a vein with a high flow. Vascular access to the superior vena cava is normally obtained directly through the internal jugular or subclavian vein, or indirectly via a peripherally inserted central (PIC) line.

Cannulae are made of silastic or polyurethane and are of fine bore. For longer-term feeding, a Hickman catheter is used; this type of silastic catheter has a Dacron cuff, which secures it in the subcutaneous fat. Before use, the position of the catheter tip in the inferior vena cava (IVC) is checked radiologically. With good care, a correctly positioned Hickman catheter can remain in place for several months or years (Fig. 5.7).

Complications of TPN

Catheter problems

Percutaneous insertion of a catheter may damage adjacent structures and can cause pneumothorax, air embolus and haematoma. Catheter placement under ultrasound guidance helps avoid such problems. Incorrect catheter positioning is excluded by taking a chest X-ray prior to commencing infusion.

Thrombophlebitis

Thrombosis is common when long lines are used, when the catheter tip is not in an area of high flow, and when very hypertonic solutions are infused. The telltale signs are redness and tenderness over the cannulated vein, together with swelling of the whole limb and engorgement of collateral veins if the thrombosis is more proximal. Occasionally, a superior mediastinal syndrome develops in patients with superior vena cava thrombosis. If major vessel occlusion is suspected, the diagnosis is confirmed by venography and anticoagulation is commenced with heparin. If vascular access has to be maintained, an attempt can be made to lyse the clot with urokinase or plasminogen activator. If the clot cannot be dissolved, the cannula must be removed and a new one positioned in an unoccluded vein. The patient may need to remain on long-term anticoagulation.

Infection

Infection and septicaemia are the most frequent complications of TPN. The usual offending organisms are coagulase-negative staphylococci, *Staphylococcus aureus* and coliforms, but the incidence of fungal infection is increasing, possibly because many of the patients requiring TPN are immunocompromised or receiving broad-spectrum antibiotics. Most catheter infections are the result of poor care of the feeding line. The insertion site must be protected with an occlusive dressing and should be cleansed on

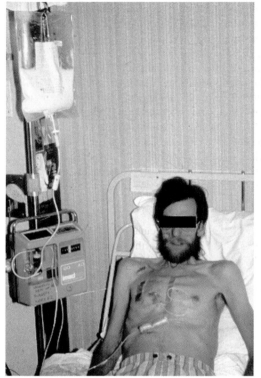
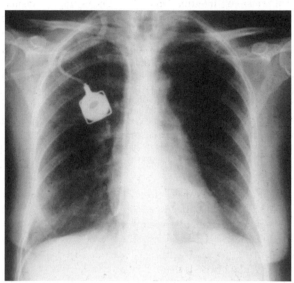

Fig. 5.7   Total parenteral nutrition (TPN).
A Malnourished patient receiving TPN. B Chest X-ray of patient with indwelling Portacath for long-term TPN. The subcutaneous catheter hub is accessed using a Huber needle.

alternate days with an antiseptic agent. The line must only be used for infusion of nutrients and never for taking or giving blood or administering drugs. Great care is taken to avoid contamination when changing bags. A nutrition support nurse is invaluable in avoiding catheter sepsis and supervising all aspects of catheter care. If the patient receiving TPN develops pyrexia, the protocol outlined in Table 5.4 should be followed.

Table 5.4   DETECTION AND TREATMENT OF CATHETER SEPSIS

If a pyrexia > 38°C develops, or there is a further rise in temperature if already pyrexial
- Stop parenteral nutrition and check for other sources of pyrexia (e.g. chest or urinary tract infection)
- Take peripheral and central blood cultures
- Administer intravenous fluids
- Heparinize catheter
- Consult senior medical staff

If blood culture is negative
- Restart parenteral nutrition

If blood culture is positive
- Remove catheter and send tip for bacteriological analysis
- Administer appropriate antibiotic therapy
- If necessary, replace catheter and restart parenteral nutrition within 24–48 hours

Where central access must be preserved
- Seek specialist advice from hospital nutrition team

Metabolic complications

Metabolic complications include under- or overhydration. Patients with coexisting medical conditions (e.g. cardiac failure) should be carefully monitored. Hyperglycaemia may occur and requires either a reduction of the glucose load or the concomitant infusion of insulin via a separate pump. Hypokalaemia and hypophosphataemia are common when severely malnourished patients are re-fed after a long period of starvation because of the large flux of potassium and phosphate into the cells; correction is by further supplementation. Abnormal liver function tests may occur in severely stressed or septic patients. If the changes are marked and progressive, the overall substrate load should be reduced and discontinuation of parenteral nutrition considered.

Peripheral vein nutrition

Lipid emulsions and isotonic solutions of amino acids are available which are less irritant than conventional TPN solutions and which can be infused into peripheral veins. Such solutions can be used in the short term, but their prolonged use is associated with thrombophlebitis and conventional techniques should be employed if long-term support is needed. Peripheral catheters require the same level of care as central catheters, and the patient must still be monitored for signs of infection or metabolic complications.

BOX 5.4 PARENTERAL NUTRITION

- Parenteral feeding is indicated if the patient cannot be fed adequately by the oral or enteral route
- The need to restrict volume when using total parenteral nutrition (TPN) means that concentrated solutions are used, which may be irritant and thrombogenic. TPN is therefore infused through a catheter in a high-flow vein (e.g. superior vena cava)
- TPN is usually given in an 'all-in-one' 3 litre bag with a mixture of glucose, fat and L-amino acids combined with fluid, electrolytes, vitamins, minerals and trace elements
- The major complications with TPN can be classed as catheter-related, septic or metabolic. A multidisciplinary approach to the management of TPN patients by a nutrition team will minimize such complications

MONITORING OF NUTRITIONAL SUPPORT

Patients receiving nutritional support are monitored to detect deficiency states, assess the adequacy of energy and protein provision, and anticipate complications. Patients receiving enteral feeding require less intense monitoring but are prone to the same metabolic complications as those who are fed intravenously.

Pulse rate, blood pressure and temperature are recorded regularly, an accurate fluid balance chart is maintained (remembering not to overlook insensible losses), and the urine is checked daily for glycosuria. Body weight is measured twice weekly.

Serum urea and electrolytes are measured daily, as are blood glucose levels if there is glycosuria. Full blood count, liver function tests, and serum albumin, calcium, magnesium and phosphate are monitored once or twice weekly. Urine is collected over one or two 24-hour periods each week to measure sodium and nitrogen losses. To maintain a positive nitrogen balance, nitrogen intake should exceed daily losses by at least 2 g. For patients on long-term enteral nutrition or TPN (i.e. longer than 2–3 weeks) less intense monitoring is appropriate once they are stable.

6

I.F. LAURENSON

Infections and antibiotics

PATHOGENIC POTENTIAL OF MICROBES

EXALTATION

When an organism is serially passaged in vivo, its virulence may be exalted (increased) and its capacity to spread from one host to another increased.

The concept of increased pathogenic potential as a result of exaltation in vivo must be linked with the ability of some commensal or opportunist bacteria to acquire and pass on new, potentially dangerous genetic information. This may affect an organism's ability to colonize, to infect, to produce toxin or to develop multiple antibiotic resistance. The 'hospital staphylococcus' illustrates some of the alarming possibilities that can result when an organism acquires new genetic material in the course of its colonization. Gram-negative bacilli, especially *Klebsiella*s, have also demonstrated a potential for dangerous genetic exchange. The extending range of β-lactamases in such widely different genera as *Haemophilus, Neisseria* and *Bacteroides* species, is a matter for concern and may lead to treatment failure with commonly used β-lactams. The transmission of organisms from patient to patient, or between staff and patients, must be rigorously avoided. Hand-washing on the ward is critical, as is the wearing and appropriate changing of disposable gloves in situations where transfer of flora from one patient to another may occur.

PATHOGENIC SYNERGY

Two or more organisms may combine forces in a mixed infection and demonstrate enhanced virulence. Examples include acute ulceromembranous gingivitis (Vincent's infection), Meleney's synergistic gangrene, and various fusospirochaetal or mixed infections with anaerobic components, all of which may lead to progressive destruction of tissue or a fulminating invasive infection. Mixed infections are common in a wide range of conditions, e.g. cerebral, dental, lung and pelvic abscess, and peritonitis. When the anaerobic *Bacteroides* spp are present in such infections, they may interfere with phagocyte function and produce detectable levels of β-lactamases in abscess fluid. These β-lactamases protect normally susceptible organisms of mixed infections from the actions of antimicrobials. These factors may explain the observed synergistic action of coexisting pathogens.

ASEPSIS

SURGICAL RITUAL

In surgical areas, clear and specific instructions must be given on pre-operative skin cleansing of the patient and on adequate disinfection of the operation site. The relative advantages of masks, gowns and drapes at operation are debated, and the limitations of these precautions should be understood. Not only may they serve to protect the patient, they can also protect the operator from fluid splashes. Only suitable protective materials should be used.

There should be a clear disinfectant policy and an antibiotic policy that ensures antimicrobial agents are used sensibly on the wards and in the operating theatres. Strict adherence to the principles of sterilization and disinfection is essential when cleansing and processing surgical instruments and anaesthetic equipment.

STERILIZATION

This is an absolute term denoting the complete removal or inactivation of viable microorganisms (protozoa, fungi, bacteria and viruses). It can only be achieved by strict attention to detail. Instruments or articles can be classified as sterile following thorough cleaning if they have been subjected to any of the following:

- wet heat in an autoclave at 121°C for 20 minutes, or at a higher temperature for a shorter time (HTST) to provide an equivalent exposure (Fig. 6.1)
- dry heat in a hot-air oven at 160°C for 1 hour (Fig. 6.1)
- irradiation under strictly controlled conditions (used predominantly in industry)
- special sterilizing chemicals, liquids or gases, such as formaldehyde, glutaraldehyde or ethylene oxide, under strictly controlled conditions.

Some transmissible agents, known as prions, challenge these conventional assumptions; an example is that respon-

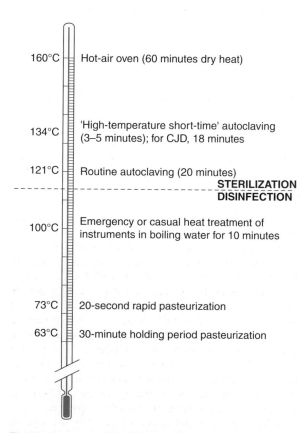

Fig. 6.1   A summary of heat-treatment temperatures.
(After Collee JG. 1981. In: Applied medical microbiology, p. 104. Blackwell, Oxford)

sible for Creutzfeldt–Jakob disease (CJD). To prevent prion transmission, instruments used in such patients should not be reused on any other patient. Prions of variant CJD (vCJD) have also been found in gut lymphoreticular tissue, raising the spectre of inadvertent transmission on instruments that have not been properly cleaned prior to standard sterilization methods, which are known to be ineffective. The use of 'once only' disposable instruments is required to prevent transmission.

DISINFECTION

This term denotes a significant reduction in the numbers of organisms present, particularly those that might cause infection. With few exceptions, chemical disinfectants are not sterilizing agents. Antiseptics are relatively mild disinfectants that can be used on living tissues without causing undue harm.

Disinfection and preparation of the skin for surgery

Pre-operative shaving at the site of incision is no longer recommended, as it leads to increased wound infection. For convenience, however, the site often has to be cleared of hairs immediately prior to the operation. This tends to be carried out in the anaesthetic room or in the operating theatre itself. Before a surgical incision is made in intact skin, the transient and resident flora at the operation site can be markedly reduced by thorough cleansing, and remaining flora largely inactivated by the application of a suitable antibacterial agent. This will inactivate vegetative forms of bacteria only; it cannot be expected to kill bacterial spores. Accessible vegetative bacteria on the skin can be quickly inactivated by applying 70% ethanol, or 70% isopropyl alcohol, in water. The addition of an antiseptic such as chlorhexidine or iodine 1–2% further enhances the bacterial kill. However, any surgery where diathermy is used has a risk of igniting any residual alcohol from the skin preparation. The aqueous solution of chlorhexidine or iodine is therefore used in most operating theatres. Without the presence of alcohol, however, the skin preparation is less effective, and this should be borne in mind by the surgeon. As its action is time-dependent, the solution should be left in contact with the skin for as long as possible before it is dried and the incision performed.

SURGICAL INFECTION

INFECTION, BACTERAEMIA AND SEPTICAEMIA

The term 'infection' means the presence of organisms in a normally sterile site, usually but not necessarily accompanied by an inflammatory host response. When bacteria are present in the blood, as shown by blood culture, the term 'bacteraemia' is used. This phenomenon may be transient. 'Septicaemia' is similar but a greater severity is implied.

MICROBIOLOGICAL DIAGNOSIS OF INFECTION

In the appropriate clinical context, symptoms and signs of infection should be sought. Before antibiotics are given, appropriate specimens of pus (in a sterile container without additives), wound swabs, blood cultures, sputum and urine should be sent rapidly to the microbiology laboratory, accompanied by a clearly completed request form with full details of the patient, the clinical situation, antibiotic allergies and any treatment. Urgent Gram staining may guide initial therapy. It should be noted if mycobacterial infection is under consideration. In some cases, serological or special techniques may be helpful. Microbiological advice should be sought.

WOUND INFECTION

The term 'contamination' usually denotes the passive presence of a relatively small number of various species of bacteria. An open wound is invariably contaminated with organisms, which may be derived endogenously from the patient's skin or exogenously from an external source such as the soil or air, or the hand of an attendant. The outcome of the microbial challenge depends on many factors, including the circumstances of contamination. When one or more contaminants has a survival advantage over the others and replicates in the wound, infection is initiated and microbial pathogenicity expressed. There may be bacterial invasion, toxin production or a combination of these. Occasionally, there may be fungal or viral infection.

If contamination is minimal, as in an elective surgical incision performed under good conditions on a patient in good general health, the defences of the host cope completely. If contamination is severe, and particularly when other adverse factors operate, the challenge may rapidly result in a fulminating and overwhelming infection unless prompt and adequate action is taken to counter it. Such conditions arise, for example, with a lacerated wound following a road accident in an elderly person, or a perforated colon in a debilitated patient.

Thus a wound infection implies the implantation of a potentially infective inoculum under conditions that allow the organism to evade or overcome host defences; it is a function of the number of organisms in the inoculum, their

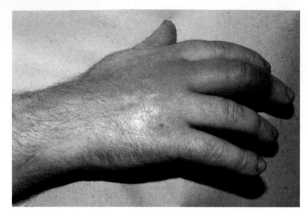

Fig. 6.2 Lymphangitis caused by *Streptococcus pyogenes* following minor trauma to the finger.
(Courtesy of Mr AS Whyte FRCS.)

quality or nature, and the efficacy of local and general host defences.

Factors predisposing to infection

In accidental wounds, several infective organisms are likely to be present, although *Staphylococcus aureus* or β-haemolytic streptococci alone may cause severe infection (Fig. 6.2). Therefore, prompt and adequate surgical treatment should be given before the stage of bacterial contamination has led to proliferation and passed into that of active infection. Ideally, this should be within 1–2 hours of injury, and must include thorough cleansing of the wound and the removal of all debris (surgical toilet), followed by the excision of all devitalized tissue (debridement). If primary surgical care is not given within 6 hours, infection must be presumed.

Factors concerned with healing, and the problems of wound management are considered in Chapter 12.

Tissue oxygenation

Primary host defences against wound infection include phagocytosis and intraleucocytic microbicidal systems. Effective phagocytosis, good tissue perfusion and oxygenation are requirements for the optimal function of these

---

BOX 6.2 PREDISPOSING FACTORS THAT ENCOURAGE OR PROMOTE INFECTION

- Contamination with potential pathogens
- Foreign material in the wound
- Virulence-enhancing effect of some materials, such as soil, calcium and iron salts
- Delay in primary attention
- Pathogenic synergy (see above)
- Devitalized tissue
- Oedema/pressure/constriction
- Impaired blood supply
- Extravasation of tissue fluids and blood
- Host factors lowering resistance, e.g. extremes of age, debility, immunocompromised states, diabetes, cigarette smoking, alcoholism, steroids, severe obesity or malnutrition, remote infection

---

defences. All wounded tissue is less aerobic than normal tissue; impaired oxygenation persists for some days until healing is established. If the patient is initially shocked, tissue perfusion is further constrained and a vicious circle may result. Post-operative hyperoxygenation of the patient lowers the incidence of infection following colorectal surgery.

Temperature

Both wound and patient hypothermia give rise to impaired tissue perfusion and oxygenation. This results in a number of adverse outcomes, such as delayed wound healing, increased infection rates, intra- and post-operative myocardial ischaemia, coagulation disturbances and prolonged hospital stay. Thus accidental hypothermia, particularly in the perioperative period, should be avoided.

Symptoms and signs of infection

It is important to detect infection in a wound early. Cardinal local symptoms and signs include pain, erythema, warmth, oedema, and possibly serous or seropurulent exudate. The patient's temperature may rise and local tenderness may increase, with muscle guarding in the affected part.

Pyogenic organisms provoke a polymorphonuclear leucocytosis. The erythrocyte sedimentation rate (ESR) and plasma viscosity increase and the level of C-reactive protein rises. In the immunocompromised or severely infected patient, some of these features, such as temperature and white cell count, may be apparently 'normal' or depressed. If the infection is severe, with early progression to bacteraemia and septicaemia, the patient may quickly and insidiously develop 'septic' shock (see below).

When an operation involves an unavoidable and significant microbial challenge to the tissues, as in colonic surgery, it is standard practice to protect the patient by giving antimicrobial prophylaxis just before or at anaesthesia induction and to cover the period of challenge. It is important that this should be for a short time to prevent the selection of resistant organisms and side-effects. For example, a suitable antibiotic may be given just before surgery and cover continued for up to 24 hours post-operatively.

Post-operative wound infection

Bacterial infection of a surgical wound is still a common post-operative complication (Fig. 6.3). It depends on a number of factors, including the type of operation and incision, the surgical team's skill, the patient's susceptibility to infection and the duration of operation. Regular surveillance and feedback of a surgical team's infection rates can result in a review of practice and lowering of such rates. The following generalizations reflect current experience:

- Clean wounds in healthy tissue should heal promptly. With adequate facilities, an infection rate of less than 2% should be the aim of a good surgical team. Infections with *Staphylococcus aureus* occur from time to time. A series of such infections in a surgical unit suggests that a member of the team may be a carrier. Infections with coagulase-negative staphylococci are particularly associated with the implantation of heart

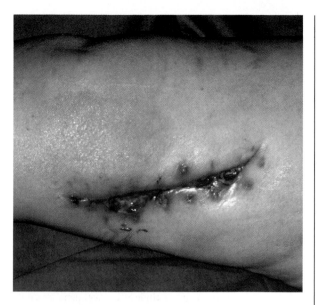

Fig. 6.3   Post-operative wound infection.
(Courtesy of Mr AS Whyte FRCS.)

valves, orthopaedic prostheses, vascular grafts, central venous catheters or other artificial materials.

- 'Clean contaminated' operations on the head and neck, oesophagus, stomach and proximal small bowel are at risk of infection with oropharyngeal flora such as cocci, oral anaerobes and coliforms. Perioperative antimicrobial prophylaxis has significantly reduced the incidence of infection in such operations. A 10% infection rate is not uncommon, especially if gastric achlorhydria allows bacterial multiplication in the stomach. This has special relevance to patients receiving drugs that raise gastric pH, such as H_2 antagonists or proton pump inhibitors. Antimicrobial prophylaxis is also important in surgery of the biliary tract, where potentially infective organisms include faecal streptococci (enterococci), coliforms, pseudomonads and *Clostridium perfringens*. Despite antimicrobial use, infection rates of 5–10% are still recorded in such patients.

- Urological surgery, such as transurethral resection of the prostate, risks infection with coliforms and enterococci, and similar post-operative infection rates.

- 'Contaminated' operations, such as colorectal surgery and those on patients with complicated appendicitis, are associated with higher post-operative infection rates, ranging from 5% to 20% or more. Coliforms and *Bacteroides* spp are common pathogens, often acting synergistically. Mixed infections with faecal streptococci and *Proteus* or pseudomonads pose special problems in clinical management. 'Dirty' operations on abscesses or infected tissue may have an incidence of post-operative wound infection as high as 40%.

- The hazard of infection can be reduced by careful choice of antimicrobial prophylactic agents, meticulous pre-operative preparation of the patient, and good anaesthetic and surgical techniques. Acute emergency cases are at special risk.

SEPSIS, SHOCK AND THE SYSTEMIC INFLAMMATORY RESPONSE SYNDROME (SIRS)

The non-microbiological term 'sepsis' implies clinical evidence of infection, plus evidence of a systemic response to infection. Gram-negative and Gram-positive sepsis may be associated with septic shock. Gram-positive shock is caused by cell-wall components and lipoteichoic acid. It is clinically indistinguishable from Gram-negative sepsis, which involves endotoxin. For further details, see Chapter 3.

HELICOBACTER PYLORI

Infection with *H. pylori* carries the risk of upper gastrointestinal inflammation and neoplastic disease. The prevalence varies with geography and increases with age. In developing countries, infection is virtually universal by the age of 20 years, whereas in more developed countries, acquisition is gradual and may reach 60% of the population by the age of 60. There are associations with peptic ulcer disease, gastric carcinoma and lymphoma. Pernicious anaemia is negatively associated, as is infection with certain (cag A^+) strains and oesophageal reflux, Barrett's oesophagus and adenocarcinoma of the stomach. Diagnosis of *H. pylori* infection can be made endoscopically by biopsy and/or culture, or non-invasively by faecal antigen testing and urease breath tests. *H. pylori* eradication with triple therapy can be used in most cases of disease caused by this organism. A proton pump inhibitor or bismuth salt with two antibiotics, such as amoxicillin with clarithromycin or metronidazole, is used. Treatment failure is usually related to compliance difficulties or antibiotic resistance.

ANAEROBIC INFECTION

TETANUS

The key features of tetanus, which is caused by *Clostridium tetani*, are given in Box 6.3. When infection is established,

---

BOX 6.3   TETANUS

- *Clostridium tetani* is an anaerobic spore-forming bacillus found in soil and faeces
- Tetanus may develop from small contaminated puncture wounds, which may be so small that they are ignored by the patient (one-third of cases)
- Survival in wounds is favoured by hypoxia and by haematoma formation, devitalized tissue, and the presence of soil and foreign bodies
- Failure to cleanse, excise and debride wounds favours multiplication of the organism and the liberation of exotoxin
- Tetanus contributes little to local inflammation but exotoxin increases muscle tone, leading to muscle spasms and exaggerated responses to trivial stimuli
- The incubation period varies from a few days to 3 months (usually less than 2 weeks); the longer the incubation period and delay to the onset of spasms, the better the prognosis
- Antibiotics (penicillin or erythromycin) are an *adjunct* to correct surgical care of wounds

6

C. tetani contributes little to local wound inflammation. However, it produces an exotoxin (tetanospasmin, commonly called tetanus toxin). This enters the pre-synaptic terminals of the lower motor neurons, producing local failure of neuromuscular transmission. Retrograde axonal transport carries the toxin to the cell bodies of these neurons in the brain stem and spinal cord.

Clinical features

The clinical presentation of tetanus is often insidious. A tingling, ache or stiffness in the wound area is usually the first symptom. Jaw movements become restricted (hence the traditional name, 'lockjaw'), facial muscle spasms produce a sardonic grin (risus sardonicus), and the muscles of the neck and back become stiff. Dysphagia, laryngeal spasm and spasm of the chest wall muscles and diaphragm can compromise ventilation and threaten life.

In severe cases, painful muscle spasms become more widespread and increase in frequency and duration. Arching of the back muscles can produce a state known as 'opisthotonos'. Sphincter spasm may cause micturition difficulties.

The patient remains conscious, although consciousness is frequently clouded. The muscle spasms are painful and exhausting, and may be triggered by minor stimuli. The temperature is normal or only slightly elevated, despite profuse sweating and tachycardia, manifestations of autonomic dysfunction. These features are due to sympathetic overactivity, which may also cause worrying swings in blood pressure.

It is important to appreciate that these are the clinical features of a severe attack. Some cases are milder and do not progress to the full spectrum of generalized muscle spasms.

Diagnosis

The diagnosis is essentially clinical. It may be supported by the demonstration of typical slender bacilli with drumstick spores in material from the devitalized wound tissue, and confirmed by the demonstration of tetanus toxin in serum.

Prevention

Tetanus is a preventable disease; some call it an 'inexcusable disease'. Its low prevalence in countries with well-developed medical services depends on prompt and adequate attention to wounds (Fig. 6.4) and programmes of active immunization.

The aim is to provide a minimum of five doses of tetanus-containing vaccine at appropriate intervals for all individuals. Intravenous drug users are at greater risk of tetanus

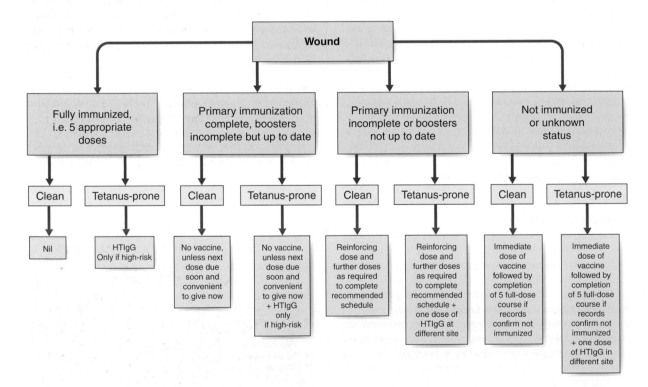

Fig. 6.4
Anti-tetanus wound management.
Tetanus-prone wounds include: (a) wounds or burns that require surgical intervention and when that treatment is delayed for > 6 hrs; (b) as (a), with significant degree of devitalized tissue or puncture-type injury, particularly in contact with soil or manure; (c) wound containing foreign bodies; (d) compound fractures; (e) wounds or burns in patients who have systemic sepsis. High risk: heavy contamination with material likely to contain tetanus spores, and/or devitalized tissue. (HTIgG = human tetanus immunoglobulin; only given where indicated)
Doses for prevention: 250 U by intramuscular injection, or 500 U if > 24 hrs since injury or risk of heavy contamination or following burns.
Treatment of tetanus: See Management below.
(Adapted from UK Department of Health Guidance as at August 2006:
www.dh.gov.uk/PolicyAndGuidance/HealthAndSocialCareTopics/GreenBook/fs/en.)

and booster doses should be given if there is any doubt about their immunization status. As a precautionary measure, travellers whose last dose of tetanus-containing vaccine was more than 10 years previously should have a further booster in case immunoglobulin is not available, should a tetanus-prone injury occur.

Human tetanus immunoglobulin (HTIgG) is available in many countries, rather than equine immunoglobulin (antitetanus serum, ATS), to give immediate transient protection to non-immune patients. Its use is reserved for those considered to be tetanus-prone, and then as an adjunct to active immunization and antibiotic treatment (see below).

Antibiotic prophylaxis

Penicillin (or, if the patient is hypersensitive, erythromycin) should be started before the wound is cleaned and explored. A 5-day course is given, the first tablet being administered just before wound toilet. It must be stressed that antibiotic treatment does not replace the need for basic surgical care of the primary wound, but it may be a necessary adjunct.

Management

Treatment of tetanus is intensive and must begin as soon as the diagnosis is made. Surgical debridement of any wounds is indicated.

Life support

The airway and ventilation must be rapidly assessed and, if necessary, endotracheal intubation performed under benzodiazepine sedation and neuromuscular blockade. The effects of toxin that has fixed to receptors in the nervous system must be countered if the patient is to survive. Muscle spasms are controlled by benzodiazepines such as diazepam, or a propofol infusion. Such sedation also helps to reduce the patient's awareness of a terrifying experience. Sometimes neuromuscular blockade is required.

Destruction of the infecting organism and neutralization of the toxin

Human tetanus immunoglobulin is given either by intravenous infusion (5000–10 000 U) or intramuscularly at multiple sites (150 U/kg). The use of 3000 U of lyophilized intrathecal HTIgG free of preservatives has recently been shown to be beneficial (EBM 6.1). The wound is excised, cleaned and left open. Metronidazole (500 mg intravenously or 1 g rectally 8-hourly by suppository) will kill surviving bacteria and prevent further production of toxin. In North America, metronidazole is thought to be more efficacious

than penicillin. Appropriate doses should be continued for 7–10 days. The first dose of antibiotic and the antitoxin should be given immediately, and before wound excision if possible. Active immunization with intramuscular tetanus toxoid should also be commenced early, and a further two doses given at monthly intervals.

GAS GANGRENE AND OTHER CLOSTRIDIAL INFECTIONS

Clostridium perfringens is the principal cause of clostridial myonecrosis or gas gangrene. The organisms form spores, which reside in soil and faeces, and contaminate skin and clothing. They are strict anaerobes and their growth is favoured by failure to debride contaminated wounds.

The spectrum of infection extends from superficial contamination of an open wound to clostridial myonecrosis and gas gangrene. Diffuse myositis and gas gangrene produce profound systemic upset and quickly threaten the affected limb, as well as the life of the patient.

Infection typically takes 2–3 days to become manifest (Fig. 6.5). The wound and surrounding tissues must be inspected. Rapid onset of pain without local findings should alert the practitioner to gas gangrene. A brown seropurulent discharge with a characteristic odour, oedema, crepitus and pain on examination support the diagnosis, confirmed microscopically by the presence of Gram-positive rods. Blood culture may help to establish the diagnosis and guide management.

Prevention

Prompt and adequate primary wound care by excision and debridement is essential. Contaminated wounds must not be closed by primary suture. Penicillin remains the prophylactic antibiotic of choice, with erythromycin as a good alternative. Polyvalent gas gangrene antitoxin is no longer used.

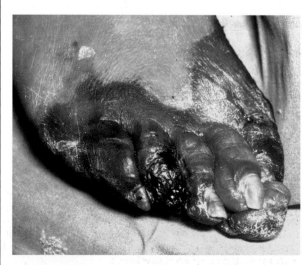

Fig. 6.5 Gangrene developing in the foot of a diabetic.
(Courtesy of Mr AS Whyte FRCS.)

EBM 6.1 INTRATHECAL IMMUNOGLOBULIN IN THE TREATMENT OF TETANUS

'One randomized controlled trial has shown that patients with tetanus treated by the intrathecal route with anti-tetanus human immunoglobulin had better clinical outcomes than those treated by the intramuscular route.'

Miranda-Filho D, et al. BMJ 2004; 328:615–617.

6

BOX 6.4 CLOSTRIDIAL INFECTION

- *Clostridium perfringens* is the principal cause of gas gangrene (clostridial myonecrosis), but other clostridial species may also be involved
- The organism is a spore-forming strict anaerobe present in soil and faeces, and its growth in a wound is favoured by failure to debride
- Toxins produced by *Clostridia* (lecithinase, collagenase, proteinases, hyaluronidase, lipase and haemolysins) devitalize cells, destroy the microcirculation, and favour the spread of infection along tissue planes
- The clinical manifestations of infection are first local (crepitus, brown seropurulent discharge and painful myositis) and then systemic (tachycardia, pallor and clouded consciousness)
- Infection may take 2–3 days to become manifest, but should be suspected if there is an unexplained deterioration in the general clinical condition
- Clostridial myonecrosis is prevented by adequate excision and debridement of contaminated wounds, the prescription of antibiotics (penicillin or erythromycin), and avoidance of inappropriate primary closure
- Established gas gangrene is managed urgently by opening the wound widely and excising all devitalized tissue, by prescribing antibiotics in very high dosage, and (possibly) by hyperbaric oxygenation. Amputation may be unavoidable

Management

Established infection is treated radically. Devitalized tissue must be excised until bleeding viable tissue is encountered. Sometimes amputation is inevitable.

Wounds are loosely packed and left open, to be closed only when they appear healthy. Amputation stumps are also left open in the first instance.

Intensive supportive therapy to correct and maintain fluid and electrolyte balance is necessary. Antibiotic therapy is essential. Penicillin is given in very high dosage, together with metronidazole to control other anaerobes. Additional antibiotics may be needed in mixed infections that may be encountered.

Hyperbaric oxygenation in a pressure chamber may have a role in clostridial myonecrosis, necrotizing fasciitis, refractory osteomyelitis and intracranial brain abscess, but remains controversial.

Following penetrating injury to the colon or rectum, mixed clostridial infection may occur. Wide debridement, free drainage, intensive broad-spectrum antibiotic therapy and a proximal colostomy are essential measures.

PROGRESSIVE BACTERIAL GANGRENE AND NECROTIZING FASCIITIS

These form a spectrum of advancing bacterial gangrene which may occur after a seemingly trivial injury or an operation, typically in the lower abdomen or perineum.

Progressive bacterial gangrene (bacterial synergistic gangrene, dermal gangrene, Meleney's gangrene) involves only the skin and advances relatively slowly. A variety of organisms have been incriminated, and synergistic action between microaerophilic streptococci and associated organisms is considered important. Predisposing factors include general debility, diabetes and hypoxia.

The syndrome of necrotizing fasciitis can be divided into two entities. Type I involves at least one anaerobic species isolated in combination with one or more facultative anaerobic species such as streptococci (other than group A) and coliforms. Type II (haemolytic streptococcal gangrene) involves group A streptococci alone or in combination with other species, such as *Staphylococcus aureus*. Necrotizing fasciitis is an uncommon severe infection affecting primarily the subcutaneous fat and deep fascia (Fig. 6.6). The skin dies as a result of thrombosis of its blood supply. It is a rapidly advancing, frequently fatal disease in which any part of the body may be involved, but most commonly the extremities. The rapidity and extent of tissue destruction are very alarming. The initial clinical feature of pain at the affected site in the setting of possible infection is key in alerting the clinician to the possible diagnosis. In 25% of patients there is no skin erythema. Initial cellulitis may be associated with the appearance of dusky purple patches in its centre, which progress to skin necrosis. There may be crepitus in 20% of cases. The patient becomes very ill and develops septic shock.

Fournier's gangrene is a term that refers to necrotizing fasciitis occurring around the male genitals. It may extend to

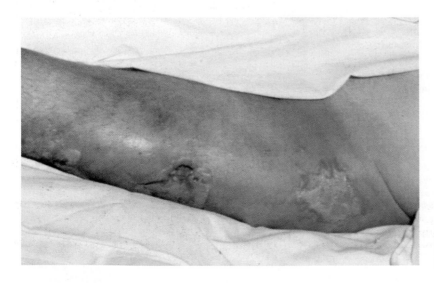

Fig. 6.6 Necrotizing fasciitis of the lower limb. (Courtesy of Medical Microbiology Department, University of Edinburgh.)

involve the abdominal wall. Typically, mixed bacterial cultures are grown.

Diagnosis and management

Prompt diagnosis should lead to the mainstay of treatment: immediate radical surgical excision of the affected area. Haemoglobin, blood glucose, blood urea and electrolyte concentrations should be determined. Haemodynamic instability must be corrected with intravenous infusions. Aspirates, swabs and excised tissue are sent for Gram filming and culture. Blood is also sampled and sent for culture. Intra-operative frozen section examination can confirm the diagnosis. Diabetes may coexist and predispose to this condition.

Intravenous antibiotics are started immediately: a combination of high-dose benzylpenicillin, metronidazole and gentamicin is recommended. Clindamycin should be included in group A streptococcal infection, as in vitro animal data show this is more effective than penicillin. Where possible, cultures should be taken before antibiotics are given. Treatment is modified in the light of patient factors such as renal function and culture reports as they become available.

Urgent surgical review and radical excision of the affected area, including skin, subcutaneous tissue and deep fascia, are performed. Amputation may be necessary. The patient returns to theatre daily for inspection and further necessary excision until the infection is under control. The resulting defect in the skin and deep fascia, which frequently is very large, may require skin grafting.

OTHER ANAEROBIC INFECTIONS

The Gram-negative non-sporing anaerobic pathogens include *Bacteroides*-like spp (*Bacteroides fragilis*, *Prevotella* (*Bacteroides*) *melaninogenica*, *Porphyromonas asaccharolytica* etc.) and fusobacteria such as *Fusobacterium necrophorum*. These often occur in association with anaerobic cocci and other facultative organisms in a wide range of mixed putrefactive infections, including cerebral abscess, periodontal disease, ulceromembranous gingivitis and dental abscess, cancrum oris, Ludwig's angina, aspiration pneumonia, lung abscess, infected bite wounds, synergistic gangrene, necrotizing fasciitis, peritonitis, pelvic abscess, perianal and ischiorectal abscess, balanoposthitis, vaginitis/vaginosis and decubitus ulcers. The most important

6

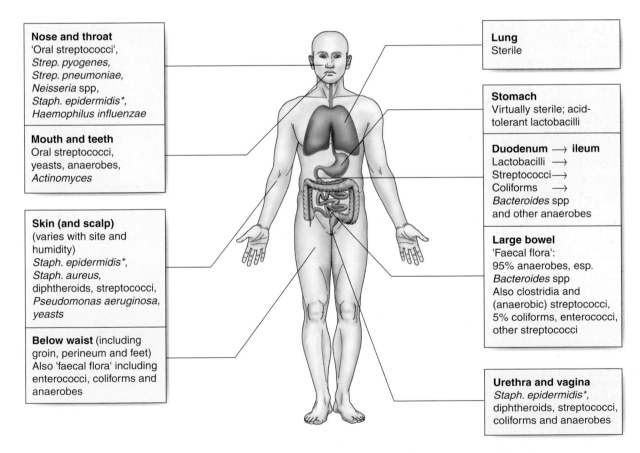

Fig. 6.7 **Distribution of normal adult flora.**
Mucosal or skin breaches may allow normal flora to infect usually sterile sites. Overgrowth by potentially pathogenic members of the normal flora may occur with changes in normal composition, e.g. after antimicrobial treatment, local changes in pH (vagina and stomach) or defective immunity (e.g. AIDS or immunosuppressive treatment). The most common yeast is *Candida albicans*.
* *Staphylococcus epidermidis* is the most common 'coagulase-negative staphylococcus' frequently found on skin. Density of colonization varies greatly with age and site.

aspect of treatment of most abscesses, particularly those in the perianal and ischiorectal region, is surgical drainage to prevent damage and sequelae, such as anal sphincter dysfunction. Some abscesses are best drained under radiological guidance.

The common anaerobic component of many of these infections must be appreciated if the results of treatment are not to be disappointing. In some cases, there is alarming pathogenic synergy, which overwhelms the patient if effective treatment is delayed.

HOSPITAL-ACQUIRED (NOSOCOMIAL) INFECTIONS

Nosocomial infection is the term used to describe infection that becomes manifest while the patient is in hospital, typically more than 48 hours after admission. Such infection may be endogenous, from the patient's own flora, or exogenous, from the hospital environment. Infection may spread from the environment, between patients, and between patients and staff. Patients who remain in hospital for some time acquire hospital organisms. Such hospital strains of bacteria may have evolved a special facility for colonization and infection. After any prolonged series of inpatient investigations it is wise to allow patients to return home before surgical treatment, so that their normal flora can be restored away from the hospital environment.

SITES OF COLONIZATION

Hospital practice often fails to recognize the significance of a patient's own endogenous flora in relation to both potential protective and pathogenic effects. For example, long-stay patients, particularly when elderly, should ideally not be treated in an acute surgical ward, as the dispersal of acquired skin flora, e.g. from an infected bedsore, into the ward environment and on to surfaces in toilet areas, poses a danger to other patients. The distribution of 'normal flora' in healthy adults is shown in Figure 6.7. The 'colonization resistance' of the gut is markedly reduced by some forms of antibiotic therapy. This allows the emergence of *Clostridium difficile*-associated diarrhoea, as well as opportunities for the exchange of antibiotic resistance between strains and species of gut bacteria.

HOSPITAL MICROBIAL CHALLENGES

Hand-borne or surface-mediated challenges

The hands of patients and staff are of great importance in conveying microbes. Compliance with hand decontamination among health-care workers is often poor, at about 40% or less. Readily available alcohol-based hand rub helps compliance, but proper hand-washing is still required where soiling has occurred. Until opinion-formers (i.e. hospital consultants) lead by example in this area, rates of hospital-acquired infection are likely to remain higher than need be. Such infection is increasingly the cause of litigation.

Airborne and ingested challenges

These also pose significant risks to the surgical patient. Adequate ventilation of theatres and wards, bed spacing, ventilator and anaesthetic equipment care, avoidance of particle (e.g. from bed making) and droplet dispersal, and water engineering maintenance (*Legionella* spp) will reduce the risk of airborne infection. Isolation of patients with diarrhoea, a high standard of hygiene in hospital catering systems and preparation of intravenous nutrition and drugs in sterile conditions will all help to reduce the risk of ingested infection.

Table 6.1 INOCULATED CHALLENGES, PROBLEMS AND POSSIBLE CONTROL MEASURES	
Hazard	**Possible control measures**
Blood-borne pathogen (e.g. viruses, protozoa—malaria, treponemes—syphilis)	'Standard precautions' Prevent inoculation of carrier's blood Immunization Exclude blood donations from high-risk donors Screen blood donations Emergency antiviral prophylaxis Routine antimalarial with blood infusion Removal of contaminated component (e.g. neutrophil filters—cytomegalovirus, variant Creutzfeldt–Jakob disease) Heat treatment of blood donation Detergent treatment of blood donation
Contaminated infusion (e.g. with staphylococci and aerobic Gram-negative bacilli)	Sterile infusion equipment and infusates Once-only needle, connectors, infusion kits Careful management of connectors etc.
Percutaneous catheter	Hand decontamination, skin preparation with iodine, chlorhexidine or alcohol Sterile technique Multidisciplinary team for management Optimal management of the insertion site and limitations of entry into the system, administration set and catheter itself Tunnelling of catheter

Inoculated challenges

Inoculated challenges and controls are of increasing clinical significance (Table 6.1). 'Standard precautions' include the concept that appropriate barrier precautions should routinely be taken to prevent skin and mucous membrane contact with any patient's blood or other body fluids. Any patient may be 'high-risk'. Infection with blood-borne viruses, such as hepatitis B (HBV), hepatitis C (HCV) and the human immunodeficiency virus (HIV), is an important example of the serious potential hazard of skin-penetrating injuries in patients and all clinical staff. This arises from cross-contamination with blood or other body fluids from someone with a recognized infection, or from someone who may be a known or unknown carrier. Following inoculation with infected blood, the risks of infection to the naive injured party are approximately 30%, 3% and 0.3% for HBV, HCV and HIV, respectively. Such an injury should be encouraged to bleed and washed immediately with soap and water. If the eye is involved, this should be copiously irrigated with water. Many other pathogenic agents, including various bacteria, *Plasmodium* spp and *Treponema pallidum*, can be transmitted by accidental inoculation of blood or blood products. Glove punctures occur in surgical staff in up to 30% of operations, and skin-penetrating injuries with needles and knives are common events, demanding constant caution. The carrier rate for hepatitis B in the UK is around 0.1%; in some countries in Africa and Asia, it is as high as 5–15%. Amongst others, surgeons are particularly at risk, and should take care to avoid skin-penetrating injuries and skin, eye and mucous membrane exposure in circumstances in which contamination with blood, blood products or other body fluids is likely.

The infective state of a patient or carrier in relation to HBV is demonstrated by the detection of hepatitis B surface antigen (HBsAg) in the serum. Detection of hepatitis B 'e' antigen (HBeAg) indicates an individual at particularly high risk of spreading infection.

At present, medical, dental, nursing and midwifery students in the UK should be immunized against hepatitis B for their own protection, and their response checked. Non-responders should be shown to be non-infective.

If a non-immune person has a skin-penetrating injury or mucosal exposure to likely hepatitis B contamination, emergency (post-exposure) passive protection can be given by intramuscular injection of hyperimmune hepatitis B immunoglobulin (HBIgG), preferably within 48 hours. Unless the non-immune person is a known non-responder, active immunization should also be commenced. In the case of penetrating HIV contamination, urgent post-exposure antiretroviral prophylaxis should be available. There are currently no such recommendations following HCV exposure. Knowledge is advancing rapidly and the detail of these recommendations may change. Should health-care workers think that they might have been exposed to a blood-borne virus such as HBV, HCV or HIV, they should be tested after counselling and followed up. Advice on how to protect sexual partners may also be required. The sensitive and confidential handling of such individuals presents a significant challenge to occupational health departments and health-care organizations.

Hazards associated with intensive care

Special infective hazards may be posed by a variety of procedures performed in an intensive care unit, including the use of ventilators, nasogastric tubes, drugs reducing gastric acid secretion, suction apparatus, intravenous lines, percutaneous needles and catheters. It is paradoxical that our most severely compromised patients should be exposed to such inadvertent challenges.

The remarks made above concerning the avoidance of hospital-acquired infection become vital in intensive care, where the patients are already critically ill. All units should have well-developed policies to avoid the transfer of organisms from staff to patients, or from patients to patients.

CONTROL OF HOSPITAL-ACQUIRED (NOSOCOMIAL) INFECTION

An effective hospital infection control programme depends above all on leadership, teamwork, conscientiousness and communication. The specialized risks of blood-borne viruses are described above. Prions such as vCJD present special difficulties.

Prompt detection and management of hospital infection

Day-to-day monitoring in the wards and related areas is essential to ensure that infections are detected quickly and recorded. Surveillance is particularly important in specialist areas with patients at high risk of infection, such as intensive care, neonatal and renal units, and in areas where neutropenic patients are nursed. There must be close liaison with the laboratory, so that early notification of a particularly dangerous pathogen is ensured and trends in antibiotic resistance are monitored. Close cooperation between the infection control team (doctors and nurses), senior ward staff and laboratories is essential.

Prevention of transmission of infectious agents

Approaches to preventing the spread of infection in a hospital range from the provision of suitable isolation and containment facilities for those with special infections or at particular risk of infection, to the prompt availability of an expert team to mount an immediate investigation and institute necessary control measures as required. Prompt diagnosis and treatment of an infection can contribute substantially to the prevention of transmission. Clear policies on the following matters are important to protect patients from cross-infection:

- recording of infection
- the correct use of disinfectants
- safe disposal of infected material
- cleaning, disinfection and sterilization of instruments
- management of patients who have infections associated with special risks
- proper use of antibiotics
- use of immunizing agents.

6

Table 6.2 ANTIBIOTICS IN SURGERY: SUGGESTIONS FOR SPECIFIC THERAPY

Organism	First choice	Alternative
Meticillin-sensitive *Staphylococcus aureus*	Flucloxacillin	Erythromycin
Meticillin-resistant *Staphylococcus aureus (MRSA)**	Vancomycin	Teicoplanin
Coagulase-negative staphylococci	Vancomycin	Teicoplanin
Streptococcus pneumoniae	Benzylpenicillin	Erythromycin
Streptococcus pyogenes (group A β-haemolytic streptococcus)	Benzylpenicillin	Erythromycin
Enterococci	Amoxicillin	Vancomycin
Bacteroides species	Metronidazole	Co-amoxiclav
Escherichia coli 1. Sepsis, including bacteraemia 2. Urinary tract infection	Cefuroxime Trimethoprim	Ceftazidime Amoxicillin
Haemophilus influenzae	Amoxicillin	Co-amoxiclav or cefuroxime
Klebsiella species	Co-amoxiclav	Cefuroxime
Proteus species	Co-amoxiclav	Cefuroxime
Pseudomonas aeruginosa	Ceftazidime	Ciprofloxacin
Clostridia	Benzylpenicillin + metronidazole	Metronidazole
Clostridium difficile	Stop predisposing antibiotic	Metronidazole (or vancomycin, oral); re-treat relapse

N.B. These suggestions should be considered in the light of local epidemiology, sensitivities, drug availability, site and severity of infection.
* Gemmell CG, et al. Guidelines for the prophylaxis and treatment of meticillin-resistant *Staphylococcus aureus* (MRSA) infections in the UK. Journal of Antimicrobial Chemotherapy 2006; 57:589–608.

Table 6.3 INITIAL ('BEST-GUESS') THERAPY FOR ACUTE INFECTIONS

Type of infection	Antimicrobial	Alternative
Chest infection Uncomplicated Community-acquired pneumonia 'Aspiration' pneumonia Hospital-acquired/post-operative	Amoxicillin Co-amoxiclav + erythromycin Co-amoxiclav Ciprofloxacin + flucloxacillin	Erythromycin Cefuroxime + erythromycin Cefuroxime + metronidazole Ceftazidime + vancomycin
Urinary tract infection 'Lower' infection Acute pyelonephritis Prostatitis	Trimethoprim Cefuroxime Ciprofloxacin	Amoxicillin Gentamicin Trimethoprim
Wound infection Cellulitis Abscess	Penicillin + flucloxacillin Drain collection	Erythromycin Flucloxacillin
Intra-abdominal	Amoxicillin + metronidazole + gentamicin	Cefuroxime + metronidazole
Cholecystitis–cholangitis	Cefuroxime + metronidazole	Piperacillin–tazobactam
Pelvic inflammatory disease	Azithromycin + metronidazole + gentamicin	Doxycycline + piperacillin–tazobactam
Amputations and gas gangrene	Benzylpenicillin + metronidazole	Metronidazole
Septicaemia and septic shock	Amoxicillin + metronidazole + gentamicin/ciprofloxacin	Piperacillin–tazobactam
Severe *Pseudomonas* infections	Ceftazidime + gentamicin	Ciprofloxacin
Candida sepsis	Fluconazole	Amphotericin B

Note These suggestions are for occasions when immediate treatment is necessary. Amendments may be necessary in the light of local epidemiology and microbiological and clinical developments.

ANTIMICROBIAL MANAGEMENT OF WOUND INFECTIONS

It is important to know when a wound is being significantly colonized by a potential pathogen. Regular inspection of wounds is essential, and microbiological assistance should be sought when necessary. The decision to treat a wound infection should be based on clinical judgement and should not be an automatic response to a positive culture report. In some cases, removal of a suture at an inflamed point (minor stitch abscess) may be all that is needed to allow host defences to operate. Similarly, the isolation of coliforms from a mild superficial infection of an abdominal wound need not call for active antimicrobial therapy if the patient's general condition does not indicate a constitutional upset. On the other hand, a positive blood culture obtained from a patient with signs of impending shock, or the isolation of a significant pathogen (e.g. *Streptococcus pyogenes*) from a wound with signs of regional lymphadenitis, calls for immediate antimicrobial treatment.

Inconsistent or incompatible findings must be discussed with senior experts. For example, a report on a secondary plate culture, obtained after a specimen of pus has been subjected to enrichment culture in cooked meat broth, might yield a profuse, almost pure growth of *Clostridium perfringens* derived from spores contaminating skin adjacent to the wound. If the wound is giving no clinical cause for alarm and the patient's general condition is satisfactory, a diagnosis of gas gangrene is most unlikely to be justified. Heroic treatment must not be instituted on the basis of such evidence.

Suggestions for specific antibiotic therapy are given in Table 6.2, and initial ('best-guess') therapy is indicated in Table 6.3. Such therapy should be guided by local epidemiology and antimicrobial sensitivity data.

PRINCIPLES GOVERNING THE CHOICE AND USE OF ANTIBIOTICS

Antibiotics should be used with care. The clinician should attempt to recognize self-limiting infections while taking account of the potential toxicity and cost of any antibiotic. As antibiotic resistance is increasing, antibiotic abuse carries collective penalties for the individual patient and for the community.

In some situations, such as in the management of an infected ingrowing toenail (Fig. 6.8), antibiotics have a minimal role. Some consider that clinicians who manage these infections with antimicrobials should be strung up by the toenails! Careful removal of the nail is the appropriate management, with antimicrobial cover. In other situations, particularly in surgery, antibiotics are merely an adjunct to definitive drainage of an abscess or the removal of devitalized tissue.

If clinically indicated, the choice of therapy should be positively determined. Some organisms associated with certain illnesses are almost invariably sensitive to certain antibiotics. For example, the group A β-haemolytic

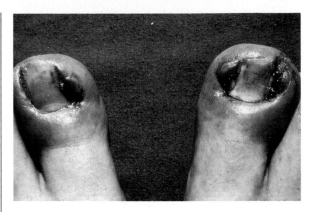

Fig. 6.8 Infected ingrown toenails.
(Courtesy of Mr AS Whyte FRCS.)

streptococcus (*Streptococcus pyogenes*) is always sensitive to benzylpenicillin. On the other hand, hospital staphylococci are virtually always resistant to penicillin. Antibiotic sensitivity tests are necessary to guide the clinician in many cases. It is reasonable to initiate therapy on clinical evidence, but the drugs selected must be reviewed once the microbiological report is available. When an antibiotic has been selected, an adequate dose must be given by the recommended route at the correct time intervals. In hospital practice, there is often a disturbing difference between the practical interpretations of '8-hourly' and 'three times a day'.

When an organism acquires resistance to an antibiotic, it has an advantage over others of the same species in the presence of the relevant antibiotic. If the antibiotic is used extensively or carelessly in a ward, resistant organisms may become predominant.

The penicillinase-producing staphylococcal menace of the last two decades has been largely controlled, but staphylococci with multiple resistance are a threat. Many other bacteria exploit mechanisms of resistance to gain inroads into the patient they invade.

In general, an effort should be made to use a single effective antibacterial agent in the treatment of a particular infection. If a combination of antibiotics is used, the decision should be based on positive evidence that this is rational. In some cases—for example, when a patient is seriously ill and a mixed infection is likely (as in acute peritonitis)—it may be necessary to give more than one antibiotic to cover a likely combination of pathogens. This blunderbuss strategy should be reserved for such desperate situations and should be rationalized at the earliest opportunity in the light of the patient's progress and available microbiological guidance.

ANTIBIOTIC POLICY

A policy for the use of antibiotics is desirable and must be kept under regular review because of continuing changes in the patterns of bacterial resistance to antibiotics. Ideally, the resistance patterns of all pathogens isolated from sputum, urine, bile, pus and blood should be regularly recorded and periodically reviewed, e.g. at 6-monthly intervals. A policy may then be devised that restricts the use of those antibiotics to which resistance is developing. Knowledge of resistance permits more appropriate use of antibiotics in circumstances where it is necessary to give 'blind' treatment: for example, in life-threatening infections where antibiotics must be prescribed before the results of culture and sensitivity tests are known. The guidelines given in Box 6.5 should be observed when prescribing antibiotics.

PROPHYLACTIC USE OF ANTIBIOTICS

For further information, see http://www.sign.ac.uk/guidelines/published/index.html#Surgery. The guideline dates from July 2000 and was under review in December 2006.

The principle of antimicrobial prophylaxis is to achieve high concentrations at the incision and site of operation at commencement of, during and immediately after surgery. Where prophylaxis is appropriate, it should normally extend for less than 24 hours. There is evidence that selective decontamination of the gut with non-absorbable anti-microbials may also help reduce some post-operative infection. The prophylactic use of antibiotics is established in the situations described below.

Tetanus

Patients with tetanus-prone accidental wounds are given prophylaxis, as described above, but the wounds must still be treated by meticulous debridement or, if treatment is delayed, by excision.

BOX 6.5 ANTIBIOTIC POLICY

- Antibiotics should be avoided in self-limiting infections and due consideration should be given to expense, toxicity and the need to avoid the emergence of resistant strains
- Choice of therapy is determined positively by knowledge of the nature and sensitivities of the infecting organism(s). Therapy may be initiated on clinical evidence, but must be reviewed in the light of culture/sensitivity reports
- Restrict the use of antibiotics to which resistance is developing (or has developed)
- Single agents are preferred to combination therapy, and narrow-spectrum agents are preferred to broad-spectrum agents whenever possible
- Adequate doses must be given by the recommended route at correct time intervals
- Antibiotics that are used systemically must not be used topically
- The side-effects of antibiotics should be known and monitored
- Expensive antibiotics are not used if equally effective and cheaper alternatives are suitable
- With few exceptions (e.g. lung abscess), antibiotics should not be used to treat abscesses unless adequate surgical or radiological drainage has been achieved
- Body fluids from patients receiving antibiotics must be disposed of carefully to avoid the emergence of antibiotic-resistant strains in staff, patients and the environment
- Some policies may include automatic 'stop' orders

Gas gangrene

Patients with ischaemic limbs that require major surgery are at considerable risk of developing gas gangrene. Benzylpenicillin is given 1 hour pre-operatively and continued 6-hourly for 3–5 days.

Endocarditis

Patients with a heart lesion, such as congenital, rheumatic or degenerative valve disease or septal defects, or with prosthetic heart valves or past endocarditis are at risk of bacterial colonization if bacteraemia occurs. Before any operation that might expose them to such a risk, they are given prophylactic antibiotics. The exact regimen depends on the predisposing risk factor, the nature of the operation, and whether there has been recent exposure to penicillin or a history of penicillin allergy.

Typical regimens include high-dose amoxicillin or clindamycin, amoxicillin with gentamicin and vancomycin, or teicoplanin with gentamicin. Prophylaxis may not be necessary for some (dermatological) procedures, but is indicated for dental, upper respiratory tract, genitourinary, obstetric, gynaecological and gastrointestinal procedures. A post-operative dose may also be required. It is advisable to consult expert guidelines, such as those in the latest edition of the *British National Formulary* (BNF), or to talk to an infection specialist for advice on a particular patient.

Clean surgery

Antibiotic prophylaxis is not routinely recommended for all cases, but may be beneficial in breast surgery and hernia repairs, especially where any artificial material is implanted.

Gastrointestinal and genitourinary surgery

Patients undergoing gastrointestinal and genitourinary surgery, whether elective or emergency, are at risk of wound infection, intra-abdominal infection and septicaemia. Many methods have been advocated in the past decade to reduce this risk. A single large dose of antibiotics appropriate for the predicted bacterial flora, administered intravenously on induction of anaesthesia, is probably the most convenient and effective method. Co-amoxiclav alone, or metron-idazole in combination with a suitable cephalosporin, has a good success record. Such regimens, particularly if prolonged or including a cephalosporin, may lead to the emergence of meticillin-resistant *Staphylococcus aureus* (MRSA) and *Clostridium difficile*-associated diarrhoea. In heavily contaminated surgery and in emergency surgery, additional doses at 8-hourly intervals post-operatively may confer further benefit. Lavage of the operative field with sterile saline is also often carried out.

Management of compound limb fractures

As a compound fracture is almost invariably associated with considerable contamination in an area of severely damaged tissue, it is reasonable to give antibiotic cover at once, and preferably before radical wound toilet and debridement if this does not delay essential surgical attention. Opinions differ on the choice of antibiotics. Staphylococci, coliform organisms and anaerobes are likely infecting organisms, often occurring together and with catastrophic potential.

Some surgeons rely on penicillin and metronidazole to control at least two of the likely components. Others would use co-amoxiclav, a second- or third-generation cephalosporin, clindamycin or erythromycin.

Prosthetic implants

Prophylactic antibiotics are obligatory when any prosthetic material is inserted. Staphylococcal infection is the most serious problem: for example, in heart valve replacement, cardiac pacemaker insertion, ventriculovenous shunts, vascular grafts, joint prostheses, mammary prostheses or polypropylene mesh repairs of massive abdominal wall defects. However, other bacteria may also be involved, and broad-spectrum cover is usually given immediately pre-operatively and 8-hourly post-operatively, to last up to 24 hours. It is important to have informed microbiological advice.

Skull fractures and meningitis

Patients with skull fractures may develop a cerebrospinal fluid (CSF) leak or communication with a sinus or the middle ear. About 11–25% of individuals with CSF leaks become infected. The delay from the time of injury to the onset of meningitis is highly variable, from days to several years. Therefore, patients and their families should be taught how to recognize the symptoms and signs of meningitis and their doctors informed of the risks. Antibiotic prophylaxis is of uncertain benefit and is not advised.

MANAGEMENT OF IMMUNOSUPPRESSED PATIENTS, INCLUDING THOSE WHO HAVE HAD SPLENECTOMY

Prophylaxis

Patients with suppressed immune mechanisms, as a result of either disease or therapy (e.g. transplant patients), should receive antibiotic prophylaxis when undergoing surgery. The choice of antibiotic is dictated by individual circumstances and expert microbiological help should be sought. Splenectomized patients are at increased risk of infection with encapsulated bacteria and protozoa. Those having elective splenectomy should be immunized with pneumococcal vaccine at least 2 weeks in advance of surgery. Penicillin or amoxicillin should be commenced and continued for some years. In addition to routine vaccinations, *Haemophilus influenzae* type B, influenza and conjugate group C meningococcal vaccine are recommended. Travellers to areas endemic for meningococcus groups A, W135 or Y infection or for malaria should take expert advice.

Management

Prompt empirical antibiotic treatment of suspected bacterial infections in immunosuppressed patients is advisable. A combination of an aminoglycoside with an antipseudomonal penicillin or cephalosporin is often relied upon to cover the range of likely organisms. In these patients it is also important to be on guard against fungal and protozoal infections, and to be aware of problems posed by viruses such as herpes simplex, varicella zoster and cytomegalovirus.

6

7

S.J. WIGMORE

Ethical and legal principles in surgical practice

INTRODUCTION

There are few circumstances in life where an individual is required to place such trust in another individual as when a patient submits himself or herself to a surgical procedure. In this context, it is quite right and proper that the practice of surgery should be subject to legislative requirements and to ethical principles. Patients hold certain rights and society has imposed certain requirements on surgeons. Within this framework there is flexibility and latitude, as is required by a system that is constantly evolving with advances in medical care and scientific innovation.

The practice of surgery requires a range of skills and a broad knowledge base. Prominent among these skills is the ability to identify, analyse and resolve ethical dilemmas. Medical ethics and the law, as it applies to medicine, have substantial overlap. In a pluralist society, individuals hold different but reasonable views on how ethical issues should be resolved. Political, cultural and legal differences between societies and the complex new issues arising from advances in biotechnology mean that medical ethics and medical law are in an ongoing state of flux.

The rights of patients are enshrined by a variety of codes of practice such as the Hippocratic Oath and the Declaration of Geneva. In addition, regulatory authorities and professional institutions such as the General Medical Council and the Royal Colleges of Surgeons provide guidance on standards of behaviour and levels of professional competence. Statutes in law provide a mechanism whereby failures in systems or in duty of care can result in financial or custodial penalties. Traditional medical ethics focuses largely upon the professional ethics of physicians and on the doctor–patient relationship. The term 'bioethics' has become popular in recent times. Traditional medical ethics is at its core, but it also acknowledges interplay with the more general ethics of biology, science, sociology and culture.

Fluency in the resolution of ethical dilemmas is not a part-time accomplishment for use only in theoretical debate; it is a full-time clinical and professional skill necessary for practical problem-solving and decision-making in the real world.

SYSTEMS AND PRINCIPLES IN MEDICAL ETHICS AND BIOETHICS

SYSTEMS OF BIOETHICS

Western medicine is characterized by a number of ethical traditions that find expression in codes of practice and in the culture of health-care workers. Among these are the deontological (duty-based) and the utilitarian (consequence-based) traditions.

The deontological tradition stresses the duties of practitioners and the rights of patients. This is often prescriptive and has much in common with the tenets of organized religion. Clinicians 'ought' to act in particular ways because this is 'right', often irrespective of the consequences. Statements such as 'Never kill,' 'Never cause pain' and 'Always tell the truth' are classic expressions in this tradition.

The deontological tradition stresses the autonomy of the patient and the primacy of the doctor–patient relationship. Individuals should always be viewed as ends in themselves, never as means to an end. Generally speaking, ethical dilemmas should be resolved by the application of principles that are 'universal'.

Sometimes, 'absolute' principles that are contradictory present as competing priorities in particular circumstances (e.g. 'Never cause pain' and 'Always preserve life'—but what if a life-saving intervention causes pain?). Real-life situations often pose these difficulties.

Utilitarians, by contrast, suggest that doctors should always do that which leads to a 'good' or the 'best' outcome. 'The greatest good of the greatest number' is commonly used as a summary of this approach. If the 'right' action does not lead to the 'best' outcome, then it should be reviewed or abandoned. Rationing of health-care resources brings utilitarian analyses into particular prominence. On occasion, the individual may be the 'loser' in the greater scheme of things, a common criticism of this approach.

Utilitarian analysis can be applied to an individual case—what is in the *patient's* best interest —as well as to a group of cases—what is in *patients'* best interests (or will lead to the best outcomes)? These are felt to be strands within the spectrum of utilitarianism.

For example, weighing up the consequences of acting according to a general moral rule (e.g. that patients over 80 years with type II diabetes should never have coronary artery bypass grafting, as the long-term survival of this group is likely to be less than that of a younger non-diabetic group) can be described as 'rule' utilitarianism. On the other hand, weighing up the consequences of a particular act (e.g. deciding not to proceed with an aggressive bowel resection in a relatively feeble man with mild dementia) could be described as 'act' utilitarianism.

These traditions are not opposite ways of viewing and acting upon ethical dilemmas. They tend to derive the same

---

BOX 7.1   GENERAL MEDICAL COUNCIL PRINCIPLES OF GOOD MEDICAL PRACTICE

- Make the care of your patient your first concern
- Treat every patient politely and considerately
- Respect patients' dignity and privacy
- Listen to patients and respect their views
- Give patients information in a way they can understand
- Respect the rights of patients to be fully involved in decisions about their care
- Keep your professional knowledge and skills up to date
- Recognize the limits of your professional competence
- Be honest and trustworthy
- Respect and protect confidential information
- Make sure that your personal beliefs do not prejudice your patients' care
- Act quickly to protect patients from risk if you have good reason to believe that you or a colleague may not be fit to practise
- Avoid abusing your position as a doctor
- Work with colleagues in the ways that best serve patients' interests

7

7

conclusions when 'working' moral issues are at stake. Both traditions have a strong flavour of universalizability. Ethical analyses, however, usually focus on particular cases. Because of this, it is often argued that the importance of context may well have been understated in the past.

Some current intellectual traditions, notably existentialism, situation ethics and post-modernism, are less convinced of the existence of general laws/principles that can be applied to particular cases. These focus more on how to solve specific problems as they arise, and are open to the insights of other religious, racial, philosophical and cultural traditions. Some doctors dislike this sense of moral relativism.

There is a spectrum between cases in which context and situation need to be the dominant consideration and those in which universally derived general principles can be applied. No one tradition or perspective is 'more correct'; they offer different perspectives to problem-solving, but often arrive at the same practical solution.

PRINCIPLES

Beneficence: doing good

A number of principles (traditionally four) are accepted as the basis of medical ethics. In individual cases, there is often conflict between simultaneous adherence to all of these. Depending on the context (and on whether a deontological or utilitarian approach is favoured), a 'least unsatisfactory' trade-off between principles must be negotiated or achieved. Skill is needed in identifying and achieving the best balance.

There is the obligation to do 'good' for the patient. Deontologists view this as a universal moral duty, utilitarians as achieving the universally desired best outcome. In the face of uncertainty, this may not be straightforward. It is worth reflecting on whose view of 'good' should be taken as the outcome of importance. In the past, medical judgement as to 'best outcome' predominated, with relatively little input from the patient. This attitude may be less prevalent today.

Beneficence demands competence. In a multidisciplinary, multi-specialist environment, doctors should not exceed their personal competence if a more appropriate practitioner or service is available. Accreditation and continuing medical education are central to this, as are elements such as professional development, research and audit.

Communication skills are vital. Weighing up possible outcomes is one thing; sharing them with the patient and negotiating choices are quite another.

Non-maleficence: avoiding harm

The principle of *Primum non nocere* ('First, do no harm') has been a central tenet of medical ethics since the days of Hippocrates. All interventions, however well intentioned, may cause harm. Making sure that the balance between benefit and harm is appropriate and proportionate is an important clinical judgement. In the past, professional decisions (i.e. that the balance achieved by a particular course of action was acceptable) often paid scant attention to the patient's perspective of the balance. This is paternalism—according overwhelming weight to clinicians' judgement on the balance between beneficence and non-maleficence, with little weight given to respect for patient autonomy.

Sometimes the opposite may occur. A patient may demand a procedure that, in the considered opinion of the practitioner, may cause more harm than good. In this setting, after appropriate discussion with the patient, the proper course of action is to refer the patient for another opinion. There is no professional obligation to respond uncritically to consumerism.

Respect for autonomy

Individuals should be treated as ends, not as means. Respect for the dignity, integrity and authenticity of the person is a basic human right. Deriving from this principle are the important issues of consent and confidentiality. As mentioned above, working through the first two principles seeks to arrive at a professional judgement as to what is in the patient's best interests. Moving from advice to action involves further consideration.

Informed consent is central to the doctor–patient relationship. Two issues arise here. The first relates to a patient's capacity to give or withhold consent. The second relates to the amount of information that needs to be shared with (or withheld from) the patient.

From both a legal and an ethical perspective, the patient retains the right to decide what is in his or her best interests. All conscious adults are held to have the capacity to make choices, unless evidence to the contrary can be advanced. Making a choice that seems irrational or is at variance with professional opinion does not alter that capacity.

Capacity to consent exists if a patient can:

- understand relevant information (explained in broad terms and with simple language)
- consider the implications of different options (in terms of his or her values)
- come to a communicable decision.

Jehovah's Witnesses illustrate this point well. Although the views of this church with regard to contact with blood products may not be in accordance with the majority view in Western society, a decision to forego red-cell concentrate transfusion in a life-threatening situation must be respected if the above circumstances exist.

There are circumstances in which the capacity to consent may not exist:

- minors
- transient or irreversible cognitive impairment
- mental illness
- undue coercion.

These groups present different challenges. The law relating to children is complex, with differences between English and Scottish law in some important interpretations. Many children will be able to understand, reflect and decide on their wishes. The scenario becomes complex if a difference develops between the views of a child and those with parental responsibility. In some instances, a competent child may refuse treatment, in contradiction to the wishes of the parents. An automatic right of the parents to overrule this may not exist. In these situations, legal advice is recommended.

Patients with mental illness may retain the capacity to consent to particular procedures. If not, treatment may be given in emergency or urgent situations with their compliance (subject to the remarks below). If the patient does not comply and is detained under the Mental Health Act 1983, then treatment for the mental disorder may be administered compulsorily, subject to the safeguards included within the Act. Treatment for other physical disorders may not be enforced on the patient against their wishes, and legal advice is strongly recommended in these circumstances.

Patients with transient or irreversible cognitive impairment frequently require medical attention (including surgical procedures). Acutely unwell patients often fall into this category. Some may have fluctuating capacity, owing to fever, drugs, anxiety etc. Regular assessment is mandatory, with clear record-keeping. In emergencies, treatment may need to be administered in the patient's best interests. Certain guidelines are helpful (although seeking further advice from professional organizations or legal sources is always prudent). Clear communication with all relevant parties, careful documentation of the process, and broad consultation are appropriate.

Where non-therapeutic or controversial treatment is proposed (e.g. sterilization or withdrawal of feeding) for a patient who does not have the capacity to consent, then even greater care, communication and consultation are needed.

Informed consent presumes information-sharing. If a patient does have the capacity to consent, then questions arise as to how much information should be provided, in what format it should be presented and recorded, and who should be responsible for this.

The legal basis of informed consent differs between states. In countries such as Australia and Canada, there is a legal duty to provide patients with the information that a prudent or reasonable patient, in that patient's particular circumstances, would wish to have in order to arrive at a decision. In the UK, the amount of information that a reasonable doctor would provide, in that patient's particular circumstances, is required (although a court might decide that, in unusual circumstances, failure to disclose certain risks of procedures might be negligent, even if this is

accepted practice as attested by a responsible body of medical opinion). As in the circumstances already discussed, further counsel should be sought if there is doubt.

Information about certain possible risks may be retained under so-called 'therapeutic privilege', if it is honestly felt that this would needlessly harm the patient psychologically (justified by an 'act' utilitarian attitude with heavy emphasis on non-maleficence). This privilege cannot be invoked when informed consent to participation in a research study is being obtained, for obvious reasons.

There should be no overt or covert pressure to consent. This may come from a variety of sources: employers, insurance companies, physicians or institutions deriving financial benefits from use of a specific therapy, or religious groups. Prisoners, other detainees and those detained under mental health legislation may be particularly vulnerable.

The process of obtaining consent should be administered by a suitably trained and competent person, with sufficient knowledge of the treatment and its possible outcomes to engage in discussion with the patient. For many routine procedures, a standardized information leaflet may be helpful. The provision of such a leaflet does not, however, obviate the doctor's responsibility of ensuring that the procedure is fully understood by the patient. Providing sufficient time for discussion and reflection is important, particularly for complex procedures of uncertain outcome.

Ideally, a written record of the patient's consent should be obtained, with sufficient detail to identify their express wishes (particularly if certain aspects of treatment have been declined). Assuming (implied) consent to a variety of procedures because of compliance with a perfunctory 'consent form signed' interaction is not a prudent course of action.

The other major principle deriving from respect for autonomy is the right to confidentiality. This is of even greater moment in an age of electronic record-holding, with multidisciplinary teams caring for patients. Information relating to patients must never be casually revealed to other persons. Within teams, only that information relevant to a team member fulfilling his or her part in the process of care should be shared. If individual cases are discussed to illustrate or inform teaching activities, then the identity of the patient must be concealed. There are some circum-

---

BOX 7.3 RESPECTING PATIENT AUTONOMY

1. Establish the various options available (including non-treatment)
2. Seek evidence of previously expressed views (e.g. advance directives)
3. Seek the opinion of third parties to whom the patient may be known (e.g. parents, partner, GP, family) as to the patient's previously expressed views
4. Administer the level of treatment that least restricts the patient's future choices (i.e. life-saving or stabilizing treatment, rather than physician-selected choice of 'definitive' treatment)
5. If substantial doubt or conflict exists, seek counsel from more experienced colleagues, from professional organizations and/or from legal sources
6. If necessary, seek advice as to whether a court ruling is necessary

7

stances (e.g. notifiable diseases) in which there is a statutory obligation to reveal details about an individual patient. In general, confidentiality is an integral part of the doctor–patient relationship; not only is it good practice to adhere to these guidelines, in some circumstances it is a legal requirement under the Data Protection Act 1998.

Justice: promoting fairness

In modern health care, demand outstrips supply. Consequently, access to health-care interventions varies (by either explicit or implicit rationing). The principle of justice is important here. The allocation of resources requires a rank-ordering system with some philosophical justification for the method chosen. There are many theories of justice, some deriving from the deontological and utilitarian traditions. If scarce resources are to be allocated, how should this be done? Discrimination based on race, gender, age or 'social worth' obviously violates the principle of justice.

A 'rule' utilitarian might suggest that we seek to maximize the overall welfare of society and minimize the waste of resources. Many surgical services have allocation systems loosely built upon the premise that selecting and organizing allocation around a limited number of criteria predictive of best outcome serves this purpose most efficiently. This disadvantages some patients. Alternative models might prioritize on the basis of degree of pain or threat to life. Operating on 100 ingrown toenails will provide substantial relief to many patients; performing five cardiac transplants will save five lives that would otherwise be lost.

One approach that may improve equity is to apply Aristotle's formal principle of justice of (Nicomachean ethics). This suggests that 'equals' should be treated 'equally', but where 'inequality' exists then 'unequal' treatment should occur to correct this imbalance. In the example, those with terminal cardiac failure clearly had a more immediate and life-threatening (unequal) need than those with ingrown toenails. Allocating resources to them acts, in part, to redress the 'inequality' in the situation.

There is usually broad societal consensus that some kind of system that seeks to balance welfare maximization with equity is acceptable, particularly if it is transparent and reactive to the identification of systematic imbalances. However, the individual patient may not share this view and may feel that his or her case is the 'most deserving'.

If there is an obligation to achieve the best outcome for each patient, how can a physician support an allocation system that does not place him or her 'top of the list'? A deontologist could argue that the patient's interests are best served by a transparent (respecting autonomy, communication, information-sharing) system with a commitment to justice (applying equally to this patient as to others). Abandoning this might lead to a free-for-all in which the patient's needs might have even less chance of being met.

The context in which these decisions need to be made is so wide-ranging that it is impossible to establish core rules. Doctors do need to be explicit when justifying why choices are made. The extreme of immediate clinical need (in which beneficence is likely to be the dominant relevant principle) is particularly challenging. Will the 'slightly less

unwell' patients always get 'shoved back in the queue' when new emergencies present? Justice and fairness need to be applied broadly. These principles apply to the individual patient, but also to other patients whose circumstances may be influenced by events relating to that patient. Similarly, we need to be fair to other members of the health-care team and to the broader needs of society.

It is probably fair to say that autonomy and justice are themes enjoying considerably more attention now than in the intermediate past, when medical paternalism may have been a more culturally dominant phenomenon than in the present.

SPECIFIC TOPICS

INCAPACITY

In 2000, the Adults with Incapacity Act was passed in Scotland. This act of parliament permits the administration of life-saving or essential treatment to adults who are unable to give consent themselves either due to an inability to communicate their wishes or an inability to understand or recall making decisions. The Act requires the minimum intervention commensurate with effective treatment and also requires consideration of advanced directives from the patient or views of relatives or guardians. This serves not only to facilitate the treatment of patients with temporary or permanent incapacity for their benefit, but also provides clear guidelines for doctors to treat patients with incapacity in an ethical way. It is likely that this Act will be extended to cover the rest of the United Kingdom.

EUTHANASIA

This term is used to describe the deliberate termination of life in circumstances where a patient suffers from an incurable, progressive and distressing (because of pain or disability) illness. Its motivation is usually compassionate, and frequently (but not always) the patient requests that it be done. It is both illegal and considered to be unethical in the UK.

It should be distinguished from other 'end-of-life' issues, such as withdrawing or withholding 'extraordinary' measures in situations where these are deemed futile, or where a patient has expressed a wish that such measures not be implemented.

Similarly, the concept of the 'double effect' is felt to be a different issue. In this scenario, an action may lead to 'good' and 'bad' outcomes (e.g. treating cancer pain with opiates in a dose that might cause the patient to die more rapidly than if they were withheld). The primary intention is to relieve pain, not to cause death. It is the *intention* that is felt to distinguish this act from euthanasia.

Discussions on the distinction between 'killing' and 'letting die' merge into those distinguishing between active and passive therapeutic decisions. With an ageing population and ever more elaborate possibilities to prolong life, it is likely that this topic will continue to be both topical and controversial.

ABORTION

Therapeutic abortion, whether legal or illegal, is the subject of extensive debate on philosophical, religious and political grounds. Currently in the UK, legal abortion is regulated by the Abortion Act 1967 (amended following the Human Fertilization and Embryology Act 1990). The broader debate on the ethics of abortion (particularly as it applies to abortion before 24 weeks' gestation, or if there is a substantial risk of severe physical or mental abnormalities in the unborn child) is beyond the scope of this chapter, but it is pertinent to note that abortion is legal in a number of circumstances that might be encountered in surgical practice.

Abortion may be performed in emergency circumstances after 24 weeks' gestation if there is a risk to the life of the pregnant woman, or if it is necessary to prevent grave permanent physical or mental injury to the woman. Furthermore, although conscientious objection to abortion normally excuses a health-care worker from participation in the process of abortion, this does not extend to the emergency situations described above.

NEGLIGENCE

This implies that a duty of care exists, that a breach of that duty of care has occurred, and that harm has occurred as a result of this. Fault is felt not to be as serious as when harm occurs as a result of either intention or recklessness. (In either of these circumstances, prosecution under criminal law is likely.)

The duty of care exists because of the nature of the professional relationship between the doctor and the patient. The standard against which performance is judged is derived from the outcome of the cases of *Bolam v Friern Hospital Management Committee (1957)* in England and Wales, and *Hunter v Hanley (1955)* in Scotland. A doctor is felt not to be negligent if his or her actions are 'in accordance with a practice accepted as proper by a responsible body of medical men skilled in that particular act' (*Bolam*), or if the actions cannot be described as those which 'no doctor of ordinary skill would be guilty of if acting with ordinary care' (*Hunter*). Many cases of negligence are pursued by patients as a consequence of their perception that the truth about mistakes concerning their care was hidden. For this reason, it is recommended that if a doctor is responsible for an error of management, the patient should be told and, if appropriate, an apology should be given. Lord Woolf recommended, in his report Access to Justice 1995, that there should be greater transparency in circumstances where negligence may have arisen and that greater efforts should be made to identify the key issues of the complainant such that earlier resolution of cases could be achieved, with many minor complaints not needing to follow a legal process.

Practical support and advice are readily available from professional organizations such as the British Medical Association, defence organizations such as the Medical Defence Union, Medical Protection Society and Medical and Dental Defence Union of Scotland, or regulatory authorities such as the General Medical Council.

HUMAN TISSUE ACT

The Human Tissue Bill was published in 2004 and came into effect as an Act of Parliament in 2006. In essence it is a response to concerns raised by the Alder Hey, Bristol and Isaacs inquiries, and seeks to remedy some of the inadequacies in the Human Tissue Act 1961. The bill contains legislation and a code of practice concerning the storage and use of tissues derived from human subjects and also their use in transplantation (replacing the Human Organ Transplant Act 1989).

COMPLETION OF A DEATH CERTIFICATE

When a patient dies, it is a legal requirement that certain details regarding the patient's time, place and cause of death are recorded. This death certificate must be completed before a body can be released to the family or their agents for disposal. The death certificate must be completed by a doctor and should state the likely cause of death and factors or concurrent illnesses that are likely to have contributed to the death. In certain circumstances, the cause of death may not be known, may be unexpected, may be associated with suspicious circumstances such as poisoning, or may occur soon after surgery. In such cases, the doctor responsible should discuss the case with staff from the Coroner's office in England, Wales and Northern Ireland, or with the Procurator Fiscal in Scotland. On such occasions, the Coroner or Procurator Fiscal may require that a post-mortem be carried out before a death certificate is issued. When it is intended to cremate a body, special regulations apply and a cremation form needs to be filled out that must also be completed by a practitioner with 5 years' or more full registration. Special attention needs to be paid to the presence of pacemakers or other potentially explosive devices in the patient's body. The cremation of fetal remains of less than 24 weeks' gestation does not require a cremation certificate.

POST-MORTEM EXAMINATION

There are two reasons for conducting a post-mortem examination. First, it may be a legal obligation to establish the cause of death prior to the issue of a death certificate, as mentioned above. Second, a post-mortem examination may not be a legal necessity but may shed light on the cause of death when this is uncertain. This may be valuable for the family to help them understand the reasons for the death of a relation, and this information may be equally valuable to the medical attendants who were responsible for the patient. In the first circumstance above, consent is not required from the deceased's next of kin; however, in the second situation consent is required. This should be obtained sensitively and may require an explanation of the procedure and of the possible outcomes of the examination. The issue of organ retention, as raised by the Alder Hey inquiry, has led to specific recommendations regarding the handling of the organs and tissues of deceased persons; these are detailed in the Human Tissue Bill but are beyond the scope of this book.

ORGAN DONATION

Solid organ transplantation has revolutionized the treatment of organ failure in a number of different systems. Clearly, the process of transplantation requires a source of organs and this in turn is subject to regulation to maintain ethical standards.

Living donor

It is possible for an individual to donate a kidney or part of the liver to another individual to be used for transplantation. Ethical practice requires that such a procedure should not harm the donor and should have a reasonable chance of success. Consent is particularly important in this context. There is no requirement for individuals to be genetically related; however, there is a legal requirement that cases in which there is no genetic relationship are reviewed by the Unrelated Live Transplant Regulatory Authority (ULTRA). (In the UK this function was taken over by the Human Tissue Authority in April 2006.) This body ensures, amongst other things, that individuals are not subjected to coercion or financial remuneration as incentives to donate. It is also considered good practice for all living donors to be assessed or reviewed by an independent medical examiner who is not connected to the transplant unit, to ensure that there is no conflict of interest.

Cadaveric heart-beating donation

Currently, most organs used for transplantation are derived from heart-beating donors who have been diagnosed as having brain-stem death, often following intracranial haemorrhage. This diagnosis is made following a series of detailed neurological tests performed by two experienced doctors on two separate occasions. Brain-stem death is an absolute condition and all of the criteria for its diagnosis must be met. Following this diagnosis, it may be possible to proceed with organ donation if the deceased has indicated prior assent through joining the organ donor register, carrying a donor card or making a pre-mortem statement to this effect. When such information is lacking, the next of kin of the deceased are approached, usually in the presence of a transplant coordinator, to ask for their lack of objection to organ donation. Transplant coordinators are also capable of informing doctors if potential donors meet legal and medical requirements for organ donation.

RESEARCH GOVERNANCE

According to the Department of Health, the purpose of research governance is to 'improve research quality and safeguard the public by: enhancing ethical and scientific quality, promoting good practice, reducing adverse incidents and ensuring lessons are learned, preventing poor perform-ance and misconduct'. These values are designed to be applied to the individual, the institution and those sponsoring research. On a practical level, adherence to the principles of research governance protects all of the interested parties, particularly the patient. Medical journals quite rightly pay a great deal of attention to research governance issues to ensure that only good-quality, reliable, ethical and safe research is published.

ETHICS COMMITTEES

Clinical trials and research on human subjects have been cornerstones in the advancement of medical and surgical disciplines. Unethical experiments performed by Nazis in the Second World War acted as a catalyst for the development of modern ethical principles applied to human research. These ideas were amalgamated into a number of declarations, named after the cities in which they were made. Two stand out: the Declaration of Geneva, made in 1948, which presents what is essentially the modern Hippocratic Oath, and the Declaration of Helsinki, made in 1964, which lays out the ethical principles that guide modern medical research. To perform research on human subjects or even on material derived from human subjects, it is necessary to apply for permission from a regional ethics committee. Such committees are composed of a number of medically qualified and lay members who study applications with reference to the principles enshrined by the Declaration of Helsinki to ensure that the proposed research is safe and in the interests of society. Such committees consider all kinds of aspects of the research, such as whether it is likely to answer or is capable of answering the question addressed, whether the planned intervention is safe, the quality of the information given to patients, the likely outcomes, and protocols for dealing with an adverse event; even aspects such as indemnity cover and data protection issues are addressed. Thus it can be seen that ethics committees in many ways provide assurance that the principles of research governance are being adhered to.

BOX 7.4   FURTHER INFORMATION

- Boyd KM, Higgs R, Pinching AJ. The new dictionary of medical ethics. London: BMJ Publishing; 1997
- Davies M. Textbook on medical law. 2nd edn. London: Blackstone; 1998
- General Medical Council. Good medical practice. 2nd edn. London: GMC; 1998
- General Medical Council. Seeking patients' consent: the ethical considerations. London: GMC; 1999
- Mason JK, McCall Smith RA. Law and medical ethics. London: Butterworth; 1994

Websites

- www.cirp.org/library/ethics/helsinki *Declaration of Helsinki*
- www.cirp.org/library/ethics/intlcode *International Code of Medical Ethics*
- www.cirp.org/library/ethics/geneva *Declaration of Geneva (the 'modern' Hippocratic Oath)*
- www.dh.gov.uk/PolicyAndGuidance/ResearchAndDevelopment/ ResearchAndDevelopmentAZ/ResearchGovernance/ fs/en *Research governance*
- www.gmc-uk.org/guidance *General Medical Council Standards of Medical Practice*
- www.parliament.the-stationery-office.co.uk/pa/cm200304/cmbills/009/2004009.htm *Human Tissue Bill*

M.A. POTTER

Principles of the surgical management of cancer

THE BIOLOGY OF CANCER

A neoplasm or new growth consists of a mass of transformed cells that does not respond in a normal way to growth regulatory systems. These transformed cells serve no useful function and proliferate in an atypical and uncontrolled way to form a benign or malignant neoplasm. In normal tissues, cell replication and death are equally balanced and under tight regulatory control. However, when a cancer arises, this is generally due to genomic abnormalities that either increase cell replication or inhibit cell death (Fig. 8.1). The mechanisms by which this abnormal growth activity is induced (carcinogenesis) are complex and can be influenced in many ways: for example, inherited genetic make-up, residential environment, exposure to ionizing radiation or carcinogens, viral infection, diet, lifestyle and hormonal imbalances. These cellular insults give rise to alterations in the genomic DNA (mutations) and it is these mutations that lead to cancer formation. Mutations can lead to disruption of

the cell replication cycle at any point and lead to either activation or over-expression of oncogenes, or the inactivation of tumour suppressor genes, or a combination of the two (Table 8.1).

Changes within the cellular genome occur frequently but do not necessarily result in a tumour. Natural protective mechanisms repair errors in DNA replication; similarly, immune surveillance, simple wastage (i.e. loss of cells from the surface) and programmed cell death (apoptosis) destroy mutant cells before they proliferate. For persistence of growth and hence cancer formation, these protective mechanisms must break down (e.g. failure of mismatch repair due to mutations in genes such as *MLHI* and *MSH2*, or failure of apoptosis). The host's internal environment may also have a role in the 'promotion' of tumour growth. Good examples are the 'hormone-dependent' cancers of the breast, prostate and endometrium, which require a 'correct' balance of hormonal secretion from the endocrine glands of the host for their continued growth. The natural history of a tumour is also related to its growth rate, which in turn is determined by the

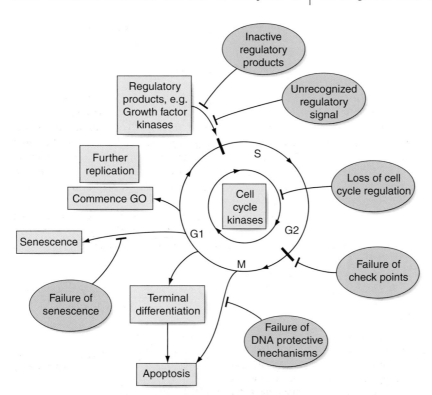

Fig. 8.1   Cell replication and cancer formation.
Normal cell replication is under tight regulation by endogenous growth factors. Mutations that result in abnormal growth factor proteins can lead to cancer formation.

Table 8.1 EXAMPLES OF GENE MUTATIONS THAT CAN LEAD TO CANCER FORMATION	
Gene	**Point of action in cell cycle**
p16, CDK4, Rb	Cell cycle check point
MSH2, MLH1	DNA replication and repair
p53, fas	Apoptosis
E cadherin	Cellular adhesion
erb-A	Cellular differentiation
Ki-ras, erb-B	Regulatory kinases
TGF-β	Growth factors

BOX 8.1   FACTORS LEADING TO LOSS OF CELL CYCLE REGULATION

Growth of a cancer is due to loss of cell cycle regulation, which is dependent on:

- Increased cell proliferation
- Decreased programmed cell death (apoptosis)
- A combination of the two

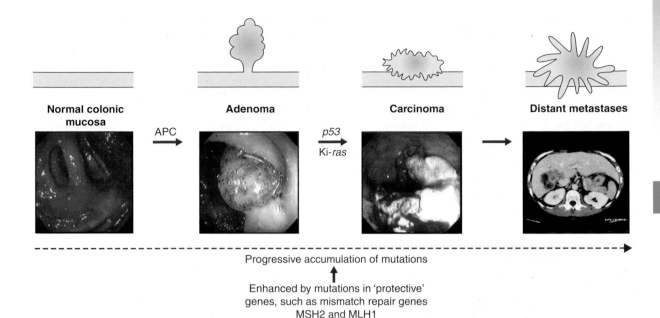

Fig. 8.2   Colorectal adenoma–carcinoma progression.
By the progressive acquisition of genetic mutations, normal colorectal epithelium forms a benign polyp, which can progress to an invasive or metastatic cancer.

balance between cell division and cell death. Some tumours are slow-growing (e.g. prostate) and years may pass before deposits reach a size that threatens normal organ function. Others grow rapidly as a result of a high rate of cell proliferation, and some expand rapidly (despite a relatively normal rate of cell proliferation) if cell death is slow to occur.

THE ADENOMA–CARCINOMA PROGRESSION

Neoplasms may be benign or malignant; the essential difference is the capacity to invade and metastasize. The cells of benign tumours do not invade surrounding tissues but remain as a local conglomerate. Malignant tumours are invasive and their cells can directly invade adjacent tissues or enter blood and lymphatic channels, to be deposited at remote sites. This malignant genotype develops as a result of the progressive acquisition of cancer mutations (by point mutation, chromosomal loss or translocation). The acquisition of the malignant phenotype can be recognized histologically as a tumour develops from a benign adenoma through to a dysplastic lesion, and finally into an invasive carcinoma (Fig. 8.2). The progression from benign to malignant cancer is sometimes observed at one of the intermediate or pre-invasive stages, known as carcinoma in situ. Although many cases of carcinoma in situ eventually progress to an invasive phase (over a period of months or years), there is evidence to suggest that this does not always happen. Nevertheless, the concept of tumour progression from a benign to malignant phenotype provides the rationale behind screening and early detection programmes; i.e. if benign or pre-invasive lesions are removed, this will prevent invasive disease.

INVASION AND METASTASIS

Benign tumours rarely threaten life but may cause a variety of cosmetic or functional abnormalities. In contrast, malignant tumours invade and relentlessly replace normal tissues, destroying supporting structures and disturbing function; they can spread to distant tissues (metastasize), eventually causing death. Metastases are cancer deposits similar in cell type to the original cancer found at remote (secondary) sites in the body.

The process of invasion and metastasis is complex (Fig. 8.3) and is dependent on the biology of the tumour. Some tumours metastasize earlier in their clinical course

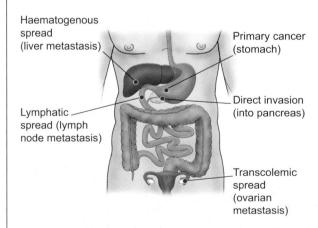

Fig. 8.3   Invasion and metastasis.
Cancers invade adjacent tissues by direct infiltration. Spread to distant sites (metastasis) is via the blood stream or lymphatics, or across body cavities (transcolemic spread). Following initial growth, cancer cells lose local adherence and invade blood vessels. They are then transported via the blood stream to adhere in distant organs and grow into secondary tumours.

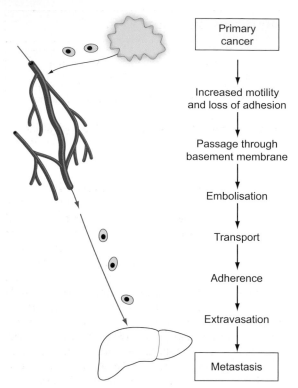

Fig. 8.4   Metastasis.
Following initial growth, cancer cells lose local adherence and invade blood vessels. They are then transported via the blood stream to adhere in distant organs and grow into secondary tumours.

than others. This variation may depend on the tissue of origin of the primary tumour, but can also vary widely according to the phenotype of individual tumours. For example, cancer of the breast is thought to metastasize early, and micrometastases are often present but not detectable when the patient first presents. Some patients with apparently localized colorectal cancer are cured by radical surgery, but others receiving the same treatment deteriorate rapidly with metastatic disease. The mechanisms that control invasion and metastasis are obscure (Fig. 8.4). Local pressure effects from the expanding tumour and the increased motility of tumour cells may play a role in local invasion. Malignant cells secrete a number of factors that may determine their biological behaviour and promote growth at both primary and metastatic sites. The matrix metalloproteinases (MMPs) are a family of zinc-dependent endoproteinases with enzymatic activity directed against components of the extracellular matrix. Their enzymatic action facilitates tumour cell invasion and metastasis by degrading extracellular collagens, laminins and proteoglycans. Other proteases, such as urokinase, plasminogen-activating factor and the cathepsins, are also involved in metastasis formation. Clumps of cancer cells can then embolize to distant tissues and form metastases. The survival of metastatic deposits depends on angiogenesis, which is mediated by an imbalance between positive and negative regulatory molecules released by the tumour cells and surrounding normal cells. Negative factors, such

as angiostatin or endostatin, will inhibit new vessel formation. Positive factors, such as vascular endothelial growth factors or fibroblast growth factors, will enhance metastasis. Cancer cells also secrete prostaglandins, which can induce osteolysis and may promote the development of skeletal deposits.

NATURAL HISTORY AND ESTIMATE OF CURE

Calculations based on an exponential model of tumour growth suggest that three-quarters of the lifespan of a tumour is spent in a 'pre-clinical' or occult stage, and that the clinical manifestations of the disease are limited to the final quarter.

For cure, every malignant cell must be eradicated. Not only should there be no recurrent tumour during the patient's lifetime, there should also be no evidence of residual tumour at death. This rigid definition of curability can rarely be applied. A normal duration of life without further clinical evidence of disease is generally accepted as evidence of cure, even though microscopic deposits of tumour may still be present.

'Cure' rates of individual cancers are assessed by survival rates at various times after treatment. Conventionally, 5- and 10-year intervals are used. Cumulative survival curves (life tables) can be constructed for individual cancers and compared with those of age-matched healthy subjects of the same population (Fig. 8.5). Divergence of survival curves indicates that patients with cancer are dying faster than their normal counterparts, whereas parallel curves indicate that patients with the disease are dying at no greater rate than their age-matched controls. The point at which these two curves become parallel is the time at which cure can be assumed.

Cure rates vary according to the aggressiveness of the disease and the success of treatment. In some patients with cancer (e.g. stomach and lung), metastases grow rapidly and cause death within a few years of clinical presentation. In others (e.g. cancer of the breast and melanoma), many years may elapse before metastatic spread becomes evident and, even when metastases have occurred, life may be long. It is for this reason that 5-year survival rates cannot provide

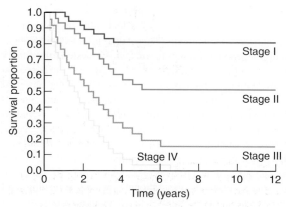

Fig. 8.5   Kaplan–Mier survival curve.

a satisfactory estimate of cure for all tumours. Many regard the treatment of a malignant tumour as a matter of extreme urgency. When one considers the natural duration of a cancer, a week or two spent in careful investigation, counselling and planning of treatment is good practice. However, this period must not be unduly delayed, as patients with cancer are naturally worried and wish to have their initial treatment completed within a reasonable time.

THE MANAGEMENT OF PATIENTS WITH CANCER

The goals of treating cancer can be broadly grouped as follows: prevention, cure and palliation. Prevention seeks to modify behaviour to prevent cancer formation. For example, the avoidance of smoking or direct sunlight may prevent the formation of lung or skin cancer. Taking a small dose of aspirin on a regular basis may protect against colorectal cancer (chemoprevention). When a cancer has formed, treatment is aimed at cure for early-stage disease. When a cancer is locally advanced or has metastasized, the chance of cure reduces. In cancers that are felt to be incurable, treatment is then aimed at palliation of troublesome symptoms.

SCREENING

If cancer can be detected before it causes symptoms, then it is generally smaller, has less chance of having metastasized and is therefore more amenable to cure. Detecting benign lesions with malignant potential, pre-invasive cancer, and invasive malignancy before it becomes symptomatic is called screening (Fig. 8.6). Screening is expensive and its effectiveness in relation to cost must be critically evaluated before routine use (EBM 8.1). Screening is most effective when targeted at specific risk groups and when

---

EBM 8.1   RECENT SCREENING TRIALS

'Studies in Sweden in the late 1980s established that screening for breast cancer allowed for early detection and improved cancer-specific survival. Recent studies have shown that these benefits can be achieved in the context of national screening programmes and for other cancers such as colorectal cancer.'

Blanks RG, et al. Br Med J 2000; 321:665–669.
Mandel JS, et al. J Natl Cancer Inst 1999; 91(5):434–437.

8

the screening test has a high level of acceptability (i.e. the vast majority of the target population accept the invitation to undergo the screening procedure). For successful screening, the test used must be able to detect the cancer at a stage when earlier treatment will lead to fewer deaths from the cancer. In any given population, the likelihood of a cancer being present is generally low (< 1%); hence, the test must be sensitive in order to detect these relatively rare lesions. The test must also be specific (i.e. have a low false-positive rate); otherwise, individuals will undergo unnecessary investigation or even inappropriate treatment. Finally, the proposed treatment of a cancer patient detected by a screening programme must be effective. In the UK, cervical cytology is offered to women on a 3-yearly basis until the age of 60, and mammographic screening (Fig. 8.7)

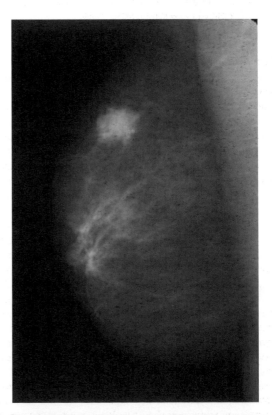

Fig. 8.7   Single mammogram showing malignancy in peripheral breast tissue.
(Illustration courtesy of Mr M. Barber, Consultant Breast Surgeon, Western General Hospital, Edinburgh.)

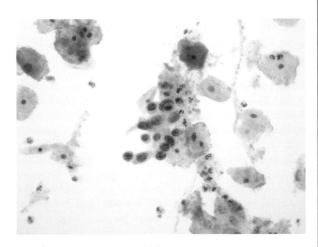

Fig. 8.6   Cervical cytology.
A group of severely dyskaryotic squamous cells in a ThinPrep liquid-based cytology preparation. (Illustration courtesy of Dr A.R.W. Williams, Senior Lecturer/Honorary Consultant in Pathology, University of Edinburgh.)

Table 8.2 EXAMPLES OF CANCER TYPES THAT ARE OR COULD BE THE SUBJECT OF SCREENING PROGRAMMES

Cancer	Screening test
Breast	Mammography
Cervix	Smear cytology
Colon	Faecal occult blood test and flexible sigmoidoscopy
	Colonoscopy
Prostate	Prostate-specific antigen (PSA)

Table 8.3 MULTIDISCIPLINARY TEAM INVOLVED IN CANCER CARE

Medical staff
- Surgeon
- Physician
- Radiologist
- Oncologist
- Radiotherapist
- Palliative care physician
- General practitioner

Nursing staff
- Ward nurse
- Chemotherapy nurse
- Clinical nurse specialist
- Hospice nurse

Paramedical staff
- Oncology dietitian
- Physiotherapist
- Occupational therapist
- Clergy

BOX 8.2 CRITERIA FOR SCREENING PROGRAMMES

A test for use in cancer screening must:

- Be sensitive
- Be specific
- Be acceptable
- Detect cancer at a stage when cure is possible
- Have a reasonable cost

8

is offered to women between 50 and 64 years on a 2-yearly basis. Acceptance rates vary, but below 60–70% the viability of the programme is questionable. Other tumour types that might be amenable to screening are listed with their relevant screening tests in Table 8.2.

Screening for inherited cancer

Some forms of cancer can be inherited; for example, about 5% of patients with colorectal cancer develop the disease because of an autosomal dominant inherited mutation either in the *APC* gene (polyposis coli) or in the mismatch repair genes such as *MSH2* and *MLH1* (hereditary non-polyposis colorectal cancer, or HNPCC). Alternatively, about 5% of women develop breast cancer as a result of an autosomal dominant inherited mutation on the *BRCA1* or *BRCA2* genes. In these instances, closely related family members should be offered the appropriate tests to detect these specific mutations. Carriers of the mutation can then be offered prophylatic surgery, e.g. bilateral mastectomy (for *BRCA1* and *BRCA2* carriers) or restorative procto-colectomy (for *APC* carriers) in an attempt to eliminate subsequent cancer development.

THE CANCER PATIENT'S JOURNEY

The management of cancer frequently involves surgery, be it radical for cure or palliative to relieve distressing symptoms. Even in patients where the primary treatment is not surgical, the surgeon can play an important role: for example, in obtaining diagnostic biopsies. Because of the complexity of modern cancer management, cancer services in a hospital are currently organized around a multi-disciplinary team approach. The team commonly includes surgeons, medical oncologists (chemotherapy), clinical oncologists (radiotherapy/chemotherapy), radiologists, pathologists and clinical nurse specialists (Table 8.3).

Individual aspects of patient care are undertaken by different members of the team, but overall staging and treatment plan are discussed on a weekly basis at the multidisciplinary team meeting.

Good communication with the patient and between team members forms the basis of optimal patient care. There are several key stages in the management of the patient with cancer, which can be regarded as a journey from the onset of symptoms to definitive treatment and subsequent follow-up (Fig. 8.8). The exact sequence of events may differ from one patient to the next. For example, it may be necessary to remove the tumour to obtain full information on staging before an adequate treatment plan can be evolved. Patients usually begin their 'cancer journey' by deciding that a symptom or symptoms they have developed are serious enough to merit consultation with their GP. These symptoms may be a result of local or systemic effects of the cancer.

SYMPTOMS THAT MAY INITIATE A PATIENT'S 'CANCER JOURNEY'

Local effects

A tumour that lies on the surface of the body may become visible, change in shape or pigmentation, bleed, or discharge mucus or pus. A hollow viscus or duct may be obstructed by a tumour, e.g. a bronchus (causing pulmonary collapse), a segment of bowel (causing intestinal obstruction) or the bile duct or pancreatic duct (causing jaundice). A tumour within a closed space may cause pressure symptoms. For example, increased intracranial pressure may complicate intracerebral tumours, and paraplegia may arise from a spinal cord tumour. Invasion of an organ by a tumour may compromise its normal functions and cause organ failure. Invasion of tissues such as the pancreas, bone or nerves can cause severe pain. A cancer can also mimic the pain of benign disease: for example, dyspeptic symptoms in stomach cancer.

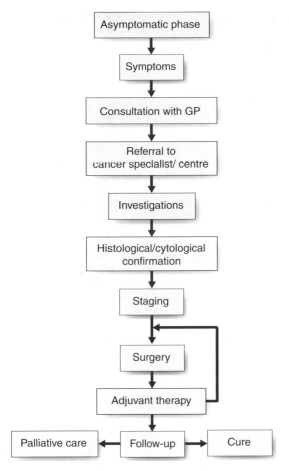

Fig. 8.8 The patient's cancer journey.
During the patient's management, several key stages are encountered, from symptoms to diagnosis and treatment.

BOX 8.3 SYMPTOMS THAT SHOULD INITIATE INVESTIGATION

- Weight loss
- Rectal bleeding/melaena
- Haemoptysis/persistent cough
- Haematuria
- Breast lump
- Dysphagia/dyspepsia
- Persistent headache
- Persistent non-specific symptoms

GP to a hospital specialist. Frequently, however, the initial presenting complaint of a patient with cancer is non-specific, e.g. general malaise. Other symptoms, such as epigastric pain, are common complaints encountered by the GP and are usually associated with benign disease. These symptoms are more challenging to the GP and it can be difficult to decide which patient needs an urgent referral and which does not. Cancer patients presenting with such non-specific symptoms may consult their GP on more than one occasion. Persistence of such non-specific symptoms should raise the index of suspicion towards neoplastic disease and lead to specialist referral.

REFERRAL TO A SPECIALIST/CANCER CENTRE

Patients who are referred with a suspected diagnosis of cancer are often seen urgently in the surgical outpatient clinic appropriate to the probable site of origin of the tumour. In practice, the time taken to see the hospital specialist is a small proportion of that taken to diagnosis when other factors, such as delay to presentation, referral and investigation, are considered. At the initial consultation, it is important to spend time taking a full and detailed history and examination. It is also important to spend time addressing any patient anxieties and in providing the patient with a clear view of any investigations that are planned. It is here that other members of the multidisciplinary team, such as the clinical nurse specialist, can help enormously. Following the initial consultation, the patient will be asked to attend for investigations as either an inpatient or an outpatient, to confirm or refute the diagnosis. Increasingly, 'one-stop' clinics are being provided, allowing the initial consultation and investigations to be performed at one clinic attendance. This approach is particularly suited to the diagnosis of breast cancer.

INVESTIGATIONS

Investigations serve two main purposes. First, they are aimed at histological or cytological confirmation of the diagnosis of cancer. Second, they are used to assess the extent of the primary disease (local invasion) and to look for evidence of metastatic spread. This is known as 'staging' the disease.

Diagnostic investigations

Initial investigations to make the diagnosis should proceed in a logical order, starting with simple blood tests (e.g.

Systemic effects

Weight loss is often the key symptom that alerts both patients and their doctor to the possibility of malignant disease. A proportion of patients become so emaciated that they appear to die of starvation. This syndrome is known as cancer cachexia, and is clinically characterized by anorexia, severe weight loss, lethargy, anaemia and oedema.

The secretory products of some tumours can produce characteristic clinical syndromes. These products may be appropriate to the organ of origin. Thus, a tumour of the adrenal cortex may secrete excess corticosteroid and cause Cushing's syndrome; a parathyroid tumour may secrete excess parathormone and cause hypercalcaemia; and an islet cell tumour of the pancreas may secrete excess insulin and cause hypoglycaemia. On the other hand, secretory products may be inappropriate to the site of a tumour. Such 'ectopic' secretion occurs predominantly in tumours of neuroendocrine origin, and produces a variety of endocrine syndromes.

CONSULTATION WITH THE GP

Distressing or dramatic presenting symptoms—for example, rectal bleeding—rightly produce a prompt referral from the

8

tumour markers) and progressing through more complex imaging investigations, with the ultimate aim of obtaining histological or cytological confirmation of the diagnosis (Table 8.4). Plain radiology may demonstrate a soft tissue tumour, e.g. tumours of the lung or bone, but for tumours of the stomach or intestine contrast studies are necessary. For some deep-seated tumours, e.g. those of the pancreas or brain, other methods of imaging are needed. These may include angiography, radioactive scintigraphy and ultrasonography (US), but increasingly CT (Fig. 8.9) and MRI are the standard forms of investigation. Neoplastic disease can be confirmed cytologically, e.g. by the demonstration of malignant cells in secretions, in washings from hollow viscera, or in needle aspirates. Biopsies obtained at either upper or lower gastrointestinal endoscopy can provide material for histology, as can ultrasound or CT-guided Tru-cut needle biopsies. In some instances, it may be necessary to perform an examination under anaesthetic or diagnostic laparoscopy (Fig. 8.10) to obtain suitable diagnostic material. In general, a treatment plan for the management of a patient cannot be formulated until a histological or cytological diagnosis has been made. However, there are circumstances in which this is not possible (e.g. in certain patients with pancreatic cancer), and then clear radiological evidence may be used instead.

Staging investigations

Staging investigations will depend on the site of the primary cancer and the relevant common sites of metastasis. Local invasion can be assessed—for example, in oesophageal

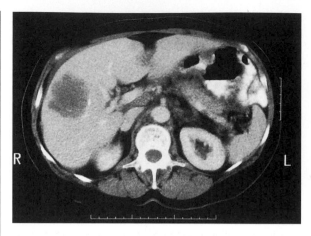

Fig. 8.9 Staging CT of the abdomen showing a large solitary liver metastasis in a patient with colorectal cancer.

cancer—by endoscopic ultrasound. CT or MRI scans can also be usefully employed to assess local invasion. Metastatic spread can be determined by a variety of investigations, e.g. bone scans, CT scans and laparoscopy. Often, staging investigations will have been undertaken as part of the diagnostic process, e.g. CT scans.

The aim of staging is to define the extent of the disease, assess its likely prognosis, and permit the development of an appropriate treatment plan by the multidisciplinary team. The International Union against Cancer (Union Internationale contre le Cancer, or UICC) has described a system of staging (TNM) in which three components are assessed. These are the extent of the primary tumour (T), the presence and extent of metastases in regional lymph nodes (N), and the presence of distant metastases (M). The addition of numbers to each component indicates the extent of the disease within that category. The bigger the number, the more advanced the disease.

In the initial TNM system, only clinical, radiological and endoscopic investigations were used. Such clinical staging is still important in defining the extent of disease and may be

Table 8.4 INVESTIGATIONS FOR THE DIAGNOSIS OF CANCER

Blood tests
 ● Haematology
      FBC
 ● Biochemistry
      LFTs
      Tumour markers

Radiology
 ● Plain X-rays
      CXR
 ● Contrast-enhanced
      Barium enema
 ● Ultrasound
 ● CT
 ● MRI

Endoscopy   ● Upper GI endoscopy   ● Colonoscopy   ● Endoscopic retrograde cholangiopancreatography (ERCP)
Cytology/histology   ● Body fluids, e.g. sputum and urine   ● Fine-needle aspiration (FNA), e.g. breast and thyroid cancer   ● Radiologically guided FNA   ● Endoscopic brushings or biopsy
Operative   ● Examination under anaesthetic and biopsy   ● Excision biopsy, e.g. lymph node   ● Diagnostic laparoscopy and biopsy   ● Laparoscopic ultrasound

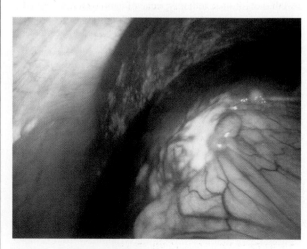

Fig. 8.10 Diagnostic laparoscopy.

used to plan the initial management of a patient. However, without histological confirmation, such clinical staging can sometimes be highly inaccurate. For example, the palpability of regional lymph nodes is a poor indicator of their involvement by tumour. Impalpable nodes may still contain metastases, whereas palpable nodes may be the seat of reactive hyperplasia (sinus histiocytosis) rather than tumour. Small deposits of tumour in viscera and bones cannot be detected by routine radiology, and thus many patients who on clinical and radiological grounds appear to have localized disease have in fact unrecognized widespread microscopic tumour deposits. For this reason, the TNM system has now been modified to include not only a pre-treatment clinical classification, but also a post-surgical pathological classification, denoted as pTNM. Excision of regional lymph nodes is one way to provide such information. In some melanomas and skin tumours, and in cancer of the bladder and large bowel, histological assessment of the depth of tumour penetration provides important information about the extent and prognosis of the disease. It must be recognized that all staging has its limitations and that microscopic tumour deposits may not be detected, particularly in terms of distant metastases. These staging systems are therefore used to provide a 'best-guess' scenario upon which to base the patient's treatment.

Prognosis is also affected by the biological characteristics of a tumour. For example, its degree of nuclear and cellular atypia and the extent of lymphocytic infiltration, inflammatory response, and perineural and vascular invasion all influence outcome. These factors, as well as biochemical indices (e.g. oestrogen receptor status in breast cancer), can all be used in the planning of a patient's treatment.

MANAGEMENT

Following the initial diagnosis and staging, the patient may be discussed by the multidisciplinary team or may proceed to surgery, where the primary tumour, surrounding tissue and locoregional lymph nodes are excised and then sent for histopathology. Thus, the clinical staging is translated into histopathological staging; the multidisciplinary team can then discuss further aspects of management with the maximum amount of information available.

Benign tumours

Provided sufficient surrounding tissue is excised to ensure its complete removal, a benign tumour is cured by local excision. Some benign tumours, e.g. pleomorphic adenomas of the parotid, extend beyond their apparent macroscopic limits. Removal of the involved segment of the gland or organ is then the only sure way to cure.

BOX 8.4 PURPOSE OF STAGING
• Define the extent of disease • Assess likely prognosis • Allow the development of a treatment plan

Malignant tumours

A radical cancer operation implies complete removal of the tissue bearing the tumour, together with a margin of unaffected surrounding tissue. In some tumours, there is sequential spread, first locally, then to lymph nodes, and then to distant organs such as the liver and lungs. In this situation, careful local removal, along with the locoregional lymph nodes (known as 'en bloc resection'), can be curative. Often, however, the spread of a tumour may be more unpredictable and in essence the removal of local lymph nodes is simply to provide information for the stage of the cancer, rather than being of true therapeutic benefit. The management of regional lymph nodes thus depends on the site and type of the tumour. With some tumours, e.g. those of the gastrointestinal tract, regional lymph nodes are routinely resected on the basis that sequential spread may have occurred. In other tumours (e.g. breast cancer), lymph node sampling or sentinel node biopsy may be more appropriate, especially if en bloc lymph node resection may be associated with significant morbidity: for example, limb lymphoedema.

Complete radical excision, which is confirmed by histological examination with no evidence of lymph node metastasis, carries a high chance of surgical cure. A good example is total mesorectal excision performed for rectal cancer (Fig. 8.11). During any operation for cancer, care is taken to try to avoid the spillage of malignant cells. In some sites (e.g. testis or large bowel), it is usual to ligate the main vessels draining the area before the tumour is mobilized, so that further malignant cells are not shed into the circulation. Care is taken to avoid handling a tumour of the bowel and to prevent spillage of cells into the lumen, which may cause cancer recurrence at the anastomosis. Many surgeons also irrigate the wound or body cavity with dilute cetrimide or betadine to destroy 'free-floating' cells and thus reduce the likelihood of local recurrence. Overall, a careful and meticulous approach to all aspects of the operation is vital. Attention to each detail improves the outcome of surgery.

There are data to suggest that surgery performed in specialist centres where surgeons are regularly performing radical operations produces better survival rates than surgery in non-specialist centres. Hence, surgeons are increasingly sub-specialized and concentrate on performing selected operations (EBM 8.2).

Adjuvant treatment

As mentioned previously, the most accurate staging of a patient with cancer is generally available after pathological evaluation of the resected specimen. Once this information is available, the patient can be discussed by the multidisciplinary team with a view to the need for further therapy.

Clearly, it is sometimes not possible to remove all the local disease. Moreover, early systemic dissemination may have occurred. Thus, an adjuvant to surgery is needed to provide both local and systemic control. For example, adjuvant chemotherapy may help prevent both local recurrence and distant metastasis, and this is commonly used in patients with colorectal or breast cancer who have lymph node involvement. However, surgical excision must be

8

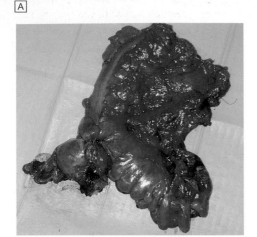

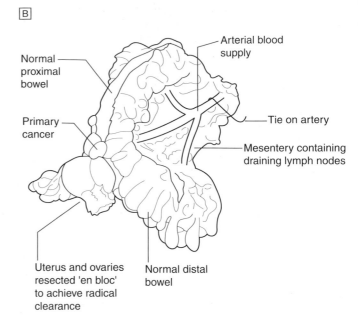

Normal proximal bowel

Arterial blood supply

Primary cancer

Tie on artery

Mesentery containing draining lymph nodes

Uterus and ovaries resected 'en bloc' to achieve radical clearance

Normal distal bowel

Fig. 8.11 Rectal cancer.
Ⓐ Operative specimen demonstrating a mesorectal excision of a rectal cancer. Ⓑ The diagram shows the structures that have been removed with this en bloc resection.

EBM 8.2 IMPROVED OUTCOME WITH SUB-SPECIALIZATION

'The treatment outcomes for cancer patients have improved with the advent of sub-specialization among cancer surgeons (e.g. specialist breast surgeons for breast cancer, colorectal surgeons for colorectal cancer etc.). This benefit seems to be due to the integration with multidisciplinary teams rather than simply due to case volume.'

*McArdle CS, Hole DJ. Br J Surg 2004; 91(5):610–617.
Parks RW, et al. Br J Cancer 2004; 91(3):459–465.
Martijn H, et al. Colorectal Cancer Study Group of the Comprehensive Cancer Centre South. Euro J Cancer 2003; 39(14):2073–2079.*

---

adequate, and adjuvant radiotherapy or chemotherapy must not be regarded as a safety net for careless surgical practice. In some cancers, such as ovarian cancer, transcolemic spread occurs early and a radical operation is impossible. Here surgical reduction of the tumour burden may contribute to the success of systemic treatment, which is aimed at controlling the disease as a whole.

Achieving a balance between the relief of symptoms and the morbidity induced by radical cancer therapy is often difficult, and it is important to remember that the quality of life is as important as the duration of survival. Chemotherapy is potentially toxic; morbidity and quality of life must always be considered before undertaking this form of treatment.

The success of adjuvant chemotherapy varies from one histological type of cancer to another. In general, drugs are given in combination over a period of 6–12 months. Toxicity, such as mouth ulcers, diarrhoea, weakness and alopecia, is common but in general tolerable. Results in colorectal and breast cancer suggest that the likelihood of death from recurrent cancer is reduced by about 20–30% in patients with evidence of lymph node metastasis.

Because of the localized nature of radiotherapy, it is administered to reduce the chances of local recurrence rather than of distant metastasis. Radiotherapy may be given prior to surgery to try to 'down-stage' or shrink a bulky and fixed tumour (e.g. rectal cancer) and thus make surgery easier to perform. Sometimes radiotherapy is given to rectal cancers pre-operatively, even if the cancer is surgically resectable, to improve subsequent local recurrence rates; this is termed neoadjuvant radiotherapy. Alternatively, it may be given to the post-operative patient in whom the chances of local recurrence are thought to be high (e.g. a patient in whom the margins at the edge of the resection specimen are involved with tumour). When tumours are relatively radiosensitive, radiotherapy can reduce the need for radical surgery and a more cosmetically acceptable conservative operation is then possible (e.g. lumpectomy and radiotherapy, as opposed to mastectomy in breast cancer).

The impact of intensive chemo- and radiotherapy on growth in children with malignant disease can be significant. The potential for cure, which is possible in many childhood malignancies, has to be balanced against the long-term morbidity of growth failure as a side-effect of such treatment.

Other modes of adjuvant therapy include less toxic therapies, such as administration of the anti-oestrogen tamoxifen in women with breast cancer. Experimental models have shown that monoclonal antibodies, synthetic peptides, antisense oligonucleotides and soluble adhesion molecules can inhibit tumour growth. Gene therapy carries the potential to restore the function of altered tumour suppressor molecules. MMP inhibitors and angiogenesis inhibitors offer other potential avenues for novel anticancer therapy.

FOLLOW-UP

In most patients with tumours amenable to surgical treatment, it is important to check subsequently that there is no local recurrence of disease and that the patient is symptom-free (EBM 8.3). In general, patients are seen more frequently in the early months after surgery, as this is the period when recurrence is most likely; it is also the period when it is necessary to detect and treat non-cancer-related post-operative complications. The nature of the surgery will influence the follow-up strategy; patients undergoing palliative surgery will have different follow-up requirements from those undergoing curative surgery. However, it is often difficult to detect recurrence or metastasis in the asymptomatic post-operative patient, and some would question the value of routine sophisticated investigations in the detection of metastatic disease in such cases. Current evidence suggests that, in some cases, once the primary therapy has been undertaken, patients may be discharged back to their GP for follow-up with re-referral to the multidisciplinary team as necessary.

PALLIATION OF ADVANCED CANCER

The management of patients with incurable disease involves the relief of distressing symptoms (palliative care). This is a specialist branch of medicine in its own right, and the palliative care physician and the associated team play an important part in the overall management of the cancer patient. The terminal stages of malignancy can be prolonged, and pain and other distressing symptoms are common. Effective palliation is achieved by a variety of means. Local and/or systemic adjuvant therapy can be used to induce tumour regression: for example, to reduce the pressure effects of cerebral metastases. Surgery can be employed to resect symptomatic metastases or bypass a malignant obstruction. When a palliative operation is performed, the patient and his or her relatives should understand that its object is to prevent additional suffering, and not to attempt cure. Medical treatments are used to relieve symptoms such as pain, nausea, depression, infections etc. A wide range of analgesic and narcotic drugs is available to relieve pain. The choice depends on the type of pain, its severity, and the stage of the illness. The aim is to achieve complete analgesia without impairing mental clarity or inducing side-effects. It is essential never to let the patient wait for the next dose of analgesic. Schedules of administration are planned to prevent rather than treat pain. When pain is severe, narcotic drugs should be used; fear of addiction is irrelevant in this context. Treatment should start with simple analgesics for mild pain (e.g. paracetamol) and move to more potent agents if the pain is not readily controlled (e.g. dihydrocodeine, co-proxamol). For severe pain, slow-release morphine sulphate tablets (MST) are usually administered 12-hourly, and can be combined with morphine elixir or dextromoramide for occasional breakthrough pain. For persistent pain, transdermal patches or continuous subcutaneous infusions of analgesics can be administered. The psychological and social aspects of care for both the patient and the family should also be addressed.

PROGNOSIS AND COUNSELLING

Honesty is the basis of the doctor–patient relationship and it is almost always best to tell patients that they have cancer. However, in doing so one should reveal as much of the truth as the patient wishes to have or can understand. When therapy is undertaken with curative intent, it is most important to emphasize that this is the goal in mind. Radical cancer surgery followed by radiotherapy or chemotherapy can be very arduous, and maintenance of morale is essential. When palliation is the objective, it is important not to remove the patient's hope, as 'the end of hope is the beginning of death.' It is usually best to speak to patients in a quiet, private room with one of the nursing staff present.

CARE OF THE DYING

Death from malignant disease is usually a gradual process of withdrawal. A sympathetic doctor can greatly help patients and their relatives. A dying patient must never feel abandoned in a surgical ward, and doctors and nursing staff must be prepared to spend time to help the patient die with dignity. In general, however, most patients die either at home (with support from palliative care nurses etc.) or in a hospice, where the level of quiet and care is appropriate to the situation. Early involvement of the hospice/palliative care team helps allay patient fears and optimize the control of distressing symptoms.

EBM 8.3   NEED FOR FOLLOW-UP

'The value of 'aggressive' follow-up of post-operative cancer patients is controversial. Some have shown that systematic post-operative follow-up using a variety of techniques such as tumour markers, regular radiology and endoscopy can increase the number of patients with recurrence that is amenable to further surgery with curative intent.'

Castells A, et al. Dis Colon and Rectum 1998; 41(6):273–714.

BOX 8.5   PRINCIPLES OF SURGERY FOR CANCER

- Multidisciplinary team approach
- Accurate pre-/post-operative staging
- En bloc radical surgery
- Appropriate pre-/post-operative adjuvant therapy
- Good communication with patient and relatives
- Audit of results

Palliative care of children with terminal malignant disease is becoming increasingly available in the UK. A number of children's hospices have now been established which offer this service and they have proven to be of great support, not only to affected children, but also to their parents and families.

9

C.E. ROBERTSON

D. MCKEOWN

Trauma and multiple injury

9

TRAUMA EPIDEMIOLOGY

The most common cause of death from birth to the fourth decade, and the fourth most common cause overall, is trauma. For individuals between 15 and 24 years, trauma leads to three times as many deaths as any other cause. On average, for individuals of working age, heart disease and cancer result in the loss of 10 years of potential life, but road traffic accidents (RTAs) alone cause the loss of 30–35 years. The economic cost is staggering. Patients with trauma occupy 10% of hospital beds and, globally, trauma accounts for 1–2% of gross national product.

However, experience of trauma cannot be extrapolated from other countries to predict events or outcomes. For example, in the UK, RTAs, falls and interpersonal violence account for the majority of major trauma (Fig. 9.1). Fewer than 1 in 10 patients with major trauma have penetrating injury, and this is usually caused by knives. In the USA, approximately 20% of the population owns a gun, and RTA deaths are matched by firearm injuries. Having a gun in the home increases the risk of homicide threefold, and that of suicide fivefold. For 15–24-year-olds, these figures increase by a factor of 10. A recent UK study found that the total number of homicides over a 2-year period for a population of 0.8 million was similar to that seen in a single day among the same-sized population of many American cities. In so-called developed countries, annually, 1 person in 50 will be involved in an RTA. Of these, 1% will die, 10% will need hospital treatment and 25% will be temporarily disabled.

It is often quoted that trauma deaths have a trimodal distribution. The first 'peak', representing deaths occurring immediately after or within a few seconds of injury, contributes up to 50% of the total. The second 'peak', up to 4 hours after injury, accounts for 30% of deaths, and the final 20% take place (usually in an intensive care unit) days or weeks after the event. Much significance has been placed upon this alleged temporal relationship, particularly the second peak. On the basis that interventions for the second group of patients offered great potential for preventing unnecessary deaths, the provision and nature of pre-hospital and hospital trauma services in the USA and the UK were changed profoundly. Unfortunately, the 'second peak' is a myth, at least in the UK, where the vast majority of deaths occur immediately after or within a very few minutes of injury. Furthermore, the subsequent deaths do not cluster into peaks. So, although attempts to improve care for those who initially survive must continue, the overwhelming message is that trauma prevention is far more important than any other aspect.

Trauma is a common cause of death and morbidity in children. After the first year of life, it is the most common cause of death in the paediatric population. The most common causes of serious injury seen in children are RTAs and falls. Non-accidental injury accounts for a significant number of the remainder.

The pattern of injury seen in children differs from that in adults. The small mass of the child is less able to disperse the kinetic energy of impact; as a consequence, multi-system injury is more common. The large paediatric head (in proportion to the rest of the body) means that head injuries are common. The larger body surface area to body mass results in increased heat loss after injury. There are often significant psychological sequelae to major trauma in children. It has been estimated that as many as 60% of such children are left with behavioural or learning difficulties after a serious accident.

INJURY BIOMECHANICS AND ACCIDENT PREVENTION

To anticipate the injuries from any given trauma event, the clinician must understand the biomechanics involved. An accurate history can identify or predict the great majority of an individual patient's injuries.

The magnitude of injury is related to the energy transferred to the victim during the event, the volume/area of tissue involved, and the time taken for the interaction. Tissue characteristics, such as elasticity, plasticity and fluid content, are also important. These factors are summarized in the formula:

$$\text{Injury magnitude} \propto C\frac{E}{TV}$$

where E = energy transfer, T = time, V = volume of tissue, and C = tissue factors (a constant).

Kinetic energy, the energy of motion, is proportional to the mass of the object but to the square of its velocity. This can have unexpected effects. For example, a pedestrian struck by a car of mass 700 kg travelling at 100 kph receives over three times more destructive energy than if hit by a heavy lorry of mass 5000 kg travelling at 40 kph. If the car travels at 160 kph, over 10 times the energy is involved. The longer the time frame during which the kinetic energy is transferred to the body, the less the acceleration/deceleration force sustained and the less the trauma that results.

These physical principles underpin strategies of accident prevention and protection. Obviously, reducing the chance

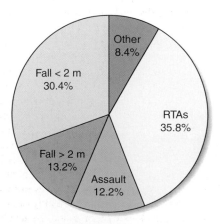

Fig. 9.1 Causes of trauma deaths.
(Data kindly provided by the Scottish Trauma Audit Group 1992–1999.)

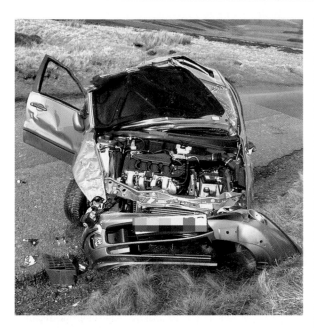

Fig. 9.2 Car involved in a high-speed, head-on collision, showing the magnitude of structural damage.

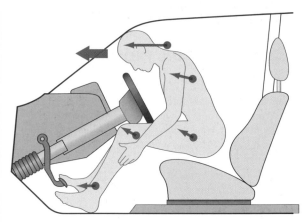

Fig. 9.3 Impact sites in an unrestrained head-on collision.

9

of direct contact helps; separating pedestrians and traffic is the single most important factor in reducing pedestrian injury rates. This is illustrated by the fact that, in the US, < 2% of traffic fatalities are pedestrians, whereas in the UK they account for 36% of the total. In a similar fashion, the central reservation barriers on motorways dramatically reduce the chances of high-speed head-on collisions (Fig. 9.2).

If impact does occur, then limitation of the velocities involved is the most important determinant in reducing injury. One in 10 drivers involved in RTAs travels inappropriately fast. Even a 1 mph (1.6 kph) reduction in *average* road speed reduces fatal accidents by 8%. The 20 mph (32 kph) zones in residential areas, together with traffic calming measures, significantly reduce deaths and serious injuries, in particular to children and the elderly.

Contact factors can be minimized by vehicle design: crumple zones, energy-absorbing materials, preventing the ejection of passengers from the vehicle and reducing intrusion into the passenger compartment. For the occupants, seatbelts, airbags, collapsible steering columns and soft fascia compartments enable contact deceleration to take place over a longer time period, reducing the potential for injury (Fig. 9.3). Properly used, seatbelts reduce the risk of death/serious injury by 45%. Airbags further reduce the risk of death by 10% for belted drivers, and by 20% for unbelted front-seat passengers, but may not provide protection from side-impact events, or if the vehicle rolls over.

These devices can also modify the patterns of injury, particularly if they are incorrectly positioned. Seatbelts and airbags do reduce deaths overall but certain injuries, e.g. sternal fractures and soft-tissue neck injuries, may be associated with their use. With lap belts, pancreatic, renal, splenic and liver injuries are increased and hyperflexion of the trunk over the belt can produce anterior compression fractures of the vertebrae. Finally, seatbelts are only protective when used. A recent study showed that 90% of rear-seat passengers were unrestrained. These passengers increase the severity of their own injuries, as well as causing injury to restrained individuals in the front seats.

ALCOHOL AND DRUGS

The message is often unwelcome, but few episodes of trauma are without direct human failing or causation (there is, for instance, a fourfold increase in the risk of being involved in an RTA while using a mobile telephone, a level similar to that seen when driving with a blood alcohol level at the legal limit).

The combination of youth, inexperienced motor skills, an innate belief in immortality and a powerful vehicle accounts for an extraordinarily high rate of events. Accident rates decline with increasing age and experience, but at the other end of the spectrum, the elderly have a disproportionately high incidence of trauma because of coexisting medical conditions and visual/motor impairments that affect judgement.

At all ages, alcohol is the major causal factor for all types of trauma; 60% of individuals sustaining trauma in assaults have consumed alcohol. For burns, homicides and drowning, alcohol is implicated in 30–50% of events. Its combination with young males and road vehicles is particularly lethal; in this group, one-third of all fatalities, and 10% of all injuries, involve alcohol consumption. Drink–driving laws do reduce the proportion of fatal crashes involving intoxicated drivers, but high-risk behaviour remains common. Although death rates from alcohol-related events have fallen, the risk of being involved in an accident with a blood alcohol at the current UK driving limit is twice that for an individual with no alcohol in their blood. At higher levels, the risk dramatically increases even further. About 20% of RTA deaths are related to drug or substance misuse, but the difficulties of testing and the involvement of prescribed medications, such as sedatives, are less completely evaluated.

WOUNDS

CLASSIFICATION AND PRODUCTION

- *Abrasions or grazes.* These are caused by the tangential application of blunt force. Dirt is often ingrained in the surface layers of skin, with the risk of short-term infection and, if untreated, later permanent 'tattooing'. The abrasion's site and nature may give useful clues as to the direction and magnitude of injury forces.
- *Contusions, ecchymoses or bruises.* These result from blunt force disrupting superficial capillaries. The overlying skin is intact. When small blood vessels are involved, a large collection of blood (haematoma) may develop. It is impossible to tell the age of a bruise accurately by its colour, but if it is yellow, the bruise is likely to be at least 18 hours old.
- *Lacerations.* Blunt forces tear, shear or crush skin and soft tissues, producing lacerations. The wound edges are irregular and often abraded or contused, as are the surrounding tissues.
- *Incised wounds or 'cuts'.* These are produced by sharp edges, such as knives or glass shards, and have characteristically clean edges with clear margins. The greatest dimension of an incised wound is its length (cf. puncture wound).
- *Puncture wounds.* Sharp points or edges produce puncture wounds, in which the greatest dimension is the depth. When the wound pierces a body cavity, it is 'penetrating'; if it passes through a viscus, it is 'perforating'.

GUNSHOT WOUNDS

Gunshot wounds (Fig. 9.4) highlight the gulf between UK and US practice. In the US, deaths from gunshot wounds are the fourth leading cause of years of potential life lost before the age of 65. Guns are used in over 60% of suicides

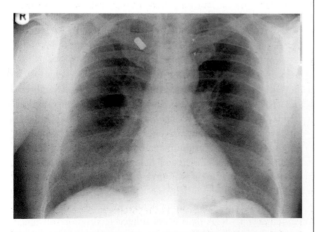

Fig. 9.4   Chest X-ray showing a bullet to the right of the upper mediastinum.
(Courtesy of Miss Kate Wilson.)

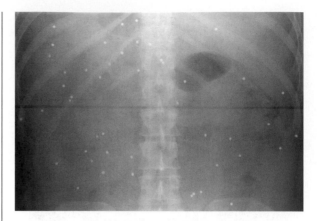

Fig. 9.5   X-ray of the lower chest and upper abdomen, showing pellets from a shotgun injury.
Note the wide dissipation of the pellets.

and 70% of all homicides. Non-fatal gunshot wounds outnumber the fatal ones two- to threefold.

As with other injury, the exchange of energy is crucial. Low-velocity missiles cause local injury, involving tissue tearing and compression. When velocities exceed 500–600 m/s, cavitation injury—a temporary space torn in tissues at right angles to the direction of travel—is also produced. This process develops in microseconds and, depending upon the body tissues involved and their elasticity, can involve a volume many times the diameter of the bullet itself. The wounding potential can be further magnified by features specifically designed to increase the area of injury and the release of energy; examples include bullets that tumble in tissues and others designed to deform or fragment on impact (dum-dum or semijacketed bullets).

Shotgun events are relatively more common in the UK than handgun or rifle injuries. The muzzle velocity of these weapons is relatively high, but dissipation of the shot and air resistance on the pellets quickly decrease their velocity and limit the wounding potential (Fig. 9.5). These weapons are lethal at close range but, unless 'choked', are relatively less wounding at greater distances, where they tend to cause superficial injury to skin and subcutaneous tissues.

FALLS

The major determinant of injury and the chance of death is directly proportional to the height fallen, as the accelerating force of gravity is constant. A body falling two storeys (10 m) has an impact velocity of ~50 kph. At impact, the deceleration forces are determined by the individual's mass, the nature of the landing surface and the body's orientation on landing. Surfaces such as mud, snow, soft earth and, to a lesser extent, water can permit an increased duration of impact, reducing deceleration forces and hence injury. For an 'average' man, a 5 m fall on to a concrete surface produces a deceleration force of approximately 700 g, but if the landing is onto a soft, yielding surface, the

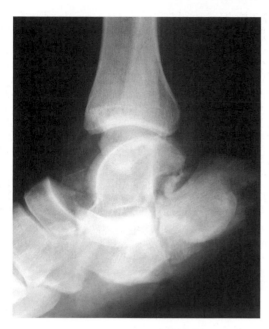

Fig. 9.6 Lateral view of ankle and grossly comminuted fracture of calcaneum, involving the subtalar joint.
The mechanism of injury was a fall on to the feet from 15 metres.

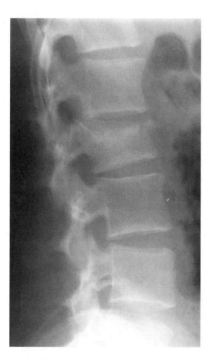

Fig. 9.7 Compression (wedge) fracture of the L2 vertebral body, caused by a fall from height.

area and hence less damage (Figs 9.6 and 9.7). Feet-first falls involve a relatively small area of contact, but deceleration forces can be reduced by flexing the knees and hips. Regardless of the position on landing, however, for falls > 5 m there is a high incidence of deceleration injuries to intrathoracic and intra-abdominal structures, particularly where these are relatively immobile or tethered: for example, the aortic root and the mesenteric arteries. Overall, a fall on to an unyielding surface from 15–20 m has a > 50% mortality.

INJURY SEVERITY ASSESSMENT

Audit of trauma patients, both individually and as a group, is essential. To allow objective comparison between systems or hospitals, injury classifications have become standardized.

Two types of classification are used. The first measures the severity of anatomical injury. The most commonly used system is the Abbreviated Injury Scale (AIS). Once the patient's injuries have all been identified (this may only be possible at discharge or autopsy), each separate injury is assessed from a scoring 'dictionary' and awarded a numerical score. The Injury Severity Score (ISS) is then derived from the three highest AIS scores within six body areas (head and neck, abdomen and pelvic contents, bony pelvis and limbs, face, chest and body surface). ISS provides an internationally recognized objective evaluation of anatomical injury.

The second type of classification is physiological. The best-known physiological scoring system is the Glasgow Coma Scale, which is used to assess the neurological state of injured patients objectively, and which also has prognostic value. The Glasgow Coma score (GCS), in conjunction with two other physiological recordings, systolic blood pressure and respiratory rate, can be used to produce the 'Revised Trauma Score'. Although widely used, physiological scoring systems have intrinsic problems. Some patients with severe injury may not be identified initially, usually because the assessment has been performed before detectable physiological compromise has had time to occur. The system may also overestimate injury severity if physiological changes occur (due, for example, to alcohol) that are not reflected in the measured parameters, or which modify these factors.

stopping distance may be several centimetres, decreasing the force 10–20-fold.

The body's position during landing affects the contact area and the propagation of energy since, if the same force is dissipated over a larger area, there is less force per unit

---

9

BOX 9.1 ACCIDENT FEATURES ASSOCIATED WITH MAJOR TRAUMA

- Death of another individual in the same accident
- High-velocity impact, e.g. pedestrian or cyclist (motor or pedal) struck at > 30 kph, or vehicle occupants in collisions with closing speeds > 60 kph
- Entrapment in or intrusion into the passenger compartment of the vehicle
- Ejection from a vehicle
- Falls from heights > 3 m
- Penetrating injury of the chest, abdomen or neck

The combination of anatomical and physiological scoring systems allows comparisons between predicted and actual patient outcomes. The impact of age, and factors such as whether the injury was blunt or penetrating, can be incorporated. This permits meaningful audit between hospitals and trauma systems.

PRE-HOSPITAL CARE AND TRANSPORT

The objective of pre-hospital care is to prevent further injury, initiate resuscitation and transport the patient safely and rapidly to the most appropriate hospital. The size and demographics of the population served, along with geographical constraints, affect this directly.

In the USA, basic trauma care is often provided by fire and police services. Emergency medical technicians and paramedics supply advanced care, with direct communication links to the receiving hospital. If their injuries are several or severe, or if there is a significant mechanism of injury, patients may bypass the nearest hospital and be taken directly to a designated trauma centre.

In the UK and Europe, ambulance services, augmented by physician-led teams, often transport the patient to the nearest hospital. In 1995, the Department of Health recommended the presence of a paramedic in each frontline ambulance. Paramedics can provide techniques such as tracheal intubation, peripheral intravenous access, and the administration of intravenous fluids and drugs. Intuitively, the use of such skills by ambulance paramedics at the scene of injury or en route to hospital should improve outcome for injured patients, but controlled studies have not demonstrated this. There are two main reasons for this surprising result. Firstly, paramedic treatment may increase pre-hospital time, delaying definitive care. Such delay is closely related to increases in mortality. Secondly, the techniques used may themselves have intrinsically adverse effects. For example, intravenous fluids given to patients in whom bleeding cannot be controlled (e.g. intraperitoneal bleeding, major vascular disruption, pelvic or long bone fractures) can precipitate additional blood loss by increasing blood pressure. Except for situations in which unavoidable delays will occur for a pre-hospital patient (usually entrapment or impalement, or rural or inaccessible locations), advanced pre-hospital techniques are inappropriate.

Transport from accident locus to hospital must be safe and rapid, with constant communication. In the UK, land-based ambulance service vehicles perform this, with additional support from helicopters and fixed-wing aircraft. Much experience has been obtained with helicopters in military medical environments, and in the USA and Australia; they dramatically increase costs and have additional risks for both patient and crew. Despite the potential to reduce journey times, the types of helicopter used in the UK have major operational difficulties with poor visibility, night-time flying, high winds and urban environments. Recent audit in an urban environment in the UK failed to show an improvement in response times, with longer on-scene times and no increase in survival for trauma patients. There is a clear justification for helicopter use in offshore and mountain rescue and in certain rural incident situations, but the majority of patients will continue to be transported by land ambulances.

TRAUMA CENTRES

A trauma patient should be provided with definitive surgical and intensive care facilities as soon as possible after injury. The problem is how to deliver this standard. In the 1970s and 1980s, trauma centres were introduced in the USA and a few European cities, where they unequivocally reduced preventable, in-hospital trauma deaths. Some of the results were remarkable, with 'avoidable' deaths reduced 5–10-fold for patients taken directly to a level 1 centre. The key elements in these systems were: transfer of patients from the accident scene directly to the centre; reception by senior staff on a 24-hour basis; the availability of all appropriate specialties on the same site; and a high throughput of patients.

Independent evaluation of the pilot trauma centre in England, however, failed to show a reduction in death rates. Two facts may explain this disappointing result. The first is the difference in trauma epidemiology, in relation to both the nature of the trauma and the volume of patients presenting. Secondly, despite having run for several years, the centre was not fully integrated into a comprehensive regionalized system (EBM 9.1). For the foreseeable future in the UK, the provision of care will be by a trauma team approach (Fig. 9.8).

RESUSCITATION IN THE ACCIDENT AND EMERGENCY DEPARTMENT

THE FIRST 10 MINUTES

The receiving department should have advance warning from ambulance control to permit an appropriate manpower and resource response. Advance information required by the trauma team includes:

- estimated time of arrival
- number, age and sex of patients
- nature of the incident and any special features, e.g. associated chemical/radioactive contamination, helicopter transportation etc.

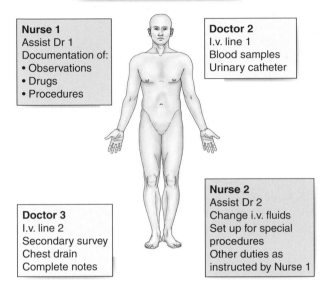

Doctor 1
Overall charge of case
Airway plus cervical spine control
Ventilation
Dictates order of priorities
Decides referral

Nurse 1
Assist Dr 1
Documentation of:
• Observations
• Drugs
• Procedures

Doctor 2
I.v. line 1
Blood samples
Urinary catheter

Doctor 3
I.v. line 2
Secondary survey
Chest drain
Complete notes

Nurse 2
Assist Dr 2
Change i.v. fluids
Set up for special
procedures
Other duties as
instructed by Nurse 1

Fig. 9.8   Trauma team organization.

• brief details of injuries, treatment given at the scene/in transit and current condition.

The resuscitation room must have all the equipment that will be needed for at least the first 1–2 hours of resuscitation. A calm, ordered approach is essential. Compliance with universal precautions for sharps/instruments disposal, and the use of gloves, face/eye protection and protective clothing is mandatory. All personnel must be appropriately immunized for hepatitis B.

If the number and severity of injured patients exceeds the facilities immediately available, the hospital's major incident plan may need to be activated. In this event, patients are triaged on arrival according to their priority for treatment.

During reception, a concise, relevant history is obtained from the ambulance crew and other emergency personnel, noting factors associated with an increased likelihood of severe injury. Digital camera images taken at the accident scene can help the receiving trauma team assess the mechanisms and forces involved and predict likely injuries.

A trauma team, consisting of 4–5 experienced doctors and nurses, is used for the patient's initial assessment and treatment (Fig. 9.8). Each team member has a pre-assigned role and performs this, unless directed otherwise by the team leader, who must have sufficient seniority and competence to direct and control the entire resuscitation process. The team members must be entirely familiar with the tasks required of them and perform them with minimal delay or questioning.

The patient's clothing is removed completely (cut off, if necessary, to avoid patient movement), allowing adequate

---

BOX 9.2   THE PRIMARY SURVEY

• **A**   Airway with cervical spine control
• **B**   Breathing with ventilation
• **C**   Circulation with haemorrhage control
• **D**   Neurological disability and pupils
• **E**   Exposure and environment

---

access for examination and to avoid missing an occult external injury. Injured patients lose their normal thermo-regulatory ability, so they must then be kept warm and excessive exposure for examination or practical procedures should be avoided.

A traditional surgical approach, with history taking, clinical examination, investigation and treatment, is inappropriate in major trauma patients. An 'ABC' approach is logical and easy to remember, but although the steps are presented here sequentially, the trauma team performs and constantly reassesses all of these aspects *simultaneously*.

Airway

The patency of the airway is first assessed by direct inspection, identifying and removing obstructions. Loose-fitting dentures or dental plates are removed. Noisy breathing, snoring or stridor implies airway obstruction. A rigid suction catheter, used carefully to avoid stimulation of the sensitive pharynx, will remove blood, vomit, secretions and other debris from the mouth and oropharynx. Larger items, e.g. lumps of food, are extracted with forceps under direct vision.

9

The most common cause of airway obstruction is a reduced conscious level, with the tongue falling back and blocking the oropharyx. Airway clearance, together with the 'chin-lift' or 'jaw-thrust' manoeuvres, will correct this in the majority of cases. The airway is then constantly reassessed by looking (to see the chest rise and fall), listening (for abnormal airway sounds) and feeling (for the patient's exhaled breath, using the side of the cheek or hand).

Assessment of conscious level helps in airway assessment. A patient speaking in complete sentences does not have an immediate airway problem (although one may develop later). The Glasgow Coma Scale can identify patients with established or potential problems and, if the score is < 8/15, usually mandates early definitive airway intervention, as the protective gag and swallow airway reflexes are likely to be absent or compromised. In the majority of cases, the upper airway is secured with simple positioning, regular suction and the use of basic adjuncts such as oro- or nasopharyngeal airways (Fig. 9.9).

Control of the cervical spine

Irrespective of the airway control technique used, the cervical cord is constantly protected by manual in-line cervical control with the neck in the neutral position, or by using a carefully fitted rigid neck collar, sandbags and tape.

Orotracheal intubation is the advanced technique of choice. It protects the airway from aspiration of vomit or blood, and allows ventilation with controlled levels of oxygen and airway suctioning to remove debris. It does, however, require expertise in using anaesthetic and neuro-muscular paralysing agents. Prior to intubation, the patient is pre-oxygenated and must be carefully monitored throughout the process. A 'surgical' airway is extremely rarely needed; if one is required, a percutaneous cricothy-rotomy is the simplest, safest and quickest surgical approach.

Advanced airway techniques

These are required when:

- protective airway reflexes are absent (usually caused by altered consciousness)
- basic techniques are unable to cope with current or predicted airway compromise (e.g. major facial or burns/inhalation injury)
- there is a need for controlled ventilation (e.g. head and/or chest injury).

Breathing

Optimal ventilation requires a patent upper and lower airway and effective function of the thoracic wall, lungs and diaphragm. Clinical assessment is extremely helpful. Respiratory compromise is characterized by tachypnoea or bradypnoea, the use of accessory muscles of respiration, and paradoxical (see-saw) movement of the chest and abdomen, indicating failure of normal diaphragmatic function. Hypoxia may be manifest by restlessness, tachycardia, confusion, agitation, pallor or sweating, but cyanosis is uncommon and difficult to detect clinically, particularly if hypovolaemia is present.

Concern about oxygen toxicity in the initial phase of resuscitation is unnecessary, and until the patient is stable and adequate tissue oxygen delivery has been confirmed, the highest possible concentration of oxygen must be given. Pulse oximeters can detect arterial desaturation, but readings are unreliable in hypovolaemic or shocked patients, or if abnormal haemoglobins (including carboxyhaemoglobin) are present. Pulse oximetry does not replace arterial blood gas analysis, as hypercapnoea can occur with normal SaO_2 levels.

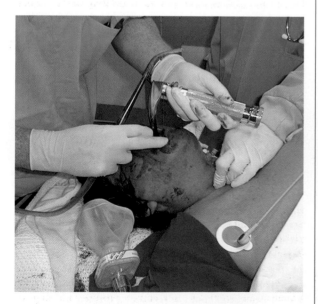

Fig. 9.9   Rapid-sequence intubation in a trauma patient.

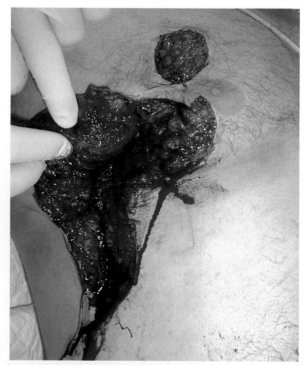

Fig. 9.10   Open (sucking) chest wound.

Clinical inspection, palpation and auscultation of the neck and chest (including the back) should detect immediately life-threatening injuries such as flail segment, penetrating wounds, tension or open pneumothoraces, major haemothorax and cardiac tamponade. These conditions need immediate treatment, e.g. needle thoracocentesis for tension pneumothorax, or the insertion of an intercostal drain for haemothorax. Open or sucking chest wounds (Fig. 9.10) are rare but, if present, allow equalization of atmospheric and intrathoracic pressures. With large defects, atmospheric air passes through the wound into the intrathoracic space with each inspiration, and the lung collapses. To prevent this, the open wound is covered with a sterile occlusive dressing, taped on three sides. This acts as a flutter valve, and formal tube thoracostomy is then performed at a separate site from the open wound.

Repeated arterial blood gas analyses are needed to ensure that hypoxia is not present and that alveolar ventilation is sufficient to prevent hypercapnoea. For patients who are intubated and ventilated, additional problems may develop. Positive-pressure ventilation may reduce cardiac output (manifest initially by tachycardia ± hypotension) because of decreased venous return to the heart, resulting from increased intrathoracic pressure during the 'inspiratory' phase of ventilation. The risk of pneumothorax (Table 9.1) in patients with coexisting chest injuries is markedly increased by positive-pressure ventilation. If a pneumothorax is already present, tension may be induced. For these reasons, tube thoracostomy is mandatory if a pneumothorax is present and positive-pressure ventilation, for whatever reason, is to be undertaken.

For patients in whom positive-pressure ventilation is instituted, the aim is to ensure adequate oxygenation (PaO_2 levels > 12 kPa) and alveolar ventilation ($PaCO_2$ levels 3.5–4 kPa). Controlled ventilation is particularly important in patients with head injury, as hypercarbia causes dilatation of the cerebral vessels and increased intracranial pressure, whereas hypocarbia produces cerebrovascular vasospasm, compromising cerebral perfusion.

The drugs needed to permit intubation and controlled ventilation may themselves obscure important clinical features, particularly of neurological or abdominal injury. Before any drugs are used, the patient's neurological status must be recorded. Additional imaging, such as computed tomography (CT), will be required if there is any suspicion of associated head injury. Abdominal injury is commonly missed in patients with altered consciousness of whatever

cause. Clinical signs are modified or absent in paralysed and sedated patients, and so additional investigations, such as ultrasound, CT or diagnostic peritoneal lavage, are important (see below).

Gastric dilatation is common in trauma patients. It results from a combination of factors, including air-swallowing (in conscious patients), bag–mask ventilation (where the airway pressure exceeds the gastro-oesophageal closing pressure), and the effects of sympathetic nervous system overactivity and electrolyte disturbance on gastric peristalsis. A distended stomach full of air, fluid and food in a patient with compromised airway protective reflexes is a situation ripe for regurgitation and potentially fatal aspiration. In addition, the distended stomach will restrict diaphragmatic movement and impair respiration. To prevent these problems, a nasogastric tube is routinely inserted and suction applied; if there is any suspicion of an anterior cranial fossa fracture, an *oro*gastric tube is used.

Circulation

The clinical detection of blood loss and the resulting haemodynamic effects is crude and non-specific. Pulse rate, cuff blood pressure and peripheral perfusion (assessed by capillary refill time) are routinely noted every 5–10 minutes in the initial stages, but these recordings have major limitations. Homeostatic mechanisms in previously fit healthy adults mean that, depending upon the rate and site of blood loss, 20% or more of total circulating blood volume can be lost without a measurable change in these recordings. Isolated readings are especially misleading. Trends in pulse rate and blood pressure are of much greater value. A rising pulse rate combined with a falling blood pressure strongly suggests uncontrolled, often occult, blood loss.

Absence of these features does not necessarily mean that all is well. The patient may not be able to respond to hypovolaemia by increasing the heart rate because of age, pre-existing cardiac disease or medications such as β-blockers. In addition, an individual's 'normal' values need to be considered. A blood pressure of 110/60 mmHg may represent severe hypotension if the patient's normal value is 190/120 mmHg, but may be normal for a healthy young adult. Unfortunately, this knowledge is rarely available in the early stages of resuscitation, and a high index of suspicion, bearing in mind the mechanism of injury, is therefore imperative.

To reduce blood loss is essential. External haemorrhage can invariably be controlled by simple direct pressure. Haemostasis from the sometimes profuse bleeding of scalp wounds is best achieved with carefully applied

---

Table 9.1 CLINICAL FEATURES OF TENSION PNEUMOTHORAX

- Cardiorespiratory distress (tachycardia, hypotension)
- Distended neck veins
- Reduced chest wall movement
- Hyper-resonant percussion note
- Absent or reduced breath sounds
- Tracheal deviation

BOX 9.3 COMMON CAUSES OF BREATHING AND VENTILATION PROBLEMS

- Airway obstruction
- Tension pneumothorax
- Massive haemothorax
- Flail chest
- Open (sucking) chest wound
- Cardiac tamponade

9

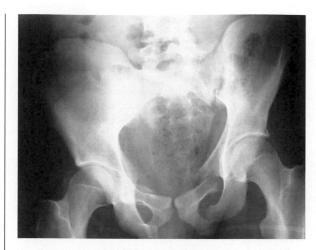

Fig. 9.12   X-ray of the pelvis, showing bilateral upper and lower pubic rami fractures, with 'butterfly' fragment and shearing injury affecting the left sacroiliac joint.

sutures. Splinting of long-bone fractures reduces blood loss from fracture sites by up to 50%, makes the patient more comfortable, and reduces analgesic requirements (Fig. 9.11). In contrast, blood loss into the peritoneal cavity, thorax or pelvis is usually concealed, can be life-threatening, and cannot be simply controlled. Patients with major pelvic fractures pose a difficult management problem, in that conventional splintage is impossible and massive and uncontrollable blood loss may result (Fig. 9.12). The optimal approach is the application of external fixator devices in the resuscitation phase, followed, if required, by angiographic embolization.

The next priority is to insert and secure two large-bore (12–14 G) intravenous cannulae. The forearms or antecubital fossae are the most accessible peripheral sites, but the nature and location of the injuries may require alternative sites, such as the femoral or external jugular veins, to be used. Central venous cannulation is difficult and potentially hazardous in shocked hypovolaemic patients, so if percutaneous access cannot be obtained, a surgical cut-down at the saphenofemoral junction at the groin is preferable, although more time-consuming. At the time of cannulation, initial venous blood samples should be taken, carefully labelled and sent for analysis, the laboratories having previously been alerted.

The effective resuscitation of the injured child requires an appreciation of the physiological differences that exist between children and adults. The normal cardiovascular and respiratory parameters vary with age. For example, the normal heart rate of a newborn infant is 160 beats/minute; the normal respiratory rate of a 1-year-old is about 30 breaths per minute. A knowledge of what is normal is required to allow the confident identification of the abnormal.

Suitable equipment is essential to resuscitate children of different ages and weights safely. Cuffed tracheal tubes are not used in small children. Small intravenous cannulae may be necessary and intraosseous needles can be used for vascular access in children under 6 years of age. Different-sized cervical collars, oxygen face masks, laryngoscopes and other equipment should be readily available in any resuscitation room receiving children.

Notwithstanding the above, the ABCDE sequence of resuscitation that is followed in the child is the same as that in the adult: *a*irway with cervical spine control, *b*reathing with oxygen, *c*irculation with control of bleeding, *d*isability, *e*xposure.

The choice of fluids for the replacement of traumatic blood loss is controversial and poorly understood. Intravenous volume replacement is begun with infusion of an isotonic crystalloid such as 0.9% saline or Ringer's lactate. In the UK, after 1000–2000 ml of crystalloid, a colloid is commonly given prior to, or together with, blood. Theoretically, colloids (such as albumin solutions, gelatins, starches or dextrans) might be expected to be more effective, but there is no good evidence to suggest this in clinical practice.

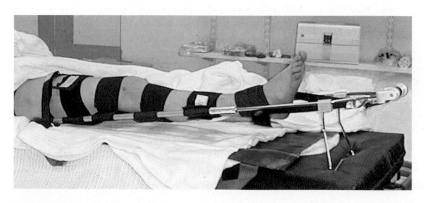

Fig. 9.11   Right lower limb in a traction device to provide splintage.

BOX 9.5   INITIAL BLOOD SAMPLES IN THE TRAUMA PATIENT

- Blood grouping and cross-matching
- Full blood count and haematocrit
- Urea and electrolytes
- Plasma glucose
- Arterial blood gases
- Kleihauer–Betke analysis (in pregnant patients)

BOX 9.6   MONITORING THE TRAUMA PATIENT

- Heart rate
- Blood pressure (cuff and intra-arterial)
- Capillary refill
- Respiratory rate
- Glasgow Coma Scale
- Urine output
- ECG
- Pulse oximetry
- Core temperature

Irrespective of the fluid chosen, it must be warmed to 37–38°C before infusion to prevent hypothermia and aggravating coagulation deficits. This is achieved with in-line warming devices that infuse the fluid at the required temperature, regardless of flow rate.

Intravenous fluid administration is initially dictated by the nature of the patient's injuries, an estimate of the current volume deficit, and the clinical and haemodynamic responses to treatment. Failure to respond to the first 1–2 litres of volume replacement suggests that the volume deficit is great (> 40% of circulating volume). It is, however, inappropriate to correct haemodynamic measurements in isolation, and there are situations where, in the presence of an uncontrolled bleeding site (for example, in the pelvis or peritoneum), increasing blood pressure will simply exacerbate blood losses.

Blood transfusion requirements depend upon the magnitude of blood loss and the physiological response. It is usual to replace losses with the aim of maintaining the patient's haematocrit at ~30%. Where there is immediately life-threatening haemorrhage, group O Rhesus-negative blood is given, but more usually fully cross-matched or type-specific blood can be supplied. Most transfusion services supply packed red cells. There is no evidence that 'fresh' whole blood is preferable. In situations of massive blood loss, where replacement of more than the equivalent of one circulating blood volume is needed, coagulation problems should be anticipated. Close liaison with the Blood Transfusion Service and haematology laboratories is essential, and platelet concentrates and coagulation factors are given on their guidance rather than purely on an empirical basis.

Measurement of urine output (> 1 ml/kg body weight/hr normally implies adequate renal perfusion), continuous intra-arterial blood pressure monitoring and serial lactate levels assist in monitoring the response to infusion. In this situation, intra-arterial blood pressure monitoring is significantly more accurate than standard cuff methods, and has the additional advantage that the in-dwelling cannula permits regular arterial blood sampling without additional patient discomfort. Continuous electrocardiogram (ECG) monitoring, oxygen saturation (by pulse oximetry), core temperature and serial blood pressure measurements are standard requirements and augment clinical judgement. A low or falling GCS may indicate cerebral hypoperfusion due to hypovolaemia or worsening intracranial injury. More sophisticated means of cardiovascular assessment can provide additional information and should be used at an early stage, but techniques such as central venous and pulmonary artery wedge pressure and cardiac output measurement are usually impracticable in the immediate resuscitative phase. They will be used later, particularly if vasoactive agents such as vasopressors or inotropes are employed.

Analgesia

A calm, gentle and reassuring approach does much to relieve anxiety and is the first step in pain relief. Adequate analgesia is often neglected—or worse, thought to be unnecessary or hazardous in trauma patients. Physiological responses to pain produce adverse effects—for example, by increasing intracranial and arterial pressure—and so analgesia is essential. Further, it must be given according to the patient's individual requirements, rather than as a rigid process.

In cooperative, fully conscious patients without respiratory problems, Entonox (50% nitrous oxide, 50% oxygen) is useful for short-duration procedures such as manipulations. Its value is limited by the need for patient cooperation (the euphoric effect may be associated with confusion and disorientation), its short duration of action and its limited analgesic effect.

Opioid drugs such as morphine or diamorphine, given in small intravenous (*never* intramuscular) doses titrated to effect, together with an anti-emetic (e.g. cyclizine), are unsurpassed for analgesia. Provided the drug is given like this, haemodynamic disturbance or respiratory depression is rare. The newer synthetic opioids have no advantages and non-steroidal analgesics are contraindicated.

Head injury or suspected head injury is not an *absolute* contraindication to opioid administration, provided that the agent is given as above and that the patient's airway, ventilation and haemodynamic status are carefully monitored. If necessary, naloxone can be given, if there is doubt as to whether alterations in conscious level are due to the opioid or to the head injury and its effects.

Local anaesthetic techniques are generally of limited value in the early management of major trauma, but an exception is the use of a femoral nerve block for patients with femoral shaft fractures. Long-bone fractures need to be immobilized to reduce pain and blood loss from the fracture site, to facilitate the taking of X-rays, patient movement and transfer, and to reduce the chances of fat embolism syndrome. Inflatable or foam-cushioned splints are suitable for upper-limb or below-knee injuries; adjustable traction splints are best for femoral fractures.

THE NEXT PHASE

The above assessments and interventions represent only the immediately life-saving procedures and should occupy just the first 10 minutes after arrival in the emergency department. Then, provided the patient's condition permits, a more detailed history and examination is undertaken, with appropriate laboratory and imaging investigations to determine the full extent of the patient's injuries and the requirement for surgery or other care. This review, or secondary survey, should enable a definitive management plan to be formulated. Throughout, the continuing priorities of *a*irway, *b*reathing and *c*irculation must be constantly reviewed and corrected as necessary.

The patient is examined from top to toe to ensure that no wound, bruise or swelling is missed. The back and spine are examined with the patient 'log-rolled', looking specifically for localized tenderness, swelling, bruising or a 'step'. The perineum is examined and a rectal examination performed (Table 9.2).

The neurological status of the patient is recorded regularly, including the GCS, pupil sizes and reactions, and any focal deficit (Table 9.3). The ears, nose and mastoid areas are carefully examined for evidence of skull-base injury, such as blood/cerebrospinal fluid otorrhoea or

BOX 9.7 CAUSES OF EARLY NEUROLOGICAL DETERIORATION IN THE TRAUMA PATIENT
Intracranial
Haematoma Cerebral oedema Fitting
Extracranial
Hypoxia Hypotension Hyper-/hypocarbia Hyper-/hypoglycaemia
Drugs

Table 9.4 ASSESSING MUSCLE POWER: THE MRC SCALE	
● No flicker of movement	0
● A flicker of contraction, but no movement	1
● Movement, with gravity neutralized	2
● Movement against gravity	3
● Movement against added resistance	4
● Normal power	5

rhinorrhoea, or bruising. Muscle power should be tested and recorded using the MRC (Medical Research Council) scale (Table 9.4), and the tendon reflexes examined. It is vital to test sensation in a methodical fashion (Fig. 9.13). The perineal area must be included (this is most easily achieved at the time of rectal examination), as the lowest (sacral) dermatomes are in this area.

Any decrease in the patient's conscious level (i.e. a numerical fall in GCS) must prompt an immediate search for, and correction of, a primary cause, such as intracranial haematoma, or secondary factors such as hypoxia, hypercarbia, hypotension or hypoglycaemia. Confounding factors may render the assessment of the GCS difficult, especially if the patient has taken alcohol or other drugs, but altered consciousness or other neurological deficit should never be assumed to be due solely to alcohol or other drugs alone until proven otherwise.

IMAGING AND OTHER DIAGNOSTIC AIDS

The radiological investigations needed in the initial phase of the management of a major trauma patient are limited but important. It is important to obtain the best-quality views, and fixed overhead X-ray facilities in the resuscitation room itself are invaluable, as transfer of the patient to a main X-ray department can be hazardous. A portable machine brought to the resuscitation room is preferable to transfer, although the images obtained will be of poorer quality.

There are three primary X-ray views in the blunt trauma patient, but these do have limitations:

● The *chest X-ray* may demonstrate thoracic injuries previously unrecognized on clinical examination, but

Table 9.2 RECTAL EXAMINATION IN THE TRAUMA PATIENT
● Anal sphincter tone ● Prostate: position, bogginess ● Blood in the rectum ● Pelvic fractures ● Perineal injury

Table 9.3 GLASGOW COMA SCALE	
Eyes open	
● Spontaneously	4
● To verbal command	3
● To pain	2
● No response	1
Best motor response **To verbal command**	
● Obeys verbal command	6
To painful stimulus	
● Localizes pain	5
● Flexion withdrawal	4
● Abnormal flexion (decorticate rigidity)	3
● Extension (decerebrate rigidity)	2
● No responses	1
Best verbal response	
● Orientated and converses	5
● Disorientated and converses	4
● Inappropriate words	3
● Incomprehensible sounds	2
● No response	1
Total number of points (minimum 3, maximum 15)	

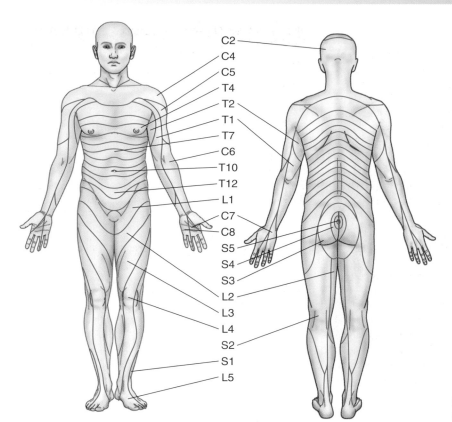

Fig. 9.13   Mannikin showing the sensory dermatomes.

9

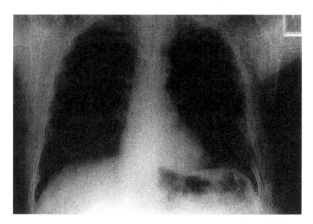

Fig. 9.14   Chest X-ray showing rib fractures and subcutaneous emphysema.

to T1. This provides valuable information on acute bony injury (Fig. 9.15), but a 'normal' neck X-ray does not exclude significant injury to soft tissues, including the cervical cord.

- On a *plain antero-posterior view of the pelvis*, injuries to the posterior elements are difficult to see (especially around the sacroiliac regions, which may lead to significant occult haemorrhage).

The use of additional imaging techniques depends upon their availability and the clinical state of the patient. For head, spinal and pelvic injury, CT is unsurpassed and rapid. In contrast to the information provided by conventional skull X-rays (Fig. 9.16), CT defines the nature and magnitude of the intracranial insult (Fig. 9.17). It is therefore invaluable in providing the information the

even on a good-quality erect view over half of the rib fractures actually present will be missed (Fig. 9.14). The patient's condition often precludes an erect film, and on a supine view pneumothoraces and/or haemothoraces are difficult to detect; even in the absence of pathology, the mediastinal contours are displaced and widened.

- The *lateral view of the cervical spine* should be a cross-table film and must include *all* of the vertebrae from C1

BOX 9.8   INITIAL X-RAYS IN THE PATIENT WITH BLUNT TRAUMA

- Chest (an *erect* film, provided that this can be performed safely)
- Cervical spine
- Pelvis
- Thoracic/lumbar spine views are indicated in patients with a mechanism of injury consistent with spinal injury, altered consciousness or distal neurological abnormality, or where other injuries or conditions, e.g. alcohol/drug use, may prevent the identification of spinal injury

9

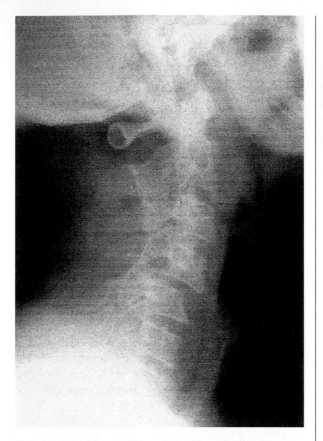

Fig. 9.15 Lateral X-ray of the cervical spine, showing C4/5 subluxation.

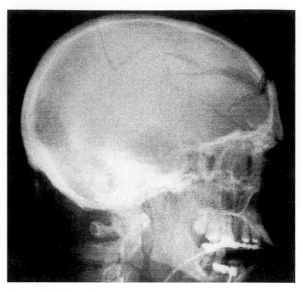

Fig. 9.16 Lateral X-ray of the skull, showing a fracture.

A

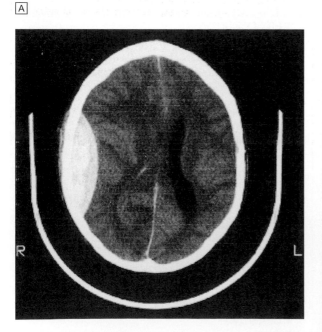

B

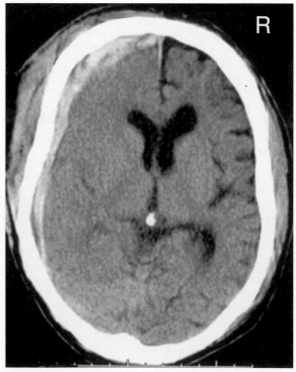

Fig. 9.17 Computed tomography in head injury.
A Right-sided extradural haematoma with midline shift. B Left-sided subdural haematoma.

physician needs to determine the requirement for neuro-surgical intervention.

In experienced hands, ultrasound examination of the abdomen is a quick, non-invasive and accurate method of detecting free intraperitoneal fluid. It can be performed in the resuscitation room and has largely supplanted diagnostic peritoneal lavage, although this technique remains a simple and rapid method for establishing the presence of intraperitoneal bleeding. Injury to some solid organs, the retroperitoneum and hollow viscera is less easily demonstrated on ultrasound, and CT—with contrast as necessary—is preferable, provided that the patient is stable and can be transferred safely to the CT suite.

AFTER THE RESUSCITATION ROOM

The immediate aim of the resuscitation team is to assess and treat life-threatening injuries. There is no absolute guide as to the length of time this process will take, but the procedures and referral must be performed expediently, without compromising patient care. The result should be a patient with a patent airway and adequate gas exchange, whose circulatory status is normal or in the process of being adequately corrected. Long-bone fractures should have been splinted appropriately and cervical spine control maintained throughout.

Continuing care then involves identifying the correct destination for the patient. The nature and extent of the injuries and the patient's physiological response to treatment dictate this. In some situations, it is impossible to 'stabilize' the patient without immediate surgical intervention. Examples include patients with exsanguinating intra-abdominal or intrathoracic haemorrhage, in whom immediate laparotomy or thoracotomy is mandated.

More commonly, the patient is, at least temporarily, stable so that further investigation can be undertaken beyond the resuscitation room prior to definitive surgical or intensive care unit admission. Senior anaesthetic and surgical staff must accompany the patient in these situations, so that, if sudden deterioration occurs, the patient can be transferred directly to theatre. Full monitoring and resuscitation equipment is mandatory for the transfer.

The subsequent destination of the patient then depends upon their overall condition and the findings of these investigations. Intensive care admission is required if ventilation is needed or anticipated, if there are multiple injuries involving main systems, or if the patient needs invasive monitoring. Stable, self-ventilating patients with less severe injuries may be managed in a high-dependency unit, but the attending staff must be familiar with multiple trauma assessment and the relevant specialties must liaise closely to ensure a multidisciplinary approach.

It may be necessary to transfer the patient to another hospital for emergency investigation not available in the receiving hospital, or as part of definitive treatment by a specialist service. Interhospital, and intrahospital, transfer is hazardous and must be performed by experienced anaesthetic and nursing staff with relevant monitoring and resuscitation equipment. The aspects of airway, ventilation and circulation control must be secured prior to transfer. The receiving unit must be informed of the relevant patient details, allowing it to prepare effectively for his or her arrival. The notes, details of investigations, X-rays, scans and observation charts must accompany the patient. The type of transport used will depend upon the distance and geography of the journey involved, but may involve air transportation with all its attendant specific considerations. Regular updates should be supplied to the receiving specialist.

BOX 9.9 INFORMATION REQUIRED BY THE RECEIVING UNIT OR HOSPITAL

- Patient's name, age and sex
- Previous health status and medications (if known)
- Pulse, blood pressure and respiratory rate (at scene, on arrival and current)
- Glasgow Coma Scale (at scene, on arrival and at present)
- Summary of injuries, including signs of head injury and any lateralizing signs
- Summary of i.v. fluids (including blood), and the haemodynamic and urine output responses
- X-ray, CT or other imaging results
- Blood grouping/cross-matching, haematology and biochemistry results
- Tetanus status/cover provided, antibiotics and other drugs given (include doses and timing)

Section 2
THE OPERATION

10

T.S. WALSH
A.J. POLLOK
J.A. WILSON

Pre-operative assessment, anaesthesia and post-operative pain control

PRE-OPERATIVE ASSESSMENT AND INVESTIGATIONS

The first part of this chapter describes the pre-operative assessment of patients undergoing surgery, and the relevance of pre-existing conditions to perioperative patient management. This includes general principles of assessment and issues specific to certain diseases.

ASSESSMENT OF FITNESS FOR OPERATION

Assessment takes place at several points. A preliminary assessment of fitness may be given by the GP in the referral letter. Thereafter, the surgeon will evaluate the patient at the outpatient clinic, when specific investigations may be organized. The surgeon may request an anaesthetic review prior to admission to hospital, particularly in patients considered to have a high perioperative risk. In some hospitals, patients are seen at a pre-admission clinic several days before surgery, where a history is taken and relevant examination and investigations are performed. The anaesthetist may review patients at the pre-admission clinic or after admission to hospital. Increasingly, patients are admitted on the day of surgery and so most assessment and preparation must be completed on an outpatient basis or during earlier hospital admissions. After admission, a further assessment of fitness for surgery and anaesthesia is made. It is important that any remaining essential investigations are performed immediately following admission to avoid delays in surgery.

The decision regarding fitness for surgery is made by the surgeon and anaesthetist. The recognition of patients with significantly increased perioperative risk is a fundamental part of pre-operative assessment. In these cases, liaison with the anaesthetist prior to admission will reduce unnecessary delays before surgery. Few patients require admission to hospital more than 24–48 hours before surgery if the appropriate investigations have been anticipated and performed.

Following hospital admission, the patient should undergo a history and clinical examination, even if these were carried out at a pre-admission clinic, in order to detect recent relevant changes in condition. The availability of the patient's notes should be checked and outstanding investigations organized. The anaesthetist should be consulted when there is uncertainty about the need for additional investigations. It is important to ensure that the patient and relatives are informed about the diagnosis and that they understand the nature and implications of the operation that is proposed. A more detailed explanation and discussion of the operation, and its associated risks and benefits, is undertaken by the surgeon prior to completion of the operation consent form.

The anaesthetist usually visits the patient on the evening before or on the day of surgery. He or she will take a history and perform a clinical examination with an emphasis on the factors most relevant to anaesthesia. An explanation of the proposed anaesthetic, along with the plan for early post-operative care and analgesia, is given. At this point, the patient should have the opportunity to voice any concerns and obtain reassurance. When appropriate, the various options for anaesthesia and post-operative analgesia can be discussed and the patient's preferences taken into account.

PERIOPERATIVE RISK

The aim of pre-operative assessment is to ensure the patient's physical condition is optimal in order to minimize risk. Patients require both physical and psychological preparation, and need to be fully informed about the procedure and its risks. For emergency surgery, compromises may have to be made for some aspects of preparation, and these should be balanced against the risks of delaying surgery.

Perioperative risk can be considered to have several components (Fig. 10.1). A logical sequence for assessment of fitness for surgery and anaesthesia is shown in Figure 10.2 and considered in detail below. Once an assessment of risk has been made by the surgeon and the anaesthetist, this needs to be balanced against the indication for and urgency of surgery, and discussed with the patient. For example, it is usual to accept a higher risk for a patient requiring urgent cancer surgery than for one requiring elective varicose vein surgery. In children, the coexistence of a congenital or genetic abnormality or the long-term effects of prematurity (including respiratory disease and cerebral palsy) may have a major impact on the safe provision of general anaesthesia.

Direct surgical risk
Technical problems with surgery and anaesthesia
Surgical complications, e.g. wound infection
Can be measured from audit of practice or from published data

---

Physiological stress of surgery
Mostly involves the cardiovascular and respiratory systems
Often difficult to predict. Depends on the nature of the surgery, the technical success of surgery, and the physiological fitness or reserve of the patient

---

Psychological
Anxiety in relation to proposed surgery and anaesthesia
Sources of anxiety may be unexpected; for example, a patient may have little concern about the surgery itself but be terrified of post-operative nausea or of being 'aware' during the operation

---

Fig. 10.1 Areas of perioperative risk.

10

10

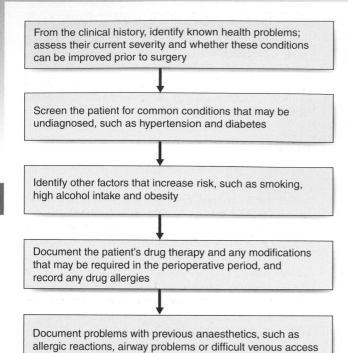

From the clinical history, identify known health problems; assess their current severity and whether these conditions can be improved prior to surgery

Screen the patient for common conditions that may be undiagnosed, such as hypertension and diabetes

Identify other factors that increase risk, such as smoking, high alcohol intake and obesity

Document the patient's drug therapy and any modifications that may be required in the perioperative period, and record any drug allergies

Document problems with previous anaesthetics, such as allergic reactions, airway problems or difficult venous access

Fig. 10.2 A logical approach to assessing perioperative and anaesthetic risk.

THE IMPORTANCE OF OXYGEN TRANSPORT TO TISSUES

Assessing cardiovascular and respiratory status is central to assessing risk, because many serious complications of anaesthesia result from inadequate supply of oxygen to tissues.

The delivery of oxygen to tissues requires the efficient transfer of oxygen from the lungs into blood, an adequate concentration of functioning haemoglobin to transport oxygen, and satisfactory cardiac output and blood pressure to transport oxygen from the lungs to the tissues. The tissue oxygen delivery of an individual can be calculated from the equation below:

$$DO_2 = CO \times CaO_2$$

where DO_2 is the oxygen delivery to tissues, CO is the cardiac output, and C_aO_2 is the oxygen content of arterial blood. The C_aO_2 can be calculated using the equation:

$$CaO_2 = (k_1 \times Hb \times SaO_2) + (k_2 \times PaO_2)$$

where Hb is the haemoglobin concentration (g/l), S_aO_2 is the arterial Hb oxygen saturation, P_aO_2 is arterial oxygen partial pressure, and k_1 and k_2 are constant values, depending what measurement units are used. These parameters are all measured by most blood gas analysis machines. In health, > 98% of oxygen is bound to haemoglobin and so the dissolved oxygen is relatively unimportant. The constant k1 is the amount of oxygen that 1 gram of pure haemoglobin can bind under ideal conditions and is usually 1.34 ml/g. It follows from this that the oxygen content of arterial blood depends on the haemoglobin concentration and arterial oxygen saturation. An average resting adult who is awake requires approximately 250 ml oxygen per minute. During anaesthesia, this decreases to about 175 ml. Oxygen delivery is normally approximately 1000 ml/min, so there is a considerable safety margin. A reduction in one parameter alone may not significantly reduce the oxygen delivery, but a reduction in all three (cardiac output, haemoglobin concentration and arterial oxygen saturation) can result in a profound decrease in oxygen delivery and cause critical organ ischaemia. The response of tissues to decreasing oxygen delivery is to compensate by increasing the amount of oxygen removed during the passage of blood through the organ (increasing oxygen extraction). Most organs can extract up to about 50–60% of the oxygen in arterial blood, but this critical oxygen extraction ratio varies widely from organ to organ. If the critical oxygen extraction ratio is exceeded, tissue hypoxia occurs, and cells must switch to anaerobic metabolism to generate energy.

Many factors alter the transport of oxygen to tissues during the perioperative period. Some cannot be anticipated, but factors such as chronic cardiovascular and respiratory disease or severe anaemia increase the likelihood of reduced oxygen delivery, particularly if these diseases are not optimally managed prior to surgery. Anaesthetic agents and techniques can alter cardiovascular function and gas exchange, and so pre-operative assessment enables the anaesthetist to choose the technique best suited to the patient.

SYSTEMATIC APPROACH TO THE INITIAL ASSESSMENT OF PATIENTS

CARDIOVASCULAR SYSTEM

History and examination

Angina indicates significant coronary artery disease. Exertional dyspnoea, orthopnoea and paroxysmal nocturnal dyspnoea suggest left ventricular failure, particularly if associated with ankle oedema. A history of blackouts or faints may indicate dysrhythmias, valvular heart disease or postural hypotension. Recent myocardial infarction is very important (see below). Routine examination should detect undiagnosed dysrhythmia (for example, atrial fibrillation), heart murmurs or hypertension.

Investigations

Patients with known cardiovascular disease should have a pre-operative electrocardiogram (ECG). ECG is worthwhile in patients at risk from cardiac disease: for example, the elderly, people with diabetes or patients with renal failure. The chance of detecting an important abnormality is low, but the pre-operative ECG provides a baseline against which to compare any subsequent tracings. There is little value in performing routine ECG examinations in other groups of patients. In some centres, pre-operative cardiopulmonary exercise testing is used to stratify perioperative risk and plan perioperative management.

In patients with symptoms of left ventricular or congestive cardiac failure, an erect postero-anterior chest X-ray (CXR) will detect cardiomegaly and left ventricular

---

BOX 10.1 HISTORY, SYMPTOMS AND SIGNS ASSOCIATED WITH HIGH PERIOPERATIVE CARDIOVASCULAR RISK

- Myocardial infarction within the past 6 months
- Poor left ventricular function
- Poorly controlled cardiac failure
- Resting diastolic blood pressure > 110 mmHg
- Poorly controlled/untreated arrhythmia
- Age > 70
- Significant aortic stenosis

---

failure. Occasionally, a transthoracic echocardiogram may be indicated to assess valve and cardiac function. Cardiac dysrhythmias that are identified during the course of the systematic enquiry or clinical examination or by ECG should be fully investigated prior to surgery, and may require a cardiologist's opinion. The significance of some common dysrhythmias is listed in Table 10.1. The perioperative management of the patient with a pacemaker is discussed below.

10

RESPIRATORY SYSTEM

History and examination

The recent onset or a change in severity of cough, sputum, wheeze or breathlessness suggests acute respiratory disease or a change in the severity of a chronic condition. In patients with known chronic obstructive pulmonary disease (COPD), asthma or fibrotic lung disease, a productive cough, increased and/or purulent sputum or fever suggests chest infection. Asthmatic patients can usually compare their current to their optimum status in terms of wheeze, dyspnoea and limitations in daily activity. It is useful to document whether patients have ever required oral steroid therapy, admission to hospital or mechanical ventilation, as these indicate more severe disease.

The severity of dyspnoea is one of the best indicators of the functional reserve of the patient's lungs. The simplest way of assessing dyspnoea is to relate it to everyday activities. It is useful to document how far patients can walk on the flat, up hills or up stairs. In patients who report significant exercise limitation, it should be confirmed that this is due to dyspnoea rather than other disease, such as angina or peripheral vascular disease. Where the history suggests significant exercise limitation due to dyspnoea, investigations of respiratory function are indicated.

Patients in the acute phase of a viral infection should have their surgical procedure delayed if possible, particularly if pyrexia, chest signs or an elevated white cell count are present. Acute viral illness is associated with an increased risk of bronchospasm in the perioperative period, and of post-operative chest infection. Chest infection is more likely because pulmonary epithelium already affected by viral infection is more susceptible to secondary bacterial infection. The majority of general anaesthetic drugs inhibit the ciliary action of the airways, predisposing the patient to post-operative pulmonary complications.

Table 10.1 SIGNIFICANCE OF COMMON ARRHYTHMIAS IN THE PERIOPERATIVE PERIOD

Arrhythmia	Significance
Uncontrolled atrial fibrillation	Exclude metabolic causes, e.g. electrolyte abnormality, thyrotoxicosis. May compromise cardiovascular function. Ventricular rate should be controlled prior to surgery
Controlled atrial fibrillation	Rarely causes severe perioperative problems unless associated with other significant heart disease. Patient may be on anticoagulants; if not, consider thromboprophylaxis
Ventricular extrasystoles	Usually of little significance. May indicate ischaemia in patients with ischaemic heart disease
First-degree heart block	Little significance
Asymptomatic bi- or trifascicular block or asymptomatic second-degree heart block	Previously considered an indication for temporary pacemaker insertion. Now usually managed by careful monitoring in the perioperative period
Third-degree heart block	Requires pacemaker insertion prior to anaesthesia

Investigations

Clear or white sputum suggests the absence of pus cells or infection, but yellow or green sputum is suspicious and should be sent for bacteriological examination. Patients are often aware themselves if sputum production is increased or more purulent. Acute exacerbations merit appropriate antibiotic therapy, chest physiotherapy and rescheduling of surgery.

In patients with known pulmonary disease, a CXR will exclude potentially serious complications such as consolidation, collapse or pleural effusion. In this situation, the pre-operative CXR also provides a useful baseline against which to compare post-operative changes. In patients without pre-existing pulmonary disease, the routine pre-operative CXR is of no value for assessing pulmonary function and rarely gives additional information. Its sensitivity for detecting undiagnosed lung conditions is also low.

Pulmonary function tests give information about the severity of lung disease and the reversibility of any obstructive component. There is no indication for pulmonary function tests in patients without lung disease or significant pulmonary symptoms, except in some specific situations, such as before thoracic surgery. The commonly performed respiratory function tests and their meaning are listed in Table 10.2. Although they are frequently used, their predictive value for post-operative complications is low.

A simple non-invasive method of assessing hypoxaemia is to measure the oxygen saturation by pulse oximetry. Because of the shape of the haemoglobin–oxygen dissociation curve, the PaO_2 is unlikely to be less than 8 kPa if the haemoglobin–oxygen saturation is > 92%. Arterial blood gases are useful for assessing some patients. Modern blood gas analysers measure the partial pressure of oxygen and carbon dioxide, and the hydrogen ion concentration. Other variables are calculated or derived (Table 10.3). Some indications for blood gas analysis in the pre-operative period are shown in Table 10.4. Perioperative risk increases with the severity of hypoxaemia. Following major surgery to the abdomen or thorax, PaO_2 decreases even in normal individuals unless supplemental oxygen is administered. Hypoxaemia is also more severe when post-operative analgesia is inadequate. The importance of adequate post-operative analgesia is discussed later in the chapter.

Patients with respiratory failure are at particular risk from anaesthesia and surgery. A minority of these patients rely on hypoxic drive rather than $PaCO_2$ for ventilation, and increased concentrations of inspired oxygen may result in hypoventilation and worsening respiratory failure. These patients have a very high risk of severe post-operative pulmonary complications such as pneumonia and respiratory failure, and frequently require ventilatory support and intensive care.

SMOKING

All patients should be informed of the risks associated with smoking and advised to stop prior to surgery, preferably at the initial clinic visit. Many patients are unwilling or unable to stop simply because a decision to operate has been made. However, there are significant benefits for the patient from even short-term cessation in the pre-operative period (Table 10.5).

Table 10.2 COMMON RESPIRATORY FUNCTION TESTS CARRIED OUT PRIOR TO SURGERY

Test	Meaning
FEV_1 (forced expiratory volume in 1 second)	Integrated measure of airflow limitation and respiratory muscle strength. If < 50% predicted or FEV_1 < 1 litre, indicates severe pulmonary disease
FVC (forced vital capacity)	Integrated measure of lung volume and respiratory muscle strength < 50% predicted values indicates severe pulmonary disease
FEV_1/FVC ratio	A measure of airway obstruction (normal value > 75%). If < 75%, reversibility to bronchodilator therapy should be tested
PEFR (peak expiratory flow rate)	Assesses airway obstruction. If < 70% predicted, suggests significant lung disease
Gas transfer factor (usually with carbon monoxide; T_{co} and K_{co})	An estimate of the lungs' overall ability to exchange gases. Any reduction over predicted values indicates reduced lung reserve

Table 10.3 BLOOD GAS PARAMETERS

	Normal range	Meaning
MEASURED VARIABLES		
PaO_2	12–15 kPa	Partial pressure of oxygen in arterial blood
$PaCO_2$	4.4–6.1 kPa	Partial pressure of carbon dioxide in arterial blood
H^+ concentration	36–44 nmol/l	Degree of acidaemia or alkalaemia
DERIVED VARIABLES		
Bicarbonate concentration (HCO_3)	21–28 mmol/l	Bicarbonate concentration in arterial plasma. Reflects respiratory and metabolic factors
Standard bicarbonate concentration (SBC) and base excess (BE)	21–28 mmol/l	Bicarbonate concentration corrected to normal $PaCO_2$
	–2 to +2 mmol/l	Only reflects metabolic factors

Table 10.4 INDICATIONS FOR BLOOD GAS ANALYSIS IN THE PRE-OPERATIVE PERIOD

Surgery type	Useful features
Elective surgery Moderate–severe COPD Fibrotic lung disease Severe chest wall deformities, e.g. ankylosing spondylitis, scoliosis Severe asthma Bronchiectasis/cystic fibrosis Lung tumour (prior to surgery)	Document the severity of hypoxaemia (PaO_2) Distinguish patients with type I failure (normal $PaCO_2$) from patients with type II failure (elevated $PaCO_2$) Distinguish patients with compensated hypercapnia (H^+ normal) from those with decompensated hypercapnia (H^+ elevated, respiratory acidosis)
Emergency surgery Known chronic lung disease Dyspnoea Shock (any form) Acute lung disease, e.g. pneumonia, pneumothorax, ARDS	Document the severity of underlying lung disease (see above) Document the magnitude of acute hypoxia and acid–base disturbance

(COPD = chronic obstructive pulmonary disease; ARDS = acute respiratory distress syndrome)

10

Table 10.5 BENEFITS OF STOPPING SMOKING PRIOR TO SURGERY

- The airway may become less hyper-reactive, reducing the incidence of bronchospasm
- Sputum production may decrease if the patient stops smoking several weeks before surgery, reducing the risk of post-operative pulmonary collapse and infection
- The ciliary function of pulmonary epithelium improves within 1–2 days, increasing sputum clearance
- The carboxyhaemoglobin concentration of blood falls within several hours, increasing the oxygen-carrying and unloading capacity of blood
- The circulating concentration of nicotine, which can cause systemic and coronary vasoconstriction, decreases within hours of stopping smoking

ALCOHOL

An assessment of alcohol intake is important in all patients presenting for surgery for the following reasons:

- Chronic alcohol excess results in the induction of liver enzymes. These enzymes are involved in the metabolism of many anaesthetic drugs. As a result, patients may have an apparent resistance to general anaesthetic agents and require larger than expected doses for the induction and maintenance of anaesthesia.
- Patients may develop an acute alcohol withdrawal syndrome in the early post-operative period.
- Patients may have alcohol-related chronic liver disease, cardiac disease or other complications.
- Patients requiring emergency surgery who are intoxicated generally require reduced doses of anaesthetic. They are at increased risk of perioperative aspiration and may require close monitoring in the post-operative period.

OBESITY

Obese patients are at increased risk from anaesthesia and surgery. This results from the technical problems caused by obesity itself, and from the increased incidence of chronic diseases and perioperative complications (Table 10.6). Obese patients require careful assessment. If the perioperative risk is considered too great, the patient should be advised to lose weight before surgery can be considered. Referral to a dietitian may be helpful.

DRUG THERAPY

All prescribed drugs being taken by the patient on admission should be recorded. In general, pre-admission drug therapy should not be stopped prior to surgery. This is particularly important for cardiovascular and respiratory medications (see later sections). The perioperative management of diabetic patients is described below. Some drug therapies that have specific relevance to the perioperative period are as follows:

Table 10.6 SIGNIFICANCE OF OBESITY IN THE PERIOPERATIVE PERIOD

Cardiovascular system
- Increased cardiac work
- Hypertension and ischaemic heart disease more common
- Accurate measurement of blood pressure difficult

Respiratory system
- Airway management often difficult
- Lung volumes reduced
- Post-operative pulmonary collapse, pneumonia and pulmonary embolism more likely
- Increased risk of perioperative hypoxia

Surgical
- Access for surgery difficult
- Increased wound infection and dehiscence

Miscellaneous
- Venous access difficult
- Increased incidence of diabetes and cardiovascular disease
- Increased incidence of hiatus hernia and aspiration

- *Long-term steroid therapy*. This may have resulted in adrenocortical suppression. For most surgery, continuation of the patient's normal dose, or an equipotent dose of hydrocortisone intravenously (5 mg prednisolone = 20 mg hydrocortisone), is adequate. For major surgery, a moderate increase in the normal dose may be given, although many anaesthetists continue the patient's normal dose or equivalent. In all patients on long-term steroids, it is important to monitor for signs of post-operative hypoadrenalism, such as hypotension/shock, hyperkalaemia and hyponatraemia. These are more likely if the patient develops other complications, notably infection.
- *Anticoagulants*. These are considered later in the chapter.
- *The oral contraceptive pill*. Oestrogen-containing medication increases the risk of venous thrombosis and should be stopped about 6 weeks prior to surgery. Progesterone-only pills do not significantly increase risk.
- *Antidepressant drugs of the monoamine oxidase inhibitor (MAOI) class*. These can interact with opioids or pressor agents, resulting in neurological and cardiovascular complications. These reactions are not universal, but ideally the drugs should be stopped 2–3 weeks prior to surgery and another agent substituted. The use of MAOIs is decreasing with the advent of newer classes of antidepressant. In an emergency, surgery can proceed, but opioids and pressor agents should be avoided.

ALLERGIES

Adverse or idiosyncratic responses to drugs or other agents (e.g. iodine or adhesive dressings) must be recorded, as a second exposure may result in a life-threatening hypersensitivity reaction. Latex allergy is increasingly recognized and is important because exposure is extremely common in the perioperative period unless special precautions are taken. In latex-allergic individuals, specific latex-free surgical and anaesthetic equipment must be used.

PREVIOUS OPERATIONS AND ANAESTHETICS

It is important to enquire into previous anaesthetics and document unexpected complications or distressing side-effects. If possible, the anaesthetic charts from previous admissions should be available for review. These will record problems such as difficult intubation and reactions to anaesthetic drugs. Major complications from previous anaesthetics or a family history of anaesthetic reactions raise the possibility of rare genetically inherited abnormalities. These are usually one of two types:

- *Pseudocholinesterase deficiency ('scoline apnoea')*. Prolonged apnoea following the administration of the short-acting depolarizing muscle relaxant suxamethonium chloride suggests a deficiency in

---

BOX 10.2   KEY FACTORS IN THE ANAESTHETIC HISTORY

- Adverse drug reactions
- Difficult intubation (more common in patients with restricted neck movement, limited mouth opening, a short neck or a receding chin)
- Damaged/loose teeth, crowns, poor dentition
- Previous post-operative nausea or vomiting
- Previous post-operative pain problems
- Needle or mask phobia
- Family history of adverse reactions to anaesthetics

---

the circulating enzyme, pseudocholinesterase. The patient may have required mechanical ventilation for several hours after previous surgery. Usually, patients should have been investigated to confirm the diagnosis. In these cases, the use of suxamethonium and some other drugs should be avoided.

- *Malignant hyperpyrexia*. An abnormality in muscle metabolism predisposes patients to this life-threatening condition when they are exposed to powerful triggers such as volatile anaesthetics and suxamethonium. In patients with the condition or when there is a family history, investigations should have been carried out in a specialist centre.

Post-operative nausea and vomiting following anaesthesia can be particularly distressing for some patients. By using short-acting agents, avoiding parenteral opiates and prescribing antiemetics, the anaesthetist can reduce the incidence and/or severity of this side-effect. Minor complications of anaesthesia are common, but may cause significant distress to patients. The risk of many of these recurring can often be reduced by modifying the anaesthetic technique.

PRE-OPERATIVE INVESTIGATIONS

The aim of pre-operative investigations is to provide the surgeon and anaesthetist with the information necessary to assess fitness for operation, and to decide whether further improvement can be made prior to surgery. Investigations relevant to specific chronic diseases have already been considered, and some are discussed in more detail below. Laboratory blood testing is the other type of pre-operative investigation frequently undertaken.

BLOOD BIOCHEMISTRY

In patients with renal dysfunction, fluid balance problems or cardiovascular disease, and in those who are receiving diuretic therapy, analysis of plasma urea and electrolytes is indicated. There is little value in checking these indices in fit patients presenting for minor elective surgery, although it is useful in the elderly or in patients undergoing major procedures. Disorders of potassium balance are the most relevant finding because both hypo- and hyperkalaemia can be associated with intra-operative dysrhythmias. Major abnormalities in electrolyte concentrations should be corrected pre-operatively. For a fuller description of the causes and management of water and electrolyte disorders, see Chapter 2.

LIVER FUNCTION TESTS

Any patient with a history of liver disease or high alcohol intake, or who on clinical examination is found to have signs of liver disease, such as jaundice, hepatomegaly or splenomegaly, should have liver function tests and a coagulation screen performed.

FULL BLOOD COUNT

Patients with a history of chronic ingestion of non-steroidal anti-inflammatory drugs (NSAIDs), upper or lower gastrointestinal tract symptoms, menorrhagia or clinical signs of anaemia should have a full blood count. The importance of functioning haemoglobin in the carriage of oxygen to tissues has already been stressed. In patients with coexisting diseases that might compromise oxygen supply to tissues, it is important to check and, if necessary, increase the haemoglobin concentration prior to surgery. In addition, patients undergoing surgery with the potential for significant blood loss should be tested.

The lowest acceptable level of haemoglobin for elective surgery is now widely accepted as about 80 g/l, unless the patient has significant cardiorespiratory comorbidity or is undergoing surgery for which significant blood loss is anticipated. The most important factor suggesting a higher haemoglobin concentration (> 90 g/l) should be present is the presence of severe ischaemic heart disease. In the case of anaemia of chronic disease, e.g. in patients with chronic renal failure, compensatory mechanisms increase tissue oxygen delivery at reduced haemoglobin concentrations. For example, the viscosity of blood is reduced and the efficiency of oxygen unloading to tissues is increased because 2,3 diphosphoglycerate (DPG) concentrations increase in red cells. There is no proven value in transfusing these patients pre-operatively (EBM 10.1).

An increased white cell count is suggestive of infection, which requires further investigation. The platelet count may be elevated in patients with chronic inflammatory or some

---

BOX 10.3 INDICATIONS FOR MEASURING COAGULATION IN THE PRE-OPERATIVE PATIENT

Patient factors

- Liver disease
- Haematological disease affecting coagulation
- Patient on heparin or warfarin
- Patient shocked or has other risk factors for disseminated intravascular coagulation (DIC), e.g. severe infection
- Patient gives a history of excessive bleeding after minor trauma (may have undiagnosed disorder)
- Patient has a history of thrombotic events, e.g. multiple deep vein thromboses (may have prothrombotic disorder)
- Hypersplenism (causes thrombocytopenia)

Surgical factors

- Major hepatobiliary surgery
- Surgery involving anticoagulation, e.g. cardiopulmonary bypass
- Surgery in which major blood loss is anticipated

---

haematological conditions. These patients are at increased risk of thromboembolic complications, and thromboprophylaxis should be administered perioperatively. Platelet counts below $100 \times 10^9/l$ may increase the risk of perioperative bleeding and are a relative contraindication to some regional anaesthetic techniques such as epidural anaesthesia. In addition to informing the anaesthetist, the physician may need to seek advice from a haematologist.

COAGULATION SCREEN

The patient's coagulation function is usually tested by measuring the prothrombin time (PT) and activated partial thromboplastin time (APTT). If disseminated intravascular coagulation (DIC) is suspected, fibrinogen concentration, fibrin degradation products or D-dimers can be measured. Coagulation should only be measured when there is clinical suspicion of an abnormality, or when the proposed surgery may alter coagulation. Some specific disorders of coagulation are considered below.

BLOOD CROSS-MATCHING

The need to group and screen or cross-match a patient's blood is dependent on the nature of the surgery. Most hospitals will have policies regarding the number of red cell units that should be available prior to particular types of surgery. For more information regarding blood and blood products, see Chapter 4.

THE HIGH-RISK PATIENT

Patients with hepatitis B or C infection and those with human immunodeficiency virus (HIV) infection represent an additional risk to medical and nursing staff. In these cases, it is essential to alert theatre staff in advance of surgery to enable appropriate precautions to be taken. In addition, laboratory staff who may receive samples taken from the patient should also be informed, and samples should be clearly labelled as high-risk.

EBM 10.1 TRANSFUSION TRIGGERS

'An RCT in anaemic critically ill patients requiring intensive care showed no increase in mortality when they were only transfused at haemoglobin < 70 g/l, and maintained at haemoglobin concentration 70–90 g/l, compared with a trigger of 100 g/l to maintain a level 100–120 g/l.'

'A systematic review of blood transfusion triggers for surgical patients concluded that transfusion was not necessary if the haemoglobin value was >100 g/l.'

Hebert PC, et al. New Engl J Med 1999; 340(6):409–417. Hill SR, et al. (Cochrane Review). Cochrane Library, issue 2, 2002. Oxford: Update Software.

10

Some patients may be at increased risk of infection but may not have been tested: for example, patients known to use intravenous drugs or who have partners known to be infected. In these cases, pre-operative testing should be considered after discussion with and consent from the patient. When hepatitis virus or HIV status is unknown, patients should be treated as high-risk.

Precautionary measures include the use of goggles to protect the eyes, covering areas of broken skin, using disposable anaesthetic circuits and filters, and double-layering gloves and gowns.

ASSESSMENT OF THE PATIENT FOR EMERGENCY SURGERY

The principles of assessment already discussed apply equally to the patient presenting for emergency surgery. The main difference from an elective procedure is that there is little time for investigations and less information may be available. Patients requiring emergency surgery may be very sick and may need basic resuscitation prior to anaesthesia and surgery. The principles of resuscitation—airway, breathing and circulation—should be followed. The correction of hypovolaemia is particularly important prior to anaesthesia because the induction of anaesthesia is associated with a significant attenuation of the normal cardiovascular compensatory mechanisms. In the hypovolaemic or inadequately resuscitated patient, in whom subclinical hypovolaemia has not been appreciated, induction may be followed by severe hypotension. Unless there is life-threatening uncontrollable haemorrhage, an adequate blood volume must be restored before anaesthesia commences.

THE PRE-OPERATIVE WARD ROUND

The purpose of the pre-operative ward round is to check that the patient has been adequately assessed and prepared. Both surgeon and anaesthetist should ensure that the patient has had a full explanation of the procedures and techniques that are planned, and has no further questions or concerns. It is important that patients know what to expect post-operatively: for example, which ward they will be in and what surgical drains or intravascular catheters will be present. They should also be clear how analgesia will be maintained, and if necessary, have had instruction in the use of patient-controlled analgesia devices.

PRE-MEDICATION

The requirement for pre-medication will be decided by the anaesthetist during the pre-operative visit. The aim is for the patient to arrive in the anaesthetic room in a relaxed and pain-free state. This can often be achieved non-pharmacologically by explanation and reassurance. Where pre-medication is considered appropriate, a benzodiazepine has the advantages of oral administration and does not require accurate timing in relation to anaesthetic induction. Where parenteral administration is the only option, and/or

the patient requires a drug with analgesic properties, an opiate such as intramuscular morphine is commonly prescribed.

FASTING

To minimize the risk of regurgitation and aspiration at induction of anaesthesia, the patient presenting for an elective procedure should have no food for 4 hours and no fluids for 2 hours before the procedure. These recommendations will result in the majority of patients arriving in the anaesthetic room with an empty stomach. However, in patients with upper gastrointestinal pathology, such as hiatus hernia, gastric outlet obstruction or delayed gastric emptying, in autonomic neuropathy (e.g. long-standing diabetes mellitus) and in the emergency situation, an empty stomach cannot be guaranteed, irrespective of the duration of fasting. This is also true of patients in acute pain and who have received opiates, both of which reduce gastric emptying. In these situations, the patient should be fasted, but the anaesthetist will assume the patient has a full stomach, modify the anaesthetic induction technique in order to reduce the risk of regurgitation, and quickly secure the airway to avoid aspiration.

IMPLICATIONS OF CHRONIC DISEASE IN THE PERIOPERATIVE PERIOD

CARDIOVASCULAR DISEASE

Ischaemic heart disease
The prevalence of ischaemic heart disease is high in developed countries, increases with age, and is more prevalent in some geographical areas than others. It is increased in patients with risk factors (Table 10.7) and may be asymptomatic. Patient assessment should therefore include not only documentation of known disease, but also consideration of the likelihood of undiagnosed disease.

Myocardial infarction
The incidence of perioperative myocardial infarction in previously healthy patients is approximately 0.2%. This contrasts with an incidence of about 6% (> 25 times higher) in patients with previous myocardial infarction. Patients with severe angina and those undergoing major surgery are at highest risk for reinfarction. The time from the last myocardial infarction has a major influence on the risk of

Table 10.7   RISK FACTORS RAISING THE SUSPICION OF ISCHAEMIC HEART DISEASE IN PATIENTS PRESENTING FOR SURGERY
<ul><li>Family history</li><li>Smoking</li><li>Hypertension</li><li>Diabetes mellitus</li><li>Obesity</li><li>Hypercholesterolaemia</li></ul>

Table 10.8   RISK OF POST-OPERATIVE MYOCARDIAL INFARCTION (MI) IN PATIENTS WITH A PREVIOUS HISTORY OF MYOCARDIAL INFARCTION

Time from MI	Incidence of post-operative MI (%)
Any previous MI	6
> 6 months	5
4–6 months	10–20
< 3 months	20–30
No previous history	0.2

Table 10.9   INCREASED PERIOPERATIVE RISK IN PATIENTS WITH CARDIAC FAILURE

Mechanism	Complication
Poor 'pump function'	Pulmonary oedema Cardiogenic shock Renal failure Organ ischaemia, e.g. bowel ischaemia Venous thrombosis
Cardiac disease	Arrhythmias Myocardial infarction Thromboembolism

10

reinfarction and should be clearly documented (Table 10.8). The mortality from post-operative myocardial infarction is higher (up to 50%) than myocardial infarction occurring outside the perioperative period. Post-operative myocardial infarction is more difficult to diagnose because the symptoms are often not typical (for example, there may be no chest pain). In addition, thrombolytic treatment is frequently contraindicated. Following myocardial infarction, elective surgery should, if possible, be delayed for at least 6 months and urgent surgery for at least 3 months. If surgery is carried out, invasive cardiovascular monitoring can reduce the risk of cardiac events (see below).

Angina

The risk of perioperative myocardial infarction in patients with angina is related to the severity of symptoms. It is important to establish and document the frequency and severity of pain, precipitating factors and the response to anti-anginal treatment. A change in symptoms over recent months is also significant. The extent to which a patient's everyday activities (for example, shopping or leisure activities) are limited is a good indication of the overall severity of disease. Many patients may have been investigated by a cardiologist and had coronary angiography. In these cases, it is important to document the length of time since these investigations were performed, along with the results.

The presence of unstable angina despite maximum medical therapy indicates very high risk. In these patients, investigation by a cardiologist should be performed prior to surgery, as symptoms may be improved by angioplasty or even coronary artery bypass surgery prior to elective surgery. In cases such as these, the surgeon and anaesthetist must balance the risk of anaesthesia and surgery against the benefits.

Coronary artery bypass graft (CABG), percutaneous angioplasty and stenting

Patients may present for surgery with a history of ischaemic heart disease treated by surgical or percutaneous techniques. The cardiovascular risk in these patients relates to the success of their surgery and whether they have developed recurrent disease. These patients should be assessed in a similar manner to those with angina.

Congestive cardiac failure

The most common cause of cardiac failure is ischaemic heart disease, but the exact cause should be identified prior to surgery. Cardiac failure is associated with increased perioperative risk via several mechanisms (Table 10.9). The risk associated with cardiac failure is linked closely to how well it is controlled prior to surgery. The presence of a third heart sound, peripheral oedema, dyspnoea or orthopnoea suggests inadequately treated cardiac failure and very high perioperative risk.

Valvular heart disease

In the perioperative patient it is important to know the severity of valvular lesions and whether the patient suffers from associated arrhythmias or ventricular dysfunction. An algorithm for managing a patient with known or suspected valvular heart disease is shown in Figure 10.3, and a summary of antibiotic prophylaxis is shown in Table 10.10.

Pacemakers

The function of some pacemakers is affected by intra-operative monitoring devices and diathermy. It is important to document the reason for pacemaker insertion, when it was inserted, what type of device is in place, and when it was last checked by a cardiologist. Cardiological review prior to surgery may be indicated, particularly if the device has not been checked in the recent past. In some cases, a pacemaker will require re-programming during the perioperative period.

Hypertension

Untreated hypertension increases perioperative risk, particularly for cerebrovascular accident and myocardial infarction. The risk relates mostly to the degree of elevation of the diastolic rather than the systolic blood pressure. The normal range for blood pressure increases with age. In a patient not known to be hypertensive, it is first important to establish the resting blood pressure unaffected by anxiety and stress. Repeated measurements over time, reference to recent medical notes, contacting the GP, or examination for the complications of hypertensive disease (such as retinopathy) are useful. Once an accurate resting blood pressure has been established, it must be interpreted with reference to the patient's age.

10

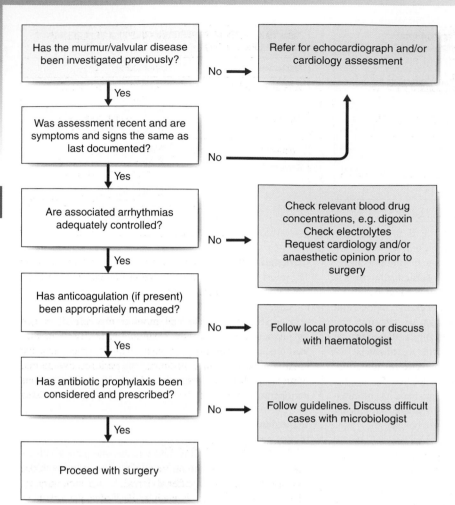

Fig. 10.3   An algorithm for managing patients with known or suspected valvular disease.

Flowchart text:

- Has the murmur/valvular disease been investigated previously? — No → Refer for echocardiograph and/or cardiology assessment
- Yes ↓
- Was assessment recent and are symptoms and signs the same as last documented? — No →
- Yes ↓
- Are associated arrhythmias adequately controlled? — No → Check relevant blood drug concentrations, e.g. digoxin / Check electrolytes / Request cardiology and/or anaesthetic opinion prior to surgery
- Yes ↓
- Has anticoagulation (if present) been appropriately managed? — No → Follow local protocols or discuss with haematologist
- Yes ↓
- Has antibiotic prophylaxis been considered and prescribed? — No → Follow guidelines. Discuss difficult cases with microbiologist
- Yes ↓
- Proceed with surgery

Table 10.10   RECOMMENDED ANTIBIOTIC PROPHYLAXIS FOR PATIENTS WITH VALVULAR HEART DISEASE
• Amoxicillin (1 g i.v./i.m. prior to induction, with 500 mg orally 6 hours later)
Prosthetic heart valve or previous endocarditis   • Amoxicillin plus gentamicin (120 mg i.m./i.v. prior to induction)
Penicillin-allergic patients   • Vancomycin (1 g i.v. over 60 mins) substituted for amoxicillin

The blood flow to organs is normally tightly regulated over a range of arterial blood pressures, in order to maintain adequate oxygen supply to cells. In untreated hypertensive patients, these auto-regulatory mechanisms become 'reset' to higher levels. This means that organ perfusion may be compromised during periods of modest hypotension. Perioperative risk can be reduced by ensuring that blood pressure has been adequately controlled for several weeks prior to surgery because, with time, auto-regulatory mechanisms return towards normal limits. As a general rule, if the resting diastolic pressure is ≥ 110 mmHg, elective surgery should be delayed.

When surgery is urgent, blood pressure should be controlled acutely using drugs that can be titrated until an appropriate diastolic pressure is achieved. As the auto-regulatory mechanisms that control organ blood flow take several days to normalize, the anaesthetist will administer sufficient drugs to achieve a moderate reduction in blood pressure, rather than completely normal values.

Perioperative management of patients with cardiovascular disease

Drug therapy

In most patients, normal cardiac drug therapy should be continued until the morning of surgery. When possible, patients should continue oral medication post-operatively. If oral intake is not possible, cardiac or antihypertensive medication can be administered intravenously if necessary. As hypotension occurs relatively frequently following major surgery, the need for intravenous therapy and the timing of reintroduction of oral medication are decided on an individual basis. The following two classes of cardiac drug merit special consideration:

- *Beta-blockers.* The perioperative use of β-blockers in patients with ischaemic heart disease has been associated with a significant reduction in cardiovascular morbidity, even if the patients were not taking these drugs prior to surgery (EBM 10.2). This probably occurs by maintaining a slow heart rate, thereby maximizing myocardial oxygen supply during diastole. Acute withdrawal of β-blockers during the perioperative period may cause rebound tachycardia and increase the risk of myocardial ischaemia.

- *Angiotensin-converting enzyme (ACE) inhibitors.* These agents are widely used to treat cardiac failure and hypertension. However, in patients taking these drugs up to the time of surgery, intra- and post-operative hypotension is common. The decision to continue or omit an ACE inhibitor in the perioperative period is usually made by the anaesthetist at the time of the pre-operative visit.

Cardiovascular management

In patients at risk from myocardial ischaemia and/or with poor cardiac function, there are two principles of management for the intra- and post-operative periods:

1. *Minimize myocardial oxygen demand.* Cardiac output can be increased via four mechanisms: increased preload, heart rate, contractility or decreased afterload. The oxygen 'cost' for each of these mechanisms differs considerably. The most efficient method of generating adequate cardiac output is to optimize preload with fluids. Tachycardia, sympathetic activation and excessive peripheral vasoconstriction all have a high oxygen 'cost' and should be avoided.
2. *Maximize myocardial oxygen supply.* Blood flow to the myocardium of the left ventricle, which has the highest myocardial oxygen demand, occurs only during diastole. It depends on the coronary perfusion pressure, which is the difference between the diastolic and the left ventricular end-diastolic pressures. Myocardial oxygen

Table 10.11   MONITORS OF CARDIOVASCULAR STATUS DURING THE PERIOPERATIVE PERIOD

Monitor	Information given
Arterial catheter	Continuous measurement of blood pressure
Central venous catheter	Central venous pressure (a measure of cardiac preload)
Pulmonary artery catheter	Pulmonary artery pressure Pulmonary capillary wedge pressure (a measure of left atrial pressure) Cardiac output (by thermodilution)
Oesophageal Doppler	Cardiac output

10

supply is therefore optimal when the heart rate is slow (when diastole is long relative to systole) and the diastolic blood pressure is high.

In order to optimize and monitor myocardial oxygen supply and demand closely, patients with severe cardiovascular or respiratory disease benefit from invasive haemodynamic monitoring during the perioperative period, particularly for major surgery (EBM 10.3). The various possible monitors, and the information they give, are listed in Table 10.11.

RESPIRATORY DISEASE

Patients with poor respiratory function require close monitoring, particularly after abdominal or thoracic surgery. They are ideally managed in a high-dependency or intensive care unit. Principles of perioperative management for the patient with chronic respiratory disease are described below.

Anaesthetic technique

General anaesthesia causes significant alterations in pulmonary function that place patients with respiratory disease at increased risk of post-operative pulmonary complications. Regional anaesthetic techniques should therefore be used whenever possible, either alone or in combination with general anaesthesia. This usually involves spinal or epidural anaesthesia or the use of nerve blocks (for example, ilio-inguinal block for hernia repair). Regional anaesthesia is discussed later in this chapter.

Post-operative analgesia

Wound pain impairs ventilation and coughing, and may result in pulmonary collapse/atelectasis, hypoxia and sputum retention. This increases the risk of post-operative infection. Effective analgesia is particularly important in the patient with respiratory disease. Systemic opiates can be used, but result in sedation and impaired coughing. Regional techniques have minimal central effects and should be considered whenever possible.

Physiotherapy

Pre- and post-operative physiotherapy is extremely important for patients with chest disease. A physiotherapist should see the patient regularly throughout the perioperative period.

Post-operative ventilation

Some patients will have insufficient reserves following surgery, or will require ventilation because of complications such as pneumonia. Post-operative ventilation of patients with respiratory disease can often be avoided by close attention to the factors described above. It is better to avoid ventilation if possible, because prolonged tracheal intubation results in an increased risk of respiratory infection. The use of non-invasive respiratory support by continuous positive airway pressure (CPAP) or non-invasive ventilation (NIV) via a face mask or hood can decrease the need for intubation and should be considered early in consultation with the intensive care unit.

JAUNDICE

Patients with jaundice pre-operatively most commonly present for biliary or hepatic surgery. However, it is important to define the aetiology of the jaundice clearly prior to surgery. Perioperative risk related to jaundice is attributable to the following:

- *Hepatitis*. Patients with clinical jaundice or biochemical evidence of liver inflammation (elevated aminotransferases) should be screened pre-operatively for hepatitis A, B and C viruses. The presence of hepatitis B or C carries the risk of transmission to medical and nursing staff. The incidence of asymptomatic hepatitis C infection is increasing in developed countries.
- *Coagulation*. Intestinal bile salts are necessary for the absorption of fat-soluble vitamins (A, D, E and K). Patients with obstructive jaundice therefore have reduced absorption of vitamin K, which is an essential co-factor for the synthesis of coagulation factors II, VII, IX and X. Vitamin K-related coagulopathy is associated with prolongation of the prothrombin time. In jaundiced patients with abnormal coagulation, surgery is best deferred until the jaundice has resolved and coagulopathy has been corrected. This is aided by relief of biliary obstruction via stenting or drainage (Ch. 18) and the administration of synthetic vitamin K for several days prior to surgery.
- *Acute renal failure*. Jaundice is associated with an increased risk of perioperative renal failure for several reasons:

  1. Dehydration commonly accompanies jaundice.
  2. Sepsis, particularly biliary sepsis, is common.
  3. A high concentration of conjugated bilirubin is toxic to renal tubular cells.

The single most important intervention to prevent renal failure in jaundiced patients is adequate hydration. Diuretic agents such as mannitol, furosemide and dopamine have been used, but there is little evidence that any agent is more effective than a volume load of 0.9% NaCl solution adequate to maintain a urine output of at least 0.5–1 ml/kg/hr.

Table 10.12 COMMON INDICATIONS FOR SURGERY IN THE DIABETIC PATIENT
Ophthalmic disease
• Proliferative retinopathy
• Cataract
Cardiovascular disease
• Peripheral vascular surgery
• Diabetic feet
• Coronary artery bypass surgery
Renal disease
• Vascular access for haemodialysis
• Renal transplantation
Infection
• Abscess drainage

Central venous pressure monitoring can assist fluid management.

DIABETES MELLITUS

About 50% of diabetic patients will require surgery at some time during their life, often for complications of their disease (Table 10.12). Perioperative risk associated with diabetes mellitus is attributable to the comorbidity associated with diabetes or to the effect of surgical stress on diabetic control.

Diabetic comorbidity

Vascular disease

Diabetics have an increased incidence of microvascular and major vessel disease. The risk of myocardial infarction, hypertension, cerebrovascular accident and thromboembolic disease is increased. Vascular disease may significantly impair wound healing.

Renal disease

Renal failure is common in diabetics and increases in frequency and severity with duration of disease, particularly if associated with hypertension. Reduced renal reserve increases the risk of perioperative acute renal failure. These patients are more likely to develop acute renal failure in response to hypotension, sepsis or nephrotoxic drugs.

Neuropathy

Patients with peripheral neuropathy are at increased risk from trivial trauma: for example, from positioning during surgery. Autonomic neuropathy may cause cardiovascular instability during and following surgery. Delayed gastric emptying increases the risk of regurgitation and aspiration during and after anaesthesia.

Infection

Infective complications are increased in diabetic patients, particularly if diabetic control is poor.

Effect of surgical stress on diabetic control

The metabolic responses to surgery, trauma and infection are described in Chapter 1. Many of the neuroendocrine responses increase glucose mobilization and lipolysis, resulting in hyperglycaemia and increased circulating free fatty acids. In addition, increased insulin release is part of the normal response to stress. In diabetic patients with decreased endogenous insulin secretion or reduced peripheral insulin sensitivity, surgery results in hyperglycaemia. Ketoacidosis may occur if insulin deficiency is severe and/or there is a major stress response. It is normal for diabetic patients to suffer increased hyperglycaemia following surgery and for insulin requirements to increase.

Principles of managing the diabetic patient

Patients with diabetes mellitus require sufficient circulating insulin and glucose to ensure an adequate supply of glucose to cells. As insulin-mediated glucose transfer into cells is linked to potassium influx, an adequate potassium supply to prevent hypokalaemia is also necessary. In general, the risk to the patient from hypoglycaemia is greater than that of mild hyperglycaemia. A blood glucose concentration of 6–10 mmol/l is a frequently used target during the perioperative period, although there is increasing evidence that tight control of blood sugar concentration is important following major surgery, especially cardiac surgery (Ch. 1). The approach used to achieve this depends on:

- whether the patient is normally managed by diet alone, oral hypoglycaemics or insulin
- the magnitude of the surgery (which relates to the anticipated stress response)
- the likely period during which the patient will be unable to take oral calories and drugs
- whether surgery is elective or emergency, and particularly if infection is present.

Typical scenarios for patients presenting for surgery are presented in Table 10.13. In practice, an appropriate regimen is best tailored to the individual patient. It is usual for diabetic patients to be placed first on an operating list, to minimize the duration of fasting.

Methods of administering insulin

Insulin, dextrose and potassium can be delivered either as a mixture or as separate infusions (Table 10.14). Generally, in straightforward cases a mixture of dextrose, insulin and potassium (often termed the Alberti regimen, Table 10.15) is simplest and safest. For more complex and less well-controlled patients, such as those with sepsis, separate infusions allow more flexibility but require more frequent monitoring of blood sugar and electrolytes.

Table 10.13 SOME TYPICAL SCENARIOS FOR DIABETIC PATIENTS PRESENTING FOR SURGERY

Patient	Procedure	Management
Diet-controlled diabetic	Elective laparoscopic cholecystectomy (moderate stress response)	Monitor blood glucose until eating
Patient on oral hypoglycaemics	Hernia repair (minor stress response)	Omit oral hypoglycaemic on morning of surgery Monitor pre-operatively for hypoglycaemia Monitor post-operatively until eating normally Restart oral hypoglycaemics when on normal diet
Normally well-controlled	Elective aortofemoral bypass (major stress response)	Omit oral hypoglycaemic on morning of surgery Monitor perioperatively for hypo or hyperglycaemia If blood glucose > 10 mmol/l, commence glucose/insulin/potassium infusion
Normally poorly controlled Blood sugar > 10 mmol/l	Emergency aortofemoral bypass (major stress response)	Commence glucose/insulin/potassium infusion prior to surgery Stop oral hypoglycaemics perioperatively
Insulin-dependent diabetic Well-controlled	Cataract surgery (minor stress response)	Omit morning insulin Monitor blood sugar for hypoglycaemia Restart regular insulin when eating
Normally well-controlled	Elective coronary artery bypass graft (major stress response)	Convert to glucose/insulin/dextrose prior to surgery Monitor blood sugar perioperatively Convert to subcutaneous short-acting insulin and then regular insulin as diet reintroduced
Blood sugar > 20 mmol/l Ketones in urine	Emergency laparotomy for diverticular abscess major stress response)	Treat as diabetic ketoacidosis and stabilize *prior* to surgery. Ensure adequate volume resuscitation Continue glucose/insulin/potassium infusion perioperatively Convert to intermittent short-acting and then normal insulin as diet reintroduced

Table 10.14   ADVANTAGES AND DISADVANTAGES OF DIFFERENT METHODS OF ADMINISTERING INSULIN AND DEXTROSE

	Advantages	Disadvantages
Combined dextrose/insulin/potassium infusions	Simple Cheap Decreased risk of hypoglycaemia Single infusion Only requires a single dedicated cannula	Bags may require frequent changes Less flexibility in poorly controlled patients
Separate infusions of dextrose and insulin	Flexible	Multiple pumps and cannulae needed Frequent blood sugar measurement required Increased risk of hypoglycaemia

10

Table 10.15   THE ALBERTI REGIMEN

- 500 ml 10% dextrose *plus* 10 U short-acting soluble insulin *plus* 10 mmol KCl
- Run 500 ml every 4–6 hours via a controlled infusion pump
- Check blood glucose every 2–6 hrs (depending on stability) and potassium 1–2 times daily
- On average, give 250 g glucose daily (1000 kcal) and 50 U insulin
- Adjust insulin and potassium according to results

Table 10.16   RISK FACTORS IN PATIENTS WITH RENAL FAILURE UNDERGOING SURGERY

Cardiovascular
- Frequently have ischaemic heart disease
- Hypertension
- Left ventricular dysfunction

Respiratory
- Pulmonary oedema and fluid overload (impaired water clearance)

Gastrointestinal
- Delayed gastric emptying

Biochemical
- Electrolyte disturbance (especially hyperkalaemia)

Haematological
- Anaemia
- Impaired coagulation (platelet dysfunction)

Miscellaneous
- Malnutrition
- Multiple drug therapies
- Abnormal drug metabolism
- Vascular access

CHRONIC RENAL FAILURE

Patients with chronic renal failure frequently present for elective or emergency surgery, and are at increased risk of perioperative complications for the reasons listed in Table 10.16. Special consideration should be given to whether patients are established on dialysis or not.

Patients not requiring dialysis

In the perioperative period, these patients are at risk of acute deterioration in renal function. This is relevant because they may become permanently dialysis-dependent. Factors that reduce the risk of deteriorating renal function are:

- *Optimizing fluid balance.* These patients are at risk from hyper- and hypovolaemia. Central venous pressure monitoring is useful, particularly for major surgery or trauma.
- *Avoiding nephrotoxic drugs.* These include NSAIDs for analgesia, and some antibiotics such as gentamicin.
- *Avoiding hypotension.* Hypotension may be related to fluid status, cardiovascular drug therapy, anaesthetic drugs or regional anaesthesia. Complications can be avoided by close monitoring and regular review.
- *Exercising caution with drugs that are excreted renally.* Some drugs used in the perioperative period will accumulate in patients with renal dysfunction not receiving dialysis. For example, morphine metabolites can accumulate, causing excessive sedation and respiratory depression.

Patients on dialysis

Particular considerations in these patients are as follows:

- Patients often pass little urine and rely on dialysis for fluid removal. Fluids should be administered cautiously, guided by central venous monitoring in complex cases.
- Patients have access devices for dialysis, such as peritoneal dialysis catheters or fistulae. A limb with a fistula should be protected during surgery to prevent thrombosis, and should never be used for vascular access or blood sampling.
- Electrolyte abnormalities are common. In particular, hyperkalaemia may develop rapidly and should be checked regularly during the perioperative period.
- Patients often require dialysis prior to surgery. This requires close communication with the nephrologist and dialysis unit.

HAEMATOLOGICAL DISEASE

Anaemia

In anaemic patients, the cause of anaemia should be investigated and rectified prior to surgery when possible: for example, using iron therapy. Anaemic patients and patients undergoing procedures associated with high blood loss, such as cardiac or major vascular surgery, are likely to require perioperative blood transfusion. In these cases, consideration should be given to perioperative blood conservation techniques such as cell salvage or the use of antifibrinolytic agents such as tranexamic acid (EBM 10.4). This requires discussion with the anaesthetist and haematologist.

ABNORMAL COAGULATION

Haemostatic disorders fall broadly into three categories: patients on anticoagulant therapy, those with inherited disorders of coagulation, and patients with acute coagulopathy.

Anticoagulant therapy

Patients receiving warfarin anticoagulation should usually stop medication 2–4 days prior to surgery to allow some correction of the anticoagulant effect. The amount required depends on the nature of the surgery and the risk to the patient from reversal of the effect. Generally speaking, a prothrombin ratio of 1.5–2:1 is acceptable for major surgery. If the warfarin effect is more completely reversed, or a greater degree of anticoagulation is required (for example, in patients with an artificial heart valve), parenteral heparin anticoagulation is substituted for warfarin during the perioperative period. When the warfarin effect requires rapid reversal—for example, when emergency surgery is needed—several options are available. Intravenous vitamin K reverses warfarin effects in most patients in 24–48 hours. In more urgent cases, fresh frozen plasma or other factor concentrates can be administered, after discussion with a haematologist. Heparin has a relatively short half-life and coagulation returns to normal within 4–6 hours of discontinuation. In rare situations where rapid reversal is required, the drug protamine can be used. This is usually done only in the setting of major vascular or cardiac surgery.

Inherited disorders of coagulation

The most important inherited disorder of coagulation is haemophilia, an impairment of factor VIII production. For major surgery, factor VIII levels should be maintained at 30–40% of normal by transfusion of factor concentrates. This is usually monitored by serial measurement of factor VIII concentrations in plasma. Haemophiliacs presenting for surgery must be managed in close collaboration with a haematologist. A significant number of haemophiliacs have been infected with hepatitis C and HIV (considered above).

Acute coagulopathy

Acute coagulopathy is most commonly thrombocytopenia and/or DIC. These conditions are often associated with life-threatening illnesses such as shock, multiple trauma, transfusion reactions and sepsis. Microvascular coagulation and activated fibrinolysis result in tissue ischaemia and simultaneous depletion of coagulation factors and platelets.

EBM 10.4 PERIOPERATIVE BLOOD CONSERVATION

'A recent evidence-based guideline recommends the use of cell salvage for surgery expected to cause blood loss > 1000 ml blood and consideration of other blood-sparing techniques.'

SIGN. Perioperative blood transfusion for elective surgery: a national clinical guideline. www.sign.ac.uk; 2003.

Table 10.17 PERIOPERATIVE RISKS ASSOCIATED WITH SURGERY IN PREGNANT PATIENTS

- Spontaneous abortion or premature labour
- Hypotension lying supine (inferior vena caval compression in second and third trimesters)
- Gastro-oesophageal reflux (increased risk of aspiration)
- Hypoxia (due to high metabolic rate and reduced lung functional residual capacity)
- Teratogenic effects of drugs (particularly in first trimester)
- Peripartum
    Massive blood loss
    Pre-eclampsia/eclampsia
    Amniotic fluid embolism

Table 10.18 RELEVANCE OF SOME MEDICAL CONDITIONS IN THE PERIOPERATIVE PERIOD

Condition	Considerations
Rheumatoid arthritis	Neck may be 'unstable'; careful positioning necessary; complex drug therapy; associated chronic diseases, e.g. renal failure, lung disease
Multiple sclerosis	Reduced respiratory reserve; stress of surgery can cause relapse or worsening of disease
Epilepsy	Drugs may interact with anaesthetics; surgical stress and some drugs may precipitate seizures
Scoliosis or spondylitis	Can significantly reduce respiratory reserve; difficult endotracheal intubation
Myasthenia gravis	Risk of respiratory failure or aspiration; anaesthetic technique needs modifying
Sickle-cell anaemia	Stress of surgery, hypoxia, hypothermia can all precipitate sickle-cell crisis

10

The coagulation screen typically shows prolonged pro-thrombin and activated partial thromboplastin times, thrombocytopenia, low fibrinogen concentration, and elevated D-dimers or fibrin degradation products. The management is complex and should involve a haematologist.

PREGNANCY

Surgery should be avoided if possible during pregnancy. The fetus is particularly sensitive to drugs, hypoxia, hypotension and infection during the first trimester. Surgery during pregnancy is usually an emergency or related to delivery itself. Many of the perioperative risks of pregnancy (Table 10.17) relate to anaesthesia, and early communication with an anaesthetist is essential when pregnant women require surgery.

MISCELLANEOUS CONDITIONS

There are many diseases that have particular relevance in the perioperative period. A detailed description is beyond the scope of this chapter, but some of those encountered most frequently are listed in Table 10.18.

ANAESTHESIA AND THE OPERATION

GENERAL ANAESTHESIA

A successful pre-operative visit from the anaesthetist, supplemented with appropriate pre-medication, should result in a patient arriving in the anaesthetic room in a relaxed state. Theatre staff and the ward nurse will check that the patient's clinical notes, a completed operation consent form, drug chart and results from pre-operative investigations are available. A pre-operative checklist is followed that includes patient identification, the procedure to be undertaken, appropriate marking of the operation site, allergies, and the presence of pacemakers or other relevant unusual factors. Anaesthesia should only be started when the checklist has been satisfactorily completed.

The overall aims of general anaesthesia are to produce a reversible and safe loss of consciousness, an attenuation of the major physiological responses to surgical stimulation (such as reflex skeletal muscle movement, tachycardia, hypertension and sweating), and optimal operating conditions. Anaesthesia is often considered to have three major components:

- *hypnosis*: the loss of consciousness and awareness
- *analgesia*: the provision of pain relief
- *relaxation*: muscle relaxation to enable surgery to take place.

LOCAL ANAESTHESIA

Local anaesthetic agents such as lidocaine and bupivacaine act by altering membrane sodium permeability, resulting in a block to the transmission of impulses along the nerve fibre. They are non-specific and therefore block all three groups of nerves (autonomic, sensory and motor). The sensitivity of an individual nerve depends on its physical properties. Size, which relates to the number of coverings and degree of myelination, is a major factor. Small unmyelinated nerves, such as sympathetic nerves, are very sensitive and are blocked early, whereas large myelinated nerves, such as motor neurons, are blocked late and recover first. The duration and intensity of the block depend on the local anaesthetic agent used (bupivacaine lasting longer than lidocaine), the total dose administered, the proximity of the injection to the nerve and the presence of a vasoconstrictor (usually adrenaline (epinephrine) 1:200 000). Adrenaline prolongs the block by producing local vasoconstriction, thereby slowing the systemic uptake and distribution of local anaesthetic, which is the main mechanism responsible for the offset of action. The most important complication of local anaesthetic injection is systemic toxicity due to high plasma concentrations resulting from either an accidental intravascular injection or rapid systemic uptake from the site.

Patients should be closely observed and have ECG, non-invasive blood pressure and pulse oximetry monitoring during the injection of large doses of local anaesthetic. In addition, there are recommended safe maximum doses of drug that should not be exceeded (Table 10.19). Major blocks using large doses of local anaesthetic should only be performed by personnel fully trained in cardiopulmonary resuscitation within an area where resuscitation equipment and drugs are readily available.

Table 10.19 SAFE MAXIMUM DOSES OF COMMONLY USED LOCAL ANAESTHETICS		
Drug	With adrenaline (epinephrine) (mg/kg)	Without adrenaline (epinephrine) (mg/kg)
Lidocaine	6	2
Bupivacaine	2	2
Prilocaine	Maximum 600 mg	

Table 10.20 SIGNS OF LOCAL ANAESTHETIC TOXICITY
Early
● Numbness/tingling of the tongue
● Perioral tingling
● Anxiety
● Lightheadedness
● Tinnitus
Late
● Loss of consciousness
● Convulsions
● Cardiovascular collapse
● Apnoea

Signs of local anaesthetic toxicity are given in Table 10.20. If toxicity occurs, the patient's airway and breathing should be secured, high-flow oxygen administered and cardiovascular collapse treated with intravenous fluids and adrenergic agents such as ephedrine. Convulsions may be controlled with small increments of intravenous benzodiazepines.

Local anaesthetics are used to block sensory nerves, allowing surgery to be performed painlessly within the area supplied by the nerve. They can be used as the sole anaesthetic in the upper limbs (brachial plexus block) and below the umbilicus (spinal—see below) where a general anaesthetic is contraindicated, or combined with general anaesthesia. Local anaesthetic techniques are also an important component of post-operative analgesic regimens.

TOPICAL ANAESTHESIA

Satisfactory mucosal absorption allows lidocaine (0.5–4%)-containing solutions, gels and creams to be used to anaesthetize the conjunctiva, and the mucosa of the mouth, pharynx, larynx and urethra. These can be applied as lozenges, sprays and gargles, and on soaked pledgets of cotton wool. Anaesthesia is rapid and usually lasts 30–60 minutes. A mixture of lidocaine and prilocaine (Emla cream) is an effective topical anaesthetic for the skin if applied 1 hour prior to venous cannulation. It is particularly useful in children and in adults with a needle phobia.

As with all local anaesthetic techniques, it is important to allow sufficient time for the local anaesthetic to be administered/take effect prior to the start of surgery.

LOCAL INFILTRATION

Local anaesthetic can be infiltrated directly into the surgical field. Injection into inflamed tissues should be avoided because alterations to drug pharmocokinetics occur. Local vasodilatation can result in rapid systemic absorption and toxicity, and the decreased local tissue pH can reduce the local anaesthetic action. In highly vascular areas, the addition of a vasoconstrictor such as adrenaline (epinephrine, 1:200 000) can prolong the duration of local infiltration anaesthesia.

Adrenaline-containing solutions should be avoided where there are end-arteries present (digits and appendages), as arterial vasoconstriction can result in a critical impairment of blood flow and ischaemia.

PERIPHERAL NERVE BLOCK

A detailed knowledge of the course of a nerve with respect to surface anatomy, its relationship to important surrounding structures and the area of body supplied allows the anaesthetist to inject local anaesthetic around the nerve in order to achieve a block. By using a nerve stimulator and insulated regional block needles, the anaesthetist can locate the nerve accurately before injection and improve the chances of a successful block. For large nerve trunks (e.g. sciatic and brachial plexus), a significant

Table 10.21 COMMONLY PERFORMED PERIPHERAL NERVE BLOCKS	
Block	**Indication**
Axillary or supraclavicular	Upper limb surgery
Interscalene	Shoulder and upper limb
Femoral	Lower limb surgery
Sciatic	Lower limb surgery
Intercostal nerves	Thoracotomy Fractured ribs Cholecystectomy
Ilio-inguinal/iliohypogastric	Inguinal hernia
Penile	Circumcision

10

volume and dose of local anaesthetic may be needed and there can be a delay of 30–40 minutes before the onset of a surgical block. Commonly performed nerve blocks, and their indications, are shown in Table 10.21.

When multiple superficial nerves supply an area (e.g. groin or scalp), a 'field block' can be achieved by a series of injections to block the nerves. During injection, attention should be paid to the total dose of drug administered in relation to the maximum recommended dose, and to the avoidance of accidental intravascular injection by repeated aspiration before injecting.

SPINAL ANAESTHESIA

Local anaesthetic can be administered into the subarachnoid (spinal) or extradural (epidural) spaces within the vertebral canal, blocking the nerves before they exit from the intervertebral foramina. In order to avoid the possibility of damaging the spinal cord, spinal anaesthesia is performed below the level at which the cord ends (L2). Similar to a lumbar puncture, a spinal needle is inserted between L3/4 or L4/5 vertebrae and the subarachnoid space is identified by the free aspiration of clear cerebrospinal fluid (CSF) (Fig. 10.4).

As the nerves of the cauda equina only receive their perineural coverings and myelin sheaths as they exit through the dura, they are very sensitive to the effects of local anaesthetics. A small volume of lidocaine or bupivacaine (2–4 ml) will usually block all the spinal nerves below T10. The addition of 6% dextrose to the local anaesthetic will render it hyperbaric with respect to CSF. The spread of this 'heavy' solution can be influenced by gravity, which gives the anaesthetist additional control over the spread of the resultant block. Spinal anaesthesia results in a reliable, rapid-onset, dense block using a small dose of local anaesthetic. With hyperbaric solutions, a reliable block to a level of T6 is usually achieved. The single injection usually gives 2–3 hours of surgical anaesthesia before sensation begins to return.

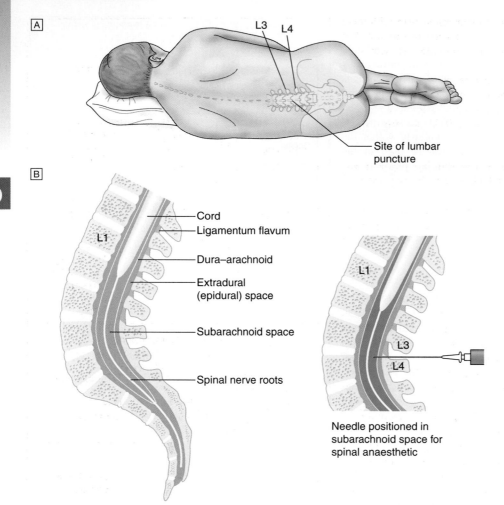

Fig. 10.4 Spinal anaesthesia.
[A] Position of the patient. [B] Position of the needle in the spinal canal.

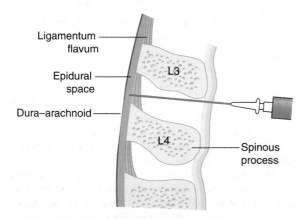

Fig. 10.5 Epidural anaesthesia.

EPIDURAL ANAESTHESIA

In epidural anaesthesia, a 'loss of resistance' technique is used to position the tip of the needle in the epidural space between the ligamentum flavum and the dura–arachnoid membrane (Fig. 10.5). This space runs the whole length of the vertebral canal and can be approached at any level from the cervical spine to the sacrum (caudal canal). The level of injection is dictated by the spinal nerves requiring blockade. Unlike nerve roots in the subarachnoid space, the nerves in the epidural space have their full complement of coverings and myelin. As a result, much larger doses of local anaesthetic are required than for spinal anaesthesia. A volume of 10–20 ml will spread upwards and downwards from the point of injection to create a band of anaesthesia that will include several dermatomes on either side of the level of injection. Commonly, a fine catheter is passed through the needle and is left in the epidural space, allowing for multiple injections or infusions of local anaesthetic solutions. Using this technique, the anaesthesia produced for the surgical procedure (either alone or in combination with a light general anaesthetic) can be continued to produce high-quality analgesia in the post-operative period (considered below).

Spinal and epidural anaesthesia also block the sympathetic outflow within the anterior nerve roots. Rapid vasomotor paralysis reflects the small unmyelinated nature of the nerves and is an early indication of a successful block. Frequently, the patient comments on warm feet, owing to cutaneous vasodilatation and an increase in blood flow through the skin. The same mechanism explains the common complication of hypotension seen with these techniques, which requires the judicious administration of intravenous fluids and/or vasoconstrictors (ephedrine or phenylephrine).

Many types of surgery can be performed using local anaesthetic techniques alone, with or without sedation. However, patients should always be fasted as for general anaesthesia, and monitoring and facilities for resuscitation should always be present.

POST-OPERATIVE ANALGESIA

Good-quality pain relief is important to patients, and failure to ensure it results in adverse physiological and psychological morbidity. Despite this, severe pain and poor or fair pain relief are experienced by approximately 20% of patients. In the UK, the Audit Commission proposed a standard that by 2002 only 5% of patients would experience severe pain. This is a difficult standard to achieve. Effective post-operative analgesia requires careful pre-operative planning, a good understanding of the proposed surgery and consideration of the patient's concurrent medical conditions. In addition, knowledge of pain physiology, pain assessment, drug delivery strategies and drug pharmacology is essential. The pain pathway is illustrated in Figure 10.6.

Many hospitals now have a dedicated acute pain service. This is a multidisciplinary team consisting of doctors, specialized nurses and other paramedical staff. They are charged not only with the delivery of post-operative pain management to individual patients, but have responsibility for institutional protocols, education of staff and patients, and quality assurance programmes to ensure service effectiveness.

PAIN PHYSIOLOGY

Sensory neurons responding to stimuli capable of producing tissue damage are termed nociceptors. Most body structures contain them. They are high-threshold polymodal receptors, meaning that they respond to a variety of noxious stimuli. Typically, they respond to noxious heat and strong mechanical and chemical stimuli, both endogenous and exogenous. In general terms, nociceptive processes begin with activation of the primary afferent nociceptor, a process known as transduction. Transduction results in the conversion of the noxious stimuli into electrochemical activity. Surgical trauma or another noxious stimulus results in an inflammatory response around the peripheral nociceptor, causing modification of its response properties. Prostaglandins are one of the many inflammatory mediators involved; hence the importance of NSAIDs in analgesic regimes.

Transmission of nociceptive activity in the peripheral nerve is via both small unmyelinated C-fibres (diameter < 2 µm; conduction speed ~1 ms^{-1}) and small myelinated Aδ-fibres (diameter 2–5 µm; conduction speed 15 ms^{-1}). This contrasts with the much larger (10 µm), rapidly conducting (> 30 ms^{-1}) Aβ-fibres, which largely terminate

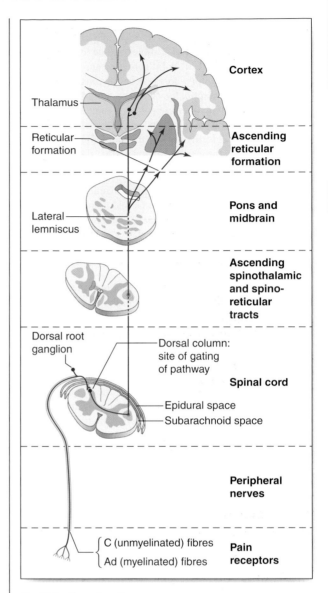

Fig. 10.6 The pain pathway.

in the superficial laminae (I and II) of the dorsal horn. Not only do primary afferent fibres synapse with second-order neurons, but there is also a complex interaction with local intrinsic spinal neurons and descending modulatory neurons coming from the brain.

The dorsal horn of the spinal cord is a key site in terms of pain transmission and modulation of activity by local intrinsic neurons and descending fibres from the brain. The predominant excitatory neurotransmitters in the spinal cord are glutamate and substance P. One of the key glutamate receptors is the N-methyl D-aspartate (NMDA) receptor. If there is sufficient afferent neuronal activity, the NMDA receptor becomes activated and this can lead to central sensitization. Central sensitization is an important factor in the development of chronic pain states. A wide range of changes can be detected in the dorsal horn, including an increase in receptive field (spatial changes), increased response to afferent activity (threshold changes),

10

increased spontaneous neuronal activity and prolonged after-discharges in response to transient stimuli.

As discussed, Aδ- and C-fibres excite centrally projecting neurons. Dorsal horn activity can, however, be modulated by inhibitory dorsal horn neurons, acting both pre- and post-synaptically. Gamma-aminobutyric acid (GABA), along with the co-agonist glycine, is the major inhibitory neurotransmitter found in the dorsal horn.

Nociceptive information is transmitted cephalad via spinal sensory neurons. In general terms, the spinal cord has three major projections to the brain. They are:

- direct thalamic projections (spinothalamic tracts)
- direct projections to the reticular and homeostatic control regions of the brain stem (spinoreticular and spinomesencephalic tracts)
- direct projections to the hypothalamus and ventral forebrain (spinohypothalamic tracts).

All nociceptive information reaching the cortex is processed and relayed by the thalamus. The thalamus then relays the information to the key areas of the brain involved in pain perception. Areas consistently found to be active in pain states are the primary and secondary somatosensory cortices (SI and SII), the insula and the anterior cingulate cortex.

Finally, descending pathways from the brain stem and other cerebral structures play an important role in modulation and integration of afferent activity in the dorsal horn. In the main, this is via the serotonergic and noradrenergic systems.

PAIN ASSESSMENT

Regular assessment of pain and pain relief is important. In the acute pain setting, unidimensional scales are usually used. Examples are simple measures such as a verbal rating scale, e.g. a four-point scale covering no pain, mild pain, moderate pain or severe pain. These are easy to use but have the disadvantage of being non-linear. Examples of linear assessment tools are numerical rating scales ranging from 0–10 or visual analogue scales of 1–100 mm. The choice of scale often falls to institutional preference. It should be remembered that the most important measure is the patient's own subjective pain experience and this should never be disregarded.

POST-OPERATIVE ANALGESIC STRATEGIES

It is important to use an evidence-based strategy when planning the post-operative pain management of patients. This area has been comprehensively reviewed by the Australian and New Zealand College of Anaesthetists and Faculty of Pain Medicine in a document entitled *Acute pain management: scientific evidence*. This document has been endorsed by the Royal College of Anaesthetists.

There is strong evidence that patients benefit from the use of multimodal analgesic strategies, i.e. different drugs or analgesic strategies that act at different parts of the pain pathway. This will result in either enhanced analgesia or a reduction in side-effects caused by some of the medications used.

For patients undergoing major surgery, a technique of either epidural analgesia or patient-controlled analgesia is employed; this should be supplemented (unless contraindicated) by regular paracetamol and NSAIDs. Appropriate step-down analgesia should be prescribed and there should be recognition that neuropathic pain can occur acutely in the perioperative period. Certain types of surgery, e.g. to the shoulder and knee, lend themselves to the use of a peripheral nerve block. For less significant surgery, a regime of 'as required' subcutaneous or oral opioid may be used. This should also be supplemented by the regular use of paracetamol and NSAIDs. These analgesic techniques will be discussed below.

EPIDURAL ANALGESIA

Epidural analgesia is the provision of pain relief by the (usually) continuous infusion of drugs into the epidural space. It is now widely used following major surgery and is particularly suited to thoracotomy, and major abdominal and lower limb surgery. The epidural is usually placed prior to surgery and continued into the post-operative period for 1–5 days.

The usual practice is the use of a low dose of local anaesthetic in combination with an opioid, typically fentanyl. This combination gives superior analgesia to either drug alone. A typical infusion mixture would be bupivacaine 0.1% with the addition of 2 µg/ml fentanyl at a rate of between 6 and 16 ml/hr.

Epidural analgesia provides improved pain relief over parenteral opioid infusion (e.g. patient-controlled analgesia), with a reduced incidence of pulmonary complications. The main disadvantages of epidural analgesia are that many institutions require patients to be in a high-dependency unit setting, expensive equipment (e.g. infusion pumps) is needed, and high levels of staff skill education are essential. The most common problems associated with epidural analgesia are hypotension, respiratory depression, analgesic failure and post-dural puncture headache.

Hypotension

This is one of the most common side-effects of epidural analgesia, occurring in around 5% of patients. In part, it is provoked by the sympathetic blockade that occurs with the epidural, but the main cause is usually hypovolaemia due either to insufficient peri- and post-operative fluid administration or to haemorrhage. If analgesia is satisfactory and the patient is well filled and not bleeding, then initially the infusion rate should be dropped. The addition of an infusion of a small dose of vasoconstrictor may be useful.

Respiratory depression

This is also common, with rates up to 15%, similar to that in patients using patient-controlled analgesia. All patients with epidural infusions should have supplementary oxygen.

Analgesic failure

Epidural may fail for reasons such as misplacement or displacement of the catheter. In addition, factors such as inadequate analgesia or intolerable side-effects—for example, hypotension, opioid-induced itch or excessive motor blockade—may cause premature discontinuation of the epidural. Patients should have an appropriate replacement technique, such as patient-controlled analgesia, instituted immediately.

Post-dural puncture headache

If the dura is inadvertently punctured during insertion of the epidural, then the patient may complain of what is classically a postural headache. It is more common in patients under 50 years of age and, although it will usually improve within 10 days, it is often treated with an epidural blood patch.

Complications such as epidural abscess (incidence 0.015–0.05%), epidural haematoma (approximately 1 in 10 000) and permanent neurological damage (incidence 0.005–0.05%) are rare but may have devastating consequences for the patient. The presence of severe back pain, with or without fever and with or without neurological signs, requires urgent investigation, usually by MRI.

PATIENT-CONTROLLED ANALGESIA (PCA)

PCA consists of a pre-programmed pump that allows a patient to self-administer a small predetermined dose of drug, usually an opioid such as morphine. When using morphine, the usual starting dose should be 1 mg, as this provides good analgesia with a lower risk of respiratory depression (than 2 mg). The dose, however, should take into consideration the patient's age, size and history of opioid exposure. Most commonly available opioids can be used in PCA form with similar efficacy. The machine has a lockout period that allows the patient to feel the effect of the dose of the drug before administering a subsequent dose. Lockouts can vary but are typically 5 minutes. Background infusions can be added but this increases the risk of respiratory depression; they should not be used routinely but have a place in patients who are chronic opioid users. PCA has been shown to be superior to standard parenteral opioid regimes such as intermittent intramuscular (IM) regimes. This may reflect inadequate IM regimes rather than a true superiority.

As with epidurals, the main drawback is the need for (often) expensive equipment. Both patients and staff need education in the use of the PCA. Errors resulting in death have been reported, involving incorrect programming and use of the wrong concentration of drug.

Side-effects

As with all opioid regimes, the main side-effects of PCA are respiratory depression and nausea. Estimates have put the incidence of respiratory depression as high as 11.5%. The incidence is, however, no worse than that of a typical intermittent IM regime and is lower than that of a continuous opioid infusion. Nausea should be treated with a standard post-operative antiemetic regime. There is no advantage to be gained by adding antiemetics directly to the pump syringe.

PARENTERAL AND ORAL OPIOID REGIMES

Strong opioids

If the surgery is of a minor nature or the patient is stepping down from an epidural or from PCA, then a parenteral or oral opioid regime may be used. It is important to avoid the so-called analgesic gap. This commonly occurs in situations when patients are stepped down from an epidural or PCA to either a weak ineffective opioid or a non-opioid regime. In most cases, patients should step down to a strong opioid-based regime, oral if possible. In most circumstances, there is little to suggest that one opioid is superior to another and so morphine is commonly used. In a typical parenteral regime, an average patient should be prescribed morphine 10 mg subcutaneously 1-hourly prn. The dose should, however, take into account the patient's age and size. Traditional regimes using 4–6-hourly IM doses should not be used, as dosing frequency is inadequate and IM injections are painful. As stated, when possible, oral analgesic regimes should be used. A typical regime would consist of oral morphine tablets at a dose of 10–20 mg 1-hourly prn. Typical opioid side-effects are nausea and vomiting, respiratory depression, altered gastrointestinal function, pruritus and urinary retention.

Weak opioids

There are many opioids on the market, many of them combined with paracetamol. Typical examples of weak opioids are codeine, and dihydrocodeine with tramadol. These may be useful in the treatment of mild pain. Drug selection is important, as some have not been shown to be particularly effective when subjected to quantitative systematic review.

Codeine 60 mg in combination with paracetamol has been shown to be an effective therapy. Dihydrocodeine, like codeine, is very commonly prescribed; however, evidence shows that a single dose of 30 mg is no more effective than placebo in relieving post-operative pain. Tramadol is both a weak opioid and a serotonin and noradrenaline (norepinephrine) re-uptake inhibitor, giving it a dual action. It is effective in both acute and neuropathic pain. Typical dosing would be 50–100 mg 1-hourly prn, with a maximum dose of 600 mg per 24 hours.

PARACETAMOL, NSAIDS AND SELECTIVE COX-2 INHIBITORS

Paracetamol is an effective drug for post-operative pain. It should be prescribed to all post-operative patients, except in the rare incidence of contraindication. Paracetamol has a morphine-sparing effect and, in combination with NSAIDs, improves analgesia.

NSAIDs have been shown to be very effective in the reduction of post-operative pain and, along with paracetamol, are a valuable component of multimodal analgesia. Their main drawback is their contraindication and side-

10

10

effect profile. NSAIDs can affect renal function, especially in dehydrated and hypovolaemic patients. Prostaglandins are important in the protection of the gastric mucosa and thus NSAIDs predispose to peptic ulceration. NSAIDs impair platelet function and may exacerbate surgical bleeding, e.g. after tonsillectomy. In certain asthmatic patients, NSAIDs can predispose to bronchospasm. Asthma is not, however, an absolute contraindication to NSAID use, as many patients with asthma can take them without problems. Providing the contraindications are respected, then NSAIDs should be used where possible.

Selective COX-2 inhibitors are as effective as conventional NSAIDs in post-operative pain. In long-term use, they have a lower incidence of peptic ulceration than conventional NSAIDs, do not seem to cause bronchospasm and do not impair platelet function. They have, probably as a class, a higher incidence of cardiovascular and thromboembolic events. They are contraindicated in patients with established ischaemic heart disease, cerebrovascular disease and heart failure. They should be used with caution in patients with risk factors for the above, e.g. diabetes, hypertension etc. Their routine use in post-operative patients is not recommended.

BOX 10.4 POST-OPERATIVE PAIN CONTROL

- Regular pain assessment is important
- Epidural analgesia provides improved pain scores with reduced pulmonary morbidity
- PCA provides superior analgesia to conventional opioid regimes
- Multimodal analgesia is essential
- Beware the 'analgesic gap'
- Be aware of the evidence base behind drugs, e.g. dihydrocodeine
- Neuropathic pain can occur in the perioperative period
- Prevention of PONV requires a multimodal approach

NEUROPATHIC PAIN

Although classically thought to be a chronic condition, neuropathic pain may occur in 1–3% of post-operative patients. Staff need to be alert for it, as it tends not to respond well to conventional post-operative regimes. Expert advice should be sought if it is suspected. In the acute phase, infusions of drugs such as ketamine or lidocaine may be required, followed by oral therapies such as a tricyclic antidepressant (e.g. amitriptyline) or an anticonvulsant (e.g. gabapentin).

POST-OPERATIVE NAUSEA AND VOMITING (PONV)

This can be a problem for as many as 30% of patients who undergo general anaesthesia. Predisposing factors include female sex, type of surgery (e.g. gynaecological surgery), previous PONV and opioid use. Some anaesthetic agents, such as propofol, have a lower incidence of PONV. Other agents, such as nitrous oxide, predispose to PONV. The use of opioid-sparing techniques and the maintenance of adequate hydration are important. Drugs proven to be effective in preventing PONV are the 5-HT$_3$ antagonists, e.g. ondansetron, droperidol and dexamethasone. As with analgesic regimes, a multimodal technique is most useful, especially in high-risk patients.

11

R.W. PARKS

Practical procedures and patient investigation

11

INTRODUCTION

Every practical procedure performed on a conscious patient should be preceded by an explanation, which should include the reasons for the procedure and what it will entail. Appropriate reassurance should always be given. Many patients find comfort in continuing reassurance throughout the procedure, and most are helped by a description of sensations they are likely to experience before these occur. Where appropriate, informed written consent should be obtained.

GENERAL PRECAUTIONS

It is important to be aware of the risk of infection or trauma to patient, operator and assistant during any practical procedure. These risks are minimized by following a few simple rules:

- Needles should not be resheathed and all disposable sharp instruments discarded by the operator should be placed in an appropriate container to minimize the risk of needle-stick injury.
- Drapes and other soiled equipment should be placed in appropriate containers.
- Gloves and gown should only be removed after all used instruments and disposable equipment have been placed in appropriate containers.

ASEPTIC TECHNIQUE

Transmission of infection is an ever-present problem, and the risk of spread should be minimized. As a minimum precaution, the skin should be cleansed with an antiseptic solution before all procedures, and sterile instruments should be used. For some procedures, such as central venous catheterization, bladder catheterization, insertion of chest drains and lumbar puncture, a full aseptic technique must be used. The steps required are outlined in Table 11.1.

LOCAL ANAESTHESIA

Local anaesthetic agents inhibit membrane depolarization and hence block the transmission of nerve impulses. They may be used topically, i.e. painted or sprayed on mucous membranes and wound surfaces, so that they are absorbed locally to produce analgesia. Areas suitable for topical analgesia include the urethra, eye, nose, throat and bronchial tree. Local anaesthesia may also be administered by local infiltration, and this is used widely for minor surgical procedures. Local anaesthetic drugs are potentially toxic and care must be taken to avoid inadvertent intravascular injection. The first sign of toxicity is often numbness or tingling of the tongue or around the mouth, followed by lightheadedness and tinnitus. At higher blood levels, there is loss of consciousness, convulsions and apnoea.

Table 11.1 ASEPTIC TECHNIQUE

- An assistant is desirable to open non-sterile packs and 'drop' required instruments or solutions on to the sterile field
- Hand-washing for aseptic techniques ('scrubbing up') should last a full 3 minutes. The hands and forearms are wetted under a running tap and thoroughly washed with an antiseptic solution such as povidone–iodine (Betadine) or chlorhexidine (Hibiscrub)
- A sterile brush is then used to scrub the hands: in particular, the ulnar border, the interdigital clefts and the nails
- After the wash is completed, the hands are rinsed and held hands up/elbows down, so that water from the hands runs from the elbows into the sink
- The hands are dried on a sterile towel and the operator puts on a sterile gown and gloves. Thereafter, the operator must not touch anything other than sterile equipment or instruments
- The operative field is now cleansed with an antiseptic solution such as povidone–iodine or chlorhexidine, using sterile instruments and swabs. The area prepared should be much greater than the anticipated operative field, and cleansing should start from the centre and work outwards
- The operative field is then encircled with sterile drapes, which are secured so as to leave the operative field at the centre and provide the operator with as wide a sterile surrounding as possible

---

Cardiovascular collapse eventually occurs as a result of myocardial depression, vasodilatation and hypoxia. In general, efficacy is related to correct placement and toxicity to total dose. Where there is doubt about placement or a wide area of infiltration is anticipated, it is safer to calculate the maximum recommended dose and dilute it to the desired volume with 0.9% saline.

Lidocaine is the most widely used local anaesthetic agent and is available in 0.5–2% solutions. The maximum recommended dose is 3 mg/kg. Lidocaine is a short-acting anaesthetic (lasting up to 2 hours), whereas bupivacaine is longer-acting (up to 8 hours). A mixture of the two can be administered.

Solutions of local anaesthetic mixed with a 1:200 000 concentration of adrenaline (epinephrine) are also available. Adrenaline acts as a vasoconstrictor. It minimizes bleeding and reduces redistribution of the anaesthetic agent, thereby increasing its efficacy and duration of action. Local anaesthetic agents with adrenaline should not be used in anatomical areas supplied by an end-artery, such as the digits, because of the risk of vasoconstriction, ischaemia and gangrene.

WOUND SUTURE

The purpose of suturing is to approximate wound edges in such a manner as to allow optimum primary healing to take place. Wounds are sutured under as near-sterile conditions as possible, using a strict aseptic technique. A few basic principles underlie good wound care:

- Tissue should be handled gently. The wound should not be rubbed with swabs. Blood in a wound is removed by pressing a swab on to it.
- Haemostasis should be meticulous to prevent wound haematoma.

- All foreign material and devitalized tissues should be removed. Where this is prevented by heavy contamination, delayed primary suture or secondary suture should be considered.
- Potential spaces (dead space) in the wound should be closed using absorbable suture material such as Vicryl. Where this is not possible, a suction drain is led from the potential space before more superficial layers are closed.
- The tension on knots is critical. If they are tied too tightly, the suture line may become ischaemic, leading to delayed healing or non-healing and an increased risk of wound infection. Equally, insufficient tension on the suture may result in failure to appose the wound edges or inadequate haemostasis.

SUTURING THE SKIN

Cutting needles are used to suture skin. Non-absorbable sutures (see below) are generally preferred, but require subsequent removal. Interrupted sutures have the advantage over a continuous suture in that the removal of one or two appropriately sited stitches may allow adequate drainage if the wound becomes infected. The sutures should be placed equidistant from one another, taking equal 'bites' on either side of the wound. A sufficient number should be inserted to maintain apposition without the skin edges gaping. The size of bite is determined by the amount of subcutaneous fat and by whether or not the fat has been separately sutured. For abdominal wounds, 5 mm bites are taken on either side of the wound, whereas on the face a 1–2 mm bite is preferred. The wound edge is picked up with toothed dissecting forceps, then the needle is introduced through the skin at an angle as close to vertical as possible and brought out on the other side at a similar angle.

Similar principles apply when using a continuous suture. A subcuticular continuous suture is preferred by some surgeons and avoids the small pinpoint scars at the site of entry and exit of interrupted sutures, or the ugly cross-hatching that results if sutures are tied too tightly or left in too long. Table 11.2 gives the suggested times for removal of sutures. Cosmetic results as good as those achieved by subcuticular suturing can be obtained by removing sutures in half the times listed in Table 11.2 and by replacing them with adhesive strips (e.g. Steristrip). Skin stapling is commonly used for closure of wounds at any site, as it can be undertaken rapidly. The staples are supplied in disposable cartridges for single patient use and are easily removed.

Table 11.2 SUGGESTED GAUGE OF SUTURE MATERIAL FOR SKIN SUTURE	
• Around the eyes	6/0 sutures
• Elsewhere on the face	5/0 sutures
• Neck, hands and digits	4/0 sutures
• Other sites	3/0 or even 2/0 suture
• Subcuticular wound closure	4/0 sutures

Table 11.3 TIMES RECOMMENDED FOR REMOVAL OF SUTURES	
• Face and neck	4 days
• Scalp	7 days
• Abdomen and chest	7–10 days
• Limbs	7 days
• Feet	10–14 days

SUTURE MATERIALS

Suggested gauges of materials for skin suture are shown in Table 11.3.

Non-absorbable sutures

Non-absorbable sutures may be classified into three groups:

1. *Natural braided sutures* (e.g. silk, linen) have good handling qualities and knot easily and securely. Their disadvantage is increased tissue reaction and suture line sepsis, caused by the capillary action of the braided material drawing microorganisms into the suture track. Such materials also lose tensile strength quickly with time, or when wet.
2. *Synthetic braided materials* (e.g. Nurolon, Ethibond, Mersilene) cause less tissue reaction than natural materials. They have good handling qualities and knot easily and securely.
3. *Synthetic monofilament materials* (e.g. nylon, polypropylene) have less drag through the tissues and cause little tissue reaction. They are free from the capillary effect of braided sutures and cause less suture track sepsis. However, they handle less well because of increased 'memory' (i.e. they retain the configuration in which they were packaged). Knots in monofilament sutures are less secure than those in braided or natural sutures, requiring multiple throws on each one.

Absorbable sutures

Absorbable sutures are generally made from synthetic materials. They cause relatively little tissue reaction, retain their tensile strength and are absorbed slowly. They can be multifilament, such as Dexon (polyglycolic acid) and Vicryl (polyglycolic plus polylactic acid), or monofilament, such as Maxon (polyglyconate) and PDS (polydioxonone). These synthetic sutures are commonly used for subcuticular wound closure. Interrupted sutures with each knot buried are used for small wounds, whereas in longer wounds a continuous subcuticular suture is employed.

AIRWAY PROCEDURES

MAINTAINING THE AIRWAY

The ability to maintain the airway is a basic skill that every doctor, nurse, paramedic and indeed member of the general public should have. Its simplicity belies its importance, but it is a life-saving skill, which must be learnt through practice.

11

11

In the unconscious patient, muscles that normally maintain a clear airway become lax. The tongue and soft tissue fall backwards, particularly in the supine patient, occluding the airway. Maintaining a clear airway allows the patient to breathe or allows the lungs to be ventilated.

Procedure

The simplest manoeuvre is to place patients on their side with the neck extended in the so-called 'recovery position'. This allows the tongue and soft tissues to fall clear of the larynx and provide a patent airway. The mouth and pharynx should be checked and cleared of debris, such as dentures, vomit or food.

When the patient has to be kept supine, the neck should be extended. The mouth is opened slightly and the mandible pulled firmly forward by pressure applied behind both angles of the jaw. The mandible is held in this position by closing the mouth and using the teeth as a splint. Forward pressure is maintained behind the angles of the jaw (jaw-thrust manoeuvre) or submentally (chin-lift manoeuvre), avoiding pressure on the soft tissues (Fig. 11.1). In some cases, particularly in edentulous patients, an oropharyngeal airway helps to maintain a patent airway.

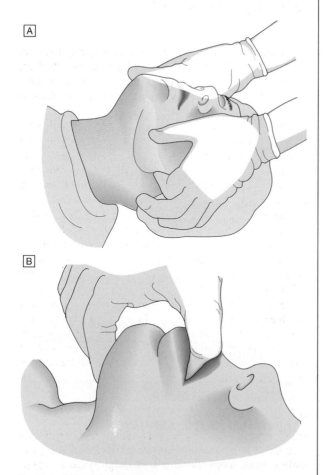

Fig. 11.1 Maintaining the airway.
A The jaw-thrust manoeuvre. B The chin-lift manoeuvre.

VENTILATION BY MASK

The lungs may be ventilated by mask and bag, using one of two systems. The first is a rebreathing bag with an adjustable valve and fresh gas supply (which should be present in each anaesthetic room, intensive therapy unit and resuscitation room). The second and more widespread is the self-reinflating type of bag, such as the 'Ambu' or 'Laerdal' bags, which do not rely on a gas supply but to which supplemental oxygen can be added. For the inexperienced, this technique is best performed with the help of an assistant.

Procedure

The airway is held patent with the patient supine, as described above. A mask is applied to the face and held in position using the thumb and index fingers of both hands. The little fingers of each hand are placed behind the angles of the jaw and used to lift the mandible forward. The ring and middle fingers are placed on the mandible to help maintain this position. The assistant squeezes the bag to ventilate the lungs. The adequacy of ventilation is assessed by observing appropriate chest movement.

With more experience, it is possible to maintain a patent airway and hold the mask on with one hand, and squeeze the bag with the other.

THE LARYNGEAL MASK AIRWAY

This recently introduced airway is designed to be inserted into the pharynx, and has a cuff that, when inflated, forms a cup around the larynx. It is not a replacement for endotracheal intubation and does not protect the airway from aspiration. It does, however, provide a patent airway when positioned correctly, and allows effective ventilation of the lungs. As with other procedures, insertion should be learned under supervision.

Procedure

For men a size 4 is suitable, and for women a size 3, with smaller sizes being available for children. The cuff should be deflated and lubricated with gel. The patient's head is maintained in an extended position using the left hand, and the airway is held in the right hand and introduced into the mouth (Fig. 11.2). The airway is passed backwards over the tongue until resistance is felt. It should then be at the level of the larynx at the upper oesophageal sphincter. The cuff is inflated and the airway should be seen to rise slightly out of the mouth. Position is confirmed by the ability to ventilate the lungs with gentle pressure on a bag system.

ENDOTRACHEAL INTUBATION

Endotracheal intubation can be life-saving; it can maintain a patent airway, facilitate oxygenation and prevent aspiration. Every opportunity should be taken to acquire this skill in the elective situation in the anaesthetic room.

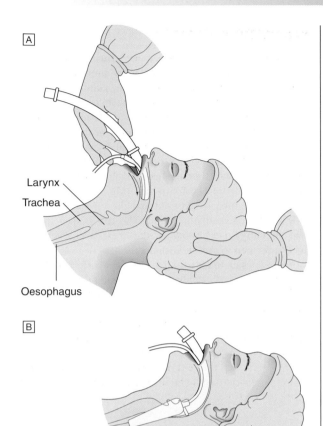

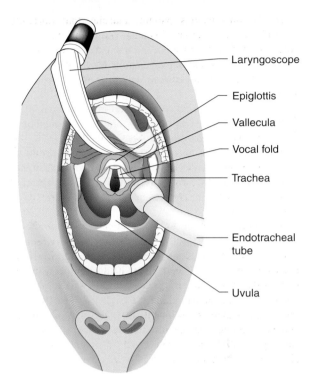

Fig. 11.3   Oral endotracheal intubation.

Fig. 11.2   Insertion of a laryngeal mask airway.
A Gentle insertion of airway with head in extended position.
B Advancement of airway.

Procedure

The patient's neck is flexed and the head extended at the atlanto-occipital joint. Retaining a pillow under the head but leaving a space free from beneath the shoulders will usually help to attain this position. Failure to position the patient correctly is one of the most common causes of difficulty in intubation.

The laryngoscope is held in the left hand; its blade is inserted into the right side of the patient's mouth and passed backwards along the side of the tongue into the oropharynx. The blade is designed to push the tongue over to the left side of the mouth. Care is taken to avoid damage to the lips and teeth. The laryngoscope is *pulled* upwards and forwards, *not* used as a lever, to lift the tongue and jaw and reveal the epiglottis (Fig. 11.3). The blade is then advanced to the base of the epiglottis.

Failure to visualize the epiglottis usually reflects the fact that the blade has not been inserted far enough, in which case only the base of the tongue will be seen. Alternatively, it may mean that it has been inserted too far, in which case the upper oesophagus will be seen. The appropriate adjustment in position should be made. The laryngoscope is pulled further upwards and forwards to reveal the vocal cords.

For men a 9 mm cuffed tube is usually appropriate, and for women an 8 mm tube is generally used. For children, a rough rule of thumb to gauge tube size is age divided by 4 + 4.5 mm. Normally, an uncuffed tube is used in children.

The endotracheal tube is passed through the vocal cords into the trachea and advanced until its cuff is about 1 cm through. Many endotracheal tubes have a mark to indicate this position. The laryngoscope blade is then withdrawn and the cuff inflated to provide an airtight seal in the trachea.

The most serious complication of endotracheal intubation is failure to recognize misplacement of the tube, particularly in the oesophagus or, to a lesser degree, in the right main bronchus. Misplacement is best avoided by direct visualization of passage of the tube between the vocal cords, inspection of the chest wall for equal movement of both sides of the chest, and auscultation for breath sounds bilaterally in the mid-axillary line. Absence of breath sounds or the presence of only quiet ones in the epigastrium is a further reassuring sign. If there is any doubt about the position of the tube, it should be removed and ventilation instituted by mask.

SURGICAL AIRWAY

Inability to intubate the trachea is an indication for creating a surgical airway. In the emergency situation, such as in patients with severe facial trauma or pharyngeal oedema secondary to burns, the insertion of a large-calibre plastic cannula through the cricothyroid membrane (needle cricothyroidotomy) below the level of the obstruction can be life-saving. Intermittent jet insufflation of oxygen at 15 litres/min (1 sec inspiration and 4 secs to allow expiration) can provide oxygenation for a limited period (30–45 minutes) until a more definitive procedure can be undertaken.

Surgical cricothyroidotomy is performed by making an incision that extends through the cricothyroid membrane and inserting a tracheostomy tube.

In children, care must be taken to avoid damage to the cricoid cartilage, which is the only circumferential support to the upper trachea. Surgical cricothyroidotomy is therefore not recommended for children under 12 years of age.

Procedure

It is important to check all equipment and connections before starting. With the patient in the supine position and the neck in a neutral position, the thyroid cartilage (Adam's apple) and cricoid cartilage are palpated. The cricothyroid membrane lies between the lower border of the thyroid cartilage and the upper border of the cricoid cartilage. The skin is cleansed with antiseptic solution and local anaesthetic infiltrated into the skin, if the patient is conscious. The thyroid cartilage is stabilized with the left hand and a small transverse skin incision made over the cricothyroid membrane. The blade of the scalpel is inserted through the membrane and then rotated through 90° to open the airway. An artery clip or tracheal spreader may be inserted to enlarge the opening enough to admit a cuffed endotracheal or tracheostomy tube (Fig. 11.4). The central trocar of the tube is removed and the tube connected to a bag-valve or ventilator circuit. The cuff is then inflated and air entry to each side of the chest is checked. The tube is secured to prevent dislodgement.

Formal open tracheostomy may be performed as an emergency procedure, but is more commonly undertaken

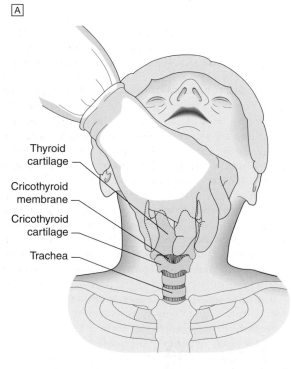

Thyroid
cartilage

Cricothyroid
membrane

Cricothyroid
cartilage

Trachea

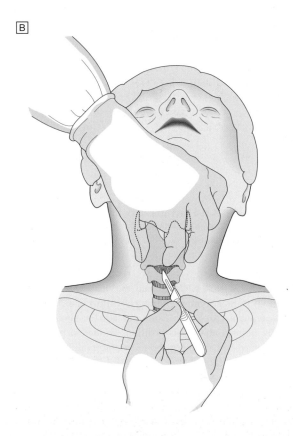

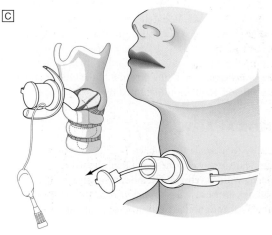

Fig. 11.4 Surgical cricothyroidotomy.
A Palpation of thyroid cartilage. B Incision through cricothyroid membrane. C Insertion of tracheostomy tube.

in critically ill patients requiring long-term ventilation. It is a procedure for an experienced clinician and involves making an inverted U-shaped opening through the second, third and fourth tracheal rings.

CHANGING A TRACHEOSTOMY TUBE

It is common practice to change a tracheostomy tube every 7 days. Suction must be available.

Procedure

If a cuffed tube is to be inserted, the integrity of the cuff is checked and it is then fully deflated. Lubricant gel is applied to both the cuff and tube. The patient is placed semi-recumbent with the neck extended. If replacement is likely to be difficult, a suction catheter inserted into the old tracheostomy tube can be used as an introducer for the new tube.

The cuff of the old tube is deflated. Secretions often collect above the cuff and enter the trachea when it is deflated, causing the patient to cough; both patient and operator should be alert to this. Because the tube is curved, it should be removed with an 'arc-like' movement. The site is then cleansed and any secretions are removed. In the spontaneously breathing stable patient, there is no need for undue haste. The new tube is inserted with a similar movement to that employed for removal, and its cuff inflated.

Any signs of respiratory distress should raise suspicion of the possibility of misplacement or occlusion of the tube. The tube and trachea are immediately checked for patency by passing a suction catheter through the tube. If the catheter passes easily into the respiratory tract, usually signified by the patient coughing as the catheter touches the carina, other causes for respiratory distress should be sought.

When the tracheostomy is no longer needed, an airtight dressing is applied over the site after removing the tube. There is no need for formal surgical closure at this stage, as in most instances the wound will close and heal spontaneously. For the first few days, patients should be encouraged to press firmly on the dressing when they wish to cough, so as to avoid air leakage through the tracheostomy site.

THORACIC PROCEDURES

INTERCOSTAL TUBE DRAINAGE

Intercostal intubation is used to drain a large pneumothorax, haemothorax or pleural effusion. To drain a pneumothorax, a size 14–16 Fr catheter is inserted, using a lateral approach in the mid-axillary line of the sixth intercostal space. Drainage of an effusion or haemothorax requires a larger drain (20–26 Fr), which should be inserted in the seventh, eighth or ninth intercostal space in the posterior axillary line. A slightly higher insertion in the mid-axillary line may be technically easier in supine, acutely ill patients.

Procedure

If a low lateral approach is to be used, reference should be made to the chest X-ray to ensure that the drain will not be inserted subdiaphragmatically. A strict aseptic technique must be used. The skin, intercostal muscles and pleura are infiltrated with local anaesthetic. If a rib is encountered by the needle, the tip is 'walked' up the rib to enter the pleura above the rib edge. The depth at which the pleural space is entered is determined by aspiration with the syringe. A 3 cm horizontal incision is now made in the skin. A tract is developed by blunt dissection through the subcutaneous tissues and the intercostal muscles are separated just superior to the top of the rib to avoid damage to the neurovascular bundle. The parietal pleura is punctured with the tip of a pair of artery forceps and a gloved finger is inserted into the pleural cavity (Fig. 11.5). This ensures the incision is correctly placed, prevents injury to other organs, and permits any adhesions or clots to be cleared. The trocar is removed from the thoracostomy tube,

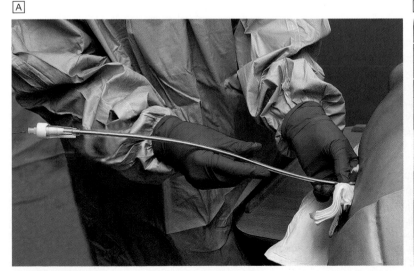
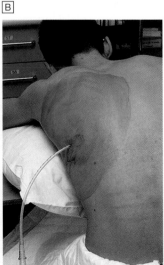

A Insertion   **B** In situ

Fig. 11.5 Chest drain.

the proximal end is clamped, and the tube is advanced into the pleural space to the desired length. The tube is sutured to the skin with a heavy suture to prevent accidental dislodgement. A 'Z' suture is placed around the incision, wrapped tightly around the drainage tube and tied, thus securing the tube. A sterile dressing and an adhesive bandage are applied to form an airtight seal and prevent aspiration of air around the tube. The drainage tube is attached to an underwater drainage system and a chest X-ray is then obtained. Low-pressure suction may be applied to the drainage bottle to assist drainage or re-expansion of the lung.

REMOVAL OF AN INTERCOSTAL DRAINAGE TUBE

The drainage tube may be removed 12–24 hours after cessation of drainage. As a precaution in the case of pneumothorax, the tube is first clamped for several hours and a chest X-ray taken to ensure that there has been no recurrence.

Procedure

The 'Z' suture is freed from the tube and can be used to close the wound. Where this is not possible, the suture should be totally removed and a new one inserted around the wound. Patients are asked to hold their breath and the tube is withdrawn, after which the skin is firmly closed with the previously inserted suture. A sterile dressing is firmly applied over the wound and a chest X-ray repeated to confirm that there is no pneumothorax.

PLEURAL ASPIRATION

Aspiration of fluid from the pleural cavity is performed for diagnostic or therapeutic purposes. Protein or amylase content, and cytological or bacteriological examination may be diagnostic. Complete aspiration of large effusions allows fuller expansion of the lungs and may improve ventilation.

Procedure

Where aspiration is to be undertaken for diagnostic purposes only, a 21-gauge needle and syringe are adequate. For therapeutic aspiration, a larger-bore needle, 50 ml syringe and three-way tap system should be used. The procedure is carried out using a strict aseptic technique.

The patient is positioned sitting up, resting the arms and elbows on a table. The position and size of the effusion should be outlined by percussion and chest X-ray. The lower border of the effusion is determined, particularly on the right to avoid puncturing the liver. In the case of small effusions, ultrasound guidance is helpful.

The skin, intercostal muscles and pleura are infiltrated with local anaesthetic in the seventh or eighth space, in line with the inferior angle of the scapula. The needle is advanced over the upper border of the rib to avoid damage to the neurovascular bundle. Continuous suction should be applied to the syringe and the needle advanced no further than is required to aspirate fluid freely, thereby avoiding damage to the underlying lung.

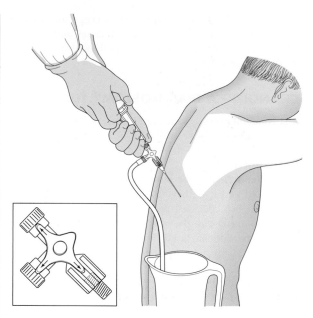

Fig. 11.6   Pleural aspiration.

If the volume of fluid to be removed is greater than the volume of the syringe being used, a three-way tap greatly reduces the risk of air entry and allows the syringe to be emptied into a collection vessel (Fig. 11.6); this avoids having to disconnect the syringe each time it is filled. It is normally recommended that no more than 1–1.5 litres of fluid be removed at any one time. This reduces the risk of sudden mediastinal shift or the development of pulmonary oedema associated with rapid re-expansion of a collapsed lung. Coughing or pain on aspiration is an indication that visceral pleura is in close contact with the end of the cannula, which should be repositioned or withdrawn.

At the end of the procedure, the needle is withdrawn and a sterile dressing applied. A chest X-ray is taken to assess the amount of residual fluid present and to exclude a pneumothorax.

ABDOMINAL PROCEDURES

NASOGASTRIC TUBE INSERTION

A nasogastric tube is inserted to drain stomach contents in conditions such as intestinal obstruction, or to administer enteral nutrition. In most situations, a 14–16 Fr single-lumen radio-opaque nasogastric tube with multiple distal openings will suffice. Double-lumen tubes are occasionally used to allow continuous low-pressure suction and to prevent the lumen from becoming blocked by gastric mucosa.

Procedure

The nose is inspected for any deformity and the more patent nasal passage is chosen for insertion. The patient is placed in the sitting position and a local anaesthetic spray may be used to anaesthetize the nasal passage. The tube is well lubricated with gel and passed backwards along the floor of the nasal passage (Fig. 11.7). A slight

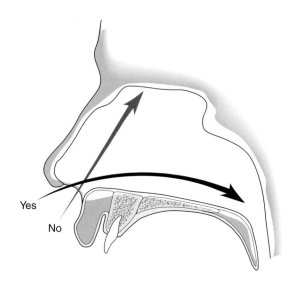

Fig. 11.7 Nasogastric intubation.
Note the correct direction for inserting the tube.

resistance may be felt as the tube passes from the nasopharynx to the oropharynx, and the patient should be warned that a retching sensation may be experienced at this point.

The patient is now asked to swallow, and with each swallow the tube is advanced down the oesophagus. It is important not to push the tube rapidly and force its insertion in a patient who is retching; rather, slow and steady progress should be sought, with small advancements made during each act of swallowing. The oesophago-gastric junction is about 40 cm from the incisor teeth, and ideally, about 10–15 cm of the tube should be placed into the stomach. Most nasogastric tubes have markings to allow measurement of the length inserted. Correct placement of the tube is confirmed by free aspiration of gastric contents, and by auscultation in the epigastrium while 20 ml of air is insufflated. Once in place, the tube is fixed to the nose with adhesive tape.

In patients with head injuries, the nasal route is avoided because of the risk of introducing infection—or even the nasogastric tube itself—into the central nervous system through an open fracture of the skull base. The oral route is also considered in patients with serious coagulopathy, as passage of the tube through the nose may result in significant haemorrhage. Finally, blind passage of a tube in the early period following oesophagectomy should never be attempted, as this may disrupt the anastomosis.

FINE-BORE NASOGASTRIC TUBES

Elemental diets tend to have an unpleasant taste and are poorly tolerated when swallowed normally. Such diets are therefore best given by infusion through a fine-bore nasogastric tube, which is more comfortable and less likely to cause oesophageal erosions than a standard nasogastric tube. It does, however, require great care in insertion, as it can easily pass into the respiratory tract.

Procedure

Fine-bore nasogastric tubes have a wire stylet to facilitate passage. The tube is passed in the same way as a standard nasogastric tube. Again, it is important not to force the tube but to advance it slowly and steadily with each swallowing action made by the patient. The position of the tube is confirmed by X-ray, and only then is the stylet removed. Once removed, it must never be reintroduced while the tube remains in place, as there is a significant risk of perforating both the tube and the oesophagus. The tube tends to collapse if aspirated, so that aspiration cannot be used to check its position.

It is often advantageous to position the fine-bore feeding tube in the jejunum. This can be achieved using a radiological imaging technique or by the use of enteral feeding tubes, which have a mercury-filled tip and are 'self-propelled' into the jejunum.

GASTRIC LAVAGE

The most common indication for gastric lavage is the removal of ingested poisons or drugs. Much less frequently, it is used to lower or raise the core body temperature.

Aspiration of gastric contents is a serious risk. If there is any doubt about the patient's ability to maintain the airway, expert assistance must be sought and endotracheal intubation considered prior to the procedure. The patient's level of consciousness, the presence of a gag reflex and the ability to cough are the most useful guides to the need for endotracheal intubation.

Procedure

After the need for endotracheal intubation is assessed, the patient is placed on the left side in the recovery position, with a 15° head-down tilt of the trolley. A large-bore gastric tube is introduced into the mouth. A mouth gag is useful to prevent the patient from biting the tube. As the tube is passed into the oropharynx and upper oesophagus, the patient is likely to gag and even to vomit. The tube is advanced into the stomach and its correct position confirmed by the free flow of gastric contents. If there is doubt, ausculation of the epigastrium during injection of air down the tube will confirm correct placement. About 100–200 ml of warm water are passed down the tube into the stomach. The end of the tube is then lowered below the level of the stomach into a collecting bucket, and gastric contents are allowed to syphon out. The manoeuvre is repeated until the returned water becomes clear. It is important to avoid over-distension of the stomach. Activated charcoal can be instilled into the stomach to act as an absorbent, if this is appropriate. On completion of lavage, the tube is removed.

OESOPHAGEAL TAMPONADE

The Sengstaken tube is a gastric aspiration tube with inflatable gastric and oesophageal balloons, which may be used for emergency treatment of bleeding oesophageal varices. A modification, the Sengstaken–Blakemore or Minnesota tube (Fig 18.10), has an additional channel

11

to allow the aspiration of saliva from the oesophagus above the level of the oesophageal balloon.

The use of a Sengstaken–Blakemore tube is generally a temporary measure to control haemorrhage prior to definitive treatment, or to allow transfer of the patient to a specialist centre. It is advisable to deflate the oesophageal balloon for 5 minutes every 6 hours to avoid the risk of ischaemic necrosis and ulceration of the oesophageal mucosa. The tube is not normally kept in place for more than 24 hours.

Procedure

The Sengstaken–Blakemore tube should be stored in a refrigerator, as this renders it less pliable and thus facilitates insertion. The oesophageal and gastric balloons are checked for leaks and then completely deflated using an aspiration syringe prior to insertion. The tube is inserted in the same way as a normal nasogastric tube. However, it is much more uncomfortable and local anaesthesia is recommended for nasal passage. A patient with bleeding varices is unlikely to cooperate fully and the tube may have to be passed with the patient on his or her side. If there is difficulty inserting the tube via the nasal route, the oral route may be used.

The tube is advanced approximately 60 cm and the gastric balloon inflated with 150–200 ml of air or water. The tube is then drawn back until this lower balloon impacts at the cardia. An assistant holds the tube in this position under slight tension, and the oesophageal balloon is inflated with air to a pressure of approximately 40 mmHg, checked by attaching a sphygmomanometer. The tube is secured in position with tape, but no additional traction is necessary.

The stomach is aspirated regularly through the main lumen of the tube to check for further bleeding. This lumen may also be used for the administration of medication, such as lactulose and neomycin. A fourth lumen allows aspiration of the upper oesophagus and pharynx and reduces the risk of bronchial aspiration. In patients who are stuporose or comatose, the airway should be protected by an endotracheal tube.

ABDOMINAL PARACENTESIS

Abdominal paracentesis is performed to relieve the discomfort caused by distension with ascitic fluid, or to obtain fluid for cytological examination. The bladder must be emptied, if necessary by preliminary catheterization. A 'Trocath' peritoneal dialysis catheter with multiple side perforations over a length of 8 cm is inserted under sterile conditions.

Procedure

The operator scrubs up and wears a gown and gloves. A site is chosen for insertion of the catheter. This can be either in the midline (one-third of the way from the umbilicus to the pubic symphysis), or in the right or left iliac fossa (at the junction of the outer and middle thirds of a line drawn from the anterior superior umbilicus to the spine) (Fig. 11.8). The vicinity of scars should be avoided, as adhesions increase the risk of bowel perforation. Local anaesthetic is infiltrated through all layers of the abdominal wall. The depth at which the peritoneum is entered is determined by aspiration with the syringe.

A 3 mm stab incision is made in the skin with a scalpel. The trocar is introduced into the catheter and the shaft of the catheter is held firmly between left thumb and index finger some 4–5 cm higher than the estimated depth of the peritoneum. This prevents 'overshoot' as the right hand inserts the trocar and catheter through the abdominal wall into the peritoneum (Fig. 11.9).

The catheter is then advanced further with the left hand while the trocar is withdrawn with the right. If any resistance is encountered, the catheter is withdrawn 2–3 cm, rotated 180° and then advanced again. The minimum final length of catheter within the peritoneal cavity must be 10 cm. If this position is not obtained, the side perforations of the catheter may lie within the abdominal wall and allow troublesome extravasation of ascitic fluid into the subcutaneous tissues. The catheter is secured to the skin and attached via a connection tube with a flow-control clamp to a sterile drainage bag.

A

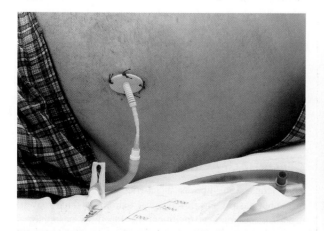

B

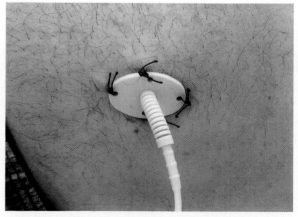

Fig. 11.8 Abdominal paracentesis catheter in situ.
A Catheter inserted in left iliac fossa. B Flange of catheter secured with sutures.

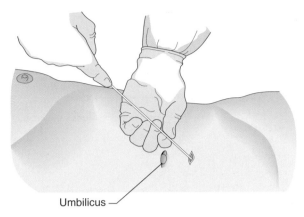

Umbilicus

Fig. 11.9   Insertion of a peritoneal dialysis catheter.

Drainage of large volumes of ascitic fluid must be accompanied by intravenous infusion of albumin in order to avoid precipitating a marked shift of fluid from the intravascular compartment into the peritoneal cavity. This prevents significant changes in haemodynamics and reduces the risk of developing cardiovascular instability, renal impairment or hepatic encephalopathy.

DIAGNOSTIC PERITONEAL LAVAGE

This procedure may be undertaken to look for the presence of blood or intestinal contents following blunt abdominal trauma. If the patient is stable, a CT scan of the abdomen is the investigation of choice; however, diagnostic peritoneal lavage (DPL) is indicated in unconscious trauma patients, in patients with multiple injuries and unexplained shock, or in patients with equivocal physical signs. The patient should have a nasogastric tube and a urethral or suprapubic catheter inserted prior to DPL, to reduce the risk of injury to the stomach or bladder.

Procedure

This procedure can be performed using a closed or open technique, the latter being favoured to minimize the risk of intra-abdominal injury. Under sterile conditions and following the instillation of local anaesthesia, a 5 cm vertical subumbilical incision is made and dissection continued through the subcutaneous tissue and linea alba. The peritoneum is opened and a cannula inserted into the peritoneal cavity and advanced into the pelvis. A syringe is connected to the dialysis catheter, and if frank blood is immediately aspirated, this is a positive DPL result. If gross blood is not obtained, 1 litre of warm sterile isotonic saline is infused and allowed to distribute evenly throughout the peritoneal cavity. The fluid is then retrieved by placing the infusion bag on the floor and allowing the effluent to drain from the abdomen by gravity. An unequivocal test will reveal gross evidence of blood, bile or faeces. If necessary, fluid can be sent to the laboratory for analysis. A positive result is obtained if the red cell count is $> 100 \times 10^9$, the white cell count is $> 0.5 \times 10^9$ or the amylase is > 175 U/ml.

VASCULAR PROCEDURES

VENEPUNCTURE

The antecubital fossa is the most convenient site, as the median cubital vein, median vein of the forearm and the cephalic vein are all easily accessible. Care must be taken to avoid the brachial artery. Sampling from smaller veins on the forearm or the back of the hand may at first sight appear more attractive, but these veins collapse easily on aspiration and adequate samples are difficult to obtain. In cases of extreme difficulty, the femoral vein should be considered. This vessel lies medial to the femoral artery, which is used as a landmark. In adults, a 21-gauge needle is used; in children, a 23- or 25-gauge will suffice.

Procedure

A venous tourniquet is applied to the upper arm and the patient is encouraged to clench the fist several times to increase venous filling. The position of the vein is identified and the skin cleansed. The needle is advanced through the skin and into the vein, with the needle bevel facing upwards. This manoeuvre is carried out in a 'two-step' fashion, first through the skin and then through the vein wall. Entry through the skin with a decisive action causes much less discomfort than a slow hesitant movement. The needle is advanced 2–3 mm into the vein and the position of the needle and syringe stabilized with one hand. The plunger of the syringe is slowly withdrawn with the other hand until the required amount of blood is obtained. The tourniquet is then released, the needle withdrawn and pressure immediately applied over the site of entry into the vein to prevent haematoma formation, which is painful for the patient and makes subsequent sampling more difficult.

The blood is placed into the appropriate sample tubes after removal of the needle from the syringe. With pre-vacuumed sample tubes, the needle should be left on the syringe in order to fill the tubes. Haemolysis invalidates some results—for example, potassium and phosphate levels—and is more likely to occur when smaller needles are used. It can be minimized by slow withdrawal of blood into the syringe.

SAFETY MEASURES

Used needles and syringes should be placed in specially reinforced carriers—'cin-bins'—to avoid the risk of needle-stick injury or blood contamination to portering or other staff. To further reduce the risk of blood spillage or contamination to medical and laboratory staff, systems have now been introduced in which the sample tubes themselves are modified so that they may be used as syringes, and sent to the laboratory without the need to transfer blood from syringe to tube (e.g. Sarstedt Monovette®).

VENEPUNCTURE FOR BLOOD CULTURE

This procedure is carried out for microbiological culture and identification of organisms that may be present in the blood. The procedure is similar to venepuncture but particular care must be taken to avoid contamination. The skin must be thoroughly cleansed and a strict 'no-touch' technique used.

Procedure

A venous tourniquet is applied, as before. The patient's skin is thoroughly cleansed with an appropriate solution, using a sterile swab or cotton wool ball. Venepuncture is performed without the operator touching the skin around the site of entry of the needle. After withdrawal, the needle is removed from the syringe and a second sterile needle substituted. This is then used to introduce the appropriate aliquot of blood into both aerobic and anaerobic culture bottles. Exact volumes of blood required and the number of bottles filled will depend on local laboratory policies. All blood culture bottles should be sent immediately to the laboratory or, if this is not possible, placed in an incubator at 37°C until transport is available.

PERIPHERAL VENOUS CANNULATION

Most intravenous infusions are given into the forearm. The veins of the leg are generally avoided because of the greater risk of thrombosis. Intravenous cannulae should not be sited over joints, if possible, as this necessitates splinting and reduces the free use of the arm by the patient. Even with splinting, cannulae are subject to more movement in these positions and are prone to more complications.

A wide range of cannulae are commercially available but all consist essentially of an outer flexible sheath and an inner metal needle. A 16- or 18-gauge cannula will suffice for most purposes in adults. Where rapid infusions of large quantities of fluid are required, a larger cannula should be used.

Procedure

A venous tourniquet is applied and the site of insertion chosen. The skin is cleansed and local anaesthetic may be infiltrated intradermally at the insertion site. Venepuncture is made in the 'two-step' fashion described above and confirmed by a 'flashback' of blood into the cannula. The cannula is initially advanced 2–3 mm into the vein, and then the cannula sheath is advanced into the vein with one hand while the metal needle is partially withdrawn with the other.

Once the cannula sheath is fully inserted into the vein, the tourniquet is released and gentle pressure applied over the vein at the tip of the cannula. The metal needle is then fully withdrawn from the cannula and the giving set, previously primed with normal saline, is connected. The cannula and distal 10–15 cm of the giving set are securely fixed to the skin with adhesive tape.

Cannulation sites should be inspected regularly for signs of swelling, erythema or tenderness, which may indicate extravasation, thrombophlebitis or infection. If any of these is present or the patient complains of pain at the site, the infusion must be stopped and the cannula resited. Extravasation may cause tissue necrosis. Thrombophlebitis occurs more readily when small veins are used, or when

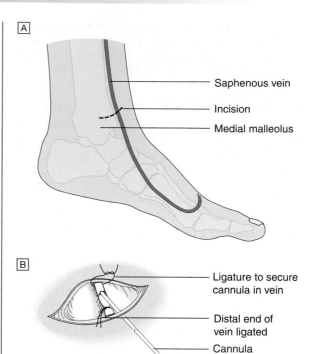

Fig. 11.10 Saphenous venous cutdown.
A Incision made anterior to the medial malleolus. B Cannula inserted in a proximal direction after ligation of the distal vein.

the pH of the infusate differs significantly from blood pH. The chances of infection increase the longer a cannula is left in situ, and infusion sites must be changed regularly.

Bolus injections through an intravenous cannula should not be made without first ensuring that the cannula is patent and that there is no extravasation.

VENOUS CUTDOWN

Venous cutdown for fluid replacement is rarely required, except in seriously hypovolaemic patients, usually following trauma. The most common site is the long saphenous vein at the ankle (Fig. 11.10). Other sites include the basilic vein in the antecubital fossa and the cephalic vein in the deltopectoral groove. It should only be regarded as a temporary measure for resuscitation.

Procedure

Venous cutdown is performed with an aseptic technique. Local anaesthetic is infiltrated over the site and a transverse incision is made in the skin over the vein, which is then identified by blunt dissection. At the ankle, the site of cutdown is 2–3 cm anterior to the medial malleolus. The vein should be cleared for a distance of 1–2 cm. The distal end of the vein is ligated with an absorbable ligature. The proximal end of the exposed vein is elevated to prevent backflow of blood, using a second absorbable ligature, and a transverse incision is then made in the vein. A large-bore cannula is passed through the skin 2 cm below the skin incision and guided into the vein. The cannula is advanced beyond the proximal ligature, which is then tied securely.

The intravenous infusion is then commenced to ensure it flows freely, and the wound is closed with non-absorbable sutures. The cannula is sutured to the skin to prevent accidental displacement and sterile dressing is applied.

CENTRAL VENOUS CATHETER INSERTION

Placement of a central venous catheter is indicated for monitoring of the central venous pressure (CVP) and for prolonged drug administration or parenteral nutrition.

Insertion is carried out using a strict aseptic technique, as infection is one of the most common complications of this procedure. If the catheter is to be used for drug therapy or parenteral nutrition, the procedure should be carried out in the operating theatre. The common sites of insertion of catheters into the superior vena cava are from the internal jugular vein in the neck, from the subclavian vein, or occasionally from a peripheral vein in the antecubital fossa. A variety of cannulae and catheters are available, but in general they are one of three types:

1. an extra-long intravenous cannula
2. a catheter inserted through a large cannula
3. a catheter inserted over a wire (Seldinger technique).
   Each has advantages and disadvantages.

Internal jugular vein cannulation

Several approaches are described, but the high approach at the level of the thyroid cartilage carries the least risk. The right internal jugular vein is preferred, as this provides a straighter route into the superior vena cava and avoids the risk of damaging the thoracic duct on the left. In general, the Seldinger technique is used; several commercial kits are available containing the necessary equipment.

Procedure

The patient is placed in a supine position, with at least 15° head-down tilt to distend the neck veins and reduce the risk of air embolism. The patient's head is turned to the left, unless there is potential for a cervical spine injury following trauma. A wide area on the right side of the neck is cleansed and draped.

The carotid artery is identified at the level of the thyroid cartilage, using the index and middle fingers of the left hand. The internal jugular vein lies just lateral and parallel to it. A bleb of 1% lidocaine is injected into the skin at the proposed puncture site.

Using an 18-gauge needle on a 10 ml syringe held in the right hand, the needle is advanced through the skin just lateral to the carotid pulsation, at an angle of 60° to the skin and in the line of the vein (Fig. 11.11). Free aspiration of blood confirms the position of the vein. This manoeuvre is repeated to place a larger (16-gauge) needle in the vein. The flexible 'J' end of the guidewire is now passed through this needle into the vein, and the needle removed over it. This leaves the guidewire in the internal jugular vein. A dilator is now passed over the wire into the vein and then withdrawn. The catheter is advanced over the wire and then the wire is removed, leaving the catheter in situ. In most adults, no more than 15 cm of catheter need be advanced into the vein to ensure correct

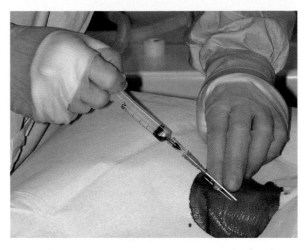

Fig. 11.11 Cannulation of the internal jugular vein.
Note the triangle between the sternal and clavicular heads of the sternocleidomastoid muscle.

placement. Blood is then aspirated from the catheter to confirm its position in the major vein. Heparinized saline (5 ml) is injected and the catheter is sutured to the skin to fix it in position. A chest X-ray is taken to check the position of the catheter and to exclude the presence of a pneumothorax, which is a recognized complication.

Subclavian vein cannulation

Several approaches to the subclavian vein are described, but usually a subclavicular one is used. Any approach to the subclavian vein carries a significant risk of causing a pneumothorax or puncturing the subclavian artery. Like all procedures, this one should be learnt under close supervision by an experienced operator.

Procedure

The Seldinger technique is generally used to insert a subclavian catheter. The patient should be placed in a supine position, with head-down tilt of at least 15°. A small pad is placed between the shoulder blades to allow the shoulders to drop backwards. Local anaesthetic is infiltrated into the skin and subcutaneous tissue. Under aseptic conditions, a large-calibre needle attached to a 10 ml syringe is introduced 1 cm below the junction of the middle and medial thirds of the clavicle. The needle is directed medially, slightly cephalad and posteriorly behind the clavicle towards the tip of a finger placed in the suprasternal notch (Fig. 11.12). Applying suction, the needle is advanced until blood is withdrawn into the syringe. The syringe is then disconnected, a flexible guidewire inserted through the needle and the needle removed. The catheter is subsequently passed over the guidewire and the latter is withdrawn. The catheter is flushed with heparinized saline and fixed in position. A chest X-ray is taken to check the position and exclude a pneumothorax.

11

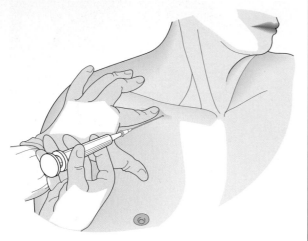

Fig. 11.12   Cannulation of the subclavian vein.

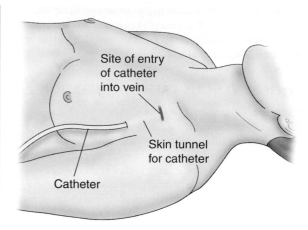

Fig. 11.13   Skin tunnel for central venous catheter.

Peripheral venous catheterization

In theory, this is the safest approach, as it avoids the risk of pneumothorax. Haemorrhage from accidental arterial puncture or as a result of a coagulopathy can be controlled by pressure. Thrombosis and thrombophlebitis are, however, more frequent compared to the subclavian or the internal jugular route. Normally, the long catheter is placed through a large cannula.

Procedure

A venous tourniquet is applied to the arm, and a suitable vein selected in the antecubital fossa through which the catheter can be passed. The area is prepared using an aseptic technique and local anaesthetic is infiltrated into the skin at an appropriate site. The cannula is inserted into the vein, as for normal intravenous cannulation, and the needle withdrawn. The long catheter is passed through the cannula into the vein and the venous tourniquet is then released.

The catheter is advanced up the basilic vein and into the superior vena cava. A guide is often provided to gauge the length of catheter inserted. Difficulty is frequently experienced in advancing the catheter past the axilla, and extension of the arm may help overcome this.

The insertion cannula is then withdrawn from the vein, leaving the long catheter in place. A chest X-ray is taken to confirm placement.

Measurement of central venous pressure (CVP)

The CVP is the pressure in the superior vena cava as it enters the right atrium. The zero point is taken as the level of the right atrium. With the patient lying supine, the mid-axillary line is the surface marking to use as the reference point and is assumed to represent zero or the level of the right atrium (Fig. 11.14). It is often convenient to mark the skin position to provide consistency in the recordings. An alternative surface reference point is the junction of the second rib and the sternum. In the supine patient, this is considered to lie 5 cm above the right atrium. Whichever reference point is used, confusion is avoided by remem-

---

BOX 11.1   CENTRAL VENOUS CANNULATION

- Air embolism is always a risk, even in the head-down position
- When using a guidewire, always hold it at some point along its length while it remains in the patient
- Blood should be easily aspirated from the catheter, if it is correctly positioned
- A chest X-ray should always be taken to confirm the absence of a pneumothorax and correct positioning. A rough guide to position is that the tip of the catheter should lie at the level of the carina on X-ray
- Cannulae inserted for intravenous nutrition are tunnelled in the subcutaneous tissue to emerge on the chest wall at a distance from the site of entry into the vein (Fig. 11.13). This minimizes the risk of sepsis spreading down the tract into the vein

---

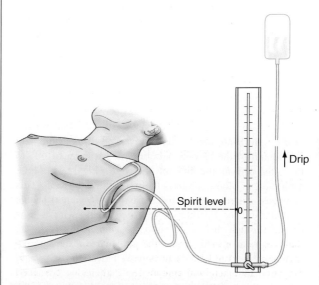

Fig. 11.14   Measurement of central venous pressure.
Note the mid-thoracic point (marked by a black dot), which is used as the zero reference point.

bering that the pressure being measured is in relation to the level of the right atrium. Consistency of recording is achieved by always using the same reference point with the patient in the supine position. A water manometer is normally used to measure this pressure.

Procedure

The water manometer system is primed with 5% dextrose prior to connection to the central venous catheter. The zero point on the manometer scale is levelled with the chosen reference point. The column is then filled to a higher level than the expected pressure and opened to the central venous catheter. The water column is allowed to fall and equilibrate. Fluctuation of the column with respiration is a reassuring sign of patency and correct positioning. The CVP is the level of the column at end-expiration.

ARTERIAL BLOOD SAMPLING

Arterial blood sampling is undertaken to measure arterial PO_2, PCO_2, $[H^+]$ and standard $[HCO_3^-]$. The radial artery at the wrist is the site of choice. The brachial artery at the elbow and the femoral artery may also be used.

A heparinized sample is required to prevent blockage in the blood gas analyser as a result of coagulation of the sample. There are several commercially available pre-heparinized syringes, but an ordinary 2 ml syringe that has been pre-heparinized as described below will suffice.

Procedure

If the syringe is not pre-heparinized, up to 0.5 ml of 1000 U/ml heparin are drawn into the syringe. The plunger is then fully withdrawn, following which the air and excess heparin are expelled from the syringe. The residual heparin will be sufficient to anticoagulate the sample. A 23-gauge needle is suitable for arterial puncture.

The course of the artery is defined by palpating the pulse between the index and middle fingers held 2 cm apart. The skin is cleansed and the needle, with its bevel upwards, introduced through the skin at an angle of about 60°. The needle is then advanced into the artery. Correct positioning is confirmed by blood pulsating into the syringe under pressure; 1–1.5 ml is normally sufficient.

The needle is withdrawn and firm pressure applied by an assistant over the puncture site for 3 minutes to avoid haematoma formation. The needle is removed from the syringe and any air bubbles expelled before capping the syringe. The syringe is gently inverted several times to ensure mixing of the heparin. The sample is sent immediately for analysis. Where delay is anticipated, it should be transported in ice.

NEEDLE PERICARDIOCENTESIS

Cardiac tamponade may result from penetrating or blunt trauma to the chest. Cardiac function may be significantly impaired by a minimal amount of blood within the fixed, fibrous pericardium. The classic signs are elevated CVP, hypotension and muffled heart sounds (Beck's triad). Immediate pericardiocentesis may be life-saving.

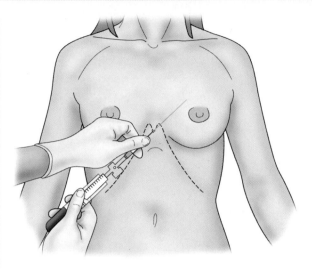

Fig. 11.15   Needle pericardiocentesis.

Procedure

The patient should be monitored throughout this procedure, with particular reference to the vital signs, CVP and electrocardiogram (ECG). An aseptic technique is used and the skin in the subxiphoid region is infiltrated with local anaesthetic. The skin is punctured 1–2 cm inferior to the left xiphochondral junction, using a wide-bore plastic-sheathed needle (at least 15 cm in length) with a syringe attached. The needle is angled at 45° and aimed towards the tip of the left scapula (Fig. 11.15). The syringe is aspirated as the needle is advanced, until it easily fills with blood. ECG changes suggest the needle has been advanced too far. Positive pericardiocentesis must be followed by surgical exploration.

URINARY PROCEDURES

URETHRAL CATHETERIZATION

This procedure may be carried out to relieve urinary retention or to determine urine output when it needs to be closely monitored. Occasionally, catheterization is necessary to facilitate nursing the incontinent patient. Anatomical obstruction may often be the cause of urinary retention in the male. It is particularly important to avoid forcing the passage of the catheter in this procedure, and if difficulty is experienced, assistance should be sought. A full aseptic technique is required for both male and female catheterization.

Procedure in the male

The shaft of the penis is held with a sterile swab and the urethral orifice cleansed with a non-alcoholic, non-iodine-containing solution. The foreskin, if present, is retracted. The shaft of the penis is held erect with a sterile swab in the left hand and traction applied to elongate the urethra. Lidocaine gel is instilled into the urethra slowly and carefully, with light but steady pressure. It is important to leave the local anaesthetic agent for a sufficient length

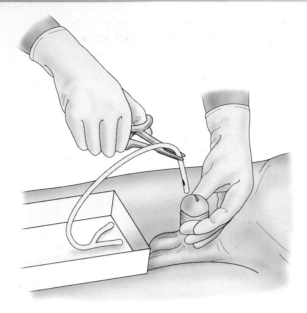

Fig. 11.16   Male catheterization.

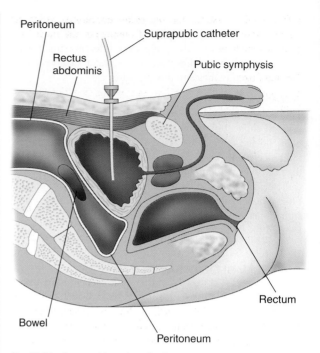

Fig. 11.17   Suprapubic catheterization.

of time before proceeding with catheterization, as difficulty in male catheterization is often caused by poor analgesia.

The urinary catheter is introduced into the urethra with a 'no-touch' technique and advanced to its full length (Fig. 11.16). Correct placement is confirmed by the passage of urine down the catheter. If this does not occur, suprapubic pressure may help. Alternatively, a bladder syringe can be attached to the catheter and aspiration used. With the passage of urine, the balloon on the catheter is inflated with the recommended volume of sterile water (generally, 10–30 ml). The catheter is gently withdrawn until the balloon engages the bladder neck, and it is then connected to the drainage tubing. The foreskin, where present, should be replaced over the glans to prevent paraphimosis.

Procedure in the female

A 16–18 Fr catheter is suitable for this procedure. The labia minora are separated with the thumb and fingers of the left hand to expose the urethral meatus on the anterior vaginal wall. The pudenda are now swabbed with antiseptic solution. Two swabs are used, each being swept once across the pudenda from anterior to posterior and then discarded.

In general, the catheter need only be inserted for half its length before the passage of urine confirms correct placement. The balloon is inflated and the catheter withdrawn until the balloon impacts in the bladder neck.

SUPRAPUBIC CATHETERIZATION

This procedure is only appropriate when the bladder is distended and urethral catheterization has failed or is contraindicated. It is carried out with a full aseptic technique.

Procedure

The position of the bladder is determined by percussion. Where available, ultrasound guidance is helpful. Generally,

the point of insertion lies two finger-breadths above the pubic symphysis in the midline.

The area is cleansed and draped. Local anaesthetic is then infiltrated through all layers of the anterior abdominal wall, using an 18-gauge needle. The depth and position of the bladder can be gauged by the free aspiration of urine through this needle. The needle is withdrawn and a stab incision made in the skin. The trocar and catheter are advanced through the incision, into the bladder (Fig. 11.17). Entry into the bladder is confirmed by the loss of resistance, at which point the catheter is advanced as the trocar is withdrawn. Free passage of urine confirms correct placement. The catheter must be advanced far enough into the bladder so that the balloon, when inflated, is well within the bladder. The balloon is then filled with 10 ml of water and a sterile dressing is applied.

CENTRAL NERVOUS SYSTEM PROCEDURES

LUMBAR PUNCTURE

Lumbar puncture is carried out to obtain a sample of cerebrospinal fluid (CSF) for diagnostic purposes, to measure the CSF pressure or to introduce materials into the CSF. It is important to examine the patient beforehand for evidence of raised intracranial pressure, examining the fundi in particular for evidence of papilloedema. Lumbar puncture is contraindicated if there is any suggestion of raised intracranial pressure, as it may result in 'coning' in such patients. The advent of computed tomography (CT) has provided a non-invasive aid to the detection of raised intracranial pressure, and in some conditions, such as subarachnoid haemorrhage, has removed the need for lumbar puncture.

Procedure

Lumbar puncture is carried out using a strict aseptic technique. Patients are placed on one side (usually the left), with their back at the edge of the bed or trolley. They are then asked to curl up as much as possible, to flex the lumbar spine and open up the interspinous spaces (Fig. 10.4).

The skin is thoroughly cleansed and drapes are applied. The space between the spinous processes of the third and fourth lumbar vertebrae is identified by the point at which a vertical line dropped from the highest point of the iliac crest crosses the spine. Local anaesthetic is infiltrated into the skin and subcutaneous tissues to a depth of about 2 cm. A small stab incision is made in the midline, midway between the two spinous processes.

For most purposes, a 22-gauge spinal needle is adequate. The needle is inserted through the stab incision and advanced in the midline in a slightly headward direction. Entry into the subarachnoid space is felt with a distinct loss of resistance, and will occur in most adults at a depth of 4–6 cm from the skin.

The stylet is withdrawn from the needle and the position confirmed by the free flow of CSF. If the subarachnoid space is not entered or bone is encountered, the position of the needle in the midline should be checked. This is best done by observing (from the side) the angle of the needle in relation to the patient's back. If the needle is in the midline, it should be withdrawn and reinserted in a slightly more headward direction. If the patient experiences pain, a nerve has been touched. The needle should be immediately withdrawn and repositioned.

Once the procedure is complete, the needle is withdrawn and a sterile dressing applied. The patient is usually advised to remain supine for at least 12 hours to minimize the risk of developing a 'spinal' headache. Persistent headache may be a result of continued CSF leakage through the puncture in the dura. In these circumstances, an anaesthetist should be asked to advise on an epidural 'blood patch'. With modern needles, the risk of CSF leakage is lessened and the advice to remain supine for 12–24 hours may be unnecessary.

DRUG ADMINISTRATION

The importance of correct prescription and administration of drugs cannot be over-emphasized (Table 11.4). Once administered, drugs can rarely be retrieved, particularly when they are administered intravenously or intra-muscularly. Very few drugs have specific antagonists, with the important exceptions of opiates and benzodiazepines. It is good clinical practice to check drugs with an assistant, particularly where dilutions are involved. Important and useful sources of information include the manufacturer's data sheet, national formulae, hospital formulae and hospital pharmacy drug information services.

Table 11.4   PRACTICE POINTS FOR DRUG ADMINISTRATION

- Use generic names wherever possible
- Print generic and, if indicated, proprietary names clearly on the prescription card
- Check that the correct drug is to be administered
- Check the patient's identity, particularly if you do not know them
- Label syringes clearly with the drug, the concentration, and the time and date drawn up
- Check the compatibility of the diluent
- Check calculations when diluting drugs or administering on a body-weight basis
- Check that the correct route of administration in the correct concentration is being used, and that the time over which the drug should be given is correct
- Carry out checks with an assistant
- It is good practice to administer only drugs you have drawn up yourself and checked with an assistant, or drugs that have been prepared under conditions that you are satisfied will result in the patient receiving the correct therapy

---

IMAGING

Radiological imaging has a central role in the management of surgical patients and may guide various therapeutic procedures. A number of imaging techniques are now available that provide information on the structure and function of systems and organs. The principal imaging techniques include radiography (including plain X-rays, contrast studies and CT), ultrasound, magnetic resonance imaging (MRI) and isotope scanning.

PLAIN RADIOGRAPHY

Radiographs account for the highest proportion of all imaging examinations. X-rays penetrate the body and cast an image either on film or on a fluorescent screen. The image is formed by the differences in attenuation of the various tissues through which the X-rays pass, producing a two-dimensional impression of a three-dimensional structure. On a plain radiograph, bone absorbs most X-rays and appears radio-opaque (white), whereas gas and fat absorb few X-rays and appear radiolucent (dark). If X-ray power (kilovoltage) and exposure time are altered, tissues of varying densities can be visualized. Other calcified tissues, such as most urinary tract stones, old tuberculous lymph nodes and calcified atheromatous plaques, are radio-opaque. Foreign materials, such as metal or glass, are also radio-opaque, but wood and plastic are radiolucent and invisible to X-rays.

Ionizing radiation is potentially harmful. Therefore, unnecessary investigations should be avoided and radiation exposure of patients and staff should be minimized. As the inverse square law determines radiation fall-off with distance, workers should maintain a good distance from the X-ray source during exposure. Radiation received by staff should be monitored by the wearing of X-ray-sensitive film badges, and protective lead aprons should be worn when staff are in exposed situations.

11

CONTRAST STUDIES

Radio-opaque contrast media may be used to demonstrate the gastrointestinal, biliary, vascular and urinary tracts. They can either be used to outline anatomical structures directly, or else be concentrated physiologically in an organ (indirect imaging). Barium sulphate is insoluble and used extensively to investigate the gastrointestinal tract. Gastrografin is a water-soluble contrast medium used if leakage from the gastrointestinal tract into the peritoneal cavity is likely. A barium swallow is used to assess the oesophagus and a barium meal to investigate the stomach and duodenum. Progress of contrast can be observed by fluoroscopic screening, using a technique known as image intensification. The large bowel is studied by giving contrast material rectally (barium enema). A single-contrast enema may be used to determine whether there is a complete mechanical obstruction in the emergency setting; however, improved mucosal detail will be obtained by using a double-contrast technique with barium and gas. Buscopan may be given at the same time to abolish spasm. In the biliary, vascular and urinary tracts, iodine-containing agents are used. The risk of life-threatening anaphylactic reactions with the newer, low-osmolar, non-ionic agents is minimal but these are still recognized complications of intravascular administration. Intravenous contrast is also potentially nephrotoxic in patients with impaired renal function.

COMPUTED TOMOGRAPHY (CT)

CT involves use of a series of X-rays directed at a narrow transverse section of the body and detected by multiple receptors. More modern machines spiral around the patient (spiral CT), resulting in more rapid image capture and higher resolution of images. Each element of the beam is attenuated according to the density of the tissue it traverses, and is converted into a grey-scale image that is displayed on a screen or printed on to a film as a two-dimensional image. Further information can be gained after adminis- tration of oral, rectal or intravenous contrast. Three- dimensional reconstruction can be performed to assess relationships between structures and aid in the discrimi- nation of abnormalities.

ULTRASONOGRAPHY

This is a safe, non-invasive, painless technique that allows the visualization of solid internal organs. Using 1–15 MHz mechanical vibrations (above the range of human hearing), generated and detected by a transducer, an image is obtained because of differences in the reflection of the transmitted sound at the interface of tissues with different impedance. For transcutaneous ultrasonography, the probe must be 'coupled' to the skin with conduction gel to exclude an air interface. Calcified tissue, such as stones, causes an abrupt and marked change in acoustic impedance, resulting in virtually complete reflection of ultrasound and a posterior acoustic shadow. For biliary ultrasound, the patient should be fasted to minimize bowel gas shadows and to reduce gallbladder contraction. Ultrasonography of the pelvis is aided by a full bladder, as this provides a fluid-filled, non-reflective window to scan the pelvic organs. Special probes have now been developed for insertion into various body orifices, such as rectum, vagina and oesophagus, and also through laparoscopic and endoscopic equipment. These probes can be placed closer to the target organ, allowing the use of higher-frequency sound that has lower penetration but greater resolution. Ultrasound can be employed to study blood flow using the Doppler principle. Ultrasound is reflected from the red blood cells, the movement of which causes a frequency shift related to the velocity. This is used to generate an audible signal that can be used to assess whether flow is normal or abnormal.

MAGNETIC RESONANCE IMAGING (MRI)

MRI, formerly known as nuclear magnetic resonance, involves the application of a powerful magnetic field to the body; this causes the protons of all hydrogen nuclei to behave like magnets. They are initially aligned and then excited by pulses of radio waves at a frequency that causes them to resonate and emit radio signals. These are recorded electronically and, using sophisticated computer technology, images can be displayed in any anatomical plane. MRI does not use ionizing radiation, is harmless and provides very good images of soft tissues. It has the disadvantages that it is expensive, time-consuming and unsuitable for patients with pacemakers or metallic implants. An exciting new application of MRI is the study of blood flow and cardiac function. Magnetic resonance angiography (MRA) avoids intravascular injections and is replacing some conventional techniques. Magnetic resonance cholangiopan- creatography (MRCP) has now replaced endoscopic retro- grade cholangiopancreatography (ERCP) for diagnostic imaging of the biliary tract, as it avoids the potential complications of pancreatitis and bleeding, although ERCP remains a valuable therapeutic tool.

RADIOISOTOPE IMAGING

Radioisotope imaging provides more information about function than structure. Suitable tracer agents combine a substance taken up by the target tissue and a radioactive label. Radioisotopes in common usage include ^{99m}Tc (technetium), ^{123}I and ^{131}I (iodine), ^{111}In (indium), ^{133}Xe (xenon), ^{67}Ga (gallium) and ^{201}Th (thallium). Distribution of radioisotopes is visualized using a gamma camera. Investigations employing radioisotope techniques include bone scanning, lung scanning to detect pulmonary emboli, renal scanning for gastrointestinal bleeding, leucocyte scanning for inflammation and infection, and thyroid scanning.

POSITRON EMISSION TOMOGRAPHY (PET)

PET is a new, more expensive radioisotope technique that is proving useful in the imaging of physiological brain metabolism, tumour detection and functional cardiac imaging.

12

R.W. PARKS

Post-operative care and complications

12

INTRODUCTION

Following an operation, there are three phases of patient care. After a short period of immediate post-operative care in a recovery room to ensure the full return of consciousness, the patient is returned to surgical ward care, unless there are indications for transfer to a high-dependency unit or intensive therapy unit. On discharge from ward care, patients may still require rehabilitation and convalescence before they are ready to resume domestic or other activities. This chapter discusses the first two phases, during which attention focuses on the regulation of homeostasis and the prevention, detection and management of complications.

The major life-threatening complications that may arise in the recovery room are airway obstruction, myocardial infarction, cardiac arrest, haemorrhage and respiratory failure. These complications can also arise during ward care, but except for haemorrhage and cardiopulmonary catastrophe, many of the problems arising in this phase do not threaten life and are often specific to the operation performed.

A timeline showing typical times for the development of post-operative complications is given in Figure 12.1.

IMMEDIATE POST-OPERATIVE CARE

Patients who have received a general anaesthetic should be observed in the recovery room until they are conscious and their vital signs are stable. Acute pulmonary, cardiovascular and fluid derangements are the major causes of life-threatening complications in the early post-operative period, and the recovery room provides specially trained personnel and equipment for the observation and treatment of these problems.

In general, the anaesthetist exercises primary responsibility for the patient's cardiopulmonary function and the surgeon is responsible for the operative site, the wound

---

> **EBM 12.1   OPTIMAL POST-OPERATIVE CARE**
>
> *'Optimal post-operative care requires clinical assessment and monitoring; respiratory management; cardiovascular management; fluid, electrolyte and renal management; control of sepsis; and nutrition.'*
>
> SIGN guideline 77 Post-operative management in adults; 2004.

and any surgically placed drains. Clinical notes should accompany the patient. These include an operation note describing the procedure performed, an anaesthetic record of the patient's progress during surgery, a post-operative instruction sheet with regard to the administration of drugs and intravenous fluids, and a fluid balance sheet.

Monitoring of airway, breathing and circulation is the main priority in the immediate post-operative period (EBM 12.1). The nature of the surgery and the patient's premorbid medical condition will determine the intensity of post-operative monitoring required; however, the patient's colour, pulse, blood pressure, respiratory rate, oxygen saturation and level of consciousness will be routinely observed. The nature and volume of drainage into collecting bags or wound dressings, and urinary output are also monitored, if appropriate. Continuous electrocardiogram (ECG) monitoring is undertaken and oxygenation is assessed by the use of a pulse oximeter. Monitoring of central venous pressure (CVP) may be indicated if the patient is hypotensive, has borderline cardiac or respiratory function, or requires large amounts of intravenous fluids.

The patient may initially remain intubated, but following extubation should receive supplemental oxygen by face mask or nasal prongs and should be encouraged to take frequent deep breaths. The patient must breathe adequately and maintain a good colour. Shallow breathing may mean that the patient is still partially paralysed. A dose of neostigmine can reverse the residual effects of curariform

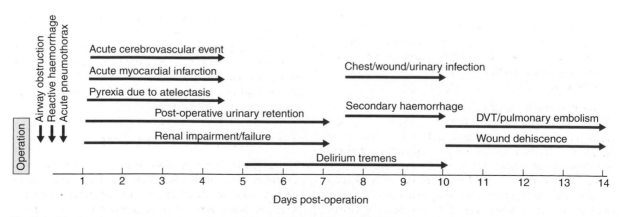

Fig. 12.1   **Timeline showing typical times for development of post-operative complications.**

BOX 12.1   IMMEDIATE POST-OPERATIVE MONITORING

- **A**irway: attention to maintenance of airway
- **B**reathing: ensure adequate ventilation
- **C**irculation: monitor for evidence of blood loss
- Assess the patient's
  - Colour
  - Pulse
  - Blood pressure
  - Respiratory rate
  - Oxygen saturation
  - Level of consciousness

agents. Cyanosis is an ominous sign indicating hypoxaemia due to inadequate oxygenation, and may be due to airway obstruction or impaired ventilation. Respiratory depression later on in the post-operative period is usually caused by over-sedation with opioid analgesic agents.

AIRWAY OBSTRUCTION

The main causes of airway obstruction are as follows:

- *Obstruction by the tongue* may occur with a depressed level of consciousness. Loss of muscle tone causes the tongue to fall back against the posterior pharyngeal wall, and may be aggravated by masseter spasm during emergence from anaesthesia. Bleeding into the tongue or soft tissues of the mouth or pharynx may be a complicating factor after operations involving these areas.
- *Obstruction by foreign bodies*, such as dentures, crowns and loose teeth. Dentures must be removed before operation and precautions taken to guard against displacement of crowns or teeth.
- *Laryngeal spasm* can occur at light levels of unconsciousness and is aggravated by stimulation.
- *Laryngeal oedema* may occur in small children after traumatic attempts at intubation, or when there is infection (epiglottitis).
- *Tracheal compression* may follow operations in the neck, and compression by haemorrhage is a particular anxiety after thyroidectomy.
- *Bronchospasm or bronchial obstruction* may follow inhalation of a foreign body or the aspiration of irritant material, such as gastric contents. It may also occur as an idiosyncratic reaction to drugs and as a complication of asthma.

Attention is directed at defining and rectifying the cause of airway obstruction as a matter of extreme urgency. Airway maintenance techniques include the chin-lift or jaw-thrust manoeuvres, which lift the mandible anteriorly and displace the tongue forward (Ch. 11). The pharynx is then sucked out, an oropharyngeal airway is inserted to maintain the airway, and supplemental oxygen is administered. If cyanosis does not improve or if stridor persists, reintubation may be necessary.

HAEMORRHAGE

Significant blood loss via a surgical drain, particularly if associated with hypovolaemic shock, is an indication for immediate transfer of the patient from the recovery room back to the operating theatre for re-exploration and control of the bleeding source. Reactive bleeding is usually caused by a slipped ligature or dislodgement of a diathermy coagulum as the blood pressure recovers from the operation. Superficial bleeding into the surgical wound rarely requires immediate action; however, patients who have undergone neck surgery must be observed for the accumulation of blood in the wound. If necessary, the wound can be reopened in the recovery room to prevent airway compression and asphyxia.

Late secondary haemorrhage typically occurs 7–10 days after an operation and is due to infection eroding a blood vessel. Rigid drain tubes may also occasionally erode a large vessel and cause dramatic late post-operative bleeding. Secondary haemorrhage associated with infection is often difficult to control. Interventional radiological techniques may achieve temporary control, but surgical re-exploration is usually indicated.

SURGICAL WARD CARE

GENERAL CARE

Monitoring of vital signs, including temperature, continues on return to the ward. In addition, output from the urinary catheter, nasogastric tube and surgical drains is monitored. The frequency of recordings or measurements can be reduced as the patient stabilizes.

Patients are normally visited morning and evening by the medical staff to ensure that there is steady progress. Anxiety, disorientation and minor changes in personality, behaviour or appearance are often the earliest manifestation of complications. The general circulatory state and adequacy of oxygenation are noted, and vital signs recorded on the nursing chart are checked. Temperature readings provide vital information regarding progress and may give early indication of potentially serious post-operative complications.

The chest is examined and all sputum inspected. Full chest expansion and coughing are encouraged. Following abdominal surgery, the abdomen is examined for evidence of excessive distension or tenderness. The return of bowel sounds and the free passage of flatus reflect recovery of gut peristalsis. The legs are checked for swelling, discoloration or calf tenderness.

TUBES, DRAINS AND CATHETERS

If a nasogastric tube is in place, it is kept open at all times to serve as a vent for swallowed air. Free drainage of gastric contents may be supplemented by intermittent manual aspiration. Nasogastric tubes are removed once the volume of aspirate diminishes. It is not always necessary to wait until bowel sounds have returned or flatus has been passed. Nasogastric tubes are uncomfortable and may prevent coughing with expectoration, and so they should not be retained for longer than necessary. Surgical drains are generally removed when the volume of effluent diminishes. If a urinary catheter has been placed, it should be removed once the patient is mobile.

FLUID BALANCE

Fluid balance is reviewed regularly. The standard intravenous fluid requirement for an adult is 3 litres/day, of which 1 litre should ordinarily be normal (isotonic) saline and 2 litres should be 5% dextrose; however, this should be judged according to the patient's general circulatory status, the observed fluid losses, and the daily measurement of serum urea and electrolyte levels. It is not necessary to replace potassium within the first 24–48 hours after surgery, as the body's store is sufficient. Potassium supplements (60–80 mmol daily) can subsequently be added to intravenous fluids, provided urinary output is adequate. Intravenous fluid therapy is discontinued once oral fluid intake has been established.

BLOOD TRANSFUSION

Haemoglobin measurement will be a guide to the need for post-operative blood transfusion. A full blood count should be undertaken within 24 hours of surgery and, as a general rule, blood is administered if the Hb is less than 80 g/l. Above this level, patients can be prescribed oral iron, unless they have cardiovascular instability or are symptomatic from their anaemia. If a blood transfusion is given, pulse, blood pressure and temperature should be recorded to detect a transfusion reaction. Major ABO incompatibility can result in an anaphylactic hypersensitivity reaction, with severe bronchospasm and hypotension, whereas incompatibility of minor factors may result in tachycardia, pyrexia and rash. Other potential complications of blood transfusion are hypothermia (if the blood has not been adequately warmed), hyperkalaemia (due to leakage of potassium from the red blood cells), acidosis (if the blood has been stored for a long period) and coagulation abnormalities (as stored blood is deficient in clotting factors).

NUTRITION

Nutrition in post-operative patients is frequently poorly managed. A few days of starvation may cause little harm, but enteral or parenteral nutrition is essential if starvation is prolonged. Enteral nutrition is preferred, as it is associated with fewer complications and is believed to augment gut barrier function. If a prolonged period of starvation is anticipated in the post-operative period, a feeding jejunostomy tube can be inserted at the time of abdominal surgery. Alternatively, a fine-bore nasogastric or nasojejunal feeding tube can be passed (Ch. 11). If the enteral route cannot be used, total parenteral nutrition can be prescribed. Dietary intake should be monitored in all patients in the post-operative period, and oral high-calorie supplements given if appropriate.

COMPLICATIONS OF ANAESTHESIA AND SURGERY

GENERAL COMPLICATIONS

Nausea and vomiting can be caused by surgery and/or anaesthesia, and an anti-emetic can prove useful. If nausea has been associated with previous anaesthetics, anti-emetic drugs should be administered prophylactically. Transient hiccups in the first few post-operative days are usually no more than a nuisance. Persistent hiccups can be a serious complication, exhausting the patient and interfering with sleep, and may be due to diaphragmatic irritation, gastric distension or metabolic causes, such as renal failure. If no precipitating cause can be found, small doses (25 mg) of intravenous chlorpromazine may be helpful.

Spinal anaesthesia may cause headache as a result of leakage of cerebrospinal fluid, and patients should remain recumbent for 12 hours after this form of anaesthesia. If headache persists, it may be necessary to seal the injection site in the dura–arachnoid with a 'blood patch' (i.e. an extradural injection of the patient's blood, which clots and so seals the leak). Myalgia affecting the chest, abdomen and neck is a specific complication of suxamethonium administration, and may last for up to a week.

Intravenous administration of irritant drugs or solutions can cause bruising, haematoma, phlebitis and venous thrombosis. Intravenous cannulae, particularly those placed in large veins, should be securely sealed to guard against air embolism. Sites of cannula insertion should be checked regularly for signs of infection, and the cannula replaced if necessary. Arterial cannulae and needle punctures are the most common cause of arterial injury, and may rarely lead to arterial occlusion and gangrene.

PULMONARY COMPLICATIONS

Respiratory complications remain the largest single cause of post-operative morbidity and the second most common cause of post-operative death in patients over 60 years of age. Pulmonary complications are more common after emergency operations. Special hazards are posed by pre-existing chronic obstructive pulmonary disease (COPD). Once a patient has fully recovered from anaesthesia, the main respiratory problems are pulmonary collapse and pulmonary infection. Pleural effusion and pneumothorax occur less commonly. Pulmonary embolism is a major complication of deep venous thrombosis, which is considered later.

Pulmonary collapse
Inability to breathe deeply and cough up bronchial secretions is the primary cause of pulmonary collapse after surgery. Contributory factors include paralysis of cilia by anaesthetic agents, impairment of diaphragmatic movement,

over-sedation, abdominal distension and wound pain. When there is complete obstruction of a bronchus or bronchiole, air in the lung distal to the obstruction is absorbed, the alveolar spaces close (atelectasis), and the affected portion of the lung contracts and becomes solid. Small bronchioles (1 mm or less) are prone to close when lung volume reaches a critical point (closing volume). The closing volume is higher in older patients and in smokers, owing to the loss of elastic recoil of the lung, which increases the risk of atelectasis. The extent of collapse varies from closure of a small segment to collapse of a lobe or, when a main bronchus is obstructed, the entire lung. Atelectasis is a very common complication of surgery and usually occurs within 24 hours. It is of clinical relevance because it leads to increased work of breathing and impaired gas exchange; if untreated, secondary bacterial infection will supervene, causing lobar or bronchopneumonia.

The clinical signs of pulmonary collapse include rapid respiration, tachycardia and mild pyrexia, with diminished breath sounds and dullness to percussion over the affected segment. Arterial PaO_2 is low and the chest X-ray shows areas of increased opacification.

Pre-operative measures to reduce the risk of pulmonary collapse following surgery include stopping smoking before the operation, physiotherapy for patients with COPD, and deferring elective surgery for at least 2 weeks in patients with a chest infection.

Post-operatively, pulmonary collapse is prevented by encouraging the patient to breathe deeply, cough and mobilize. Adequate analgesia and regular chest physiotherapy are of great importance in the post-operative period. Placement of an epidural catheter in patients undergoing major abdominal surgery may help alleviate post-operative wound pain. Hypoxia is treated by giving oxygen by mask or nasal prongs, and bronchospasm is relieved by inhalation of salbutamol.

When hypoxia is severe, endotracheal intubation, assisted ventilation and repeated bronchial aspiration may be needed. Posture is important and the patient should initially be placed on the unaffected side to aid expansion of the collapsed lung. Bronchoscopy may be needed to suck out a plug of inspissated secretion.

Pulmonary infection

Pulmonary infection commonly follows pulmonary collapse or the aspiration of gastric secretions. Pyrexia, tachypnoea and green sputum are typical. The chest signs are those of collapse with absent or diminished breath sounds, often in association with bronchial breathing and coarse crepitations from surrounding areas of partial bronchial occlusion. Chest X-ray usually demonstrates patchy fluffy opacities.

The patient is encouraged to cough, and antibiotics are prescribed after sputum is sent for bacteriological examination. Most pulmonary infections are caused by the respiratory commensals, *Streptococcus pneumoniae* and *Haemophilus influenzae*, but many post-operative pulmonary infections are caused by Gram-negative bacilli acquired by aspiration of oropharyngeal secretions. Antibiotics provide the mainstay of treatment. Oxygen is given if there is hypoxia, and more intensive measures,

including bronchoscopy and assisted ventilation, are instituted if respiratory function continues to deteriorate.

Respiratory failure

Respiratory failure is defined as an inability to maintain normal partial pressures of oxygen and carbon dioxide (PaO_2 and $PaCO_2$) in arterial blood. Blood gas determinations are the key to its early recognition and should be repeated frequently in patients with previous respiratory problems. The normal PaO_2 is > 13 kPa at the age of 20 years, falling to around 11.6 kPa at 60 years; respiratory failure is denoted by a value of less than 6.7 kPa. Severe hypoxaemia may result in visible central cyanosis.

Acute respiratory distress syndrome (ARDS)

ARDS is characterized by impaired oxygenation, diffuse lung opacification on chest X-ray and an increasing 'stiffness' of the lungs (decreased compliance). It may result from pulmonary or systemic sepsis, following massive blood transfusion, or as a consequence of aspiration of gastric contents. The syndrome displays a wide spectrum of severity. Many minor and transient cases recover spontaneously, whereas in a proportion of cases, progressive respiratory insufficiency occurs. Tachypnoea with increasing ventilatory effort, restlessness and confusion develop. Hypoxia initially responds to an increase in the oxygen content of inspired air, but progressively increasing concentrations are required to prevent the PaO_2 from falling. The pathophysiology is unclear, but endotoxin-activated leucocytes are thought to be deposited in the pulmonary capillaries, releasing oxygen-derived free radicals, cytokines and other chemical mediators. Damage to the vascular endothelium results in increased capillary permeability and leakage of fluid, causing widespread interstitial and alveolar oedema. This is seen as bilateral diffuse fluffy opacities on chest X-ray. The lungs become increasingly stiff and difficult to ventilate.

Management includes supportive measures in the form of ventilation with positive end-expiratory pressure (PEEP) and treatment of the underlying condition, i.e. control of infection by antibiotics, drainage of any source of pus and correction of hypovolaemia. The mortality rate of severe ARDS is approximately 50%.

Pleural effusion

Small pleural effusions (Fig. 12.2) are not uncommon following upper abdominal surgery, but are usually of no clinical significance. They may be secondary to other pulmonary pathology, such as collapse/consolidation, pulmonary infarction or secondary tumour deposits. The appearance of a pleural effusion 2–3 weeks after an abdominal operation may suggest the presence of a subphrenic abscess. Small effusions may be left alone to reabsorb if they do not interfere with respiration. Alternatively, pleural aspiration is performed and the fluid sent for bacteriological culture.

Pneumothorax

The most common cause of post-operative pneumothorax is the insertion of a central venous line, and a chest X-ray

12

12

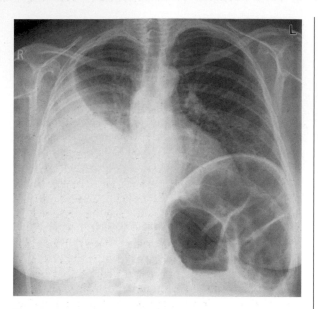

Fig. 12.2 Post-operative pleural effusion.

is necessary after this procedure to exclude this potential complication. There is also an enhanced risk of pneumothorax in patients on positive-pressure ventilation, presumably owing to rupture of pre-existing bullae. The insertion of an underwater seal drain is usually followed by rapid expansion of the lung.

CARDIAC COMPLICATIONS

The risks of anaesthesia and surgery are increased in patients suffering from cardiovascular disease. Whenever possible, arrhythmias, unstable angina, heart failure or hypertension should be corrected before surgery. Valvular disease, especially aortic stenosis, impairs the ability of the heart to respond to the increased demand of the post-operative period. The administration of fluids to patients with severe aortic or mitral valve disease should be carefully monitored.

Myocardial ischaemia/infarction
Although in most cases there is a history of preceding cardiac disease, myocardial ischaemia or cardiac arrest can occur in an otherwise fit patient. Patients with ischaemia may complain of gripping chest pain, but this is not invariable (particularly in the elderly diabetic patient or in the early post-operative period) and hypotension may be the only sign. The absence of symptoms after operation is thought to be due to the residual effects of anaesthesia and to the administration of post-operative analgesia. If ischaemia is suspected, an ECG is performed urgently and arrangements are made for cardiac monitoring. A sample of blood is withdrawn to estimate concentrations of cardiac enzymes. One-third of post-operative myocardial infarctions are fatal.

Cardiac failure
Although acute cardiac failure occurs most often in the immediate post-operative period, patients with ischaemic or valvular heart disease, arrhythmias or major surgical insult can also go into failure in the subsequent recovery period. Clinical manifestations are progressive dyspnoea, hypoxaemia and diffuse congestion on chest X-ray. Excessive administration of fluid in the early post-operative period in patients with limited myocardial reserve is a common cause, which can be avoided by monitoring CVP. Treatment consists of avoiding further fluid overload, and the administration of diuretics and cardiac inotropes.

Arrhythmias
Sinus tachycardia is common and may be a physiological response to hypovolaemia or hypotension. It is also caused by pain, fever, shivering or restlessness. Tachycardia increases myocardial oxygen consumption and may decrease coronary artery perfusion. Sinus bradycardia may be due to vagal stimulation by neostigmine, pharyngeal irritation during suction, or the residual effects of anaesthetic agents. Atrial fibrillation is the most common post-operative arrhythmia. Fast atrial fibrillation may result in haemodynamic disturbances and may require pharmacological intervention. Refractory cases may require cardioversion.

Post-operative shock
Shock is defined as a failure to maintain adequate tissue perfusion. The three main types are hypovolaemic, cardiogenic and septic shock. Hypovolaemic shock may be caused by inadequate replacement of pre- or perioperative fluid losses or post-operative haemorrhage, whereas cardiogenic shock is usually secondary to acute myocardial ischaemia/infarction or an arrhythmia. Hypovolaemic and cardiogenic shock are characterized by tachycardia, hypotension, sweating, pallor and vasoconstriction. Septic shock is characterized in the early stages by a hyperdynamic circulation with fever, rigors, a warm vasodilated periphery and a bounding pulse. Later features include hypotension and peripheral vasoconstriction. Without appropriate management, shock will result in oliguria and the development of multisystem organ failure, and may lead to death.

URINARY COMPLICATIONS

Post-operative urinary retention
Inability to void post-operatively is common, especially after groin, pelvic or perineal operations, or operations under spinal/epidural anaesthesia (Fig. 12.3). Post-operative pain, the effects of anaesthesia and drugs, and difficulties in initiating micturition while lying or sitting in bed may all contribute. Males tend to be more commonly affected than females. When its normal capacity of approximately 500 ml is exceeded, the bladder may be unable to contract and empty itself. Frequent dribbling or the passage of small volumes of urine may indicate overflow incontinence, and examination may reveal a distended bladder. The

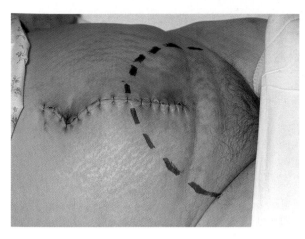

Fig. 12.3 Post-operative urinary retention.

management of acute urinary retention is catheterization of the bladder, with removal of the catheter after 2–3 days (Ch. 11).

Urinary tract infection
Urinary tract infections are most common after urological or gynaecological operations. Pre-existing contamination of the urinary tract, urinary retention and instrumentation are the principal factors contributing to post-operative urinary infection. Cystitis is manifested by frequency, dysuria and mild fever, and pyelonephritis by high fever and flank tenderness. Treatment involves adequate hydration, proper drainage of the bladder and appropriate antibiotics.

Renal failure
Acute renal failure after surgery results from protracted inadequate perfusion of the kidneys. The most common cause of post-operative oliguria is pre-renal vascular insufficiency from hypovolaemia, water depletion or extracellular fluid depletion. Hypoperfusion of the kidney may be aggravated by hypoxia, sepsis and nephrotoxic drugs. Patients with pre-existing renal disease and jaundice are particularly susceptible to hypoperfusion, and are more likely to develop acute renal failure.

The complication can largely be prevented by adequate fluid replacement before, during and after surgery, so that urine output is maintained at 0.5 ml/kg/hr or more. The importance of monitoring hourly urine output means that bladder catheterization is needed in all patients undergoing major surgery, and in those at risk of renal failure. Early recognition and treatment of bacterial and fungal infections is also important in the prevention of renal failure.

Urine output below 700 ml in 24 hours (or less than 0.5 ml/kg/hr for several hours on catheter drainage) should be considered pathological oliguria. Management involves the restoration of an adequate circulating intravascular compartment by the administration of intravenous fluids. A CVP line is usually required to measure circulating blood volume. Diuretics may be administered only if the patient is well hydrated; however, they should not be continually prescribed if the patient remains oliguric. Low-dose dopamine may increase renal blood flow.

Acute post-operative renal failure occurs when the reversible stage of acute renal insufficiency progresses to acute tubular necrosis. Volume loading becomes potentially dangerous with established renal failure, and the mainstays of treatment at this stage are the replacement of observed fluid loss, plus an allowance of approximately 500 ml/day for insensible loss, and restriction of dietary protein intake to less than 20 g/day. Biochemical status is checked by frequent estimations of serum urea and electrolytes. Hyperkalaemia can be treated by intravenous administration of insulin and glucose or cation exchange resins. Haemofiltration or haemodialysis may be indicated if conservative measures fail to prevent rapid rises in serum concentrations of urea and potassium. Recovery from acute tubular necrosis can be anticipated in survivors after 2–4 weeks. The patient will then enter a polyuric phase, in which fluid and electrolyte balance requires careful monitoring. The mortality rate in patients who develop post-operative renal failure is 50%.

CEREBRAL COMPLICATIONS

Cerebrovascular accidents (CVA)
These are usually precipitated by sudden hypotension during or after surgery in elderly hypertensive patients with severe atherosclerosis. They are a specific complication of carotid endarterectomy, occurring in 1–3% of cases, but may also complicate cardiac surgery.

Neuropsychiatric disturbances
These occur frequently and cover a wide spectrum of disorders. The most common is mental confusion with agitation, restlessness and disorientation, and is known as delirium. It usually occurs in the elderly and may arise on a background of dementia due to cerebral atrophy, but is often precipitated by the use of sedative or hypnotic drugs.

Acute toxic confusion state is a well-recognized acute psychiatric disorder that occurs in some patients during a serious illness or after a major surgical intervention. Many factors can contribute, and it is important to look for a treatable cause, such as hypoxia, sepsis, or a metabolic disturbance such as uraemia or electrolyte imbalance. Sleep deprivation, particularly in intensive care units, can also cause severe mental disturbance.

Delirium tremens (acute alcohol withdrawal syndrome)
Delirium tremens occurs in alcoholics who stop drinking suddenly. In most instances, this can be predicted from a detailed history. Prodromal symptoms include personality changes, anxiety and tremors. The fully developed condition is characterized by extreme agitation, visual hallucinations, restlessness, confusion and, rarely, convulsions and hyperthermia. If symptoms are mild, treatment involves the prescription of oral diazepam and vitamin B. Control of extreme agitation may require intravenous administration of diazepam, or haloperidol.

12

VENOUS THROMBOSIS AND PULMONARY EMBOLISM

These complications are discussed in detail in Chapter 25, but the essential details are summarized here for convenience.

Deep venous thrombosis (DVT)

The pathogenesis of venous thrombosis involves stasis, increased blood coagulability and damage to the blood vessel wall (Virchow's triad). The incidence of DVT varies with the type of operation and the associated risk factors, which include increasing age, obesity, prolonged operations, pelvic and hip surgery, malignant disease, previous DVT or pulmonary embolism (PE), varicose veins, pregnancy, and use of the oral contraceptive pill.

Measures to prevent DVT include taking care to avoid prolonged compression of the leg veins during and after the operation; the use of graded compression support stockings (TED stockings); mechanical or electrical compression of the calf muscles during surgery; and subcutaneous heparin (5000 U 12-hourly). Many surgeons use low molecular weight heparin (at doses recommended by the manufacturer) in all patients over 40 who require a general anaesthetic.

DVT is frequently asymptomatic, but may present with a painful, tender swollen calf. It may be the cause of a post-operative fever. Duplex ultrasonography is now the investigation of choice for diagnosing DVT. Ascending venography may be used to confirm the presence and extent of thrombosis, and is particularly useful for iliofemoral thrombosis. Radiolabelled fibrinogen uptake can also be used to detect DVT, but at present its use is limited to patients being screened for DVT.

An established DVT is treated by immediate anticoagulation with an intravenous bolus of heparin (5000 U), followed by a continuous intravenous heparin infusion. An alternative regimen is the use of low molecular weight heparin given as a once-daily dose. Heparin therapy is stopped once the patient is on full oral anticoagulation using warfarin, which is then normally continued for 3–6 months. The dose of warfarin is adjusted to maintain a prothrombin time (now reported as the international normalized ratio, or INR) at 2–3 times normal.

Pulmonary embolism

Massive pulmonary embolus with severe chest pain, pallor and shock demands immediate cardiopulmonary resuscitation, heparinization and urgent CT pulmonary angiography. Fibrinolytic agents, such as streptokinase or urokinase, can be infused intravenously to encourage clot lysis if it is at least 6 days after surgical intervention, or in extreme cases the clot can be removed at open pulmonary embolectomy under cardiopulmonary bypass.

If a small embolus is suspected in a patient complaining of chest pain, sometimes in association with tachypnoea, haemoptysis and a pleural rub and effusion, a radioisotope perfusion–ventilation lung scan ($\dot{V}/\dot{Q}$ scan) is the key investigation. A chest X-ray and ECG are advisable, mainly

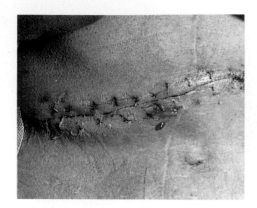

Fig. 12.4 Wound infection.

to rule out alternative causes of pain and collapse. If the $\dot{V}/\dot{Q}$ scan reveals lobar or segmental perfusion defects, the patient is heparinized and monitored carefully. In such cases, it is also important to search for the source of the embolus; if phlebography reveals thrombus in the iliofemoral segments, then a filter can be inserted into the inferior vena cava to prevent further pulmonary emboli.

Warfarin therapy is recommended in all patients who have sustained a pulmonary embolus, and therapy is normally continued for 3–6 months.

WOUND COMPLICATIONS

Infection

Infection (Fig. 12.4) is the most common complication in surgery. The incidence varies from less than 1% in clean operations to 20–30% in dirty cases. Subcutaneous haematoma is a common prelude to a wound infection, and large haematomas may require evacuation. The onset is usually within 7 days of operation. Symptoms include malaise, anorexia, and pain or discomfort at the operation site. Signs include local erythema, tenderness, swelling, cellulitis, wound discharge or frank abscess formation, as

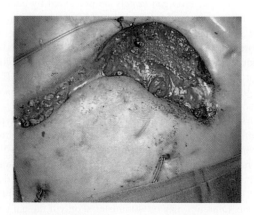

Fig. 12.5 Wound dehiscence.

well as an elevated temperature and pulse rate. If a wound becomes infected, it may be necessary to remove one or more sutures or staples prematurely to allow the egress of infected material. The wound is then allowed to heal by secondary intention. Antibiotics are only required if there is evidence of associated cellulitis or septicaemia. If the wound infection is chronic, the presence of a suture sinus or an enterocutaneous fistula must be excluded.

Dehiscence

The incidence of abdominal wound dehiscence should be less than 1%. Wound dehiscence (Fig. 12.5) may be partial (deep layers only) or complete (all layers, including skin). A serosanguinous discharge is characteristic of partial wound dehiscence. The extrusion of abdominal viscera through a complete abdominal wound dehiscence is known as evisceration. This rare complication usually occurs within the first 2 weeks after operation. Risk factors include obesity, smoking, respiratory disease, obstructive jaundice, nutritional deficiencies, renal failure, malignancy, diabetes and steroid therapy; however, the most important causes are poor surgical technique, persistently increased intra-abdominal pressure, and local tissue necrosis due to infection. The wound should be resutured under general anaesthesia. Incisional herniation complicates approximately 25% of cases.

BOX 12.2 COMPLICATIONS OF ANAESTHESIA AND SURGERY

General complications

- Nausea and vomiting
- Hiccups
- Headache

Pulmonary complications

- Pulmonary collapse
- Pulmonary infection
- Respiratory failure
- Acute respiratory distress syndrome (ARDS)
- Pleural effusion
- Pneumothorax

Cardiac complications

- Myocardial ischaemia/infarction
- Cardiac failure
- Arrhythmias
- Post-operative shock

Urinary complications

- Urinary retention
- Urinary tract infection
- Renal failure

Cerebral complications

- Cerebrovascular accidents (CVA)
- Neuropsychiatric disturbances
- Delirium tremens

Venous thromboembolism

- Deep venous thrombosis
- Pulmonary embolism

Wound complications

- Wound infection
- Wound dehiscence

12

13

S. PATERSON-BROWN

Day-case surgery

INTRODUCTION

Although day-case surgery has been performed for over 50 years, it has taken the increasing economic constraints on health care over the last 15 years to produce the changes in culture that have resulted in as many as 75% of general surgical procedures being performed as day cases in some hospitals. This chapter will attempt to outline some of the reasons behind these changes, to describe the types of patient and procedure suitable for day-case surgery, and to explore the process involved in the delivery of surgical care.

The Royal College of Surgeons of England published guidelines on day-case surgery in 1985, and subsequent support from the government followed in 1990. The definition of a surgical day case, according to these guidelines, is a patient who is admitted for investigation or operation on a planned, non-resident basis (i.e. goes home in the evening), and who occupies, for a period, a bed or unit set aside for this purpose. This definition should exclude those patients who can be dealt with competently on an ambulatory basis in accident and emergency or outpatient departments. Recently, there have been increasing moves to extend the role of 'day-case' surgery to include those patients who have their operation in a day-case unit but who stay overnight (extended day-case or 23-hour surgery). This allows patients operated on in the late afternoon to remain overnight, along with those who cannot go home for social reasons, and prevents them having to occupy inpatient beds.

Ambulatory surgery, if the American definition is used, includes all patients who leave hospital within 23 hours. It is more than 'day surgery' and represents an approach to health care that capitalizes on technological developments and optimizes the service delivered to patients. It encompasses the patient's journey from GP consultation, through treatment and care on a 23-hour basis, to discharge or ongoing care in a primary-care setting. Care packages are run according to strictly tailored protocols understood by all and agreed with GPs to ensure appropriate referral and levels of treatment.

The aims of ambulatory care are:

- to maximize one-stop, minimal-stop and locally accessible services wherever possible
- to increase day surgery and direct access to secondary care services from primary care
- to utilize advances in medical and information technology to promote flexibility in service provision and accessibility.

There has been a move throughout the UK, following similar initiatives in Europe and North America, to develop stand-alone centres where simple hospital-based investigations and uncomplicated procedures can be carried out (Independent Diagnostic and Treatment Centres). The aim is obviously to reduce the workload on the regional hospitals, while at the same time allowing patients to be treated nearer home. The most common procedures carried out in these centres are minor ones (local anaesthetic surgery—'lumps and bumps'), and both upper and lower gastrointestinal endoscopy.

Table 13.1	ADVANTAGES AND DISADVANTAGES OF DAY SURGERY
Advantages	
• More cost-efficient	
• Reduction of waiting lists for certain procedures	
• Consultant-based service	
• Reduced patient stress from being in hospital	
• Quicker, e.g. GP fast-tracking	
Disadvantages	
• Less immediate follow-up	
• Unexpected need for inpatient care post-operatively	
• Dependence on other services, e.g. A&E, GP, if problems occur	
• Not all patients suitable	
• Not all specialties available on site	

REASONS FOR DAY-CASE SURGERY

It is clear that the ability to perform a procedure as a day case has many advantages. These are highlighted in Table 13.1, along with some of the disadvantages.

COST EFFICIENCY

In terms of cost efficiency, many factors must be taken into consideration. Day surgery is not cheap and the emphasis should be put on efficiency of expenditure rather than overall cost. Day surgery should aim to provide an intensive, efficient service with high turnover and minimal disruption to patients. For these reasons, day-surgery units should be well equipped with up-to-date facilities, and should also be diverse enough to allow utilization by many specialties for a wide spectrum of patients. Many hospitals have now decided to invest in independent day-surgery units, which prevent beds from being used by emergency patients.

Major cost-saving areas have been identified, including the reduction in routine inappropriate pre-operative investigations and excessive and repetitive documentation. As the majority of units run on a 5-day basis, this also allows a reduction in nursing and medical staffing costs at night-time and weekends. Although it is difficult to quantify the added expenditure in terms of reliance on other services (such as A&E, GP and district nurses) in the event of a problem arising outside the hospital setting, it is generally agreed that this adds up to considerably less than inpatient hospital care.

ACCOMMODATION FACTORS

Patients utilize a bed for only a short period of time, and when procedures are performed in specialist day-surgery units, beds in the general hospital wards are left available for others who require more specialist input. This has the advantage of improved continuity of care for the inpatient, but also allows the continuation of elective surgery in times of inpatient bed shortage. Some units are now able to sustain a rate of service that allows two patients to use a bed in

13

the same day. All this has a significant impact on inpatient waiting lists, and allows both groups of patients to be treated more quickly.

The other main advantage of short-term care is early mobilization and a reduction in the subsequent risk of thromboembolic disease, as patients are increasingly encouraged to begin mobilizing as early as possible following their surgery.

PSYCHOLOGICAL ASPECTS

The psychological benefits of day-case surgery are apparent from patient questionnaires, which have consistently revealed that the majority prefer day care to inpatient care. This is particularly relevant in children, for whom the stresses of being in hospital can be overwhelming. The ambience of a specialist day unit and the ability to return home to a familiar environment soon after surgery go a long way towards alleviating these stresses, and also reduce any anxieties regarding future hospital visits. Another positive feature from the patients' viewpoint is the fact that services are generally consultant-led, although nurse-run, and any contact is usually with a specialist. The majority of patients are given a date for their surgery on the day of their clinic visit, allowing planning around the procedure. Patients with certain conditions, particularly lesions amenable to local anaesthetic removal, do not require clinic review and can be added straight to a list, thereby reducing the clinic waiting list and inconvenience to the patient.

DISADVANTAGES

Unfortunately, day-case surgery does have certain disadvantages. Not all procedures are suitable for the day-case unit and not all patients are suitable for day-case surgery. Some considered suitable may turn out to require ongoing investigation or care after surgery. Furthermore, because patients enter hospital on the morning of surgery, some operations may have to be cancelled for a number of reasons, including uncontrolled hypertension, new-onset disease such as diabetes, or abnormal results of investi-

gations performed at booking that have not been reviewed before admission. However, careful pre-operative assessment and efficient planning should keep these cancellations to a minimum. As mentioned earlier, extending the role of the day-case unit to include an overnight stay for some patients allows a significant number of patients to be managed through the 'day-case' unit who would normally have been treated in an inpatient bed.

REFERRAL FOR DAY-CASE SURGERY

Referral for day surgery can come about in a number of ways and the common methods will be discussed (Fig. 13.1).

REFERRAL FROM CLINIC

This is the most conventional method of referral. The patient is seen in the outpatient clinic, considered suitable for day-case surgery and referred directly to the day unit for pre-assessment. This is advantageous, as it allows all the necessary details to be discussed and planned in a single trip, and means that if the strict criteria for suitability are not met, the patient can be referred back to the surgeon for alternative arrangements to be made. It also allows for any investigations that are required to be performed that day, so that the results can be reviewed in time for surgery.

WAITING-LIST ADMISSION

Patients who require a procedure that is suitable for being performed as a day case may be added to a day-case surgery waiting list. Following discussion with the appropriate clinicians, the bed manager takes patients from this list and invites them for pre-assessment. Patients are given a date for surgery and an appointment for pre-assessment.

This produces a structured operating list using the 'first come, first served' principle. However, this system has inherent flaws. Patients are invited for pre-assessment with little knowledge of their pre-existing medical and social circumstances. This often means that they are unsuitable for day-case surgery, thus wasting valuable pre-assessment time as well as inconveniencing the patient. Patients may also fail to attend their pre-assessment appointment.

OUTREACH CLINICS

Many consultants provide clinics in peripheral settings, such as local cottage hospitals or health centres, and many of the patients seen in these clinics are suitable for day surgery. These patients can then be referred to the day surgery unit for pre-assessment, or can be seen in these outreach clinics by pre-assessment nurses.

DIRECT GP REFERRAL

This is a relatively new method of referring patients for a day-case procedure and is usually reserved for the more

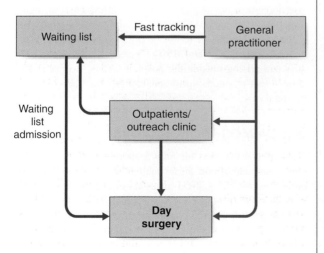

Fig. 13.1 Flowchart for day-surgery referral.

minor procedures carried out under local anaesthesia. It is the process whereby patients visit their GP with a problem remediable by day-case surgery and are added directly to a day-case list following discussion with the unit manager. These patients will not meet their consultant until the day of operation, and will only have received postal or telephone information regarding their procedure and the unit. No formal pre-assessment is usually required.

With increasing demand for integrated care pathways, this method of referral might become increasingly popular for other procedures, such as hernia repair, provided clear protocols are established between GPs and surgeons.

PRE-ASSESSMENT

Pre-assessment is one of the most important aspects of day-case surgery. It identifies concurrent diseases, and therefore the appropriate pre-operative investigations, and at the same time provides an opportunity to explain the procedure to the patient.

All patients having general anaesthesia require pre-assessment, and it may also be necessary for patients undergoing certain local anaesthetic procedures when additional investigations might be required, such as for liver biopsy. Patients undergoing most local anaesthetic procedures do not require a detailed pre-assessment.

THE INTERVIEW

Patients deemed suitable for a day-case procedure by the surgeon undergo an interview with the pre-assessment nurse. This usually takes the form of a sit-down discussion in the same outpatient clinic or in the day-surgery unit, but can often be conducted at another mutually convenient time or over the telephone. At this interview, a number of important points are covered; some of these are outlined in Table 13.2.

The interview is usually led by a senior member of the nursing staff with experience in day-case surgery, and is conducted according to protocols and a unit operational policy. These protocols should be agreed on and reviewed regularly by managers, anaesthetists, surgeons, physicians and nurses.

Ideally, all details are kept in a unitary record that will follow the patient through surgery, acting as a quick and easy reference and avoiding unnecessary replication. An example is given in Figure 13.2.

Table 13.2 IMPORTANT POINTS COVERED AT PRE-ASSESSMENT

- Date of procedure
- Attendance details and transport arrangements
- Unit procedure
- Detailed explanation of surgery, including patient information sheets
- Description of likely post-operative experiences
- Procedure-specific post-operative instructions
- Questions outside outpatient clinic setting

At the beginning of the interview, a patient's personal details are taken, including a telephone number in case of a short-notice cancellation. Details of past medical history and previous surgery are obtained, as well as a list of medications and any allergies. All patients have their height, weight, pulse and blood pressure recorded, along with a urinalysis. Their body mass index (BMI) is then calculated using the following equation:

$$BMI = \frac{Weight\ (kg)}{Height\ (m^2)}$$

- A BMI of 25–29.9 signifies that the patient is overweight.
- A BMI of 30–39.9 signifies that the patient is obese.
- A BMI > 40 signifies that the patient is very obese.

The values and answers obtained are then checked against the protocols and anyone not fulfilling the desired criteria is returned to the referring surgeon with an explanation. The surgeon can then add that patient to their inpatient waiting list or contact the GP to arrange treatment prior to reassessment.

INVESTIGATIONS

If the criteria are fulfilled, the patient then undergoes any appropriate investigations according to the individual hospital's protocol, which is usually agreed between the surgeons, anaesthetists and day-case nursing staff. These investigations should be minimal. A possible protocol would be:

- *electrocardiogram*: all patients over 60 years old and those with heart disease, hypertension or long-term diabetes
- *urea and electrolyte estimations*: all patients taking diuretics
- *sickle test*: all Afro-Caribbean patients.

Other pre-operative investigations should be performed as clinically indicated, but should again be kept to a minimum.

INFORMATION

One of the keys to a successful pre-assessment interview is the transfer of information to the patient. This should be done in a relaxed atmosphere, so that on the day of their operation patients will understand what is happening and why. Patients will often take little away from their consultation with the doctor, owing to a combination of anxiety and pressure on time. The pre-assessment interview should cover all the relevant points relating to the patient's procedure and anticipated experience, as well as allowing them time to ask questions. Relatives should be encouraged to participate in this process. Invariably, people will forget what has been discussed or be unable to explain to relatives what is wrong with them. For this reason, many units provide patient information sheets, which give a brief description of the procedure and the post-operative instructions (Fig. 13.3). This document should also include

13

13

DAY-CASE SURGERY ASSESSMENT FORM
PATIENT SELF-ASSESSMENT
Please answer the following questions

Have you ever had:	Yes/No
1. Any surgical operations? Please list:	p/p
2. Any anaesthetic or surgical problems? Please list:	p/p
3. Is there a family history of anaesthetic problems? Please list:	p/p
4. Any other serious illnesses? Please list:	p/p

Please tick the box if you suffer from any of the following conditions:

1. Chest pain on exercise or at night	p
2. Asthma, bronchitis or significant breathing problems	p
3. High blood pressure	p
4. Heart murmur	p
5. Fits or faints	p
6. Yellow jaundice	p
7. Indigestion, heartburn or acid reflux	p
8. Diabetes	p
9. Arthritis or neck problems	p
10. Anaemia or other blood problems	p
11. Excessive bleeding or bruising	p
12. Kidney or waterwork problems	p
13. Weakness of muscles	p
14. Do you have a pacemaker?	p

What medicines do you take?
Please list:

Do you have any allergies?
Please list:

Social history:	Yes/No
1. Can someone accompany you home in a car or taxi?	p/p
2. Does/can someone responsible stay in the house with you post-surgery?	p/p
3. Do you have a telephone?	p/p
4. Do you have easy access to a toilet?	p/p
5. How many flights of stairs do you have to climb to get to your front door?	p
6. Do you smoke? 1 = never 2 = stopped > 6 months 3 = stopped < 6 months 4 = current	p/p
(How many per day?)	p
7. Do you drink alcohol? If you answered yes, how much per week?	p/p

Surgeon's assessment

1. Diagnosis?

2. Proposed procedure?

3. Anaesthetic proposed?

4. Pre-operative investigations required?
Please tick those required:

ECG (over 60 years old or ischaemic heart disease, hypertension or long-term diabetes)	p
U&Es (on diuretic therapy)	p
FBC (history of anaemia/menorrhagia)	p
Sickle (Afro-Caribbean)	p
Other (please specify)	p
Considered suitable for day-case procedure?	p/p

Fig. 13.2 Day-case surgery assessment form.

a number to call in case of emergencies or should further questions arise. Informed consent should be obtained by the surgeon undertaking the procedure, either in the clinic or on the day of surgery, depending on whether there is likely to be a significant delay.

PATIENT SELECTION

Day surgery is expanding in terms of the procedures available and the spectrum of patients on whom they can be performed, and this growth is expected to continue. The

DAY-CASE SURGERY: PATIENT INFORMATION SHEET

HERNIA
A hernia is a bulge in the abdominal wall due to a weakness in the muscle wall. At your operation, the weakness will be identified and repaired, using either stitches or a nylon mesh. This procedure is often carried out as a day case, but even when you go home there will still be discomfort in your groin for 5–7 days. You may go back to normal activities as soon as you feel able, and this will usually depend on pain.

Wound/stitches/dressings
The skin will have been closed with either a long continuous stitch visible only at either end of the wound, or with separate individual or dissolvable stitches. We will let you know if and when they are to be removed. The wound may bleed a little; if it does, press firmly over the wound for 5 minutes. If the wound becomes hot, red, swollen or painful, go to your GP or Accident and Emergency.

Pain
We will give you a supply of pain killers. Take these regularly for the first 24–48 hours, then after that as necessary. Do not wait until you have pain.

Working/driving/exercise
You should plan to take the first 2 weeks after surgery relatively quietly. The amount of exercise is limited by discomfort but, once this has settled, normal activities including lifting can be resumed. You should not drive until you are able to do an emergency stop comfortably–practise this before driving!

Bathing/showering
Avoid bathing/showering for a couple of days. Your dressing may come off the first time you have a bath. This is all right and it does not need to be replaced.

Follow-up
A follow-up appointment will not normally be made to see the surgeon again but one can be arranged via your GP or the day surgery unit. There is a small incidence of recurrent hernias, i.e. a hernia reappearing over the following years. This only occurs in approximately 2–5% of cases; if it does happen, you should contact your GP. There is a small chance of a degree of numbness below the wound. This should not cause undue concern and usually settles in time.

Fig. 13.3 Day-case surgery patient information sheet: hernia.

13

decision to refer a patient for a day-case procedure ultimately lies with the surgeon who reviews the patient in the outpatient clinic and who will be performing the operation. Certain standards should be met to ensure that the patients will undergo operation with minimal upset, and ultimately that the procedure will be safe. A number of social and medical factors influence this decision, and a few of these are outlined in Table 13.3. Many of these will directly influence:

- suitability for a day-case procedure
- the type of operation performed
- the type of anaesthetic used
- the need for special precautions.

CONTRAINDICATIONS TO DAY SURGERY

It is generally accepted that the following factors are contraindications to day surgery, but some of these may be considered only relative contraindications, depending on whether an extended 23-hour overnight service is available:

- patients with unstable/significant medical conditions that will usually put them in categories 3 and 4 of the

Table 13.3 PATIENT FACTORS INFLUENCING SUITABILITY FOR DAY-CASE SURGERY

- Age
- Demographics
- Past medical history
- Medications
- Convenience and patient preference
- Transport availability
- Home circumstances
- Anaesthetic considerations and American Society of Anesthesiologists (ASA) status

13

Table 13.4	AMERICAN SOCIETY OF ANESTHESIOLOGISTS (ASA): NEW CLASSIFICATION OF PHYSICAL STATUS

Class 1

- The patient has no organic, physiological, biochemical or psychiatric disturbance. The pathological process for which operation is to be performed is localized and does not entail a systemic disturbance

Class 2

- Mild to moderate systemic disturbance, caused either by the condition to be treated surgically or by other pathophysiological processes

Class 3

- Severe systemic disturbance or disease, from whatever cause, even though it may not be possible to define the degree of disability with finality

Class 4

- Severe systemic disorders that are already life-threatening, not always correctable by operation

Class 5

- The morbid patient who has little chance of survival but is submitted to operation in desperation

American Society of Anesthesiologists (ASA) classification (Table 13.4)

- gross obesity (BMI > 41)
- operation likely to exceed 2 hours
- type of procedure unsuitable (as defined by each specialty)
- hypertension (diastolic > 100 mmHg)
- severe gastro-oesophageal reflux disease (lying flat or bending)
- poorly controlled diabetes
- history of anaesthetic complications and certain drugs, e.g. warfarin (see below)
- poorly controlled asthma
- sickle-positive (sickle trait is acceptable)
- cervical spine or mandible problems
- patients live > 1 hour's travelling time away/do not have someone responsible to take them home
- no responsible person living in the same house
- no access to a telephone
- difficult access to the house (too many stairs to the front door).

Social factors

Social problems are the most common reason for a patient being deemed unsuitable for day-case surgery. Conditions in the patient's home should be suitable for a speedy and comfortable recovery, and the absence of a responsible adult at home in case of problems, an accessible toilet and access to a telephone in case of an emergency are all contraindications to day-case surgery.

Age

Age should not be an absolute discriminating factor and no age at present signals a cut-off in most units. However, elderly patients are more likely to have social and medical issues that will exclude them from consideration. Recovery of fine motor skills and cognitive functions is slowed with increasing age, and this necessitates a longer period of post-operative supervision. At the other end of the spectrum, the very young (less than 6 months) are reported to have an increased incidence of post-operative apnoeic episodes and should be observed overnight.

Demographics

The distance a patient lives from the day-surgery unit is very important. It is recommended that the journey home take no more than 90 minutes and that the house is accessible to emergency services, should these be required. For this reason, people living in isolated areas cannot be considered.

Patients' demographic details are also relevant in terms of where their surgery is carried out. This may ultimately influence their waiting time for surgery, owing to the difference in waiting-list size between units.

Medications

It is important to identify those drugs that might have an adverse effect on the outcome of the anaesthetic or the procedure itself. Protocols must be drawn up, in conjunction with the anaesthetists, highlighting any drugs of particular concern so that appropriate action can be taken at an early stage. The use of anticoagulants is not necessarily a contraindication to day-case surgery, depending on why the patient requires anticoagulation. For conditions such as atrial fibrillation, warfarin can safely be stopped 3–5 days before surgery and restarted the day after surgery. When anticoagulation is required for prosthetic heart valves, a short stay in hospital is usually required, with conversion to intravenous heparin over the perioperative period. Many surgeons also prefer aspirin to be stopped 10 days before surgery. For certain procedures, women who take the oral contraceptive pill are recommended to stop doing so 6 weeks before surgery to reduce the risk of thromboembolic disease. Those taking oral hypoglycaemics should be told to omit them on the morning of surgery, but otherwise patients should be instructed to take all regular medications as normal, unless contraindicated.

The use of certain medications, such as diuretics and lithium, will necessitate the patient undergoing certain pre-operative investigations. Provided the results are normal, this should not serve to exclude them from a day-case procedure.

Past medical history

Clues from the patient's past medical history should become apparent at the initial consultation as to their suitability for day surgery. If something is missed, there are safety nets further down the line to prevent unsuitable patients being referred, and this will be discussed in a later section. Insulin-dependent diabetics are not generally considered suitable for day-case surgery, unless they are very well controlled. Most other comorbid conditions should not serve to exclude a candidate, provided control of these conditions is satisfactory; if necessary, a decision can be made following discussion with the appropriate specialists (e.g. cardiologist,

Table 13.5 FACTORS THAT MIGHT INFLUENCE DAY-CASE SURGERY: SPECIAL CONSIDERATIONS

- Previous anaesthetic problems
- Previous surgery
- Children
- Infections, e.g. human immunodeficiency virus (HIV), hepatitis B or C, meticillin-resistant *Staphylococcus aureus* (MRSA)
- Religious beliefs, e.g. Jehovah's Witness
- Sickle-cell disease
- Cardiac pacemakers and use of bipolar diathermy
- Psychiatric conditions

respiratory physician, endocrinologist and anaesthetist) before the day of surgery. However, the anaesthetist will have the final say.

Anaesthetic considerations

It is generally agreed that those patients not falling into classes 1 or 2 of the ASA classification of physical status should not be considered for day surgery (Table 13.4). Some units allow certain ASA class 3 patients to undergo day surgery, provided their condition is not maintained by medication. Past anaesthetic reactions are also very important for obvious reasons, and if anaesthetic complications are suspected, inpatient facilities should be easily available.

Special considerations

Other important points that may influence decisions regarding the patient's suitability for surgery and the nature of surgery to be performed are listed in Table 13.5. As discussed earlier, day-case surgery may be ideal for children, provided parents are willing to accept the responsibility of aftercare. The provision of the service for children should allow for the fact that nurses with paediatric training are required, and that the ward area should have facilities for the accommodation of both child *and* parent. The unit must also have facilities available for paediatric anaesthesia and cardiopulmonary resuscitation.

Finally, patient preference should be one of the most important discriminatory factors. Following a careful explanation of procedure at pre-assessment, the patient should be allowed to make an informed decision. The other advantage of this process is that patients have the opportunity broadly to select a date that is convenient for them in terms of work or travel, and which allows them to make early preparations for their surgery.

PROCEDURES

In its guidelines on day-case surgery, the Royal College of Surgeons of England suggests a number of procedures that should be suitable. However, the final choice will depend on clinical judgement and the facilities available. Some of the principles to be considered when carrying out an operation as a day case are shown in Table 13.6. Table 13.7 gives examples of general surgical procedures that are currently carried out as day cases.

Certain general surgical procedures merit further discussion, owing to the increasing trend of performing them as day cases. Laparoscopic cholecystectomy, one of the more common operations performed in general surgical units, is currently under review regarding its feasibility as a day-case procedure. Early studies are encouraging and there is no doubt that it is indeed feasible; however, some studies have reported a high (20% or more) rate of planned day cases requiring overnight care owing to post-operative nausea, vomiting and pain, or because of conversion to an open procedure. A small number of patients also require readmission following complications, but it has been shown that readmission is no more frequent than in those operated on as inpatients. Laparoscopic hernia repair is also feasible as a day-case procedure, particularly for bilateral or recurrent hernias. Again, there is no reason why most, if not all but the most complicated, of these laparoscopic procedures cannot be carried out within the day-surgery unit, as long as there is an overnight facility. Even laparoscopic anti-reflux procedures can be performed on a day-case basis, although a high proportion of patients do end up staying overnight.

Table 13.6 PRINCIPLES APPLIED WHEN CONSIDERING A PROCEDURE FOR DAY SURGERY

- Duration (not absolute)
- Minimal risk
- Low complication rate
- Possibility of early mobilization
- Minimal post-operative pain
- Experience of surgeon
- Facilities available
- Type of anaesthetic

Table 13.7 GENERAL SURGICAL PROCEDURES PERFORMED AS DAY CASES

Procedures now performed almost entirely as day cases

- Minor anal procedures, e.g. lateral sphincterotomy
- Laparoscopy: diagnostic and therapeutic
- Hernia: unilateral or bilateral laparoscopically
- Varicose veins
- Minor oral surgery, e.g. release tongue tie, biopsies
- Family planning: vasectomy, female sterilization
- Excision of skin lesions
- Minor breast surgery
- Endoscopy

Other procedures that may be performed as day/23-hour cases

Laparoscopic cholecystectomy
Laparoscopic fundoplication
Haemorrhoidectomy
Thyroid lobectomy
Thoracoscopic sympathectomy
Wide excision of breast lump with axillary clearance

13

13

Another common general surgical procedure worthy of mention is day-case haemorrhoidectomy. Previous practice has been to monitor these cases as inpatients until their bowels have opened, and only then allowing discharge home. Recent studies have shown that haemorrhoidectomy is feasible and safe when performed as a day case, with little difference in post-operative pain or complication rates compared with inpatient care. A small readmission rate is to be expected, usually secondary to bleeding or pain, and some series have shown that only a minority of patients said that they would prefer inpatient care if they had to undergo a subsequent haemorrhoidectomy.

Many other specialties utilize day-surgery facilities and each has its own recommended procedures. Some of these merit mention because they are common procedures that until recently would have placed a large strain on inpatient facilities. They include:

- *ophthalmology*: cataract correctional surgery, correction of strabismus
- *orthopaedics*: arthroscopy, carpal tunnel release, Dupuytren's contracture release, manipulations and plaster changes
- *gynaecology*: surgical termination of pregnancy, hysteroscopy, diagnostic laparoscopy, laparoscopic sterilization
- *ear, nose and throat*: removal of foreign bodies and examination under anaesthesia, insertion of grommets, nasal polypectomy, manipulation of nasal fractures, diagnostic laryngoscopy, pharyngoscopy and oesophagoscopy (rigid and flexible), removal of vocal cord lesions.

Recent attention has also been directed towards the possibility of day-case tonsillectomy. As one of the most common childhood operations, day-case tonsillectomy is already popular in the USA. Some early UK studies suggest that it is feasible in children, with no increase in reactionary haemorrhage rates or post-operative pain compared with inpatients. However, studies carried out on adult populations have shown that a high proportion of patients preferred to stay overnight for analgesia and control of nausea and vomiting.

DECISION TO UNDERTAKE SURGERY

The decision to undertake a procedure as a day case should involve a number of factors, of which the length of time the procedure will take is one of the most important. The Royal College of Surgeons of England guidelines suggest no more than 30 minutes per case, although with recent advances in day-case anaesthesia and antiemetics this can be extended, in some units to 2 hours. The complexity of the procedure should be appropriate to the experience of the surgeon and the facilities of the unit, as well as the experience of the nursing staff. The likelihood of complications should be seriously considered, as those that require other specialists or facilities not available on site should lead to that procedure not being performed as a day case.

TRAINING OPPORTUNITIES

For the above reasons, many day-case procedures are for common conditions and so provide excellent training opportunities for junior staff. As much day surgery is consultant-led, this provides an opportunity for intensive one-on-one teaching and demonstration of basic skills. Day surgery provides a setting for a sound practical education, with expert assistance should problems be encountered.

DAY-CASE ANAESTHESIA AND POST-OPERATIVE CARE

Anaesthetic considerations and the anticipated degree of post-operative pain and nausea are important factors that make a procedure suitable or unsuitable for day-case operation.

For all procedures, the patient should be fasted from the previous night; if the procedure is to take place in the afternoon, the patient should be fasted from early on the morning of operation. Before surgery, the anaesthetist reviews all patients, as well as the results of any pre-operative investigations, and at this time any previous anaesthetic problems can be discussed and pre-medication prescribed.

Day-case anaesthesia should ideally include :

- a rapid and smooth onset of action, particularly in the absence of pre-medication
- rapid recovery without residual side-effects and active metabolites
- absence of adverse effects, such as nausea and vomiting.

Day-case surgery can be conducted under general, regional or local anaesthesia (with or without sedation). The choice of anaesthetic depends on the patient and on surgical factors, including previous anaesthetic reactions and any requirement for paralysis.

GENERAL ANAESTHESIA

General anaesthesia remains the most popular technique, especially with the newer agents that cause less of a 'hangover' effect. Intravenous agents are generally used for induction; maintenance is usually performed with an inhalational agent, although for some cases intravenous maintenance is used. The risks of day-case general anaesthesia are the same as for any general anaesthetic.

Airway control is secured with an endotracheal tube or laryngeal mask. The latter has a lower incidence of post-operative sore throat and fewer requirements for muscle relaxation, as well as avoiding some of the haemodynamic responses encountered when inserting endotracheal tubes. There is, however, an increased risk of gastric aspiration with laryngeal masks, compared with endotracheal intubation. For other procedures, especially those that are very short, some anaesthetists use only a face mask and an oropharyngeal airway.

LOCAL AND REGIONAL ANAESTHESIA

Many day-case procedures are performed under local anaesthesia. This avoids the potential hazards and side-effects of general anaesthesia, while at the same time resulting in fewer requirements for post-operative nursing and a faster return home.

Simple procedures may be performed using only local infiltration, whereas others may require a field block. Epidural and spinal anaesthesia are occasionally used for lower-extremity operations, but their use is limited by persisting sympathetic blockade requiring longer post-operative observation.

PAIN

The minimization of post-operative pain is of paramount importance in day-case surgery. Ideally, pain should be controllable using conventional oral analgesia before discharge. Potent opioid analgesics, e.g. fentanyl, alfentanyl and morphine, are still used but cause a significant increase in nausea and vomiting. Another technique employed to reduce post-operative pain is the infiltration of the wound with local anaesthetic, or a regional block while the patient is still under general anaesthesia. This means that the patient is comfortable on coming round from the anaesthetic, and works on the basis that preventing pain is superior to treating it.

Patients should be discharged with a small supply of take-home medication, usually combining a paracetamol-based compound with a potent non-steroidal anti-inflammatory agent.

NAUSEA AND VOMITING

Nausea and vomiting remain the most troublesome side-effects following day-case anaesthesia and are a common cause of unexpected overnight admission. A variety of agents, used both prophylactically and therapeutically, have been employed to combat nausea, including metoclopramide and droperidol, but these unfortunately have significant psychomotor side-effects. Use of the newer agent, ondansetron, has improved the treatment of drug-induced post-operative vomiting and also has fewer side-effects. However, it is significantly more expensive than other more conventional agents.

DISCHARGE ARRANGEMENTS

All patients are seen after surgery by both anaesthetist and surgeon. Once they are fully recovered, the procedure is explained to them and instructions are given regarding further follow-up, including arrangements for removal of sutures, wound review, and what to do if there are any problems. Although these should all have been covered in the pre-operative assessment and patient information sheet, it is best to go over them again with each patient before discharge.

Day-case surgery has been well established in paediatric practice for longer than in adult practice. Children requiring minor operative procedures under general anaesthetic recover well at home in a familiar and friendly environment. The provision of local anaesthetic regional blocks using long-acting local anaesthetic agents has had a major impact on the acceptability of such surgery in children. Home visits by suitably trained paediatric nursing staff in the post-operative period provide both patients and parents with the necessary reassurance and support to allow such surgery to be undertaken successfully.

Conditions that are suitable for day-case surgery in children include inguinal herniotomy, ligation of a patent processus vaginalis (hydrocoele), release of tongue tie, umbilical herniorraphy, circumcision, orchidopexy, minor plastic surgery procedures (including laser therapy for pigmented skin lesions), upper gastrointestinal endoscopy, diagnostic cystoscopy and surgery to correct bat ears.

13

Table 13.8 AREAS WHERE DAY SURGERY IS UNDER-UTILIZED		
Procedure	**Management executive targets for 1997 (%)**	**Accounts Commission proposed targets (%)**
Inguinal hernia—adults	10	20
Inguinal hernia—children	60	80
Breast lumpectomy	60	65
Anal fissure operation	70	75
Varicose veins	20	40
Cystoscopy	80	80
Circumcision	60	80
Dupuytren's contracture	20	50
Carpal tunnel release	80	85
Arthroscopy	65	75
Ganglion	85	90
Orchidopexy	25	60
Cataracts	1	80
Squint correction	25	80

THE FUTURE

The Accounts Commission undertook an audit of day-case surgical services in 1998. This revealed that a higher percentage of elective surgery was being performed on a day-case basis and that more dedicated day-surgery units had been set up since 1991. However, areas were identified where day-case surgery was still under-utilized and recommendations were made to the different health authorities and trusts to review and implement changes (Table 13.8). With the increase of minimally invasive surgery and superior anaesthesic techniques, it has now become clear that the majority of operations can be performed on a day-case, ambulatory or 23-hour basis.

BOX 13.1   DAY-CASE SURGERY

- The use of day-case surgery has been dramatically increasing over recent years
- Not all patients are suitable for day-case surgery and carefully designed protocols are required to prevent late cancellations
- An increasing number of procedures are now being performed on a day-case basis, in particular minimally invasive procedures
- Facilities must be available for inpatient care, if required
- There are still opportunities to increase the provision of day-case surgery in order to come into line with recent government recommendations
- Ambulatory or 23-hour surgery is one way to increase the provision of current day surgical services

Section 3
UPPER GASTROINTESTINAL SURGERY

14

R.W. PARKS

The abdominal wall and hernia

UMBILICUS

DEVELOPMENTAL ABNORMALITIES

Persistent vitello-intestinal duct

The vitello-intestinal duct runs in intrauterine life from the apex of the midgut loop to the yolk sac. It is normally obliterated long before birth, but part of it may persist as a Meckel's diverticulum on the anti-mesenteric border of the ileum. Rarer abnormalities include persistence of a band attaching the umbilicus to a Meckel's diverticulum or a loop of ileum; a patent communication (fistula) between the ileum and umbilicus; an encysted portion of the duct that does not connect with the ileum (enterocystoma); an umbilical sinus; and a persistent umbilical portion of the duct, which forms a polypoidal raspberry-like tumour of the umbilicus (enteroteratoma) (Fig. 14.1). Symptomatic remnants may have to be excised, although a broad-based Meckel's diverticulum is usually left alone if found incidentally at laparotomy. Persisting bands can cause intestinal obstruction.

Urachus

The urachus runs from the apex of the bladder to the umbilicus. It is normally obliterated at birth but may give rise to cysts, a urinary fistula, or a discharging umbilical

sinus if parts of it remain patent. Symptomatic remnants require excision.

UMBILICAL SEPSIS

Umbilical sepsis in neonates may give rise to portal thrombophlebitis, liver abscess formation, jaundice and portal vein thrombosis, which may result in portal hypertension. Tetanus can follow the application of cow dung to the umbilicus, as was once practised in some underdeveloped societies.

In adults, sepsis can result from retention of inspissated sebum within the folds of the umbilicus, and from infection of a pilonidal sinus of the umbilicus. Infection is usually mixed staphylococcal and streptococcal, characterized by erythema, tenderness and swelling. Treatment involves drainage of any pus and the prescription of systemic antibiotics.

UMBILICAL TUMOURS

The umbilicus may rarely be involved by primary neoplasms (e.g. squamous carcinoma or melanoma), or by secondary tumour that has tracked along the ligamentum teres from the liver or lymph nodes in the porta hepatis. Neoplasia is an occasional unexpected finding in an umbilicus that has been excised because of persistent discharge.

10

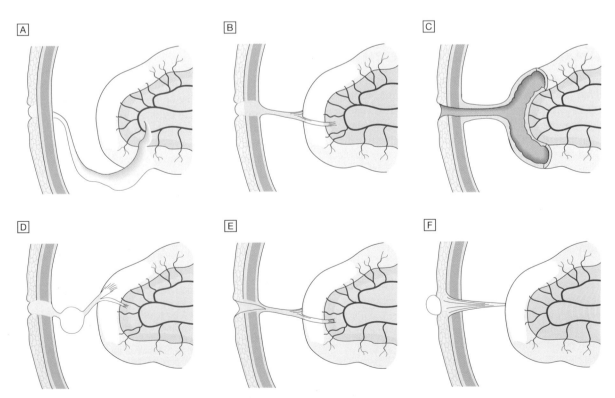

Fig. 14.1   Persistence of the vitello-intestinal duct, giving rise to developmental abnormalities.
A A Meckel's diverticulum. B A fibrous cord to the ileum. C An umbilical intestinal fistula. D An enterocystoma. E An umbilical sinus.
F An enteroteratoma.

14

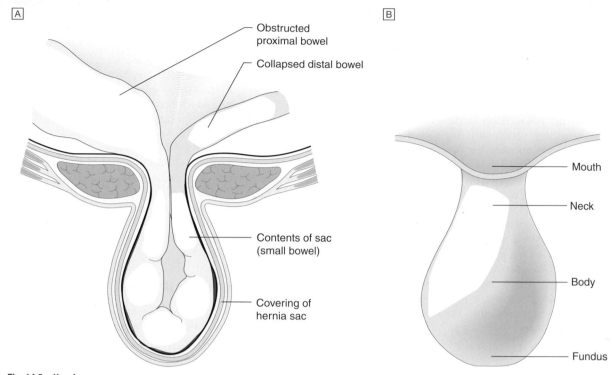

Fig. 14.2 Hernia.
A Anatomical structure. B Parts of the hernial sac.

DISORDERS OF THE RECTUS MUSCLE

HAEMATOMA OF THE RECTUS SHEATH

Spontaneous or traumatic rupture of a branch of the inferior epigastric artery occasionally produces a painful swelling of the rectus sheath in association with rigidity. This condition is not commonly diagnosed, but may represent an unusual presentation of acute abdominal pain in the elderly patient. A history of excessive physical exertion may precede the onset of symptoms. Ultrasonography can be used to confirm the diagnosis. Spontaneous resolution is typical; occasionally, however, ligation of the bleeding artery with evacuation of clot may be indicated.

DESMOID TUMOUR

This rare tumour is thought to arise from fibrous intramuscular septa in the lower rectus abdominis muscle. It is more common in women of child-bearing age and can be associated with intestinal polyposis in Gardner's syndrome. The lesion must be excised widely, as it is prone to recur and can become malignant (fibrosarcoma).

ABDOMINAL HERNIA

A hernia is an abnormal protrusion of an organ (e.g. intestine, brain) or tissue (e.g. muscle, fat) outside its normal body cavity or constraining sheath. Hernias of the abdominal wall are common. They may exploit natural openings such as the inguinal and femoral canals, umbilicus, obturator canal or oesophageal hiatus, or protrude through areas weakened by stretching (e.g. epigastric hernia) or surgical incision. The hernia is immediately invested by a peritoneal sac drawn from the lining of the abdominal wall (Fig. 14.2). The sac is covered in turn by those tissues that are stretched in front of it as the hernia enlarges (i.e. the coverings). The neck of the sac is the constriction formed by the orifice in the abdominal wall through which the hernia passes.

BOX 14.1 HERNIA

- A hernia is an abnormal protrusion of an organ or tissue outside its normal body cavity or restraining sheath
- Hernias of the abdominal wall are common and may exploit natural openings (inguinal, femoral and obturator canals, umbilicus and oesophageal hiatus) or weak areas caused by stretching or surgical incisions
- Abdominal hernias have a peritoneal sac, the neck of which is often unyielding and constitutes a potential source of compression of the hernial contents
- Hernia may be classified as reducible or irreducible, and the contents (e.g. bowel) may become obstructed or strangulated
- Strangulation denotes compromise of the blood supply of the contents and its development significantly increases morbidity and mortality. The low-pressure venous drainage is occluded first and then the arterial supply becomes occluded, with the development of gangrene

---

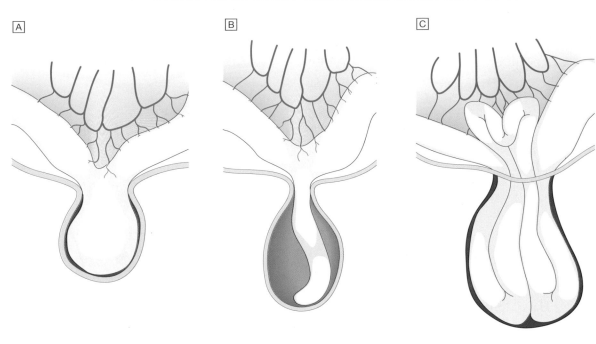

Fig. 14.3 Unusual inguinal hernias.
A Richter's hernia. B Littré's hernia. C Maydl's hernia.

A hernia may contain any intra-abdominal structure but most commonly contains omentum and/or small bowel. A hernia may involve only part of the circumference of the bowel (Richter's hernia), a Meckel's diverticulum (Littré's hernia) or two involved loops of bowel (Maydl's hernia) (Fig. 14.3). A sliding inguinal hernia is defined as one in which a viscus forms a portion of the wall of the hernia sac. Most commonly, the viscus involved is caecum, sigmoid colon or urinary bladder.

INGUINAL HERNIA

Groin hernias account for three-quarters of all abdominal wall hernias, and inguinal herniorrhaphy is one of the most frequently performed minor operative procedures. The most common types of groin hernia are indirect inguinal (60%), direct inguinal (25%) and femoral (15%). Most (85%) groin hernias occur in males. Inguinal hernias occur in 1–3% of all newborn males. The incidence in premature infants is 30 times that seen at term. In early life, an indirect inguinal hernia is by far the most common variety. After middle age, weakness of the abdominal musculature leads to an increasing incidence of direct inguinal hernias. Femoral hernias are relatively more common in females (possibly because of stretching of ligaments and widening of the femoral ring in pregnancy), but an indirect inguinal hernia is still the most common type of groin hernia in women.

Surgical anatomy

The inguinal canal is an oblique passage in the lower anterior abdominal wall, through which the spermatic cord passes to the testis in the male, or the round ligament to the labium majus in the female. The processus vaginalis traversing the canal is normally obliterated at birth (Fig. 14.4), but persistence in whole or in part presents an anatomical predisposition to an indirect inguinal hernia. The openings of the canal are formed by the internal and external rings. The internal (deep) inguinal ring is an opening in the transversalis fascia, which lies 1 cm above the mid-inguinal point (midway between the pubic tubercle and the anterior superior iliac spine). The internal inguinal ring is bounded medially by the inferior epigastric artery (Fig. 14.5). The inguinal canal ends at the external (superficial) inguinal ring, which is an opening in the aponeurosis of the external oblique muscle just above and medial to the pubic tubercle. At birth, the internal and external rings lie on top of each other, so that the inguinal canal is short and straight; with growth, the two rings move apart so that the canal becomes longer and oblique.

The testis and spermatic cord receive a covering from each of the layers as they pass through the abdominal wall. The innermost layer is derived from the transversalis fascia (the internal spermatic fascia), the middle layer from the internal oblique muscle (the cremasteric muscle and fascia), and the outer layer from the external oblique aponeurosis (the external spermatic fascia). Within the inguinal canal, the spermatic cord is covered only by the cremasteric and internal spermatic fasciae. The spermatic cord consists of the vas deferens, the artery of the vas (branch of the inferior vesical artery), the testicular artery (branch of the aorta on the right and renal artery on the left), the cremasteric artery (branch of the inferior epigastric artery), the pampiniform plexus of veins, the ilio-inguinal nerve, the genital branch of the genitofemoral nerve and lymphatics.

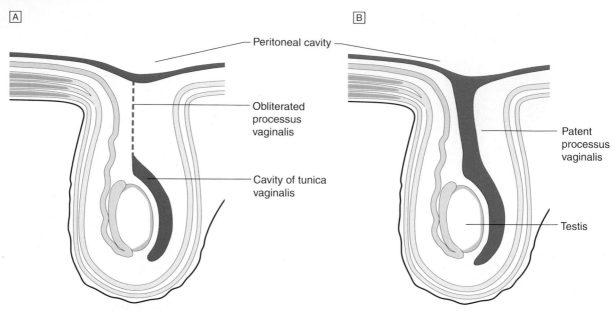

Fig. 14.4 Processus vaginalis testis.
A Normal obliteration of processus vaginalis. B Persistence of patent processus.

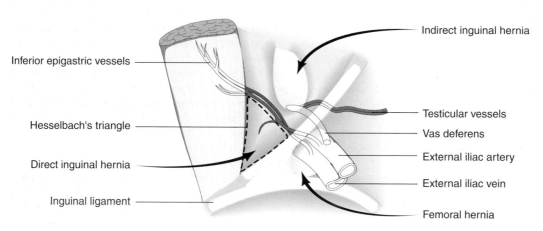

Fig. 14.5 Anatomy of the internal inguinal ring, showing sites of herniation from within.

Indirect inguinal hernia

Many indirect inguinal hernias are probably the result of failure of obliteration of the processus vaginalis. An indirect inguinal hernia enters the internal (deep) inguinal ring and descends within the coverings of the spermatic cord so that it can pass on down into the scrotum. The hernia may remain within the inguinal canal (bubonocoele), protrude through the external (superficial) inguinal ring (funicular), or extend into the scrotum (complete or scrotal) (Fig. 14.6). Very occasionally, it enlarges between the muscle layers of the abdominal wall to form an interstitial hernia.

Clinical features

The moment of herniation (or rupture) may be associated with sudden groin pain, or may pass unnoticed. Thereafter, there may be a dragging discomfort in the groin, particularly during lifting or straining, but in the absence of strangulation further pain is unusual.

The hernia forms a swelling in the inguinal canal, which may extend into the scrotum. It is often readily visible when the patient stands or is asked to cough. An inguinal hernia, which passes into the scrotum, passes above and medial to the pubic tubercle, in contrast to a femoral hernia, which bulges below and lateral to the tubercle (Fig. 14.7). A cough impulse is normally palpable, and bowel sounds can often be heard within the hernia on auscultation. If there is no visible swelling, a cough impulse is sought with the patient standing.

The hernia often reduces spontaneously when the patient lies down, or it may be reduced by gentle pressure applied in an upward and lateral direction. It may be possible to control the hernia, once reduced, by placing a finger over the internal (deep) inguinal ring.

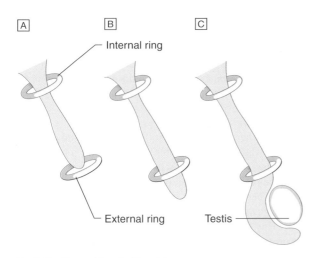

Fig. 14.6   Types of inguinal hernial sac.
[A] Bubonocoele. [B] Funicular. [C] Complete or scrotal. (IR = internal ring; ER = external ring; T = testis)

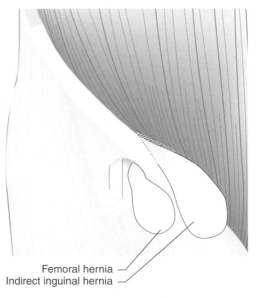

Fig. 14.7   Exit of femoral and inguinal hernias.

Direct inguinal hernia

Direct hernias are due to weakness of the abdominal wall and may be precipitated by increases in intra-abdominal pressure (e.g. obstructive airways disease, prostatism or chronic constipation). The hernia protrudes through the transversalis fascia in the posterior wall of the inguinal canal. The defect is bounded above by the conjoint tendon, below by the inguinal ligament, and laterally by the inferior epigastric vessels (Fig. 14.5). These boundaries mark the area known as Hesselbach's triangle. The hernia occasionally bulges through the external (superficial) inguinal ring, but the transversalis fascia cannot stretch sufficiently to allow it to descend down into the scrotum. The sac has a wide neck, so that the hernia seldom becomes irreducible, obstructs or strangulates. As shown in Figure 14.5, the neck of the sac of a direct inguinal hernia lies medial to the inferior epigastric vessels, whereas that of an indirect hernia lies lateral to them. Both indirect and direct hernias may occur on the same side (pantaloon or saddle-bag hernia), with sacs straddling the inferior epigastric vessels.

Clinical features

The hernia forms a diffuse bulge in the region of the medial part of the inguinal canal. It is usually readily reduced by backward pressure, and the edges of the defect may then be palpable. Clinically, it is frequently impossible to determine whether a hernia confined to the inguinal canal is of the direct or the indirect variety.

Management of uncomplicated inguinal hernia

The identification of an inguinal hernia in any child is *always* an indication to operate. In newborns, the procedure must be carried out with some urgency because of the risk of stangulation. In very premature infants, the procedure may need to be done under regional block alone, and where general anaesthesia is used, elective post-operative ven-

tilation may be required. In older children, elective surgery is usually undertaken on a day-case basis, with liberal use of local anaesthetic blocks for post-operative pain relief.

Adults with a symptomatic inguinal hernia should be offered surgery. Open mesh repair or laparoscopic repair aims to reduce post-operative pain to a minimum, enabling most procedures to be undertaken as day cases. Inguinal hernias can be controlled by a truss, but this is uncomfortable and is now seldom indicated, as repair using local or regional anaesthestic techniques can be employed in higher-risk patients.

Indirect inguinal hernia

The first step in the open approach is to open the inguinal canal, free the hernial sac from the spermatic cord (Fig. 14.8) and excise it after transfixing and ligating its neck.

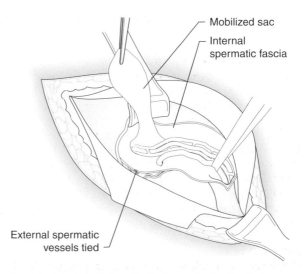

Fig. 14.8   Principle of dissection in the repair of an inguinal hernia.

14

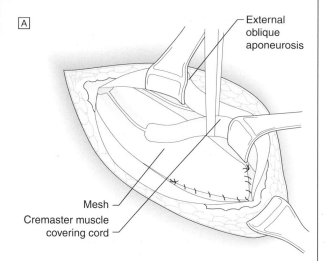

External
oblique
aponeurosis

Mesh
Cremaster muscle
covering cord

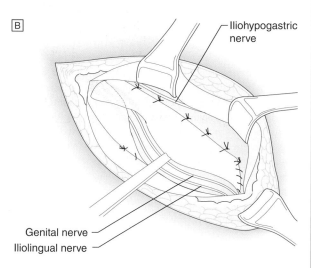

Iliohypogastric
nerve

Genital nerve
Iliolingual nerve

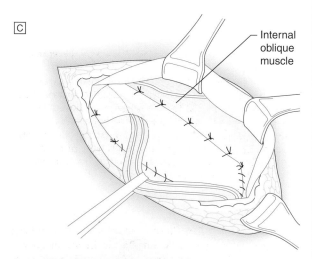

Internal
oblique
muscle

Fig. 14.9 Lichtenstein open mesh repair.
A The lower border of the mesh is secured in place with a continuous suture to the inguinal ligament. B Interrupted sutures are placed between the upper edge of the mesh and the underlying aponeurosis.
C A suture is placed laterally to close the two tails around the internal ring.

Simple excision of the sac (herniotomy) is all that is needed in young children. In older children and adults, the internal ring is usually stretched and widened, and therefore after herniotomy it is necessary to tighten the deep ring and strengthen the posterior wall (herniorrhaphy or hernioplasty).

Direct hernia

In a direct hernia, the sac is not normally excised and it is simply invaginated by sutures placed in the transversalis fascia. Insertion of a synthetic mesh is currently used to reinforce the posterior wall of the inguinal canal.

In all hernia repairs, it is important to avoid constricting the spermatic cord by making the deep inguinal ring too tight. This may compromise repair, particularly in large or recurrent hernias, and in older patients removal of the testis may be considered so that the inguinal canal can be completely obliterated.

The simplest and most common surgical procedure now performed is the Lichtenstein open tension-free repair, which involves the insertion of a synthetic mesh underneath the spermatic cord (Fig. 14.9). The mesh is secured to the aponeurotic tissue overlying the pubic bone medially, the inguinal ligament inferiorly, and the internal oblique aponeurosis and conjoint tendon superiorly. Laterally, the mesh is divided and its two sides wrapped around the spermatic cord and sutured in place.

Laparoscopic hernia repair, using a transperitoneal or pre-peritoneal (Fig. 14.10) approach, is increasing in popularity. The technique involves excising or reducing the hernial sac and inserting a mesh. Proponents of these techniques emphasize minimal pain, a more rapid return to normal activities, improved cosmesis and fewer infective complications; however, critics emphasize the necessity for a general anaesthetic, the violation of the peritoneal cavity (with the transperitoneal approach), increased costs and lack of long-term follow-up (EBM 14.1). It is generally accepted that the laparoscopic approach is particularly useful for patients with recurrent inguinal hernias or bilateral inguinal hernias.

Approximately 5% of hernias will recur. Early recurrence within 2 years is usually a result of an inadequate primary operation, whereas late recurrence reflects progression of the underlying muscular weakness. Recurrent hernias can be difficult to repair and the laparoscopic approach may be of particular benefit to these patients.

EBM 14.1 LAPAROSCOPIC INGUINAL HERNIA REPAIR

'Laparoscopic inguinal hernia repair is associated with earlier discharge from hospital, quicker return to normal activity and work, and significantly fewer post-operative complications than open inguinal hernia repair. However, the operating time is significantly longer and there is a trend towards an increase in the risk of recurrence.'

Memon MA, et al. Br J Surg 2003; 90:1479–1492

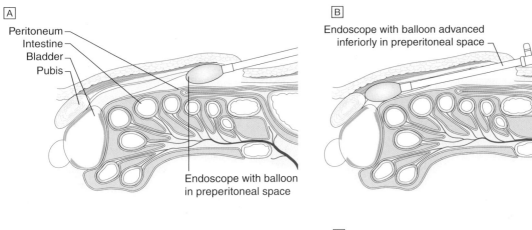

A
Peritoneum
Intestine
Bladder
Pubis

Endoscope with balloon
in preperitoneal space

B
Endoscope with balloon advanced
inferiorly in preperitoneal space

14

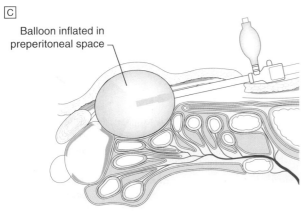

C
Balloon inflated in
preperitoneal space

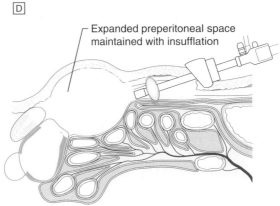

D
Expanded preperitoneal space
maintained with insufflation

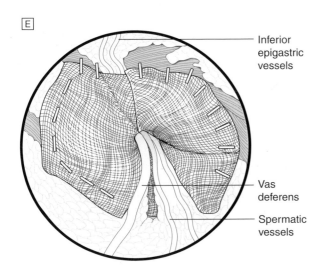

E
Inferior
epigastric
vessels

Vas
deferens

Spermatic
vessels

Fig. 14.10 A pre-peritoneal approach for laparoscopic inguinal hernia repair.
Access to the posterior rectus sheath is gained in the periumbilical region. [A] A balloon dissector is placed on the anterior surface of the posterior rectus sheath. [B] The balloon dissector is advanced to the posterior surface of the pubis in the pre-peritoneal space. [C] The balloon is inflated, thereby creating an optical cavity. [D] The cavity is insufflated by carbon dioxide. [E] Placement of the mesh. Some surgeons prefer to place the spermatic cord structures and/or the epigastric vessels through a slit in the mesh.

Sportsman's hernia

Groin injury leading to chronic groin pain is often referred to as the sportsman's hernia. However, the definition, investigation and treatment of this condition remain controversial. The differential diagnosis includes musculotendinous injuries, osteitis pubis, nerve entrapment, urological pathology or bone and joint disease. In many cases, clinical signs are lacking, despite the patient's symptoms.

Herniography studies have demonstrated a significant incidence of symptomatic impalpable hernia in patients presenting with obscure groin pain. A deficiency of the posterior inguinal wall is the most common operative finding in patients with chronic groin pain. Some authors have described a tear in the conjoint tendon as the cause of the pain, whereas in Gilmore's description, a tear in the external oblique aponeurosis, causing dilatation of the

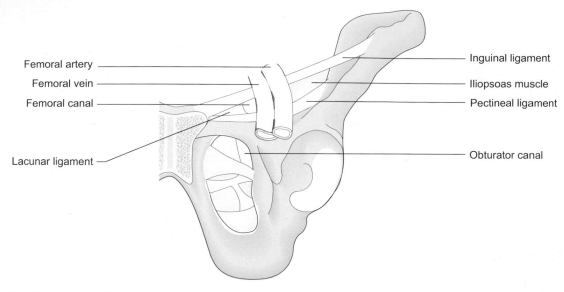

Femoral artery
Femoral vein
Femoral canal

Lacunar ligament

Inguinal ligament
Iliopsoas muscle
Pectineal ligament

Obturator canal

Fig. 14.11   Anatomy of the femoral ring.

external (superficial) inguinal ring, was implicated. Surgical intervention is recommended only when conservative management has failed. Appropriate repair of the posterior wall of the inguinal canal has proved to be of therapeutic benefit in selected patients.

Femoral hernia

A femoral hernia projects through the femoral ring and passes down the femoral canal. The ring is bounded laterally by the femoral vein, anteriorly by the inguinal ligament, medially by the lacunar ligament, and posteriorly by the superior ramus of the pubis and the reflected part of the inguinal ligament (pectineal ligament of Astley Cooper) (Fig. 14.11). As the hernia enlarges, it passes through the saphenous opening in the deep fascia of the thigh (the site of penetration of the long saphenous vein to join the femoral vein) and then turns upwards to lie in front of the inguinal ligament. The hernia has many coverings and may be deceptively small, sometimes escaping detection. It frequently contains omentum or small bowel, but the urinary bladder can 'slide' into the medial wall of the sac.

Clinical features

The hernia forms a bulge in the upper inner aspect of the thigh. It can sometimes be difficult to differentiate between an inguinal and a femoral hernia, but as indicated earlier, the former passes above and medial to the pubic tubercle as it enters the groin, whereas the latter passes below and lateral to it. Tracing the tendon of adductor longus upwards to its insertion is a useful guide to the position of the pubic tubercle.

A femoral hernia is frequently difficult or impossible to reduce because of its J-shaped course and the tight neck of the sac. As well as needing to be differentiated from inguinal hernia, it can be confused with an inguinal lymph node (no cough impulse, irreducible), saphenous varix (positive cough impulse or 'saphenous thrill', which is

prominent on standing but disappears on elevating the leg), ectopic testis, psoas abscess, hydrocoele of the spermatic cord or a lipoma.

Surgical repair of femoral hernia

A femoral hernia is particularly likely to obstruct and strangulate, and therefore surgical intervention is indicated. As with inguinal hernia, repair can be carried out under local or general anaesthesia.

The aim of operation is to excise the sac and obliterate the femoral ring by suturing the inguinal ligament to the pectineal ligament. The femoral canal can be approached from below the inguinal ligament, through the inguinal canal, or from above by entering the rectus sheath and displacing the rectus abdominis medially. The approach from above (McEvedy approach) gives the best access, and is particularly useful if the hernia contains strangulated bowel and intestinal resection is required.

BOX 14.2   GROIN HERNIAS

- Indirect inguinal hernias comprise 60% of all groin hernias and commence at the deep inguinal ring, lateral to the inferior epigastric vessels
- Direct inguinal hernias account for 25% of all groin hernias and bulge through a weakness in the back wall of the inguinal canal, medial to the inferior epigastric vessels. They rarely obstruct or strangulate
- Indirect inguinal hernias may pass down within the coverings of the spermatic cord to the scrotum; direct hernias do not descend into the scrotum
- Femoral hernias account for 15% of all groin hernias and pass through the femoral canal, emerging below and lateral to the pubic tubercle (in contrast to inguinal hernias, which pass medially to the tubercle and may descend to the scrotum)
- Femoral hernias are often small and easy to miss on clinical examination, but are prone to obstruct and strangulate

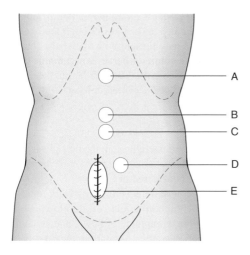

Fig. 14.12   Types of ventral hernia.
[A] Epigastric : through the linea alba. [B] Umbilical: through an umbilical scar. [C] Para-umbilical: above or below the umbilicus. [D] Spigelian: adjacent to the rectus sheath. [E] Incisional: anywhere.

VENTRAL HERNIA

Ventral hernias occur through areas of weakness in the anterior abdominal wall (Fig. 14.12): namely, the linea alba (epigastric hernia), the umbilicus (umbilical and para-umbilical hernia), the lateral border of the rectus sheath (Spigelian hernia), and the scar tissue of surgical incisions (incisional hernia).

Epigastric hernia

Epigastric hernias protrude through the linea alba above the level of the umbilicus. The herniation may consist of extraperitoneal fat or may be a protrusion of peritoneum containing omentum. The hernia is common in thin individuals and can cause local discomfort. It is repaired by closing the defect with interrupted non-absorbable sutures.

Umbilical hernia

True umbilical hernias occur in infants. The small sac protrudes through the umbilicus, particularly as the child cries, but is easily reduced. Over 95% of these hernias close spontaneously in the first 3 years of life. Persistence after the third birthday is an indication for elective repair. Surgery involves excision of the hernial sac and closure of the defect in the fascia of the abdominal wall.

Para-umbilical hernia

This hernia is caused by gradual weakening of the tissues around the umbilicus. It most often affects obese multiparous women, and passes through the attenuated linea alba just above or below the umbilicus. The peritoneal sac is often preceded by the extrusion of a small knuckle of extraperitoneal fat through the linea alba. The hernia gradually enlarges, the covering tissues become stretched and thin, and eventually loops of bowel may become visible under parchment-like skin. The sac is often multilocular and may be irreducible because of adhesions that form between omentum and loops of bowel. The skin may

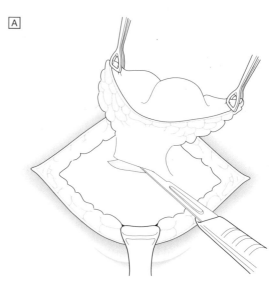

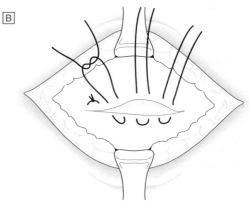

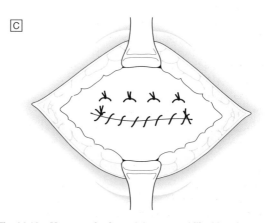

Fig. 14.13   Mayo repair of an adult para-umbilical hernia.
[A] Excision of the sac after reduction of its contents. [B] Insertion of overlapping sutures into the rectus sheath. [C] Final appearance.

become reddened, excoriated and ulcerated, and rarely an intestinal fistula may even develop.

Operation is advised because of the risk of obstruction and strangulation. Unless there is a large protrusion of the umbilicus itself, most surgical repairs can be performed

181

preserving the umbilicus. Through a transverse subumbilical incision, the anterior layer of the rectus sheath is exposed. The sac is opened and the contents are reduced. The classic Mayo repair involves the development of a flap of rectus sheath and linea alba above and below the hernial defect. The defect is closed by overlapping the layers, using mattress sutures of non-absorbable material in a 'double-breasted' fashion (Fig. 14.13). Alternatively, the defect can be closed using interrupted transverse sutures. If apposition of the hernia edges without tension is not possible, a non-absorbable mesh can be used.

Incisional hernia

Incisional hernias occur after 3–5% of all abdominal operations. Midline vertical incisions are most often affected, and poor surgical technique, wound infection, obesity and chest infection are important predisposing factors. The diffuse bulge in the wound is best seen when the patient coughs or raises the head and shoulders from a pillow, thereby contracting the abdominal muscles. Strangulation is rare, but surgical repair is usually advised. Some patients prefer to wear an abdominal support to control the hernia.

The skin wound is excised and flaps are elevated to expose the aponeurosis. The sac can be invaginated or excised, and the edges of the defect may be repaired with overlapping sutures, but repair with the insertion of a synthetic mesh is preferred.

RARE EXTERNAL HERNIA

- A *Spigelian hernia* occurs through the linea semilunaris at the outer border of the rectus abdominis muscle. Treatment is surgical, as the hernia is liable to strangulate.
- A *lumbar hernia* forms a diffuse bulge above the iliac crest between the posterior borders of the external oblique and latissimus dorsi muscles. It seldom requires treatment.

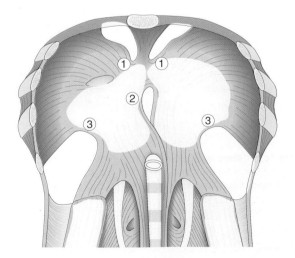

Fig. 14.14   Sites of diaphragmatic herniation.
(1) Parasternal, between the sternal and costal slips of the diaphragm (foramen of Morgagni). (2) Oesophageal hiatus. (3) Pleuroperitoneal canal (foramen of Bochdalek).

- An *obturator hernia* is a rare hernia that is more common in women and passes through the obturator canal. Patients may present with knee pain owing to pressure on the obturator nerve; however, the diagnosis is frequently made only when the hernia has strangulated and is discovered at laparotomy.

INTERNAL HERNIA

Herniation of the stomach through the oesophageal hiatus in the diaphragm (hiatus hernia) is a common cause of internal herniation and is considered in Chapter 17. A variety of cul-de-sacs and peritoneal defects resulting from rotation of the bowel and other abnormalities of development may be responsible for the entrapment of bowel and acute intestinal obstruction. For example, herniation may occur through the foramen of Winslow (opening of the lesser sac) and through various openings in the diaphragm, including the oesophageal hiatus (Fig. 14.14).

COMPLICATIONS OF HERNIA

Irreducibility

An irreducible hernia is one in which the contents cannot be manipulated back into the abdominal cavity. This may be due to narrowing of the neck of the sac by fibrosis, distension of the contained bowel, or adhesions to the walls of the sac.

Obstruction

An irreducible hernia may progress to intestinal obstruction. Abdominal pain, vomiting and distension signal the need for urgent operation *before* strangulation supervenes.

Strangulation

The vessels supplying the bowel within a hernia may be compressed by the neck of the sac or by the constricting ring through which the hernia passes. The contents initially become swollen as a result of venous congestion, and there is exudation of a blood-stained fluid. The arterial supply is subsequently compromised and gangrene follows. Organisms and toxins pass out through the bowel wall, causing local peritonitis.

The patient complains of pain in the hernia and usually has features of intestinal obstruction. The hernia is tender, the cough impulse is lost, and there may be increasing evidence of circulatory collapse and sepsis. In a Richter's hernia, only part of the circumference of the bowel is strangulated, and there may be no evidence of intestinal obstruction.

MANAGEMENT OF COMPLICATED HERNIA

If there is no evidence of strangulation, an attempt can be made to reduce an apparently irreducible hernia by giving analgesia, putting the patient to bed with the foot of the bed elevated, and applying gentle pressure. Undue force must never be used for fear of rupturing the bowel or returning the entire hernia to the abdomen with the bowel still trapped

14

within it (reduction en masse). If the hernia does not reduce readily, surgery is advised to avoid further complications.

In infants and children, the majority of 'irreducible' inguinal hernias can, in fact, be safely reduced by a suitably trained clinician. Small doses of intravenous opiate analgesia administered in the presence of suitably trained paediatric nursing staff can relax the child and assist with the reduction process. The hernia can then be repaired within 72 hours on the next available operating list. The child should be detained in hospital pending repair to allow early detection of further episodes of incarceration. Failure to reduce a hernia in this manner necessitates emergency surgery. This is usually extremely difficult and should only be attempted by experienced surgeons.

Urgent operation is indicated for all obstructed hernias, as one can never be certain that strangulation is not present. The hernial sac is opened and the contents are inspected carefully. If they are viable, they can be returned to the abdominal cavity and the hernia repaired. If there is doubt about the viability of a loop of bowel or omentum, the devitalized tissue must be resected before proceeding to repair.

14

15

S. PATERSON-BROWN

The acute abdomen and intestinal obstruction

INTRODUCTION

The 'acute abdomen' is a term used to encompass a spectrum of surgical, medical and gynaecological conditions, ranging from the trivial to the life-threatening, which require hospital admission, investigation and treatment. The primary symptom of the condition is abdominal pain.

For the purposes of multicentre studies looking at acute abdominal pain, the definition is taken as 'abdominal pain of less than 1 week's duration requiring admission to hospital, which has not been previously investigated or treated'. Acute abdominal pain following trauma is usually considered separately.

The acute abdomen is a very common clinical entity. It has been estimated that at least 50% of general surgical admissions are emergencies and, of these, 50% present with acute abdominal pain. The acute abdomen therefore represents a significant part of the general surgical work-load. Furthermore, patients with acute abdominal pain have a significant morbidity and mortality. Studies have shown a 30-day mortality of 4% among patients admitted with acute abdominal pain, rising to 8% in those who undergo operative treatment. Not surprisingly, the mortality rate varies with age, being the highest at the extremes of age. The highest mortality rates are associated with laparotomy for unresectable cancer, ruptured abdominal aortic aneurysm and perforated peptic ulcer.

Individual conditions presenting with acute abdominal pain will not be dealt with in depth in this chapter, but will be covered elsewhere.

AETIOLOGY

The causes of the acute abdomen may be subdivided into surgical, medical and gynaecological disorders. Surgical causes may be classified according to the organ involved,

15

Table 15.1 POSSIBLE CAUSES OF ACUTE ABDOMINAL PAIN

Surgical
Inflammation

- Inflammatory bowel disease
- Acute appendicitis
- Acute diverticulitis
- Acute pancreatitis
- Acute cholecystitis
- Acute cholangitis
- Meckel's diverticulitis

Obstruction

- Intestinal obstruction
- Biliary colic
- Ureteric colic
- Acute retention of urine

Ischaemia

- Mesenteric ischaemia
- Torsion of a viscus

Perforation

- Perforated peptic ulcer disease
- Perforated diverticular disease
- Perforated appendix
- Toxic megacolon with perforation
- Acute cholecystitis and perforation
- Perforated oesophagus
- Perforated bladder
- Perforation of a length of strangulated bowel
- Ruptured abdominal aortic aneurysm

Medical
Cardiovascular

- Myocardial ischaemia
- Myocardial infarction (inferior)

Gastrointestinal

- Gastritis
- Gastroenteritis
- Mesenteric adenitis
- Hepatitis
- Hepatic abscess
- Curtis–FitzHugh syndrome
- Primary peritonitis

Abdominal wall conditions

- Rectus sheath haematoma

Genitourinary

- Urinary tract infection
- Pyelonephritis

Neurological

- Tabes dorsalis

Haematological

- Sickle cell disease
- Malaria
- Hereditary spherocytosis

Endocrine

- Diabetes mellitus
- Thyrotoxicosis
- Addison's disease

Metabolic

- Uraemia
- Hypercalcaemia
- Porphyria

Infective

- Herpes zoster

Gynaecological

- Ectopic pregnancy
- Ovarian cyst
    Torsion
    Rupture
    Haemorrhage
    Infarction
    Infection
- Pelvic inflammatory disease
- Fibroid degeneration
- Salpingitis
- Mittelschmerz
- Endometriosis

15

Table 15.2 COMMON CAUSES OF ACUTE ABDOMINAL PAIN IN UK ADULTS REQUIRING ADMISSION TO HOSPITAL	
Condition	**Approximate incidence (%)**
Non-specific abdominal pain	35
Acute appendicitis	30
Acute cholecystitis and biliary colic	10
Peptic ulcer disease	5
Small bowel obstruction	5
Gynaecological disorders	5
Acute pancreatitis	2
Renal and ureteric colic	2
Malignant disease	2
Acute diverticulitis	2
Dyspepsia	1
Miscellaneous	5

Table 15.3   COMMON CAUSES OF ACUTE ABDOMINAL PAIN IN UK CHILDREN

- Acute appendicitis
- Urinary tract infection
- Mesenteric adenitis
- Gastroenteritis

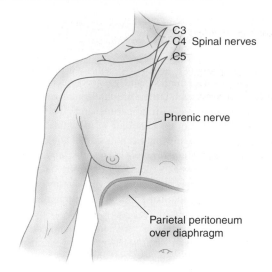

Fig. 15.1   The shared sensory innervation of the shoulder and diaphragm.

as well as the underlying pathological process. The most common causes in any population will vary according to age, sex and race, as well as genetic and environmental factors (Tables 15.1–15.3).

The remainder of this chapter will be concerned principally with surgical conditions, although it should be borne in mind that medical and gynaecological conditions may present with acute abdominal pain.

PATHOPHYSIOLOGY OF ABDOMINAL PAIN

To be able to make an accurate clinical assessment of the patient presenting with acute abdominal pain, it is necessary to understand the pathophysiology. Abdominal pain can be divided into visceral and somatic types.

SOMATIC PAIN

The parietal peritoneum covers the anterior and posterior abdominal walls, the undersurface of the diaphragm and the pelvic cavity. It develops from the somatopleural layer of the lateral plate mesoderm and its nerve supply is therefore derived from somatic nerves supplying the abdominal wall musculature and the skin (T5–L2). The exception to this is the diaphragmatic portion, which is supplied centrally by afferent nerves in the phrenic nerve (C3–C5), and peripherally in the lower six intercostal and subcostal nerves

The parietal peritoneum is sensitive to mechanical, thermal or chemical stimulation, and cannot be handled, cut or cauterized painlessly. As a result of its innervation, when the parietal peritoneum is irritated, there is reflex contraction of the corresponding segmental area of muscle, causing rigidity of the abdominal wall (guarding) and hyperaesthesia of the overlying skin.

When the diaphragmatic portion of the parietal peritoneum is irritated peripherally, there will be pain, tenderness and rigidity in the distribution of the lower spinal nerves, but when it is irritated centrally, pain is referred to the cutaneous distribution of C3, 4 and 5 (i.e. the shoulder area, Fig. 15.1). Somatic pain is classically described as sharp or knife-like in nature, and is usually well localized to the affected area.

VISCERAL PAIN

The visceral peritoneum forms a partial or complete investment of the intra-abdominal viscera. It is derived from the splanchnopleural layer of the lateral plate mesoderm, and shares its nerve supply with the viscera (i.e. the autonomic nerves). Visceral pain is mediated through the sympathetic branches of the autonomic nervous system, with afferent nerves joining the pre-sacral and splanchnic nerves, which eventually join thoracic (T6–T12) and lumbar (L1–L2) segments of the spinal cord. The visceral peritoneum and the viscera are insensitive to mechanical, thermal or chemical stimulation, and can therefore be handled, cut or cauterized painlessly. However, they are sensitive to tension, when applied by overdistension or traction on mesenteries, visceral muscle spasm and ischaemia.

Visceral pain is typically described as dull and deep-seated. It is usually localized vaguely to the area occupied by the viscus during development, and is referred to the overlying skin of the abdominal wall according to the dermatome level with the sympathetic supply, as mentioned above. Therefore, pain arising from the intestine and its outgrowths (the liver, biliary system and pancreas) is usually felt in the midline. Irritation of foregut structures (the lower oesophagus to the second part of the duodenum) is usually felt in the epigastric area. Pain from midgut structures (the second part of the duodenum to the splenic flexure) is felt around the umbilicus. Pain from hindgut structures (the splenic flexure to the rectum) is felt in the hypogastrium.

Although the division of abdominal pain into visceral and somatic pain is useful, it is important to realize that

---

BOX 15.1   ABDOMINAL PAIN

- Visceral abdominal pain is mediated by the sympathetic nervous system and is typically deep-seated and ill localized to the area originally occupied by the viscus during intrauterine life
- Colic is a form of visceral pain that arises from a hollow viscus with muscle in its walls (e.g. gut, gallbladder, ureter), and results from excessive muscle contraction, often against an obstructing agent
- Patients experiencing colic are usually unable to remain still during the bout of pain but are pain-free between attacks. 'Biliary colic' is an exception (and the term colic may be a misnomer), in that pain often waxes and wanes on a plateau and there are no pain-free intervals
- Parietal pain, such as that caused by parietal peritonitis, is mediated by somatic nerves and is localized to the area of inflammation
- Reflex guarding and rigidity of the overlying muscles is usually present, and the patient is reluctant to move for fear of exacerbating the pain
- Some areas of the peritoneum (e.g. the pelvis, posterior abdominal wall) are 'non-demonstrative' in that parietal peritonitis may be present without tenderness or guarding of overlying muscles

---

Table 15.4   INJURIOUS AGENTS CAUSING INFLAMMATION

Infective
- Bacterial
- Viral
- Fungal
- Parasitic

Non-infective
- Chemical
- Ischaemic
- Physical
  - Trauma
  - Heat
  - Cold
  - Radiation
  - Immune mechanisms

---

some pathological conditions will result in a mixed picture. For example, acute appendicitis classically presents with acute abdominal pain that is initially felt in the umbilical area resulting from appendicular obstruction, which gradually localizes to the right iliac fossa and becomes sharper in nature as the overlying parietal peritoneum becomes inflamed.

PATHOGENESIS

As one can see from the list of surgical conditions that may present with acute abdominal pain (Table 15.1), there are two main underlying pathological processes involved: inflammation and obstruction. These processes may be triggered by a variety of underlying abnormalities. It is important to realize that in any one patient a combination of abnormalities and processes may be involved.

INFLAMMATION

Acute inflammation of an intra-abdominal organ or the peritoneum may occur as a result of a variety of irritants. These may be broadly classified into infective or non-infective in nature (Table 15.4).

No matter what the trigger of the inflammation, the subsequent pathological process is the same. There is reactive hyperaemia of the injured tissue as a result of capillary and arteriolar dilatation; exudation of fluid into the tissues as a result of an increase in the permeability of the vascular endothelium; and an increase in filtration pressure. Finally, there is emigration of leucocytes from the vessels into the inflamed tissues.

The clinical consequences of the inflammatory process depend upon a multitude of factors, the most important being the underlying condition, its severity and duration, the organ involved, the patient's age and comorbidity. In general, the patient will complain of abdominal pain and tenderness, which occurs as a result of tissue stretching and distortion and is due to the release of inflammatory mediators, some of which also mediate pain. On general examination, the patient may be pyrexial and have a tachycardia; investigations may reveal a raised white cell count. Examination of the abdomen will reveal tenderness in the affected area, with guarding and rigidity if the parietal peritoneum is involved.

Peritonitis

Inflammation of the peritoneum may result from a variety of injuries and, as described in Table 15.4, they may be divided into infective or non-infective in nature. Peritonitis may be classified according to extent (either localized or generalized) and aetiology (Table 15.5). In a surgical setting, the most common cause of generalized peritonitis is perforation of an intra-abdominal viscus. Inflammation of the peritoneum results in an increase in its blood supply

---

Table 15.5   CLASSIFICATION OF PERITONITIS

Generalized peritonitis

Primary: infection of the peritoneal fluid without intra-abdominal disease
- Haematogenous spread
- Lymphatic spread
- Direct spread: usually associated with continuous ambulatory peritoneal dialysis (CAPD) catheters
- Ascending infection: from the female genital tract

Secondary: inflammation of the peritoneum arising from an intra-abdominal source
- Infectious
- Non-infectious
  - Blood
  - Ischaemia
  - Bile
  - Chemical
  - Foreign body
- Perforation

Localized peritonitis
- Usually due to spreading inflammation across the wall of an intra-abdominal viscus

---

15

and local oedema formation. There is transudation of fluid into the peritoneal cavity, followed by the accumulation of a protein-rich fibrinous exudate. In the normal state, the greater omentum constantly alters its position within the abdominal cavity as a result of intestinal peristalsis and abdominal muscle contraction. In the presence of an inflammation, the greater omentum will adhere to and surround the abnormal organ. The fibrinous exudate effectively glues the omentum to the inflamed viscus, walling it off and preventing the further spread of inflammation. In addition, the exudate inhibits intestinal peristalsis, resulting in a paralytic ileus which also limits the spread of the inflammation and infection. As a result of the ileus, fluid accumulates within the lumen of the intestine and, along with the formation of large volumes of intraperitoneal transudate and exudate, this will lead to a decrease in the intravascular volume, producing the clinical features of hypovolaemia.

The clinical features of peritonitis will again vary according to a wide variety of factors. The most common symptom is abdominal pain, which is constant and often described as sharp. The pain is usually well localized if it is secondary to inflammation of an intra-abdominal viscus, but may spread to involve the whole peritoneal cavity. Primary peritonitis can present rather more subtly, and as many as 30% of affected individuals may be asymptomatic.

The term 'peritonitis or peritonism detected on clinical examination' is used to describe the collection of signs associated with inflammation of the parietal peritoneum, and includes 'guarding' and 'rebound' tenderness. Evidence of inflammation of the parietal peritoneum in association with inflammation of an intra-abdominal viscus is often a strong indication that the patient requires some form of surgical intervention.

Infarction

An infarct is an area of ischaemic necrosis caused either by an occlusion of the arterial supply or the venous drainage in a particular tissue, or by a generalized hypoperfusion in the context of shock (Table 15.6). The typical histological feature of infarction is ischaemic coagulative necrosis. An inflammatory response begins to develop along the margins

of an infarct within a few hours, stimulated by the presence of the necrotic tissue.

The consequences of decreased perfusion of a tissue depend on several factors: the availability of an alternative vascular supply, the rate of development of the hypoperfusion, the vulnerability of the tissue to hypoxia, and the blood oxygen content. In the context of acute abdominal pain, intestinal infarction is the most common cause. Other organs that may infarct include the ovaries, kidneys, testes, liver, spleen and pancreas.

In general, the patient will complain of severe abdominal pain and the onset will depend on the nature of the underlying process. Embolization will result in a sudden onset of pain, whereas the onset in thrombosis is likely to be more gradual. Infarction and ischaemia are potent triggers of inflammation of the affected structure, and the clinical features reflect this.

Perforation

Spontaneous perforation of an intra-abdominal viscus may be the result of a range of pathological processes. Weakening of the wall of the viscus, which might follow degeneration, inflammation, infection or ischaemia, will predispose to perforation. An increase in the intraluminal pressure of a viscus, such as occurs in a closed-loop obstruction (Fig 15.2), will predispose to perforation, as will peptic ulceration, acute appendicitis and acute diverticulitis. Other less common causes are carcinoma of the colon, inflammatory bowel disease and acute cholecystitis.

Perforation can also be iatrogenic, and may occur during the insertion of a Verress needle at laparoscopy, because of a careless cut or suture placement during surgery, and during the course of an endoscopic procedure.

Spontaneous perforation of a viscus usually results in the sudden onset of severe abdominal pain, which is usually

Table 15.6   AETIOLOGY OF INFARCTION
Occlusive
Arterial
● Embolism
● Thrombosis
● Extrinsic compression
Venous
● Thrombosis
● Extrinsic compression
Non-occlusive
Shock
● Hypovolaemia
● Cardiogenic
● Sepsis
Vasoconstrictor drugs

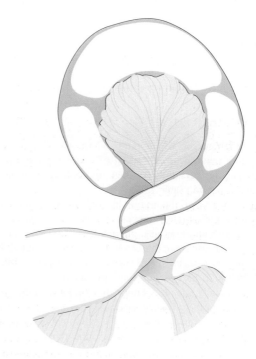

Fig. 15.2   Volvulus: an example of closed-loop obstruction.

well localized to the affected area. The resultant clinical picture depends on the nature of the perforated viscus and the relative sterility and toxicity of the material that is spilt into the abdominal cavity, in addition to the speed with which the perforation is surrounded and sealed (if at all) by the adjacent structures and omentum. The inevitable peritoneal contamination will lead to either localized or generalized peritonitis, and the associated symptoms and signs, as already discussed.

OBSTRUCTION

The term 'obstruction' refers to impedance of the normal flow of material through a hollow viscus. It may be caused by the presence of a lesion within the lumen of the viscus, an abnormality in its wall, or a lesion outside the viscus causing extrinsic compression.

The smooth muscle in the wall of the obstructed viscus will contract reflexly in an effort to overcome the impedance. This reflex contraction produces colicky abdominal pain. The exception to this rule is 'biliary colic'. The gallbladder and biliary system has little smooth muscle in its wall and attempts at contraction tend to be more continuous than 'colicky'.

If the obstruction is not overcome, there will be an increase in intraluminal pressure and proximal dilatation. The end result depends on the anatomical location of the obstruction, whether it is partial or complete, and whether the blood supply to the organ is compromised. For example, a urinary bladder calculus causing partial urinary outflow obstruction may result in a dilatation of the ureter and renal pelvis, and subsequent 'post-renal' renal failure. An obstructed inguinal hernia, on the other hand, not only will produce proximal dilatation of the intestine (usually associated with vomiting) but may also result in ischaemia of the bowel wall, leading to infarction and perforation.

CLINICAL ASSESSMENT

The ability to make an accurate assessment by taking a good history and performing an appropriate examination is a vital skill in the management of the patient with acute abdominal pain. Although an exact diagnosis is often impossible to make after the initial assessment and often relies on further investigations, it is the formulation of an appropriate, safe and effective management plan that is the most important issue. In most cases, it is possible to take a full history and perform a thorough examination, but this is not always so, and occasionally a rapid evaluation followed by immediate resuscitation is required.

HISTORY

The main presenting complaint of patients with an acute abdomen is pain. The characteristics of the pain (Table 15.7) give important clues to the likely underlying diagnosis, and these should be explored in depth. However, the importance of a full history cannot be overemphasized and is essential in all patients.

Table 15.7	CHARACTERISTICS OF ABDOMINAL PAIN

- Site
- Nature
- Radiation
- Time and mode of onset
- Severity
- Progression
- Duration
- Exacerbating/relieving factors

15

Site of pain

The site of abdominal pain is perhaps the most valuable pointer to the underlying diagnosis. In order to describe the site of pain, the abdomen is traditionally divided into either quarters or ninths (Figs 15.3 and 15.4).

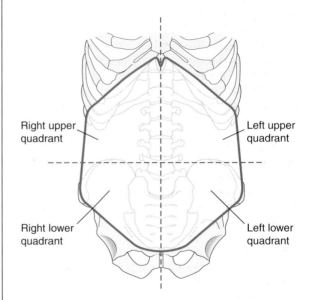

Fig. 15.3   The four quadrants of the abdomen.

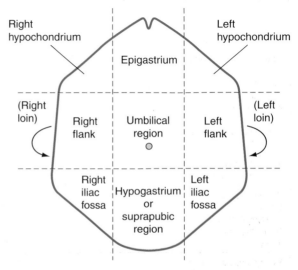

Fig. 15.4   The abdomen divided into ninths.

15

Nature of pain

As discussed above, there are two main pathological mechanisms in the development of abdominal pain: obstruction and inflammation.

Inflammation produces a constant pain made worse by local or general disturbance, and pain which is made worse by movement or coughing suggests inflammation of the parietal peritoneum. In this situation, the patient will often be seen to lie very still in order not to exacerbate the pain.

Obstruction of a muscular viscus produces a colicky pain. This pain comes and goes in 'spasms', often only lasting a few minutes at a time but returning at frequent intervals. It may be described as 'gripping' in nature, and between spasms the patient is usually pain-free. The pain itself is severe and may be helped by moving around or drawing the knees up towards the chest. Underlying inflammation must be suspected when a colicky pain does not disappear between spasms, or becomes continuous. In the case of intestinal obstruction, this might mean strangulation, for which urgent surgery is required.

Radiation of pain

Radiation is the process whereby pain extends directly from one place to another, while usually remaining present at the site of onset. When a pain radiates, it signifies that other structures are becoming involved. For example, pain from a duodenal ulcer may radiate through to the back, indicating that inflammation has occurred through the wall of the duodenum to involve structures of the posterior abdominal wall, such as the pancreas. Ureteric pain radiates to the tip of the penis in men and to the labium majoris in women.

Onset of pain

The onset of pain can be sudden or gradual. Typically, pain from a perforation is sudden and that from inflammation is gradual. Patients with the former can usually remember exactly what they were doing at the time of onset, whereas in the latter localization in time is more difficult.

Severity of pain

A patient's description of the severity of pain is very subjective. Every individual has a different reaction to pain, and this is often more reflective of the patient's personality than of the underlying pathology. A better indication is to assess the affect of the pain on the patients' lives. For example, did they call their GP? Were they unable to attend work? Did the pain interfere with their sleep? Furthermore, it is often useful to ask the patient to rate pain severity using a score on a numerical or pictorial scale.

Progression of pain

Once a pain has occurred, it may remain exactly the same, may gradually improve or worsen, or may fluctuate.

Movement of pain

It is also useful to note whether the pain moves. Acute appendicitis is a classic example of pain that moves, starting as a vague central 'referred' pain and then moving to the right iliac fossa as the adjacent parietal peritoneum becomes inflamed.

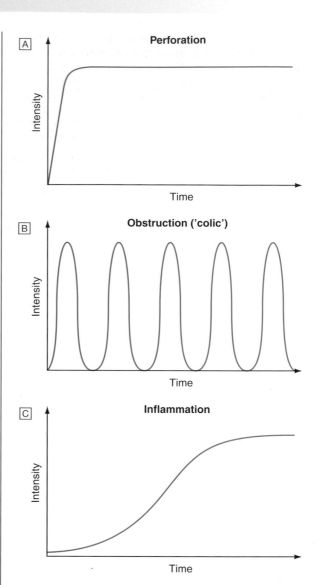

Fig. 15.5   Time vs intensity graphs for acute abdominal pain.

The various characteristics of abdominal pain, as shown in Figure 15.5, are essential in helping the clinician formulate a differential diagnosis.

EXAMINATION

During the course of taking a history it is possible to form a general impression of the state of the patient. The unwell patient with acute abdominal pain may look pale and sweaty, lie flat on the bed, be cerebrally obtunded, and be unable to move without experiencing pain. Others, however, may look surprisingly well, have a good colour, sit up in bed, talk normally and be able to move freely. All these observations should be noted and recorded, along with the temperature, pulse, blood pressure and respiratory rate.

Other important features to look for on general examination include clinical evidence of anaemia, jaundice, cyanosis and dehydration. It is important to bear in mind that physical signs are often less obvious than might be

Table 15.8 CHECKLIST FOR EXAMINATION OF THE ACUTE ABDOMEN

Method	Question	Significance
Inspection	What is the abdominal contour?	Distension: intestinal obstruction or ascites
	Does the abdomen move with respiration?	Rigid abdomen: peritonitis
	Can the patient blow out/suck in the abdomen?	Rigid abdomen: peritonitis
	Does the patient lie still or writhe about?	Fear of movement: peritonitis Writhes about: colic
	Are there visible abnormalities?	Scars: relevant previous illness, adhesions Hernia: intestinal obstruction Visible peristalsis: intestinal obstruction Visible masses: relevant pathology
Gentle palpation	Is there tenderness, guarding or rigidity?	Tenderness/guarding: inflamed parietal peritoneum Rigidity: peritonitis
Deep palpation	Are there abnormal masses/palpable organs?	Palpable organs/masses: relevant pathology
	Is there rebound tenderness?	Rebound tenderness: peritonitis
Percussion	Is the percussion note abnormal?	Resonance: intestinal obstruction Loss of liver dullness: gastrointestinal perforation Dullness: free fluid, full bladder Shifting dullness: free fluid
Auscultation	Are bowel sounds present/abnormal?	Absent sounds: paralytic ileus Hyperactive sounds: mechanical obstruction, gastroenteritis
	Is there a bruit?	Bruit: vascular disease

Do not forget to:
Examine the groin
Do a digital rectal examination
Do a vaginal examination when appropriate
Examine the chest

15

expected in the elderly, the obese, the generally unwell and those taking steroids. As in every emergency patient, a full examination, including the cardiovascular, respiratory and neurological systems, in addition to the abdomen and pelvis, must be carried out and the results documented. Specific details relating to the abdominal examination are described below and in Table 15.8.

In small children with abdominal pain, it is useful to ask the child to 'blow out' and 'suck in' their abdomen and to cough. These three movements will usually elicit pain in the presence of peritonism without laying a hand on the child's abdomen. Rebound tenderness should *never* be elicited in children. Gentle tapping with the percussing finger will elicit the same information (tap tenderness) in a much less cruel way.

Inspection of the abdomen

In order to examine the abdomen, the patient must be adequately exposed and positioned. The full extent of the abdomen should be visible, and by convention the patient should be exposed from 'nipples to knees'. This prevents the common mistake of not examining the breasts, groins and external genitalia. Patient dignity should be maintained and the breasts and genitalia covered once assessed. Patients should be positioned supine on a couch with a single pillow behind the head and shoulders and with the arms resting by their side.

Inspection of the abdomen may reveal a wealth of information. Abdominal swellings due to abnormal enlargement of the liver, kidneys or spleen, and tumours of the bowel, ovaries or other intra-abdominal or retroperitoneal structures may be visible. Scars from previous abdominal or pelvic surgery may be observed, and are of importance in the presence of bowel obstruction, which may be secondary to adhesions. All scars should be tested for the presence of herniation. Distended veins on the abdominal wall may be secondary to portal hypertension or occlusion of the inferior vena cava. The abdomen may be generally distended by intra-abdominal blood or fluid, or as a result of intestinal obstruction. In cases of obstruction, intestinal peristalsis may be visible, if the patient is thin.

Palpation

Palpation of the abdomen should be carried out in a systematic manner, beginning with gentle superficial examination of the whole abdomen looking for tenderness. This should start away from the site of maximum pain and move towards the tender site, encompassing all areas, as shown in Figures 15.3 and 15.4. Palpation over an area of tenderness will cause pain, which in turn will stimulate the patient to contract the overlying muscles (voluntary guarding). If the pain is due to inflammation, the approximation of the parietal peritoneum on to the inflammatory area will result in a reflex contraction of the overlying muscles (involuntary guarding). If the whole peritoneal cavity is inflamed, then there will be generalized peritonitis and the abdominal wall will be rigid (board-like rigidity). When the palpating hand, which has been pushing the parietal peritoneum against the inflamed viscus, is suddenly released, the viscus will bounce back and hit the parietal peritoneum, causing an additional sharp pain (rebound tenderness). This is an excellent indication of underlying peritoneal inflammation (peritonism) but is very painful and is better tested by light percussion. A history of pain on coughing is also a good indication of peritoneal inflammation.

If light palpation of the whole abdomen elicits no pain, the process is repeated pressing more firmly to detect deep tenderness. This will allow for the detection of organomegaly and the presence of any masses.

In the past, opiate analgesia was traditionally withheld from patients with acute abdominal pain on the assumption that it might mask important clinical signs, particularly of localized tenderness. This has now been shown not to be the case, and analgesia should never be withheld from a patient pending formal examination. Indeed, the administration of analgesia relaxes the patient and may often help the examination. However, repeated administration of opiate analgesia to a patient with abdominal pain in whom a definite diagnosis has not been made cannot be supported without regular reassessment, as this suggests progression of the disease process and that surgical intervention may be indicated.

During the general examination, particular attention should be paid to the supraclavicular fossae, axillae and cervical regions for the presence of lymphadenopathy. The hernial orifices must also be specifically examined, as must the male external genitalia, looking for tenderness and masses within the scrotum.

Percussion

Percussion is useful in the localization and assessment of tenderness, particularly in the assessment of rebound tenderness, in addition to determining the presence of fluid within the peritoneal cavity. The normal abdomen is universally resonant because of the presence of gas-containing bowel lying in front of the solid retroperitoneal structures, and because the normal pelvic viscera lie entirely within the bony pelvis.

The liver gives a dull note to percussion anteriorly from the level of the right fifth rib to the right costal margin, and loss of liver dullness to percussion may represent free intra-peritoneal gas. The presence of suprapubic dullness may indicate a full bladder due to urinary retention. If there is free intraperitoneal fluid, the percussion note will be dull in the flanks. The site of the dullness moves as the patient rolls on to his or her side (shifting dullness). One litre or more of fluid is required before this sign can be elicited.

Auscultation

Bowel will only produce gurgling noises if it contains a mixture of fluid and gas. Normal bowel sounds are low-pitched and occur every few seconds. Their absence over a 30-second period suggests that peristalsis has ceased, a condition termed ileus. This may be due to generalized peritonitis or atony of the bowel smooth muscle, such as might follow a prolonged period of obstruction. Increased peristalsis produces a higher volume, pitch and frequency of the bowel sounds and can be heard in mechanical obstruction (often described as 'tinkling'), in addition to conditions such as gastroenteritis. In general, bowel sounds should be described as present and normal, present and abnormal, or absent.

Auscultation should continue over the course of the aorta and the iliac arteries, listening for the presence of bruits, which are indicative of turbulent flow.

If gastric outlet obstruction is clinically suspected, the patient's abdomen may be shaken from side to side in an attempt to elicit a succussion splash.

Finally, a rectal examination is performed to assess the pelvis and, if a gynaecological disorder is suspected, a vaginal examination is indicated. Examination of the rectum is 'routine' but may be omitted, particularly in young patients, when a diagnosis and management plan have already been made and are unlikely to be influenced by any information obtained. Useful information that might be obtained from a rectal examination includes the presence of masses, tenderness and blood.

Specific clinical signs in acute abdominal pain

Murphy's sign

In acute cholecystitis, a deep breath taken by the patient elicits acute pain when the examiner presses downwards into the right upper quadrant. This is caused by the movement of the inflamed gallbladder striking the examining hand.

Boas's sign

In acute cholecystitis, pain radiates to the tip of the scapula and there is a tender area of skin just below the scapula, which is hyperaesthetic.

Grey Turner's and Cullen's signs

In patients with severe advanced cases of acute pancreatitis, bruising and discoloration can be seen around the umbilicus (Cullen's sign) and in the left flank (Grey Turner's sign). Cullen's sign was actually first described in relation to ruptured ectopic pregnancy, but is now often also associated with acute pancreatitis.

Rovsing's sign

In acute appendicitis, palpation in the left iliac fossa produces pain in the right iliac fossa.

INVESTIGATIONS

Following initial clinical assessment, and during assessment in the critically ill, measures should be taken to resuscitate the patient. During this period, further investigations can be organized to help in the diagnostic process. It is important to remember that in all patients a working list of differential diagnoses must be made after clinical assessment so that only appropriate investigations are instituted. There is no point in organizing investigations the results of which will not influence the clinical management.

The most common investigations carried out on the patient with acute abdominal pain include full blood count (FBC), urea and electrolytes (U&Es), amylase, plain radiology (erect chest and supine abdominal X-rays) and an ultrasound scan.

Blood tests

Blood tests, with the exception of a serum amylase level (which is the best diagnostic test for acute pancreatitis), rarely influence the clinical decision in patients with acute abdominal pain. However, FBC and U&Es are often taken as a baseline for future reference.

FBC and U&Es

A single reading of a raised white cell count taken on its own is fairly non-discriminatory, but a persistent elevation or a rise suggests underlying inflammation and/or infection. Obviously U&Es are essential in patients who might be hypovolaemic in order to monitor fluid replacement, particularly if surgery is being considered. Similarly, an abnormal haemoglobin level may be significant and require correction.

Serum amylase

A serum amylase greater than the upper limit of normal is highly suggestive of acute pancreatitis. Lesser values are non-specific and can be the result of a wide range of conditions. However, as many as 20% of patients with acute pancreatitis may have normal amylase levels on admission. Other causes of a raised amylase are shown in Table 15.9. In

Table 15.9   CAUSES OF HYPERAMYLASAEMIA
Pancreatic conditions
● Acute pancreatitis
● Pancreatic cancer
● Pancreatic trauma
Other intra-abdominal pathology
● Perforated peptic ulcer
● Acute appendicitis
● Ectopic pregnancy
● Intestinal infarction
● Acute cholecystitis
Decreased clearance of amylase
● Renal failure
● Macroamylasaemia
Miscellaneous
● Head injury
● Diabetic ketoacidosis
● Drugs (e.g. opiates)

patients with acute pancreatitis who present more than 48 hours after the onset of pain, the serum amylase may have returned to normal. In these patients, measurement of the urinary amylase may be of value.

Liver function tests

Liver function tests are increasingly becoming available on an emergency rather than a routine basis in many hospitals, as clinicians have recognized their value in the assessment and subsequent management of acute hepatobiliary and pancreatic disorders.

Inflammatory markers

C-reactive protein (CRP), an acute-phase protein, and the erythrocyte sedimentation rate (ESR) are both markers of acute inflammation when raised but, like the white cell count, tend to be of most value if trends rather than one-off results are observed.

Blood gas analysis

Arterial blood sampling is often used to monitor the acid–base status and the efficacy of gas exchange in the seriously ill patient. Patients with sepsis and intestinal ischaemia are likely to demonstrate a metabolic acidosis.

Serum calcium

Patients with hypercalcaemia may complain of abdominal pain as a result of abnormal gastrointestinal motility, nephrolithiasis, peptic ulcer disease, pancreatitis or malignancy. A low calcium level is one of the poor prognostic factors in patients with severe acute pancreatitis.

Sickle tests

Sickle cell crises are a rare cause of acute abdominal pain. Blood should be sent for testing on all at-risk patients.

Blood glucose

Measurement of blood glucose is important, as diabetic ketoacidosis may present with acute abdominal pain, and also because any serious illness can result in poor glycaemic control, particularly in diabetic patients.

Urinalysis

Dipstick testing

Haematuria may result from a wide range of conditions but in the context of acute abdominal pain may indicate a urinary tract tumour, infection or nephrolithiasis. Glucose or ketones in the urine indicate recent starvation or possible diabetic ketoacidosis. Protein, bilirubin or casts in the urine suggest renal or liver disease. In patients with an inflamed retrocaecal appendix, urine testing may demonstrate the presence of protein, and urgent microscopy (which will confirm or refute the presence of bacteria) should be arranged to determine whether there is an underlying urinary tract infection or whether another condition, such as appendicitis, might be the cause.

Bacteriology

If the clinical picture is suggestive of a urinary tract infection and the urine dipstick demonstrates blood or protein, urgent microscopy and culture should be requested. Specimens from any other potential sites of infection

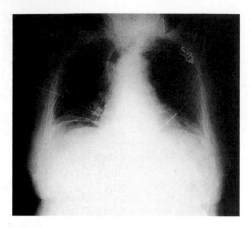

Fig. 15.6   Gas under the diaphragm seen on the erect chest X-ray in a patient with a perforated peptic ulcer.

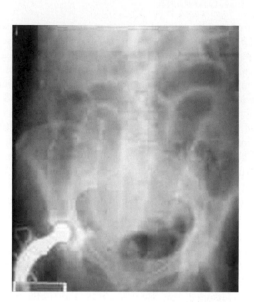

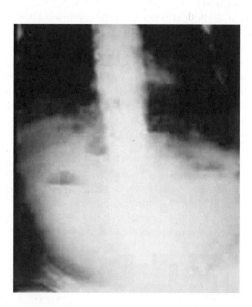

Fig. 15.7   Abdominal X-rays in small bowel obstruction.
A Supine film in a patient with small bowel obstruction due to an obstructed right femoral hernia. B Erect film in the same patient demonstrating multiple fluid levels.

should also be submitted for bacteriological analysis (stool, blood, pus etc.).

Pregnancy test

A pregnancy test should be performed in all women of childbearing age who present with acute abdominal pain and in whom the chance of pregnancy cannot be excluded. Not only is this important if X-rays are to be taken, but it will also reveal the possibility of an ectopic pregnancy if positive.

Urinary porphobilinogen

Quantitative assay of urinary porphobilinogen is the most important diagnostic test for porphyria, which may present with acute abdominal pain and should be considered in difficult cases.

Radiological investigations

Plain X-rays

The role of plain radiography in the investigation of the patient with acute abdominal pain has been well studied. The erect chest X-ray (CXR) is the most appropriate investigation for the detection of free intraperitoneal gas (Fig. 15.6) and should be carried out in any patient who might have a perforation. If the condition of the patient prevents an erect film being taken, then a left lateral abdominal decubitus film might be helpful. Although a visceral perforation is the most common cause of free intraperitoneal gas, other causes exist and should be considered where appropriate (Table 15.10).

Table 15.10   CAUSES OF FREE SUBDIAPHRAGMATIC GAS ON ABDOMINAL X-RAY
• Perforation of an intra-abdominal viscus • Gas-forming infection • Pleuroperitoneal fistula • Iatrogenic: laparoscopy, laparotomy • Gas introduced per vaginam: post-partum • Interposition of bowel between liver and diaphragm

The role of plain abdominal radiographs remains controversial despite many studies that have demonstrated that, with the exception of suspected intestinal obstruction (Fig. 15.7A), they rarely help in the diagnosis and have even less role in altering the clinical decision (EBM 15.1). However, the supine abdominal X-ray (AXR) can be of use in patients whose diagnosis is unclear and in whom the presence of calcification (e.g. ureteric colic) and abnormal gas shadows (e.g. possible intestinal ischaemia) may be helpful.

EBM 15.1 ABDOMINAL RADIOGRAPHY

'Plain abdominal radiography has a limited role in the assessment of the acute abdomen, particularly when the diagnosis is likely to be peptic ulcer disease, acute biliary disease or acute appendicitis. It is valuable when the diagnosis is uncertain and in patients with other suspected acute gastrointestinal conditions such as obstruction.'

Paterson-Brown S. In: Paterson-Brown S, ed. A companion to specialist surgical practice: core topics in general and emergency surgery, 3rd edn. London: Elsevier; 2005: 81–96.

An erect AXR is only of value in patients with intestinal obstruction, although it is well known that even then the information obtained over and above that from the supine film is small. In patients with suspected obstruction whose supine film does not show significant bowel dilatation, an erect film might reveal fluid levels (Fig. 15.7B).

Contrast radiology

Contrast may be administered orally, down a nasogastric or nasojejunal tube, or per rectum to examine the bowel in patients with acute abdominal pain. In the emergency setting, the contrast used is usually water-soluble, as free egress of barium into the peritoneal cavity can cause inflammatory reactions and makes subsequent surgery more difficult. As water-soluble contrast does not adhere well to the bowel mucosa, the information obtained is less specific and detailed than with barium, but in the patient with acute abdominal pain, the main issue that requires the use of contrast X-rays is determining the presence or absence of obstruction.

In up to 50% of patients with a perforated peptic ulcer, no free gas can be identified on plain radiography. If the diagnosis remains uncertain based on clinical assessment, a water-soluble contrast meal might be diagnostic (Fig. 15.8). In patients with small bowel obstruction, a

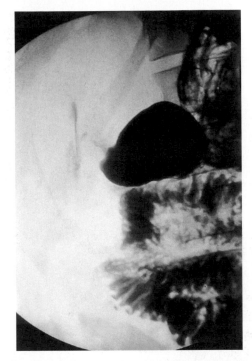

Fig. 15.8 Supine abdominal radiograph taken 20 minutes after the oral administration of 50 ml of water-soluble contrast material in a patient with a suspected perforated peptic ulcer in whom the erect chest radiograph was normal.
Note the small trickle of contrast through the perforation. These findings were confirmed at laparotomy. (From Hamilton Bailey's Emergency Surgery, 13th edn, reproduced by permission of Hodder Murray)

water-soluble small bowel follow-up can help not only in confirming or refuting obstruction, but also in predicting which patient is likely to require surgery. Failure of contrast to reach the caecum by 4 hours suggests complete obstruction, and these patients will not usually settle with non-operative management (Fig. 15.9).

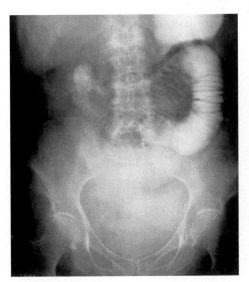

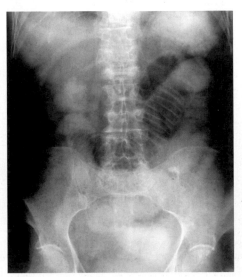

Fig. 15.9 Supine abdominal radiographs taken after oral administration of 50 ml of water-soluble contrast material.
A 90 minutes after administration. B 4 hours after. Note failure of contrast to reach the caecum and the obvious small bowel obstruction. These findings were not obvious on plain radiographs. Laparotomy confirmed small bowel obstruction due to adhesions.

15

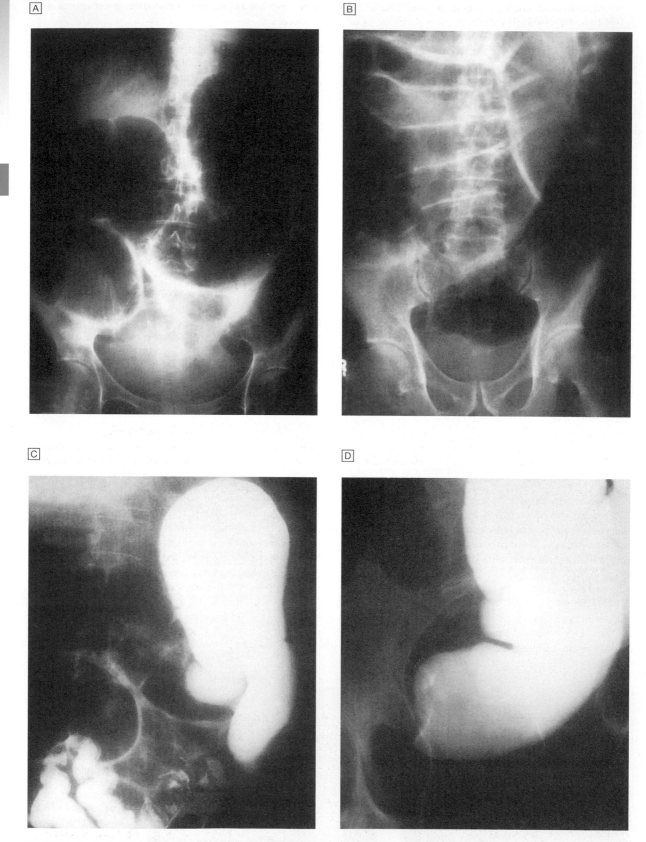

Fig. 15.10 Contrast radiology in the diagnosis of large bowel obstruction.
A and B Supine abdominal X-rays in patients with large bowel obstruction. C Contrast enema in patient A shows no mechanical cause, i.e.
pseudo-obstruction. D An obstructing carcinoma of the sigmoid colon in patient B.

A water-soluble contrast enema is now considered essential in the assessment of patients with large bowel obstruction in order to differentiate between pseudo-obstruction and an obstruction caused by a mechanical problem (Fig. 15.10). Carrying out an unnecessary operation on a patient with pseudo-obstruction is associated with a high morbidity and mortality and cannot be defended.

Intravenous pyelography confirms the diagnosis of renal obstruction by calculi and may be helpful in the diagnosis of other types of renal pain.

Ultrasonography

Ultrasound is increasingly being used in the investigation of patients with acute abdominal pain. As a general investigation it might reveal small amounts of intraperitoneal fluid in conditions such as perforation and infection, whereas in specific conditions such as acute cholecystitis, biliary obstruction, aortic aneurysms and ovarian cysts it can be diagnostic. Some studies have reported high levels of sensitivity and specificity in the diagnosis of acute appendicitis, but ultrasonography in these cases is highly operator-dependent and a negative result cannot be relied upon, particularly if the clinical picture suggests otherwise.

Computed tomography (CT)

The current multislice CT machines have such good organ definition that they are increasingly being used early in the investigation of the acute abdomen where they can reliably identify free intra-abdominal gas, ischaemic bowel, acute inflammation such as appendicitis and diverticulitis. In general, however, the main role of CT in the emergency situation is to evaluate traumatic injuries and intra-abdominal sepsis in cases where intra-abdominal collections might exist, in addition to suspected leaking abdominal aortic aneurysms. Contrast-enhanced CT is also used routinely to detect pancreatic necrosis in patients with severe acute pancreatitis.

Angiography

Mesenteric angiography used to be the investigation of choice in suspected mesenteric ischaemia, but has now been superseded by CT angiography, which can also reliably differentiate arterial from venous causes, and distinguish occlusive from non-occlusive disease. CT angiography can also be used in the diagnosis and management of lower gastrointestinal haemorrhage, although this rarely presents with acute abdominal pain. Obviously, if embolization is required, formal angiography is necessary.

Endoscopic investigations

Rigid sigmoidoscopy should be routine in all patients who present with an acute abdomen associated with rectal bleeding, and in those patients with large bowel obstruction to evaluate the anorectum. Additional information can be obtained from a flexible sigmoidoscopy or colonoscopy. Furthermore, a sigmoid volvulus can often be deflated by careful sigmoidoscopy. Upper gastrointestinal endoscopy is used to investigate patients with acute upper abdominal pain in whom a perforated peptic ulcer has been excluded, as discussed above.

Peritoneal investigations

Peritoneal lavage

Peritoneal lavage has been used for many years as a first-line investigation in patients suspected of having intra-abdominal haemorrhage from trauma, although its use has been increasingly overtaken by CT. It has also been used sparingly, but with some success, to evaluate the acute abdomen, and in those patients who present a diagnostic dilemma it can be helpful. It is carried out by inserting a dialysis catheter into the peritoneal cavity under local anaesthetic and infusing 1 litre of normal saline. The effluent is removed and examined for white cell count, amylase, bacteria and bile.

Fine catheter aspiration peritoneal cytology

This technique works on a similar principle to peritoneal lavage, except that a much smaller catheter is inserted (4.5Ch umbilical catheter through a 14G venous cannula). Any fluid aspirated is deposited on to a slide and stained for white cells. A high percentage of polymorphs confirms underlying inflammation, but does not reveal the cause.

Laparoscopy

Many studies have demonstrated that laparoscopy (Fig. 15.11) can significantly improve surgical decision-making in patients with acute abdominal pain. It is particularly useful in patients for whom the decision to operate is in doubt, and in the elderly when findings from the history and examination can be misleading. Young women probably benefit the most from laparoscopy, as it

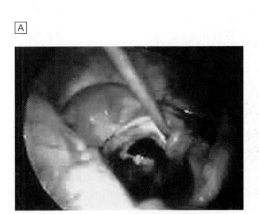

A

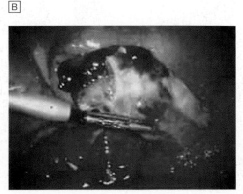

B

Fig. 15.11 Diagnostic laparoscopy
A Bleeding ovarian cyst.
B Acute appendicitis.

is so difficult in this group to differentiate acute appendicitis from acute gynaecological conditions, many of which do not require surgery.

MANAGEMENT

All patients admitted with acute abdominal pain require resuscitation and close monitoring, with regular re-evaluation. It is a good clinical rule that initial treatment should be based around the ABC principle (airway, breathing and circulation). Except in the management of overwhelming haemorrhage (e.g. ruptured abdominal aortic aneurysm and ruptured ectopic pregnancy), when resuscitation takes place on the way to the operating theatre, all patients with acute abdominal pain, including those requiring urgent surgery, benefit from adequate resuscitation. This will usually involve the administration of several litres of normal saline, intravenous antibiotics and oxygen by face mask. Monitoring by means of temperature, pulse, blood pressure, urine output and central venous pressure will depend on the clinical circumstances and will not be detailed further here. Suffice to say that good pre-operative assessment, resuscitation, monitoring and regular reviewing of the patient with acute abdominal pain (initially every 30 minutes to 2 hours, depending on the state of the patient) is a prerequisite for a satisfactory clinical outcome. Indeed, following the first assessment, close observation and regular reassessment should be carried out on *all* patients without a definitive diagnosis, as their condition may well change and the underlying cause or the correct management may become more obvious. Until this time, it is common practice to keep the patient fasted; if there are signs or symptoms of obstruction, a nasogastric tube is inserted. Appropriate analgesia should be administered early to keep the patient as comfortable as possible. Deep venous thrombosis prophylaxis should also be commenced as a routine.

The management of most conditions presenting as an acute abdomen will be covered in detail in the relevant chapters. The remainder of this chapter will cover the principles that underpin the management of peritonitis, intestinal obstruction, acute appendicitis, non-specific abdominal pain and gynaecological causes of the acute abdomen.

PERITONITIS

As discussed above, inflammation of the peritoneum is a common feature of the acute abdomen. It can be classified as acute or chronic, septic or aseptic, and primary or secondary. Acute suppurative peritonitis secondary to visceral disease is the most common form of peritonitis in surgical practice and primary peritonitis is rare. Chronic peritonitis due to tuberculosis is now rare, but can cause abdominal pain, ascites or obstruction due to matting of the bowel by dense adhesions. Aseptic peritonitis is generally due to chemical (e.g. bile, urine, blood, gastric contents, meconium) or foreign-body irritants (e.g. starch, talc,

cellulose), and is frequently followed by secondary bacterial peritonitis.

The primary objective is to deal promptly and effectively with the underlying cause. For example, perforation of a viscus must be repaired, infarcted bowel must be resected, and infective foci should be removed or drained. Operation is undertaken with minimal delay. The only time that should be spent before operation is that needed to resuscitate an ill patient. It is imperative that extracellular fluid volume is replaced adequately, and central venous pressure monitoring is essential in critically ill and elderly patients. A nasogastric tube should be inserted to empty the stomach and prevent further vomiting, and a urinary catheter should also be placed to monitor urinary output. Antibiotic cover is indicated early in all patients with established secondary peritonitis and is directed against gut flora in the first instance (e.g. a third-generation cephalosporin and metronidazole). Thorough peritoneal lavage is an essential adjunct to operation, and some surgeons employ an antibiotic-containing solution.

PRIMARY PERITONITIS

Primary peritonitis is uncommon, although in childhood it can account for up to 15% of acute abdominal emergencies. The condition used to be common in young girls following the ascent of pneumococcal or streptococcal infection from the genital tract.

Escherichia coli is now the predominant causal organism and probably gains access through the gut wall, or rarely by blood-borne spread from a distant focus. In adults, spontaneous bacterial peritonitis (SBP) may occur in patients with the nephrotic syndrome, but is more frequently seen with liver cirrhosis or chronic renal failure (particularly in those on chronic peritoneal dialysis). The mortality rate for patients with primary bacterial peritonitis varies from 20 to 80%.

Classically, diffuse peritonitis with generalized abdominal tenderness and rigidity develops within 24 hours. Fever and leucocytosis occur early. Abdominal rigidity is relatively uncommon. A sample of peritoneal fluid, which is usually turbid, is sent for Gram staining and bacterial culture. Antibiotic therapy is the mainstay of treatment, but either laparoscopy or laparotomy may be needed to rule out a surgical cause, if this is suggested by the culture of enteric organisms.

POST-OPERATIVE PERITONITIS

Peritonitis after abdominal surgery may be a residual effect of the original disease or a direct complication of its operative management (e.g. anastomotic leakage). Diagnosis is difficult, as:

- the patient is usually receiving analgesia and/or sedation, and may not complain of pain
- any pain and tenderness may be attributed to the wound
- there is often a 24–48-hour period after abdominal surgery when bowel sounds are absent and the abdomen is distended.

15

Persisting abdominal distension or the development of vomiting and distension after an initial return to normality should raise the suspicion of peritoneal infection. Suspicion is heightened if the patient looks unwell and has fever, tachycardia and an altered mental state. Plain abdominal films may merely show dilatation of the intestine, but ultrasonography can be used to detect collections. Anastomotic leakage can be demonstrated radiologically using water-soluble contrast.

Fluid and electrolyte replacement, nasogastric suction and broad-spectrum antibiotic therapy are instituted, and the need for reoperation is considered. In those patients managed conservatively, intraperitoneal collections may form or abscesses develop, but operation can sometimes be avoided by percutaneous drainage under radiological guidance.

INTRA-ABDOMINAL ABSCESS

An intra-abdominal abscess may develop in conjunction with an underlying inflammatory process or be a complication of peritonitis or intra-abdominal surgery. The abscess gives rise to pyrexia, tachycardia and clinical signs of toxicity. Leucocytosis is usual. Common sites for abscess formation are the subphrenic and subhepatic spaces, the pelvis, and between loops of bowel. Complications include rupture with generalized peritonitis, the erosion of blood vessels with potentially catastrophic bleeding, and septicaemia. Occasionally, subphrenic abscesses rupture into the pleural cavity, and pelvic abscesses sometimes discharge spontaneously through the rectum.

The site of the abscess may be suspected from the history and clinical examination, but localizing signs can be surprisingly few (particularly with subphrenic abscess, hence the expression 'pus somewhere, pus nowhere else, pus under the diaphragm'). Unexplained fever after peritoneal infection or operation should always raise the suspicion of abscess formation. Tachycardia is usual. Pain and tenderness over the ribcage, shoulder-tip pain and a 'sympathetic'

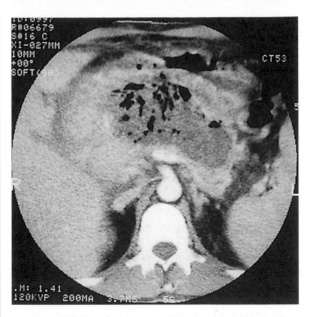

Fig. 15.13 CT scan of upper abdomen showing pancreatic abscess containing streaks of gas.

pleural effusion strengthen the suspicion of subphrenic abscess, whereas urgency of defaecation, diarrhoea and a boggy swelling in the pouch of Douglas on rectal examination are features of a pelvic abscess (Fig. 15.12).

Ultrasound and/or CT are of immense value in diagnosis (Fig. 15.13). Isotope scans following injection of ^{111}In-labelled leucocytes are now used infrequently. Ultrasonography or CT may also be used to guide percutaneous drain insertion and to obtain material for bacteriological culture. However, surgical drainage may still be needed to ensure effective drainage, particularly if the collection is loculated. Pelvic abscesses frequently rupture spontaneously into the rectum, but may require incision and drainage through the anterior rectal wall. Antibiotic therapy is used in conjunction with drainage of the abscess. Signs usually resolve rapidly following effective drainage, but female patients may be left infertile if the ostia of the fallopian tubes have been involved in a large pelvic collection.

INTESTINAL OBSTRUCTION

The term 'intestinal obstruction' refers to any form of impedance to the normal passage of bowel content through the small or large intestine. Intestinal obstruction is a common cause of acute abdominal pain, and is associated with a high morbidity and mortality if managed incorrectly. Intestinal obstruction is broadly classified as shown in Table 15.11, but the main differentiation lies between the small and the large bowel. The two entities are usually considered separately because the aetiologies and clinical presentations differ, as does their management. However, they do share some basic principles, which will be discussed here.

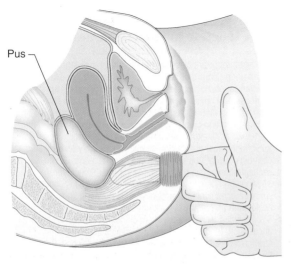

Pus

Fig. 15.12 Rectal examination for pelvic abscess.

Table 15.11	CLASSIFICATION OF INTESTINAL OBSTRUCTION

Small bowel
- High/low

Large bowel
- Mechanical/functional
- Simple/strangulated
- Partial/complete
- Acute/subacute/acute-on-chronic/chronic

Pathophysiology

Mechanical obstruction

A physical blockage causing impedance to the passage of bowel contents results in mechanical obstruction. These causes are usually divided into those that compress the bowel from the outside (extrinsic), those that arise from the wall of the bowel and obstruct the lumen (intrinsic), and those that arise within the lumen (Table 15.12). Adhesions remain the most common cause of small bowel obstruction in the UK (60%), followed by hernias (20%) and malignancy (both primary and secondary — 10%). In the large bowel, malignancy is the most common cause (65%), followed by complicated diverticular disease (10%) and volvulus (5%).

Adhesions are thought to result from a reduction in peritoneal plasminogen-activating activity (PAA), which in turn leads to a failure to break down the post-operative fibrinous adhesions that follow all intra-abdominal operations. This reduction in PAA is increased by drying and abrasion of the peritoneum during laparotomy, in addition to foreign substances such as talc (which has now been removed from surgical gloves).

Table 15.12	CAUSES OF MECHANICAL OBSTRUCTION

Intrinsic
- Congenital atresia
- Inflammatory strictures
    Crohn's disease
    Tuberculosis
- Tumours
    Benign
    Malignant

Extrinsic
- Adhesions
- Hernias
- Volvulus
- Intussusception
- Congenital bands
- Inflammatory masses
- Tumours
    Benign
    Malignant

Luminal
- Foreign bodies
- Gallstones
- Parasites
- Bezoars

Table 15.13	CAUSES OF FUNCTIONAL OBSTRUCTION

Systemic
Metabolic
- Hypokalaemia
- Hyponatraemia
- Hypothermia
- Hypoxia
- Diabetic ketoacidosis
- Uraemia
- Dehydration

Drugs
- Tricyclic antidepressants
- General anaesthesia

Sepsis (acute pancreatitis)
Retroperitoneal malignancy (Ogilvie's syndrome)
Trauma
- Head injury
- Spinal injury
- Pelvic surgery

Local (affecting bowel motility)
- Intra-abdominal infection/peritonitis
- *Strongyloides*
- Post-operative ileus

Functional obstruction

This form of obstruction results from atony of the intestine with loss of normal peristalsis, in the absence of a mechanical cause. In the small bowel it is usually referred to as paralytic ileus, whereas in the large bowel the term pseudo-obstruction is used. The atony of the bowel may be localized to one segment or may be generalized. The pathophysiology is complex, but in essence results locally from an abnormality within the myenteric plexus of the bowel wall, and generally from an imbalance between sympathetic and parasympathetic nerve supply. A wide variety of underlying causal conditions is recognized (Table 15.13).

BOX 15.2	CAUSES OF INTESTINAL OBSTRUCTION

- The most important classification of intestinal obstruction is based on the nature of the pathological process: simple mechanical obstruction, strangulation and paralytic ileus
- In mechanical obstruction distension of the proximal bowel produces marked peristalsis and colic, whereas impairment of mucosal function causes net loss of water and electrolytes into the lumen (with extracellular fluid (ECF) depletion)
- In high intestinal obstruction vomiting is an early feature. In distal obstruction, vomiting may be a late manifestation, but fluid sequestration within the gut still leads to ECF depletion
- Strangulation denotes loss of blood supply and may complicate simple mechanical obstruction. Venous drainage is usually occluded first, followed by arterial occlusion
- Strangulation increases the morbidity and mortality of intestinal obstruction. Blood and plasma are sequestered in the strangulated intestine, and bacteria and their toxins migrate through the devitalized gut wall

15

Clinical features and management

General

The bowel proximal to the physical obstruction dilates as a result of the accumulation of fluid and gas. The amount of fluid sequestrated in the bowel can be large, particularly in distal small bowel obstruction, and the gas that accumulates is mainly swallowed air, with luminal putrefaction making a small contribution. Absorption from the lumen is diminished and there is a net loss of water and electrolytes into the bowel lumen, some of which may then be lost in vomiting. The patient will therefore show signs of dehydration and hypovolaemia, with a decreased skin turgor, dry tongue, hypotension and tachycardia. The dilatation of the bowel activates stretch receptors in the wall, resulting in reflex contraction of smooth muscle. This produces colicky abdominal pain and abdominal distension. The bowel distal to the obstruction collapses as gas and fluid no longer pass into it, and as a result peristalsis within it eventually ceases. If the obstruction is not overcome, the reflex activity proximal to the obstruction will eventually cease and the bowel becomes atonic, unless strangulation or perforation intervenes. In the absence of strangulation or perforation, hypovolaemia and ultimately starvation are the main factors that threaten life. As already discussed, fluid replacement is the mainstay of early treatment, and subsequent management will depend on other factors, as detailed below.

Small bowel obstruction

Colicky pain and vomiting are early features of small bowel obstruction, with constipation appearing late and distension only really occurring if the obstruction is fairly distal. Patients usually give a short history, but the presenting event may not be the first, especially in those who have had previous abdominal surgery. Adhesions are the most common cause of small bowel obstruction (60%) in the UK. In distal small bowel obstruction, the onset may be more insidious and the vomiting may become faeculant (obstructed and stagnant small bowel contents, with resultant bacterial proliferation and overgrowth). Hernial orifices must be carefully examined and bowel sounds are likely to be high-pitched and tinkling. A full examination should be carried out. Rectal examination may reveal faecal impaction or the presence of a rectal tumour, diverticular masses or malignant deposits in the pouch of Douglas.

The major concern for the attending clinician is to exclude the possibility of strangulation. Although it is difficult to be certain, this is unlikely if abdominal tenderness (guarding or rebound) on palpation, tachycardia (after any associated hypovolaemia has been treated by rehydration), pyrexia or an elevated white cell count is absent. If any of these signs is present, then the possibility of strangulation rises accordingly, and operative treatment must be considered early. Similarly, if the colicky pain either is replaced by a continuous dull ache or is associated with a background constant pain, the possibility of strangulation increases. Strangulation is much more likely to occur if there is a closed-loop obstruction (Fig. 15.2) within which the intraluminal pressure cannot be decompressed. Strangulation follows impairment of the blood supply to and from the bowel wall and leads to infarction. It is a surgical emergency and requires urgent operative intervention.

Following clinical assessment, appropriate X-rays are organized. Small bowel distension (> 2.5 cm in diameter) confirms the diagnosis and resuscitation is instituted. Small bowel can be differentiated from the colon by the 'valvulae conniventes', which completely cross the bowel wall (unlike the taeniae coli of the large bowel, which are incomplete), their relatively central position and their diameter (the small bowel rarely distends to more than 4–5 cm in diameter, whereas the colon can distend to 10 cm and more in severe cases). If strangulation is not suspected, a period of non-operative treatment is then commenced. This will involve intestinal decompression by means of a nasogastric tube and intravenous fluid replacement. Quite marked hypokalaemia can occur in addition to the hypovolaemia, due primarily to the renal preservation of sodium, and this needs to be closely monitored and corrected.

The period of non-operative treatment varies from patient to patient and can extend to many days. Care must be taken to ensure that strangulation or starvation does not occur, and therefore most surgeons would consider 2–3 days as the limit. A water-soluble small bowel contrast follow-through (as shown in Fig. 15.9) can be helpful in determining whether there is complete or incomplete obstruction. Failure of contrast to reach the caecum within 4 hours generally implies that surgery will be required.

Intussusception

Intussusception is a common cause of intestinal obstruction in the first year of life. The terminal ileum is peristalsed into the caecum and ascending colon, thus causing intestinal obstruction (ileo-colic intussusception). This most commonly occurs after a viral illness, which is thought to lead to enlargement of the Peyer's patches in the terminal small intestine. These patches become the lead point in the intussusception. In older children, small bowel polyps, tumours, intestinal wall haematomas seen in Henoch–Schönlein purpura and Meckel's diverticula can act as lead points in an intussusception (ileo-colic, ileo-ileal or ileo-ileo-colic).

Affected children present with a short history of screaming attacks, often said to be associated with attacks of pallor and drawing up of the knees. Anorexia and vomiting are common and the normal pattern of stooling can be disrupted. The abdomen becomes distended and tender and the child may pass the classic 'redcurrant jelly' stool. Dehydration is common and affected infants may become drowsy and unrousable.

Initial management of affected infants must pay attention to rehydration. Intravenous access is essential (and often very difficult to obtain) and resuscitation with crystalloid or colloid solutions should be initiated. The history is often very characteristic, but differentiation from gastroenteritis can sometimes be difficult.

Abdominal examination may reveal a relatively 'empty' right iliac fossa, and a sausage-shaped mass may be felt in the right upper quadrant. Abdominal X-rays may help

15

15

clinch the diagnosis but may also be unhelpful. Abdominal ultrasound scan has now become one of the main methods used to confirm the diagnosis. A target sign is seen when the intussusception is scanned transversely (the rings of the target representing the various layers of the bowel wall).

Treatment involves an attempt at pneumatic reduction of the intussusception using an air enema. A small tube is passed into the rectum and air is pumped in using a pressure-limited valve. The reduction is monitored using X-ray screening. A second or third attempt, after a delay of an hour or so between efforts, may succeed where the initial attempt fails. Overall success rates for pneumatic reduction in excess of 80% have been reported. Failure to reduce the intussusception in this way requires laparotomy and reduction or resection of the affected intestine.

Large bowel obstruction

Although large bowel obstruction is 3–4 times less common than small bowel obstruction, it is more likely to require surgery and carries much higher associated morbidity and mortality. Malignancy is the most common cause of mechanical large bowel obstruction in the UK, but in

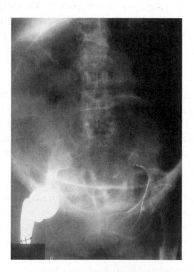

A

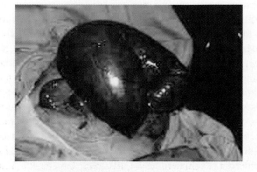

B

Fig. 15.14 A huge sigmoid volvulus.
Ⓐ Supine abdominal X-ray. Ⓑ Operative findings, with tiny pinhole volvulus visible (arrow).

> **BOX 15.3 TREATMENT OF INTESTINAL OBSTRUCTION**
>
> - In paralytic ileus, treatment is directed at the underlying cause (e.g. peritonitis, pancreatitis)
> - In mechanical obstruction, prompt diagnosis and management are normally essential to avoid the danger of strangulation. Management consists of vigorous restoration of fluid and electrolyte balance, followed by prompt surgical intervention
> - Strangulated bowel is blue or black, lacks sheen and peristaltic activity, and has no arterial pulsation in the adjacent mesentery. Strangulated bowel has to be resected with end-to-end anastomosis or exteriorization of the ends of the divided intestine
> - Situations in which conservative treatment of mechanical intestinal obstruction may sometimes be justifiable include adhesion obstruction, widespread intra-abdominal malignancy, Crohn's disease and post-operative obstruction

developing countries volvulus is more frequently encountered, and carcinoma and diverticulitis are rare. In the UK, volvulus is predominantly a disease of the elderly and the mentally impaired. It is predisposed to by the presence of a large redundant sigmoid loop based on a narrow mesentery. Most patients have a history of chronic constipation and laxative abuse.

Compared to small bowel obstruction, abdominal distension and constipation are common early features of large bowel obstruction, with colicky pain being less marked and vomiting only appearing very late. Although the rectum may be empty and complete obstruction results in absolute constipation (failure to pass faeces or flatus), a partial obstruction may result in the frequent passage of soft or liquid stools as a result of proximal peristaltic activity. These episodes of spurious diarrhoea often alternate with periods of constipation. Rectal examination is mandatory, although a cause for the obstruction is rarely palpable with the examining finger. However, the presence of blood and mucus on the glove is suggestive of a distal neoplasm. Sigmoidoscopy should be performed for two reasons: first, the obstructing lesion may be visible, and second, a sigmoid volvulus (Fig. 15.14) might be decompressed.

If the ileocaecal valve is competent, a closed-loop obstruction exists and perforation of the caecum becomes a real possibility, particularly if its diameter measures 10 cm or more on plain X-rays. In such cases, following resuscitation and confirmation of the diagnosis with a water-soluble contrast enema, urgent laparotomy is carried out. The procedure performed varies according to the condition of the patient, the extent and site of the disease, and the experience of the operating surgeon. All these factors are discussed in more detail in Chapter 20. If the ileocaecal valve is incompetent, there is less urgency to perform surgery but similar principles apply.

Pseudo-obstruction

This term refers to the presence of colonic obstruction for which no mechanical cause can be found. A wide variety of causes predisposes to this condition (Table 15.13), and once diagnosis has been established by water-soluble contrast enema, treatment is based on correction of the underlying disorder. Occasionally, in exceptional circum-

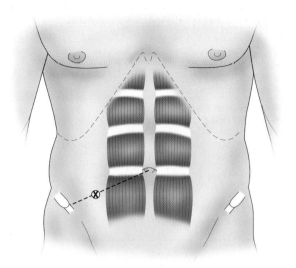

Fig. 15.15 McBurney's point.

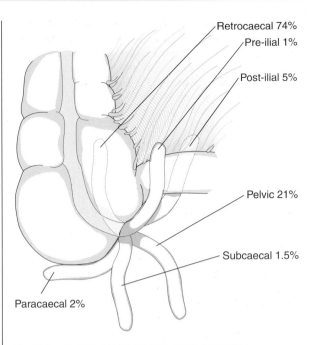

Retrocaecal 74%
Pre-ilial 1%
Post-ilial 5%
Pelvic 21%
Subcaecal 1.5%
Paracaecal 2%

Fig. 15.16 Variations in the position of the appendix.

15

stances, decompression is required, and this is carried out colonoscopically where possible. Operative decompression is rarely required.

ACUTE APPENDICITIS

Anatomy

The appendix is a worm-shaped blind-ending tube that arises from the posteromedial wall of the caecum 2 cm below the ileocaecal valve. It varies in length from 2 to 25 cm, but is most commonly 6–9 cm long. Externally, the base of the appendix is found at the point of convergence of the three taeniae coli of the caecum. On the surface of the abdomen, this point lies one-third of the way along a line drawn between the right anterior superior iliac spine and the umbilicus (McBurney's point; Fig. 15.15). The appendix has its own mesentery, the mesoappendix, and its blood supply comes from the appendicular artery, a branch of the ileocolic artery. The position of the appendix is variable, depending on its length and mobility. In cadaveric dissections the most common site is retrocaecal, but data from diagnostic laparoscopy indicate that the pelvic position is probably more common (Fig. 15.16). In children, there are abundant lymphoid follicles in the submucosa, but these atrophy with age.

Epidemiology

In the UK, appendicitis is the most common cause of acute abdominal pain requiring surgery, and it has been estimated that 16% of the population of developed countries will undergo appendicectomy for presumed appendicitis during their lifetime. There has been a decline in the incidence of appendicitis over the last 20 years, but the reason for this is unknown. There is an equal incidence in males and females. Appendicitis is uncommon in patients below the age of 2 and above the age of 65, and is most common in the under-40s, with a peak incidence between 8 and 14

years. There is a geographical variation in the incidence, being rare in Asia and Central Africa, which is thought to be due to environmental factors. In Western countries, it is seen more frequently in cities than in rural areas.

Aetiology

Despite its prevalence, the aetiology of acute appendicitis remains unclear. Several different mechanisms have been proposed, one of the more popular causes being a diet lacking in fibre and a consequent slow transit time and alteration in bacterial flora. However, this theory is challenged by a decline in incidence of appendicitis over recent years that has not been matched by an increase in dietary fibre intake. Others have suggested that viral infection may be an aetiological agent, as there is an association between appendicitis and concurrent viral illness and because there is a seasonal variation in the incidence of appendicitis.

Pathogenesis

Obstruction of the lumen of the appendix is thought to play the main role in the initiation of inflammation. Faecoliths, lymphoid hyperplasia, foreign bodies, carcinoid tumours and strictures may all cause luminal obstruction and subsequently lead to acute appendicitis. Following obstruction, the wall of the appendix becomes inflamed, commencing in the mucosa and spreading to involve the submucosa, muscular and serosal layers. A fibrinopurulent exudate forms on the serosal surface and extends to any adjacent peritoneal surface. Inflammation of the wall of the appendix causes venous congestion, which may compromise arterial inflow, leading to ischaemia and infarction. Organisms from the lumen of the appendix enter the submucosa through an ischaemic ulcer, causing liquefaction of the wall and ultimately perforation.

As a result of the transmural inflammation, small bowel and omentum adhere to the appendix, creating a localized area of sepsis. If left untreated, this may progress to form an appendix mass or even an abscess. If perforation occurs early in the clinical course, the inflamed area will not have had time to be walled off, and generalized peritonitis follows.

Clinical features

History

Classically, the onset of acute appendicitis is associated with the gradual onset of poorly localized central abdominal pain. After a variable amount of time, the pain moves to the right iliac fossa and changes in character, to become sharper, constant and well localized. It is aggravated by movement and coughing. As described earlier, this change in the nature of the pain occurs when the parietal peritoneum overlying the appendix becomes involved in the inflammatory process. In general, most patients present within 24 hours of the onset of the central abdominal pain. Many patients also admit to anorexia and occasional vomiting.

In children, the classic history and physical findings of appendicitis are often not seen. Non-specific symptoms (anorexia, nausea, vomiting, diarrhoea) and signs (fever, fetor, pallor, abdominal distension) can confuse the inexperienced clinician. The finding of tenderness and guarding in the right iliac fossa usually makes the diagnosis without the need for other investigations.

Examination

The patient with established acute appendicitis looks unwell, is flushed and has a dry furred tongue with a fetor. The temperature is usually only mildly elevated (37.3–38.5 °C) and there is often a tachycardia. Classically, the area of maximal tenderness is over McBurney's point, with guarding and rebound (percussion) tenderness. Palpation in the left iliac fossa may reproduce the pain in the right iliac fossa (Rovsing's sign) and the patient may find it painful to extend the right hip owing to irritation of the psoas muscle (psoas stretch sign). Although rectal and vaginal examinations are frequently normal, they can be useful when the abdominal signs are vague, particularly if the acutely inflamed appendix lies within the pelvis, when tenderness may be elicited with the examining finger. In young women, either rectal or vaginal examination is extremely useful in helping to differentiate acute appendicitis from acute gynaecological disorders.

Variations in clinical features

The symptoms and signs of acute appendicitis are influenced by a variety of factors, which include age, sex, personality and the position of the appendix. Only 50% of patients with acute appendicitis give a typical history. An inflamed retrocaecal appendix may produce poorly localized abdominal pain, and an inflamed pelvic appendix lying close to the bladder may produce symptoms of frequency and dysuria. In this scenario, as with a retrocaecal appendix that overlies the ureter, it may be quite difficult to differentiate between urinary infection and acute appendicitis. Dipstick examination of the urine may reveal

---

Table 15.14   DIFFERENTIAL DIAGNOSIS OF ACUTE APPENDICITIS

- Mesenteric adenitis
- Meckel's diverticulitis
- Regional ileitis (Crohn's disease)
- Carcinoma of the caecum

Gynaecological disorders
- Ruptured ovarian follicle (Mittelschmerz)
- Acute salpingitis
- Ruptured ectopic pregnancy
- Torsion of an ovarian cyst

Genitourinary
- Pyelonephritis
- Ureteric colic
- Urinary tract infection
- Right-sided testicular torsion

---

microscopic haematuria and proteinuria in both cases. However, urgent microscopy and Gram stain of the urine will demonstrate bacteria in urinary tract infection. An inflamed pelvic appendix lying near the rectum causes irritation and diarrhoea, and is commonly mistaken for gastroenteritis. However, gastroenteritis is a dangerous diagnosis to make in the acute abdomen as it almost never causes abdominal tenderness (compared to abdominal pain). A very long appendix extending up to the right upper quadrant might even mimic acute cholecystitis.

Acute appendicitis is most dangerous in the very young, the very old and pregnant women. As it is uncommon under the age of 2 years, when it does occur, it is often incorrectly diagnosed as gastroenteritis. The symptoms and signs are atypical and generalized peritonitis quickly develops. In contrast, in elderly patients, the onset is more insidious. The inflamed area tends to wall off, with the development of a mass, and symptoms and signs of obstruction may be present. In the pregnant patient, the appendix is displaced upwards by the enlarged uterus, and the site of the pain and tenderness is high in the abdomen. Appendicitis in pregnancy carries a high rate of morbidity and mortality for both mother and fetus.

A list of conditions that should be considered in the differential diagnosis of acute appendicitis is given in Table 15.14.

Complications

Gangrenous appendicitis and perforation tend to occur after a significantly more prolonged period of pain than uncomplicated appendicitis. Generalized peritonitis results if the inflamed area is not walled off by omentum and loops of bowel. If walling off does occur, either an appendix mass or an abscess will develop. A perforated pelvic appendix will lead to a pelvic abcess, and on examination there may be very little in the way of abdominal signs.

Investigations

The various investigations used in patients with suspected appendicitis have already been discussed earlier in the chapter. However, the diagnosis of acute appendicitis is

---

EBM 15.2   ACUTE APPENDICITIS

'Patients with symptoms and signs consistent with appendicitis should undergo appendicectomy. If laparoscopy has been performed first to confirm the diagnosis, then it is reasonable to proceed with laparoscopic appendicectomy.'

Paterson-Brown S. In: Paterson-Brown S, ed. A companion to specialist surgical practice: core topics in general and emergency surgery, 3rd edn. London: Elsevier; 2005: 165–182.

EBM 15.3   APPENDIX MASS OR ABSCESS

'The diagnosis should be confirmed using ultrasonography or CT scan. Patients with an appendix mass/abscess should be treated non-operatively with antibiotics and intravenous fluids. Any abscess should be drained by percutaneous means. Routine examination of the colon should be carried out 6 weeks following initial presentation to exclude a colonic cause, using either barium enema or colonoscopy. Interval appendicectomy should be reserved for those patients with recurrent symptoms, and can be carried out using the laparoscopic approach.'

Paterson-Brown S. In: Paterson-Brown S, ed. A companion to specialist surgical practice: core topics in general and emergency surgery, 3rd edn. London: Elsevier; 2005: 165–182.

BOX 15.4   APPENDICITIS

- Incidence has declined, but appendicitis is still the most common acute abdominal condition in childhood, adolescence and early adulthood
- The typical history of periumbilical colic (visceral midgut pain), followed within several hours by right iliac fossa pain (somatic pain from parietal peritonitis), is not always present
- Tenderness and muscle guarding in the right iliac fossa are the most reliable signs of acute appendicitis. Leucocytosis, high temperature and radiological signs are manifestations that may denote gangrene and perforation
- The diagnosis should be made and appendicectomy undertaken before gangrene and perforation supervene
- Gangrene and perforation are common and/or particularly dangerous in infants, during pregnancy and in the elderly

---

based on clinical assessment and there are no specific diagnostic tests. Ultrasonography in skilled hands might demonstrate a swollen non-compressible appendix, free fluid or even a mass in the right iliac fossa. If, after clinical assessment, the diagnosis remains in doubt, the clinician must proceed along one of two lines: either to carry out laparoscopy and undertake appendicectomy if indicated, or to institute a short policy of close and repeated observation with reassessment every hour.

Management

The treatment of appendicitis is almost always surgical; increasingly, laparoscopic appendicectomy is being carried out, especially if a diagnostic laparoscopy has been performed first to establish the diagnosis (EBM 15.2). Although the laparoscopic approach is undoubtedly associated with less post-operative pain, most studies have so far failed to show significant advantages in shortening hospital stay or returning to normal activities. This is probably because of the underlying sepsis, which slows recovery. It is also possible to treat patients who do not have overt peritonitis non-operatively with antibiotics, and this is often done in areas of the world where ready access to surgery is impossible. In these conditions, there is a high incidence of recurrent problems and as such this practice is not favoured. If, by the time the patient presents, a mass can be felt, non-operative management with intravenous fluids and antibiotics is the treatment of choice, provided there are no signs of peritonitis (when an operation should be carried out). In these patients, an ultrasound scan should be arranged to look for an underlying abscess; if one is present, it should be drained either under radiological guidance or surgically.

Following successful non-operative treatment of an appendix mass, it used to be traditional practice to carry out an interval appendicectomy 6–12 weeks later. This prevents further attacks, and in the elderly makes sure that there is no underlying carcinoma of the caecum. However, several studies have now confirmed that after the successful non-operative treatment of either an appendix mass or an abscess, only a few patients develop recurrent problems, and most of them do so within the first few months. It is therefore reasonable not to carry out an interval appendicectomy unless the patient experiences further symptoms or complications (EBM 15.3). It is still important, especially in older patients, to exclude a carcinoma of the caecum by either double-contrast barium enema or colonoscopy. An interval appendicectomy should be undertaken if this course is not pursued.

Prognosis

The overall mortality of appendicitis is less than 1%, rising to 5% if perforation occurs and increasing with age. The post-operative morbidity is mainly related to wound infection and late-onset intestinal obstruction from adhesions. The former can be kept to a minimum by perioperative prophylactic antibiotics (metronidazole), and the latter by careful surgery and perhaps the increasing use of laparoscopic appendicectomy. It used to be thought that fertility in female patients was adversely affected by appendicectomy, but this no longer seems to be the case; even in cases of perforated appendicitis, there appears to be no increased risk of infertility.

NON-SPECIFIC ABDOMINAL PAIN (NSAP)

This term is often applied to patients in whom no cause can be found for their abdominal pain. In studies, its incidence has been found to be around 40% for all patients admitted with acute abdominal pain, dropping to around 25% if investigations such as laparoscopy are used to improve diagnostic accuracy. The major concern in reaching a

15

15

diagnosis of NSAP is that a serious underlying condition has been missed. It has been reported that 10% of patients over 50 years of age who are discharged with NSAP from hospital after an acute admission with abdominal pain have an underlying malignancy, of which half are colonic. Another group of patients who tend to be diagnosed with NSAP are young females who may have a gynaecological condition, such as pelvic inflammatory disease or ovarian cyst pathology. With the more widespread use of laparoscopy in the investigation of patients with acute abdominal pain, the incidence of NSAP will continue to fall.

GYNAECOLOGICAL CAUSES OF THE ACUTE ABDOMEN

MITTELSCHMERZ AND RUPTURED CORPUS LUTEUM

The Graafian follicle normally ruptures 14 days after the start of the last menstrual period, and release of the ovum may be complicated by bleeding. The follicle normally becomes a corpus luteum, which degenerates before the start of the next period unless conception occurs. Bleeding from the corpus luteum is an occasional cause of pain in the late stages of the menstrual cycle.

Patients with these causes of pain are usually between 15 and 25 years of age, and experience sudden pain in one or other iliac fossa. Tenderness and guarding in the right iliac fossa can simulate acute appendicitis, and a few patients bleed sufficiently to suggest rupture of an ectopic pregnancy. Rectal or vaginal examination may reveal tenderness in the rectovaginal pouch.

The patient is treated conservatively, unless appendicitis or ruptured ectopic pregnancy cannot be excluded. Laparoscopy may help to avoid unnecessary surgery, as ultrasonography alone will not be diagnostic.

RUPTURED ECTOPIC PREGNANCY

A fertilized ovum implants at an abnormal site in 1 in 200 pregnancies; the fallopian tube is by far the most common site. The erosive trophoblast may penetrate the wall of the tube, and often ruptures after about 6 weeks. Alternatively, the conceptus may be extruded from the fimbrial end of the tube.

Bouts of cramping iliac fossa pain may be associated with fainting and vaginal bleeding. Rupture produces sudden severe pain, bleeding and circulatory collapse. The abdominal pain often becomes generalized. A missed period is reported by most patients.

TORSION OF AN OVARIAN CYST

Benign ovarian cysts are a common cause of torsion. Dermoid cysts often have a long pedicle and account for 50% of torsions in young women.

Severe cramping lower abdominal pain is often associated with a smooth round mobile mass that lies higher in the abdomen than might be expected. Tenderness and guarding may be present, particularly if there is leakage, and rupture results in diffuse peritonism. Torsion of a fallopian tube or fibroid may produce a similar picture.

At laparoscopy the twisted pedicle is transfixed and ligated and the cyst is removed. Care must be taken to avoid rupture in case the cyst is malignant. Further radical surgery may be needed if histological examination reveals malignancy.

ACUTE SALPINGITIS

Acute salpingitis may be due to streptococcal infection, but gonococcal or tuberculous infection can also be responsible. Both tubes are often involved and adhesions may seal the fimbriated end, producing a pyosalpinx.

Bilateral pain is felt just above the pubis and inguinal ligaments. There may be urinary frequency, irregular menstruation, pyrexia and leucocytosis. Vaginal examination reveals unusual warmth, a tender cervix and a vaginal discharge. The cervix appears red and inflamed, and a swab reveals the causative organism. Vaginal findings may be less marked when there is a closed pyosalpinx.

Treatment consists of antibiotic therapy. Laparoscopy is used increasingly to avoid unnecessary laparotomy if acute appendicitis cannot be ruled out. The tubes appear inflamed and oedematous, and 'milking' them gently produces a purulent discharge from which a bacteriological swab is taken.

BOX 15.5   GYNAECOLOGICAL CAUSES OF PAIN AND THE ACUTE ABDOMEN

- Non-specific abdominal pain (i.e. pain for which no cause is defined) is particularly common in female adolescents and young women, and often mimics acute appendicitis. Laparoscopy may prove increasingly valuable when the diagnosis is in doubt and the need for surgery cannot be excluded
- Minor intraperitoneal bleeding at the time of rupture of the Graafian follicle may cause mid-cycle pain (Mittelschmerz) in the iliac fossa in young girls
- Rupture of an ectopic pregnancy causes intraperitoneal bleeding and more severe abdominal pain, with circulatory collapse. Signs of pregnancy are seldom present and pregnancy testing may be unhelpful. Elevation of the foot of the bed may produce shoulder-tip pain and underline the need for laparotomy
- Torsion of an ovarian cyst often causes cramping lower abdominal pain. Ovarian cysts can become very large and produce visible abdominal swellings which lie higher than might be expected. Some cysts prove to be malignant and care must be taken to avoid rupture at operation
- Acute salpingitis is often due to gonococcal infection and produces bilateral suprapubic pain which is often associated with urinary frequency, a tender cervix and vaginal discharge

16

S. PATERSON-BROWN

The oesophagus

SURGICAL ANATOMY

The oesophagus extends from the cricoid cartilage (at the level of vertebra C6) to the gastric cardia and is 25 cm long. It has cervical, thoracic and abdominal portions. The oesophagus passes through the diaphragm at the level of the 10th thoracic vertebra and the final 2–4 cm lie within the peritoneal cavity. The relationships are shown in Figure 16.1.

The oesophagus has an upper sphincter, the cricopharyngeus, and a lower sphincter that cannot be defined anatomically but is a 3–5 cm high-pressure area located in the region of the oesophageal hiatus of the diaphragm. The oesophagus is held loosely in the hiatus by a thickening of fascia, the phreno-oesophageal ligament.

The oesophageal wall can be divided into several layers:

- an outer adventitial connective tissue layer
- an outer longitudinal muscle layer
- an inner circular muscle layer, the upper third consisting of striated muscle and the lower part of smooth muscle
- Auerbach's neural plexus, which lies between the two muscle layers
- the submucosa, which consists of mucous glands, lymphatics and Meissner's neural plexus
- the mucosa, which consists of stratified squamous epithelium, except for the distal 1–2 cm, which are lined by columnar epithelium.

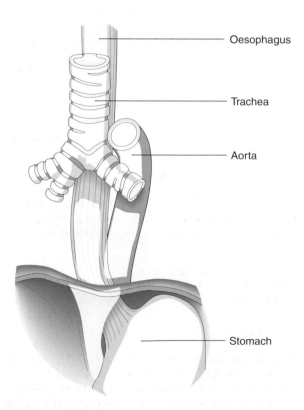

Oesophagus

Trachea

Aorta

Stomach

Fig. 16.1   Anatomical relationships of the oesophagus.

The oesophagus receives its blood supply from the inferior thyroid artery in the cervical region, the bronchial arteries and branches from the thoracic aorta in the thorax, and the inferior phrenic and left gastric arteries in the abdomen.

Venous drainage is to the inferior thyroid veins in the neck, the hemi-azygous and azygous veins (systemic circulation) in the thorax, and the left gastric (portal circulation) in the abdomen. The connection between these veins is important in the development of varices in patients with portal hypertension.

Sympathetic nerve supply is derived from pre-ganglionic fibres from spinal cord segments T5 and T6, and post-ganglionic fibres from the cervical vertebral and coeliac ganglia. Parasympathetic supply comes from the glosso-pharyngeal, recurrent laryngeal and vagus nerves.

The lymphatics run in the submucosa and drain to the regional lymph nodes, and subsequently to the posterior mediastinal, supraclavicular and coeliac lymph nodes.

SYMPTOMS OF OESOPHAGEAL DISORDERS

DYSPHAGIA

Dysphagia is defined as difficulty in swallowing. It is a serious symptom and requires assessment. Certain points in the history are helpful in leading to a diagnosis:

- *Onset.* Sudden onset suggests a foreign body. In carcinoma, the dysphagia occurs over a period of weeks, whereas in achalasia and benign strictures, symptoms tend to develop over a number of years.
- *Site.* The actual site of obstruction correlates poorly in general to where the patient feels the discomfort, although some patients who feel the obstruction to be high may have a pharyngeal pouch.
- *Progression.* Dysphagia progresses rapidly in carcinoma and slowly in benign strictures and achalasia.
- *Severity.* Difficulty in swallowing solids is initially typical of carcinoma, whereas achalasia tends to be associated with dysphagia to liquids at first.
- *Causes.* A list of the common causes of dysphagia is shown in Table 16.1.

PAIN

Heartburn is a retrosternal burning sensation, and is associated with reflux of acid into the mouth. It tends to occur after eating and is exacerbated by bending and lying down. It can be relieved with antacids and is associated with gastro-oesophageal reflux disease, peptic ulcer disease, benign strictures and primary motility disorders. Carcinoma of the oesophagus may progress to produce a constant central chest pain, which can be referred to the back between the shoulder blades. Retrosternal chest pain radiating to the back can also be a symptom of oesophageal perforation following recent instrumentation or vomiting. Achalasia tends to be painless. Angina is a differential

Table 16.1 CAUSES OF DYSPHAGIA

	Intraluminal	Intramural	Extrinsic
Pharynx/upper oesophagus	Foreign body	Pharyngitis/tonsillitis Moniliasis Sideropenic web Corrosives Carcinoma Myasthenia gravis Bulbar palsy	Thyroid enlargement Pharyngeal pouch
Body of oesophagus	Foreign body	Corrosives Peptic oesophagitis Carcinoma	Mediastinal lymph nodes Aortic aneurysm
Lower oesophagus	Foreign body	Corrosives Peptic oesophagitis Carcinoma Diffuse oesophageal spasm Systemic sclerosis Achalasia Post-vagotomy	Para-oesophageal hernia

diagnosis of retrosternal chest pain. Odynophagia is pain on swallowing, and may coexist with dysphagia.

REGURGITATION

This is an effortless process whereby food is regurgitated into the mouth. There is no associated nausea and the patient does not vomit. It is associated with achalasia, hiatus hernia and pharyngeal pouches, in which regurgitation can lead to coughing and aspiration pneumonia.

EXAMINATION

Physical examination might reveal signs that will aid in the diagnosis of oesophageal disorders. A smooth tongue, pallor and koilonychia are signs of iron deficiency anaemia, which can be present in oesophageal carcinoma, oesophagitis and Plummer–Vinson syndrome.

Lymphadenopathy, particularly in the supraclavicular region, hepatomegaly, abdominal mass, ascites and evidence of weight loss are associated with malignancy. Crepitus in the neck is a sign of surgical emphysema, which would suggest an oesophageal perforation. Neurological examination may reveal a neurological cause for the symptoms.

INVESTIGATIONS

BLOOD TESTS

A full blood count may exclude anaemia. Serum urea and electrolytes may show dehydration secondary to dysphagia. Liver function tests might show low plasma proteins, abnormal clotting and elevated enzymes in the presence of metastatic disease, and portal hypertension.

RADIOLOGY

Chest X-ray

A chest X-ray may show any of the following signs:

- consolidation and fibrosis following aspiration in patients with oesophageal motility disorders and oesophageal carcinoma
- air–fluid level behind the heart shadow from a large hiatus hernia with intra-thoracic stomach
- mediastinal mass of lymph nodes and pulmonary metastases in oesophageal carcinoma
- an indented gastric air bubble caused by a carcinoma of the cardia
- air in the mediastinum and neck after perforation of the oesophagus.

Barium swallow

A barium swallow may provide the following information:

- reflux in the head-down position
- smooth benign strictures
- irregular malignant strictures
- a fusiform dilatation with a tapered lower end, which may be evident in achalasia; the normal gas bubble in the stomach is also absent, as the oesophagus never completely empties.

Water-soluble contrast is used if perforation of the oesophagus is suspected, as barium is irritant to the mediastinum.

ENDOSCOPY

Flexible oesophagogastroduodenoscopy (OGD) is now the first-line investigation for almost all oesophageal disorders, particularly those that present with symptoms of dyspepsia, dysphagia, haematemesis, atypical chest pain and weight loss. Flexible OGD is carried out either under light intra-

16

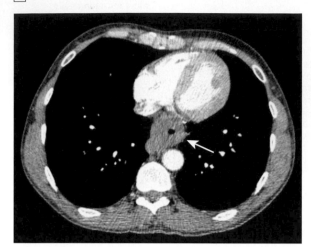

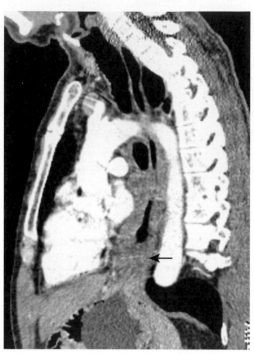

Fig. 16.2 Computed tomography (CT)
[A] Cross-sectional CT demonstrating a bulky carcinoma of the lower oesophagus (arrow). [B] Sagittal section CT demonstrating the same tumour (arrow) .

venous sedation or using a local anaesthetic throat spray. The patient should be fasted for 4 hours before the procedure. It is important to monitor pulse and oxygen saturation throughout the procedure to identify and rectify any possible respiratory depression that might follow sedation.

The technique of OGD is used to inspect the oesophageal mucosa and allows biopsies to be taken. Therapeutic procedures, such as dilatation of strictures, insertion of stents, thermal ablation of tumours (using laser or argon beam coagulation), removal of foreign bodies and control of bleeding varices and ulcers by injection of adrenaline (epinephrine), sclerotherapy, banding and thermocoagulation, can also be carried out.

Endoscopy can be complicated by perforation of the oesophagus, mainly associated with stricture dilatation.

COMPUTED TOMOGRAPHY (CT)

CT is used most commonly to investigate and stage oesophageal tumours (Fig. 16.2). Although the most modern types of multi-slice CT scanner are much better at staging malignancy than the previous ones, they can still both over- and understage tumours. As a result, endoscopic ultrasound is used as a complementary modality.

ULTRASONOGRAPHY

Percutaneous abdominal ultrasound is a relatively inexpensive and simple method for detecting liver metastases,

which can be biopsied if required. Similarly, there have been several recent reports on the use of ultrasonography in the neck to identify metastatic lymphadenopathy from oesophageal tumours. However, endoscopic ultrasonography (EUS) has revolutionized the investigation of oesophageal disorders, particularly carcinoma (Fig. 16.3). Not only can all the layers of the oesophagus be clearly seen, with excellent assessment of any tumours, but invasion outside the lumen and adjacent lymph node enlargement can also be identified and biopsied if necessary.

LAPAROSCOPY

Laparoscopy, which can be combined with laparoscopic ultrasound, is useful to exclude liver and peritoneal metastases from lower oesophageal carcinoma before surgical resection is undertaken.

MANOMETRY AND PH STUDIES

Measurements of lower oesophageal pH, using intraluminal electrodes, and of pressure, obtained from a series of saline-perfused tubes connected to pressure transducers passed down the oesophagus, can be used to investigate various motility disorders of the oesophagus, in addition to gastro-oesophageal reflux disease (Fig. 16.4).

The main tools for the investigation of oesophageal disease in children are contrast radiology, pH studies and upper gastrointestinal endoscopy.

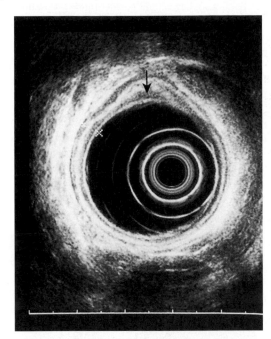

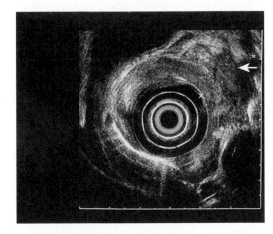

Fig. 16.3 Endoscopic ultrasonography (EUS).
[A] The normal layers of the oesophagus and a small carcinoma at 12 o'clock (arrow). [B] A large carcinoma of the oesophagus extending outside the muscle layer (arrow).

IMPACTED FOREIGN BODIES

Swallowed foreign bodies are particularly common in children after accidental ingestion, and obstruction of the oropharynx and tracheal opening by a large food bolus can rapidly be fatal. The obstruction can usually be removed by asking patients to cough or giving them a sharp blow to the back, or alternatively by using the Heimlich manoeuvre (Fig. 16.5). The level at which foreign bodies tend to stick correlates with anatomical areas of narrowing, which can be found at:

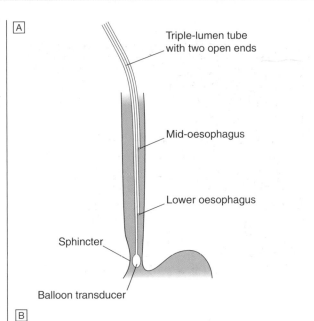

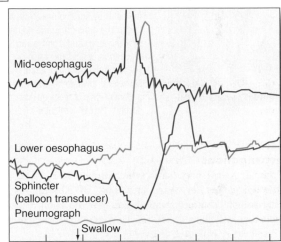

Fig. 16.4 Recording of the luminal pressure within the oesophagus.
[A] Balloon pressure transducer and open-tipped catheter assembly in place. [B] Pressure recordings of swallowing responses in a healthy subject. Note that relaxation of the lower oesophageal sphincter precedes the arrival of the peristaltic wave.

- arches of the fauces
- vallecula
- piriform fossae
- cricopharyngeus
- where the left main bronchus crosses the oesophagus
- where the arch of the aorta crosses the oesophagus
- diaphragm
- gastro-oesophageal junction.

Foreign bodies can, however, become lodged at any level where there is a benign or a malignant stricture. Patients can present in severe distress, with chest pain and retching. In severe cases, there may be a perforation, resulting in mediastinitis and haematemesis.

16

16

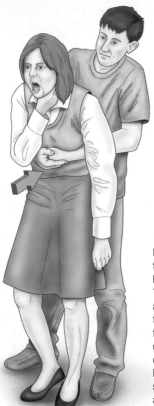

Fig. 16.5 Heimlich manoeuvre to remove an impacted foreign body in the pharynx.
The patient's dentures are removed and an attempt is made to remove the bolus by hooking it out with a finger. The arms are grasped firmly over the epigastrium and lower chest from behind the patient. Following the last gasp, a firm squeeze is given to the upper abdomen. This is repeated every 10 seconds for half a minute.

Investigations

A chest X-ray may show the foreign body if it is radio-opaque and/or there are signs of perforation. A water-soluble contrast swallow can provide confirmation. Endoscopy will allow direct visualization of the foreign body.

Management

Some patients can be treated conservatively and observed until the foreign body has passed, but in the majority endoscopic removal is advisable. This can be carried out using either flexible endoscopy under sedation or rigid oesophagoscopy under general anaesthesia.

CORROSIVE OESOPHAGITIS

Ingestion of strong acid or alkali occurs accidentally, especially in children, and deliberately in attempted suicide. It results in severe chemical burns to the mouth, pharynx and oesophageal mucosa, particularly at the sites of anatomical narrowing, owing to hold-up of the flow. Oedema, ulceration and inflammation follow, which in turn can lead to acute obstruction and perforation. The inflamed tissue then heals by fibrosis and stricture formation. Patients complain of severe continuous pain, which is exacerbated by swallowing. On examination, the oropharynx may be inflamed, the patient may be shocked and the oesophagus may have perforated.

Alkaline solutions are the most common cause of corrosive oesophageal injuries in children, particularly in the

Middle East and in developing countries. Acid ingestion causes both oesophageal and gastric injuries. Careful, early upper gastrointestinal endoscopy under general anaesthesia is essential to assess the extent and severity of the injury. Passage of a nasogastric or nasojejunal tube under the same anaesthetic will allow enteral feeding to commence and provide a passage for a guidewire, should subsequent balloon dilatation for stricture formation be necessary.

Investigations

Endoscopy or barium swallow will demonstrate the extent and severity of the injury at the time of the acute event, and later can assess stricture formation (Fig. 16.6).

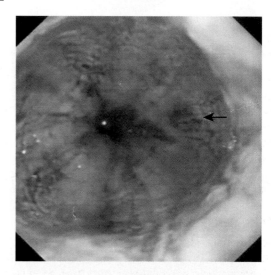

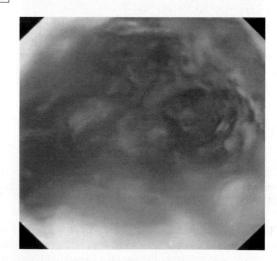

Fig. 16.6 Corrosive oesophagitis.
[A] Endoscopic view of the lower oesophagus and oesophago-gastric junction 12 hours after inadvertent ingestion of acid. The arrow shows the area of superficial necrosis involving the proximal stomach at the level of the oesophago-gastric junction. [B] The same endoscopic view after 36 hours, demonstrating mucosal inflammation but no evidence of ongoing necrosis. This patient was lucky and went on to make a full recovery without late stricture formation.

Management

In the first instance, an accurate history should be obtained and a detailed examination undertaken. Patients should be resuscitated and given appropriate opiate analgesia. They should also be encouraged to drink water to dilute the corrosive. Thereafter, the oesophagus should be rested and the patient kept nil by mouth and commenced on intravenous fluids and antibiotics. The use of steroids to reduce the extent of the inflammation and subsequent stricture formation remains controversial. Vomiting should be actively discouraged, as this can cause further burns and risks perforation. If the patient's oropharynx is severely inflamed, an artificial airway (tracheostomy) may be required. Feeding is usually established with total parenteral nutrition (TPN) or a feeding jejunostomy or gastrostomy. The patient is observed for perforation and later for stricture formation.

Strictures will usually require treatment with balloon dilatation. Long-term management may involve local resection of the stricture and primary anastomosis, or a more extensive resection with reconstruction using stomach, jejunum or colon. The stomach is often also damaged in the same disease process and, if so, cannot be used for reconstruction. Regular endoscopic surveillance will be required, as corrosive injury predisposes the oesophagus to malignant change.

PERFORATION

Aetiology

Intraluminal

This is caused by a swallowed foreign body or by removal of a foreign body during instrumentation, with rigid endoscopy carrying a much greater risk than flexible. The most common sites of perforation tend to coincide with the sites of anatomical narrowing. Perforation most commonly occurs during balloon dilatation of malignant or benign strictures.

Outside the wall

This is caused by penetrating injuries (rare).

Spontaneous

This follows episodes of violent vomiting (Boerhaave's syndrome). The perforation is frequently on the left posterolateral aspect of the lower oesophagus. A tear to the oesophageal mucosa only, following vomiting, is known as a Mallory–Weiss tear and tends to cause haematemesis.

Clinical features

The clinical symptoms depend to some extent on the site and size of the perforation. If the perforation is in the cervical region, the patient complains of pain in the neck and local tenderness, and surgical emphysema is present. Perforation of the thoracic oesophagus causes retrosternal chest pain and dysphagia. Clinically, the patient may be shocked, short of breath and cyanosed owing to a pneumothorax or pleural effusion, if the pleural space is involved. Perforation in this area can lead to mediastinitis

and septic shock. Perforation of the abdominal oesophagus can lead to peritonitis and a rigid abdomen.

Investigations

The differential diagnosis of a perforated oesophagus includes myocardial infarction and duodenal ulceration. Investigations therefore need to exclude these two diagnoses in particular, at the same time including examination of the oesophagus for perforation.

Erect chest X-ray

In addition to excluding a perforated duodenal ulcer (air under the diaphragm; Ch. 16), an erect chest X-ray may show surgical emphysema with gas in the soft tissues of the mediastinum, often extending up to the neck. The mediastinum may also be widened, and if the pleural cavity has also been ruptured, there will be a hydropneumothorax (Fig. 16.7).

Contrast swallow

The diagnosis is confirmed by a water-soluble contrast swallow, which will also demonstrate whether the perforation is localized to the mediastinum or open to the pleural or peritoneal cavities. If there is any doubt on contrast swallow, a contrast-enhanced CT scan should be arranged.

Management

Perforation of the cervical oesophagus can be treated non-operatively with intravenous fluids, withdrawal of oral fluid and diet, and the administration of antibiotics. If an abscess develops in the superior mediastinum, this will require surgical drainage.

Perforation of the thoracic oesophagus has a much higher morbidity and mortality. Localized and small perforations that do not communicate with either pleural cavity can be treated non-operatively, as outlined above. However, if the perforation follows the dilatation of a carcinoma in a patient suitable for resection, emergency oesophagogastrectomy

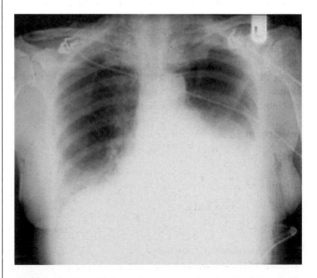

Fig. 16.7   Erect chest X-ray in a patient with Boerhaave's syndrome.
Note the left-sided hydropneumothorax.

is indicated following appropriate resuscitation. In other situations, perforation into either pleural cavity will usually require thoractomy, drainage and surgical repair.

MOTILITY DISORDERS

The most common motility disorders of the oesophagus are the non-specific variety commonly found in gastro-oesophageal reflux disease (which will be discussed later), achalasia, diffuse oesophageal spasm, nutcracker oesophagus, those associated with connective tissue disorders such as systemic sclerosis, and neuromuscular diseases.

ACHALASIA

This disorder affects the whole oesophagus. The main feature is failure of relaxation of the lower oesophageal sphincter; as the disease progresses, the obstructed lower oesophagus dilates and peristalsis becomes uncoordinated.

Achalasia is thought to be due to a partial or complete degeneration of the myenteric plexus of Auerbach, and in the later stages of the disease loss of the dorsal vagal nuclei within the brain stem can be demonstrated.

Infestation with the protozoon, *Trypanosoma cruzi*, which occurs in South America (Chagas' disease), also causes degeneration of the myenteric plexus, leading to a motor disorder of the oesophagus that is indistinguishable from achalasia.

Clinical features

The disease affects 1 in 100 000 of the population of developed countries. The patient is typically aged between 30 and 40 years, and females are affected more often than males (3:2).

There is progressive dysphagia over several years, often for both solids and liquids. Gravity rather than peristalsis is responsible for food leaving the oesophagus and the patient finds it easier to eat when standing. There may also be retrosternal pain, which gradually decreases in severity as the oesophagus loses peristaltic activity.

Other common symptoms include weight loss, halitosis and regurgitation of undigested food, which can lead to aspiration pneumonia, particularly at night, resulting in bouts of coughing and recurrent chest infections. In the longer term, achalasia can predispose to squamous cell carcinoma of the oesophagus.

Investigations

Chest X-ray

An erect chest X-ray might demonstrate a widened medi-stinum, produced by the dilated oesophagus. A fluid level behind the heart may also be seen, sometimes with evidence of aspiration pneumonia. The gastric air bubble is usually absent as a result of incomplete emptying of the oesophagus.

Barium swallow

A barium swallow will show dilatation of the oesophagus, leading to a tapered narrowing at the lower end (Fig. 16.8). As the disease progresses, there will be absent peristalsis in the body of the oesophagus.

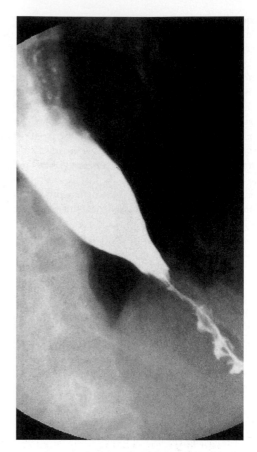

Fig. 16.8 Barium swallow demonstrating achalasia.

Endoscopy

OGD is essential to exclude other causes of lower oesophageal narrowing, in particular carcinoma.

Oesophageal manometry

The demonstration of a high-pressure non-relaxing lower oesophageal sphincter, with poor or absent peristalsis of the oesophageal body, is diagnostic of achalasia.

Management

Treatment involves either balloon dilatation of the lower oesophageal sphincter or surgical myotomy (division of the muscles over the lower oesophagus and proximal stomach). Endoscopic injection of the gastro-oesophageal junction with botulinum toxin has been shown to improve symptoms in a small group of patients, but recurrent problems occur. Balloon dilatation of the gastro-oesophageal junction disrupts the lower oesophageal sphincter (Fig. 16.9) and improves symptoms in 80–90% of patients, but carries with it the risk of oesophageal perforation. Patients who require more than two dilatations should be considered for surgery.

Operative treatment involves a Heller's cardiomyotomy. The lower oesophagus is exposed by either an abdominal or a left thoracic approach, and increasingly both procedures are being carried out using laparoscopy. The lower oesophageal sphincter is divided down to the mucosa for

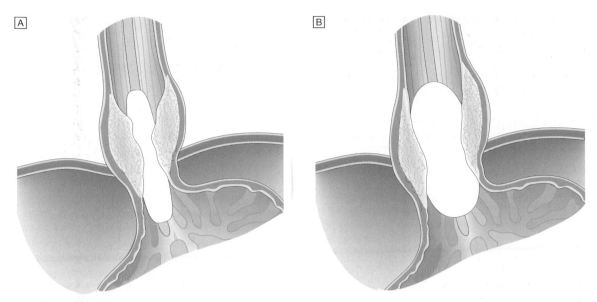

16

Fig. 16.9 Hydrostatic dilatation of achalasia.
A Balloon placed across the high-pressure zone at the oesophago-gastric junction. B Balloon expanded to disrupt the hypertonic muscle.

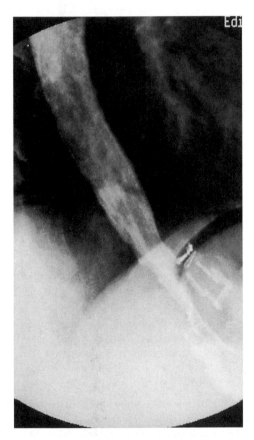

Fig. 16.10   Barium swallow after laparoscopic cardiomyotomy (Heller's procedure), with an anterior fundoplication in the same patient with achalasia, as shown before surgery in Figure 16.8.

5 cm above the oesophago-gastric junction and 3 cm down the stomach. Early complications include perforation and late complications include reflux oesophagitis, stricture formation, the development of an oesophageal diverticulum

and recurrent dysphagia from an inadequate myotomy. In order to reduce the risks of perforation and the development of reflux, most surgeons now prefer the abdominal route and carry out a partial anterior fundoplication at the same time. This helps to protect the area of the myotomy if there has been a small perforation of the mucosa, keeps the edges of the muscle apart and reduces post-operative gastro-oesophageal reflux (Fig. 16.10).

DIFFUSE OESOPHAGEAL SPASM

This disorder tends to occur in middle-aged to elderly patients. Complaints are of intermittent dysphagia and retrosternal pain, which can mimic angina. The symptoms are caused by repetitive irregular peristalsis of the oesophageal body.

Investigations
Barium swallow shows a characteristic corkscrew oesophagus, caused by the contracted muscle indenting the lumen (Fig. 16.11), and oesophageal manometry confirms the diagnosis.

Management
Medical treatment includes calcium channel blockers and proton pump inhibitors. Surgical treatment involves a long myotomy.

NUTCRACKER OESOPHAGUS

In this uncommon disorder, the symptoms are caused by repetitive forceful peristalsis. Manometry demonstrates normal peristalsis but with excessive amplitudes and pressures exceeding 150 mmHg. Medical treatment is similar to that of diffuse oesophageal spasm, but the results are disappointing. Dilatation and surgical myotomy also have poor results.

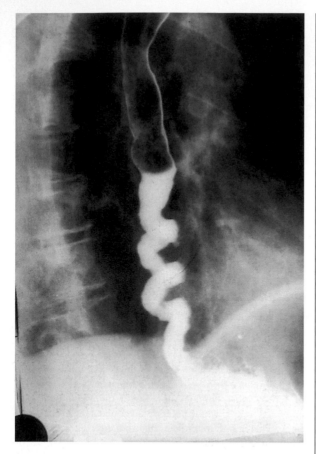

Fig. 16.11 Barium swallow showing appearances of diffuse oesophageal spasm.

PLUMMER–VINSON SYNDROME

This syndrome, first described by Paterson and Brown Kelly, is characterized by a post-cricoid web that results in dysphagia. The web is related to iron deficiency anaemia, but may be congenital or traumatic in origin. The squamous epithelium becomes hyperplastic and there is hyperkeratosis and desquamation, which leads to web formation.

Clinical features
Patients are commonly middle-aged women. Dysphagia is the main presenting complaint, but there may also be symptoms and signs of anaemia, including koilonychia, smooth tongue and angular stomatitis.

Investigations
A full blood count will show hypochromic microcytic anaemia and serum ferritin levels will be low. Barium swallow demonstrates a narrowing of the upper oesophagus with a web in the anterior wall; this is confirmed by endoscopy, during which a friable web can be seen across the lumen of the oesophagus.

Management
The web is dilated endoscopically and biopsies should also be taken, as there is an association with post-cricoid

carcinoma. The iron deficiency status is corrected by oral iron therapy.

POUCHES

Pouches are protrusions of mucosa through a weak area in the muscle wall. The best-known pouch lies in the pharynx and is associated with raised cricopharyngeal pressure, with the pouch developing through Killan's dehiscence, between the thyropharyngeus and cricopharyngeus muscles. Incoordination of swallowing and failure of relaxation of the cricopharyngeus muscle cause the herniation. The pharyngeal pouch usually develops posteriorly and is then forced by the vertebral column to deviate to the side, usually the left. Oesophageal pouches can occur around the tracheo-bronchial tree in relation to pressure from adjacent lymph nodes, if enlarged, and also just above the gastro-oeso-phageal junction in patients with raised lower oesophageal sphincter pressure.

Clinical features
Most patients are elderly and males are more commonly affected. Symptoms include regurgitation of food, halitosis, dysphagia, gurgling in the throat, aspiration and a lump in the neck (pharyngeal pouch); alternatively, the patient may be asymptomatic.

Investigations
Barium swallow demonstrates the pouch and the unco-ordinated swallowing. Endoscopy also confirms the diagnosis but must be performed with care to avoid accidental perforation of the pouch.

Management
Surgical myotomy of the cricopharyngeus and resection of the pouch used to be the surgical treatment of choice, but endoscopic stapling is now more common.

GASTRO-OESOPHAGEAL REFLUX

Gastro-oesophageal reflux is the most common cause of dyspepsia, affecting up to 30% of the population. It is caused by the retrograde flow of gastric acid through an incompetent cardiac sphincter into the lower oesophagus. The cardiac sphincter usually prevents reflux by the following mechanisms:

- a physiological high-pressure zone (not a true sphincter) in the lower end of the oesophagus
- the mucosal rosette at the cardia, which acts like a plug
- the angle at which the oesophagus joins the stomach between the left border of the oesophagus and the fundus (angle of His)
- the diaphragmatic sling (crura), which acts like a pinchcock at the lower end of the oesophagus
- the high-pressure area at the lower end of the oesophagus, caused by the positive intra-abdominal pressure.

Clinical features

The reflux of acid causes inflammation and ulceration to the oesophageal mucosa, which manifests as:

- *heartburn*, which is retrosternal burning pain, radiating to the epigastrium and through to the back
- *regurgitation* of acid stomach contents into the mouth (waterbrash)
- *dysphagia* from benign strictures or the development of non-specific motility disorders, both of which follow chronic reflux oesophagitis.

Investigations

The differential diagnosis includes myocardial ischaemia, peptic ulcer disease, cholecystitis and carcinoma of the oesophagus, and appropriate investigations are undertaken to exclude these other disorders.

Barium swallow and meal

A barium study might demonstrate a hiatus hernia, the possible presence of severe ulceration, benign strictures and reflux of contrast from the stomach into the oesophagus in the head-down position (Fig. 16.12).

Endoscopy

OGD will confirm reflux if oesophagitis is seen. Biopsies should be taken to establish the presence of inflammation and identify whether Barrett's metaplasia exists. Strictures can be dilated, but must also be biopsied to exclude malignancy.

pH monitoring and oesophageal manometry

Ambulatory 24-hour pH monitoring is the gold standard in establishing the diagnosis of acid reflux, although patients must have been off all proton pump inhibitor therapy for 7 days. Manometry is carried out at the same time to exclude

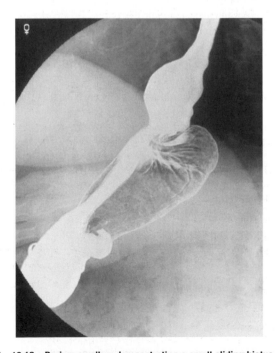

Fig. 16.12 Barium swallow demonstrating a small sliding hiatus hernia with gastro-oesophageal reflux.

> **EBM 16.1 SURGERY FOR GASTRO-OESOPHAGEAL REFLUX DISEASE**
>
> *'It has been shown that, following anti-reflux surgery, quality of life is improved and costs are reduced significantly compared with medical treatment. Anti-reflux surgery should be offered to patients with proven symptomatic reflux that cannot be controlled symptomatically with medical therapy.'*
>
> For further information:
> www.acg.gi.org/physicians/guidelines/GERDTreatment.pdf

16

other motility disorders, in particular achalasia, and to ensure that there is adequate muscular contraction in the lower oesophagus to prevent post-operative dysphagia if surgery is being considered.

Management

General treatment includes weight loss, sleeping with additional pillows and raising the head of the bed, and the avoidance of smoking, coffee, fatty foods and alcohol.

Medical treatment

Pharmacological treatment is extremely effective; it involves H_2-receptor antagonists or proton pump inhibitors to reduce gastric acid production, alginates to coat the oesophagus, and prokinetic agents such as metoclopramide to improve the lower oesophageal muscle tone and promote gastric emptying.

Anti-reflux surgery

Although surgical treatment of patients with severe anti-reflux disease has always been associated with good long-term outcomes, it has taken the introduction and refinements of laparoscopic techniques to bring the surgical option to more patients. The indications for surgery include those whose symptoms cannot be controlled by medical therapy, those with recurrent strictures despite treatment, and young patients who do not wish to continue taking acid suppression therapy for several decades. Symptoms that fail to be brought under control with acid suppression therapy are usually due to high-volume alkaline reflux, and surgery is an extremely effective cure (EBM 16.1). The presence of Barrett's metaplasia alone is not considered a suitable indication for anti-reflux surgery.

Surgery involves reduction of the hiatus hernia, if present, approximation of the crura around the lower oesophagus, and some form of fundoplication. This takes the form of mobilizing the fundus of the stomach from its attachments to the undersurface of the left hemidiaphragm and the left crus, and then wrapping it around the oesophagus, either anteriorly or posteriorly. The most common procedure currently performed is the Nissen fundoplication, in which the fundoplication is taken posteriorly around the lower oesophagus and sutured to the left anterior surface of the left side of the proximal stomach as a 360° wrap (Fig 16.13). Other procedures involving a partial (incomplete) fundoplication include the Toupet (posterior 270° wrap) and the Watson (anterior 180° wrap) repairs. Current data do not demonstrate much difference between the various approaches, provided the surgeon is experienced in the technique. All procedures have a success rate in

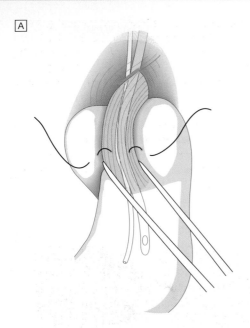

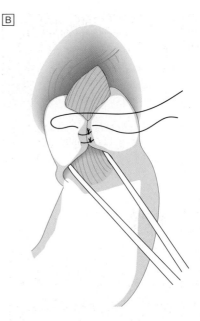

Fig. 16.13 Fundoplication for reflux oesophagitis. A Gastric fundus wrapped around the lower oesophagus. B Fundal wrap sutured in position.

curing the symptoms of reflux of around 95%. Unwanted complications after surgery (compared with those occurring in the perioperative period) include gas bloat (inability to belch) and dysphagia. These usually follow the formation of a wrap that is too tight, and are more likely after a complete fundoplication. These operations are now carried out laparoscopically, with excellent results in skilled hands.

Gastro-oesophageal reflux disease is one of the most common causes of vomiting in the first few months of life. In the majority of affected infants, simple measures, including the addition of thickening agents to milk feeds, the administration of alginates (e.g. Gaviscon) with or after feeds and the use of H_2-receptor blockers, will control symptoms. Most affected children outgrow this form of

reflux disease. In a small minority, surgery is required. The indications for fundoplication include failure to thrive despite optimal medical therapy, recurrent aspiration and chest infections, oesophageal stricture and haemorrhage from severe oesophagitis.

HIATUS HERNIA

A hiatus hernia is an abnormal protrusion of the stomach through the oesophageal diaphragmatic hiatus into the thorax. There are two types (Fig. 16.14): sliding (90%) and rolling (10%). A sliding hernia occurs when the stomach slides through the diaphragmatic hiatus, so that the gastro-oesophageal junction lies within the chest cavity. It is covered anteriorly by peritoneum, and posteriorly is

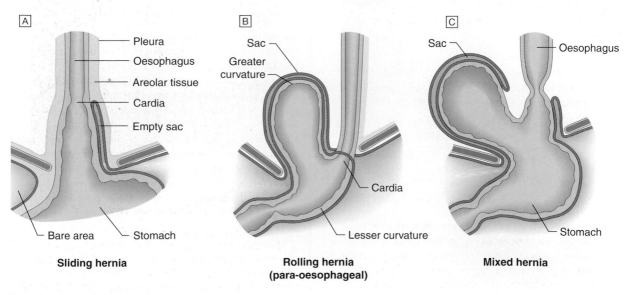

Sliding hernia

Rolling hernia (para-oesophageal)

Mixed hernia

Fig. 16.14   Types of hiatus hernia.

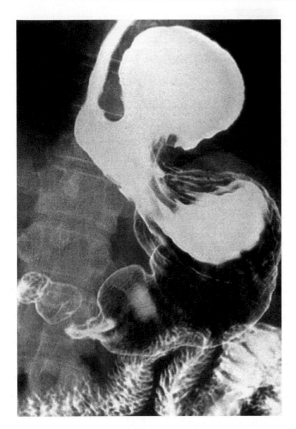

Fig. 16.15 Barium meal demonstrating a para-oesophageal hiatus hernia.

extraperitoneal. A rolling or para-oesophageal hernia is formed when the stomach rolls up anteriorly through the hiatus (Fig. 16.15); the cardia remains in its normal position and therefore the cardio-oesophageal sphincter remains intact.

Rolling and sliding hernias are caused by weakness of the muscles around the hiatus. They tend to occur in middle-aged and elderly patients. Women are affected more frequently than men and there is a higher incidence in the obese.

Clinical features

Hiatus hernias are often asymptomatic, but can produce some of or all the following symptoms:

- *Heartburn and regurgitation* owing to an incompetent lower oesophageal sphincter, which is aggravated by stooping and lying flat at night, and can be relieved by antacids.
- *Oesophagitis* resulting from persistent acid reflux, which leads to ulceration, bleeding with anaemia, fibrosis and stricture formation.
- *Epigastric and lower chest pain,* especially in para-oesophageal hernias, as the herniated part of the stomach (usually the fundus) becomes trapped in the hiatus. This can be a surgical emergency owing to the obstruction and strangulation of the stomach.
- *Palpitations and hiccups,* symptoms caused by the mass

effect of the hernia in the thoracic cavity irritating the pericardium and the diaphragm. In patients with a large rolling hiatus hernia, displacement of the whole stomach may result in a volvulus into the chest, producing symptoms of vomiting from gastric outflow obstruction.

Investigations

The diagnosis of hiatus hernia may be confirmed by performing a barium swallow and meal (Figs 16.12 and 16.15), or by upper gastrointestinal endoscopy. A chest X-ray may show a fluid level behind the heart and a widened mediastinum (Fig. 16.16).

16

A

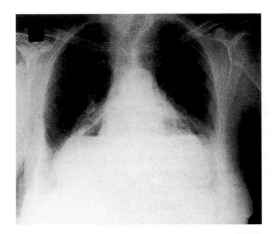

B

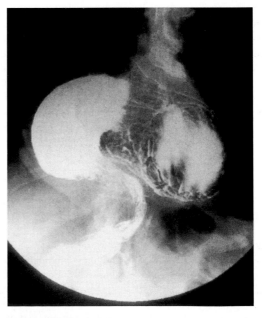

Fig. 16.16   Radiography in hiatus hernia.
[A] Erect chest X-ray in a patient with a large hiatus hernia with intrathoracic stomach. Note the air–fluid level behind the heart and the widened mediastinum. [B] Barium meal in the same patient.
(Reproduced from Hamilton Bailey's Emergency Surgery, 13th edn, with permission from Butterworth–Heinemann.)

BOX 16.1   HIATUS HERNIA

- Almost 95% of hiatus hernias are of the sliding type. Para-oesophageal (rolling) hernias are rare and mixed hernias are exceptional
- Sliding hernias are often associated with reflux oesophagitis and heartburn, but reflux can occur in the absence of herniation
- Symptomatic sliding hiatus hernias can be managed non-operatively in 85% of cases; some form of fundoplication is indicated if symptoms cannot be controlled by conservative measures
- Long-standing reflux may give rise to ulceration (with risk of bleeding, perforation and stenosis), and metaplasia may produce a Barrett's oesophagus and the risk of developing adenocarcinoma
- Para-oesophageal hernias are not normally associated with reflux, but frequently give rise to symptoms and may strangulate, so that surgical correction is advisable

Management

Treatment is as for gastro-oesophageal reflux disease; however, surgical repair of para-oesophageal hernias to prevent strangulation should always be considered in patients who are symptomatic.

BARRETT'S OESOPHAGUS

Barrett's oesophagus is columnar metaplasia of the lower oesophagus, which extends at least 3 cm above the gastro-oesophageal junction. It results from chronic damage by acid and bile reflux. The risk of adenocarcinoma is increased 40–90-fold by Barrett's oesophagus, and is particularly high in the presence of intestinal metaplasia. Patients discovered to have Barrett's oesophagus during endoscopy should be considered for endoscopic surveillance programmes. If severe dysplasia or carcinoma in situ is detected, and confirmed with repeat biopsies and review by a second pathologist, subtotal oesophagectomy should be considered. Current data suggest that, in this group of patients, an underlying carcinoma is detected in up to 50% of surgical resections.

Investigations

The diagnosis is made at endoscopy and confirmed histologically.

Management

Repeat biopsies after a course of proton pump inhibitors are recommended when a new diagnosis of Barrett's oeso-phagus has been made, as it is sometimes difficult for the pathologist to assess dysplasia in the presence of severe inflammation. There is no evidence at present that either long-term proton pump inhibitor therapy or anti-reflux surgery results in regression of Barrett's oesophagus, although they might prevent the subsequent development of dysplasia. This is currently an area of great interest and research.

TUMOURS OF THE OESOPHAGUS

BENIGN TUMOURS

These account for less than 1% of oesophageal neoplasms. The most common is the benign mixed stromal cell tumour (gastrointestinal stromal tumour, or GIST, all of which used to be called leiomyoma). This is usually asymptomatic, but may cause bleeding or dysphagia. It is best treated by local enucleation, with good results.

CARCINOMA OF THE OESOPHAGUS

The incidence of carcinoma of the oesophagus has risen in populations of developed countries over the last two decades to a figure of around 15/100 000 in parts of the UK, due primarily to an increase in adenocarcinoma. The male to female ratio is 3:1 and adenocarcinoma is predominantly a disease of Western white males. In the Far East and other parts of the world, particularly among some black males, there is a greater incidence of squamous cell carcinoma.

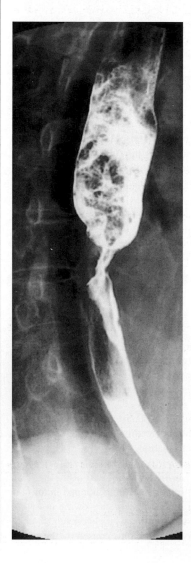

Fig. 16.17   Barium swallow in a patient with a carcinoma of the mid-oesophagus.

The most important risk factors for adenocarcinoma of the oesophagus are reflux and obesity, with a slightly increased risk of cardia tumours with smoking. Risk factors for squamous cell carcinoma include alcohol, smoking, leucoplakia, achalasia, the consumption of salted fish or pickled vegetables, and chewing tobacco and betel nuts.

Clinical features

Dysphagia that progresses from solids to liquids is one of the most common presentations. The average duration of symptoms at the time of presentation is between 3 and 9 months, and as a result, around 70% of patients are not operable at the time of diagnosis. Retrosternal pain on swallowing (odynophagia), regurgitation and aspiration pneumonitis are other forms of presentation.

Occasionally, patients may present with metastatic disease, including enlarged cervical lymph nodes, jaundice, hepatomegaly, hoarseness from recurrent laryngeal nerve involvement, and chest pain from mediastinal invasion. Other general features of malignancy include weight loss, anorexia, anaemia and lassitude.

Investigations

Even if the diagnosis is made initially by barium swallow (Fig. 16.17), it must always be confirmed by endoscopy and biopsy. For this reason, endoscopy is the best first-line investigation for anyone with dysphagia. Thereafter, investigations are aimed at accurate staging of the disease (Table 16.2) so as to assess resectability, determine a prognosis and identify patients who might benefit from neoadjuvant therapy. Local T (tumour) stage and N (nodal) spread are best assessed by endoscopic ultrasonography (Fig. 16.3). M (metastases) stage can be assessed with chest X-ray (lung secondaries), abdominal ultrasound (liver metastases and ascites), CT of the chest and abdomen (lung and liver metastases, distant lymphadenopathy) and laparoscopy (peritoneal metastases). Routine blood tests may reveal anaemia, liver disease and malnutrition, all of which require full assessment if surgery is to be considered. In those patients with proximal and middle-third tumours adjacent to the tracheobronchial tree, bronchoscopy can be a valuable investigation to assess airway invasion. If enlarged distant lymph nodes are detected, these should be aspirated for cytology, as surgical resection is contraindicated if they are positive for malignancy.

EBM 16.2   OESOPHAGEAL CANCER

'Morbidity, mortality and long-term survival rates are improved when patients are managed in high-volume centres offering major oesophageal resection. Recent studies have suggested that pre-operative chemotherapy improves survival in a small number of parients.'

For further information: 🖥 www.sign.ac.uk/guidelines
🖥 www.bsg.org.uk/pdf_word_docs/ogcancer.pdf

16

Management

The aim of treatment is to cure those with potentially curable disease and restore swallowing in the remainder. The overall 5-year survival rate remains very low (< 10%), although in patients who are suitable for resection, 5-year survival figures of 20–30% are possible (EBM 16.2).

Surgical resection

Patients with disease confined to the oesophagus and who are fit for surgery should be considered for resection. A certain proportion will be found to have more extensive disease at operation, but with better pre-operative staging, this figure should be small. Although surgical resection can provide reasonable palliation in some patients, setting out to perform a palliative resection is now not indicated because of the improvements in non-surgical palliative techniques.

There are several methods currently used to resect the oesophagus:

- *Ivor Lewis two-phase oesophagectomy.* This involves a laparotomy during which the stomach is fully mobilized on its vascular pedicles, along with the lower oesophagus. A right thoracotomy is then carried out to resect the oesophagus, and the mobilized stomach is brought up into the chest and anastomosed to the

---

Table 16.2   TNM STAGING OF OESOPHAGEAL CARCINOMA

T (Tumour)
- T_1 Tumour confined to submucosa
- T_2 Tumour extends into muscularis propria
- T_3 Tumour extends outside muscle layers
- T_4 Tumour invades adjacent structures (bronchus, aorta etc.)

N (Node)
- N_1 Lymph node metastases to para-oesophageal, cardia or left gastric regions

M (Metastases)
- M_0 No other metastatic spread
- M_1 Lymph node metastases to all other areas
  Metastases to liver, lung, brain, bone etc.

16

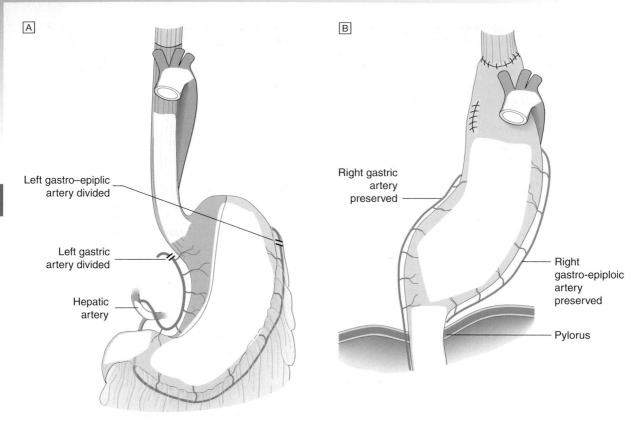

Left gastro–epiplic artery divided

Left gastric artery divided

Hepatic artery

Right gastric artery preserved

Right gastro-epiploic artery preserved

Pylorus

Fig. 16.18   Reconstruction after subtotal oesophagectomy.
Ⓐ Shaded area of oesophagus and proximal stomach to be resected. Ⓑ The remaining part of the stomach brought up to the level of the aortic arch and anastomosed to the proximal oesophagus.

proximal oesophagus. This is the preferred choice for middle and lower-third tumours (Fig. 16.18).

- *Left thoracolaparotomy.* This is a good approach for tumours around the oesophago-gastric junction, particularly when the tumour extends down into the proximal stomach and a more extensive gastric resection is required.
- *Transhiatal oesophagectomy.* This approach involves two surgeons, one operating through the abdomen and the other in the neck. The stomach is mobilized as for the Ivor Lewis procedure and the oesophagus is mobilized through the hiatus. The surgeon operating in the neck mobilizes the upper oesophagus and extends the dissection into the chest. The stomach is brought up into the neck and anastomosed to the proximal oesophagus. This technique is best suited to elderly patients with lower oesophageal tumours, in whom a thoracotomy should be avoided if possible. Patients in whom endoscopic ultrasound has demonstrated early tumours with no obvious lymph node metastases, particularly those with severe dysplasia in Barrett's oesophagus, are also suitable for this approach.

A segment of colon or small bowel can be used if it is not possible to reconstruct the oesophagus with stomach for any of these three techniques.

Post-operative care

In the early post-operative period, patients are managed in a high-dependency or intensive care unit. Nutrition can be provided by means of a feeding jejunostomy inserted at the same time as the resection.

Complications

Chest infections are the most common complication associated with pulmonary collapse and pneumothorax after thoracotomy. Adequate chest drainage, good analgesia and chest physiotherapy are all important in reducing this complication.

Anastomotic leakage occurs in 5–10% of patients and is the single most common reason for perioperative mortality, which should be less than 10% and is approximately 5% or lower in most specialist units. Anastomotic breakdown in the first few days after surgery represents a technical failure and usually results from ischaemia in the proximal part of the mobilized stomach. Early re-operation and revision of the anastomosis is the treatment of choice. Leaks that occur later are often well controlled by the chest drains, and provided the patient remains stable, can be managed non-operatively by nutritional support, antibiotics and nasogastric drainage. Assessment of the anastomosis is obtained by water-soluble contrast swallow and/or careful endoscopy.

BOX 16.2   CARCINOMA OF THE OESOPHAGUS

- Risk factors include chronic irritation (smoking, alcohol, betel nut, spices), obesity, nutritional deficiencies and environmental carcinogens (nitrosamines, *Aspergillus flavus*)
- Pre-malignant conditions include achalasia, Barrett's oesophagus, Plummer–Vinson syndrome, hiatus hernia and corrosive strictures
- World-wide, more oesophageal cancers are histologically squamous carcinomas and fewer are adenocarcinomas, which arise from columnar epithelium in the lower third (or extend upwards from the stomach). In the UK, adenocarcinoma is more common
- Late presentation with obstruction (dysphagia and regurgitation), aspiration pneumonitis, local invasion (recurrent laryngeal nerve, bronchus, mediastinum) and metastases is common
- Approximately 30% of oesophageal cancers are resectable. Squamous carcinomas may be radiosensitive
- Dysphagia in patients with unresectable cancers can be relieved by endoscopic or surgical intubation, laser treatment or surgical bypass (now rarely used)
- Overall 5-year survival rates are only 5%

Radiotherapy and chemotherapy

Radical chemoradiation can be used with curative intent on both adenocarcinoma and squamous cell carcinoma in patients not suitable for surgical resection. Although post-operative radiotherapy and/or chemotherapy (adjuvant therapy) have been shown to provide no additional survival advantage in patients with resectable disease, neoadjuvant therapy (pre-operative treatment) has produced encouraging results in recent randomized controlled clinical trials, and further developments can be expected in this area.

Palliation

Palliative treatment is used for patients with extensive disease and in those who are unfit for surgery. Treatment is aimed at the relief of symptoms, particularly dysphagia:

- *Endoscopic dilatation may* provide short-term relief and must be repeated at ever-shortening intervals.
- *Stent insertion* using expandable metal or rigid plastic stents (Fig. 16.19) provides good relief of dysphagia.

These can be inserted at surgery when an unresectable tumour is found, at endoscopy, or by interventional radiologists. The main problems include perforation during insertion, migration of the tube, blockage and tumour ingrowth. The latter can be rectified by laser ablation.

- *Laser ablation* can be carried out endoscopically and provides very good palliation of dysphagia, but does require to be repeated at regular intervals of 1–2 months. Perforation can result.
- *Radiotherapy and chemotherapy* have been used for palliation with limited success, although intra-luminal radiotherapy (brachytherapy) can be quite effective.
- *Analgesia and terminal care* are extremely important areas in palliation and are best provided by a multidisciplinary palliative care team.

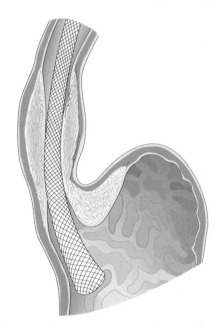

Fig. 16.19   Insertion of a metal stent to relieve dysphagia caused by obstructing cancer of the lower oesophagus.

A.C. DE BEAUX

Gastroduodenal disorders

SURGICAL ANATOMY

STOMACH

The stomach is an easily distensible viscus partly covered by the left costal margin. The diaphragm and left lobe of the liver lie on its anterior surface. Posteriorly, the stomach bed is formed by the diaphragm, spleen, left adrenal, upper part of the left kidney, splenic artery and pancreas. The greater and lesser curvatures correspond to the long and short borders of the stomach respectively, and the organ can be further divided anatomically into four distinct areas based on the microscopic mucosal appearance: namely, the cardia, fundus, body and antrum (Fig. 17.1). The stomach is limited at its proximal end by the oesophagogastric junction just below the lower oesophageal sphincter, a physiological sphincter that prevents stomach contents from regurgitating into the oesophagus. Distally, the stomach is limited by the pylorus, a true anatomical sphincter. It is composed of greatly thickened inner circular muscle and helps to regulate the emptying of stomach contents into the duodenum.

DUODENUM

The duodenum is divided into four parts, which are closely applied to the head of the pancreas. The first part is approximately 5 cm in length; its importance lies in the fact that it is the most common site for peptic ulceration to occur. The second part has on its medial wall the ampulla of Vater, where the conjoined pancreatic duct and common bile duct deliver their contents to the gastrointestinal tract. The third and fourth parts pass behind the transverse mesocolon into the infracolic compartment.

BLOOD SUPPLY

The stomach has an extensive blood supply (Fig. 17.1) derived from the coeliac axis. When the stomach is used as a conduit in the chest, as in an oesophagectomy, the left gastric, left gastroepiploic and short gastric vessels are divided, and the stomach then relies on the right gastric and right gastroepiploic vessels for viability. Ischaemia does not usually result because of the free communication between the vessels supplying the stomach. The blood supply to the duodenum is derived from both the coeliac axis (via the gastroduodenal artery) and branches from the superior mesenteric artery.

The veins from the stomach and the duodenum accompany the arteries and drain into the portal venous system.

LYMPHATICS

The lymphatics from the stomach accompany the arteries and drainage is to nodes around these vessels. Thereafter, drainage is to other groups around the aorta, liver, splenic hilum and pancreas, and then to the coeliac nodes. The lymphatics of the duodenum drain into the nodes located at the coeliac axis and superior mesenteric vessels.

NERVE SUPPLY

The parasympathetic nerve supply to the stomach is derived from the anterior and posterior vagal trunks. These pass through the diaphragm with the oesophagus. The anterior trunk gives off branches to the liver and gallbladder and descends along the lesser curvature. The posterior trunk gives off a coeliac branch and descends along the lesser curvature of the stomach, going on to supply the pancreas,

17

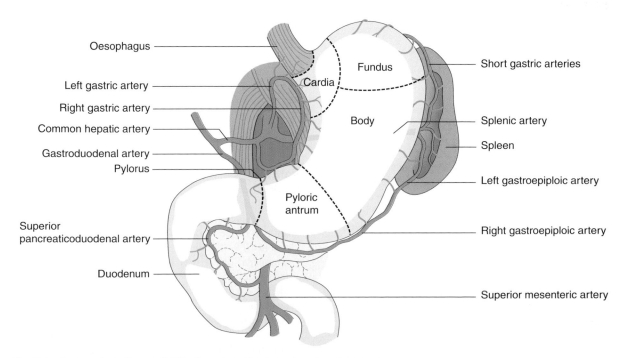

Fig. 17.1   Anatomy, including arterial blood supply to the stomach and proximal duodenum.

small intestine and large intestine as far as the distal transverse colon. The parasympathetic system supplies motor fibres to the stomach wall, inhibitory fibres to the pyloric sphincter (thus effecting relaxation of the sphincter), and secretomotor fibres to the glands of the stomach. Sympathetic fibres accompany the gastric arteries to reach the stomach from the coeliac ganglion. These provide motor fibres to the pyloric sphincter. The duodenum receives a sympathetic and parasympathetic supply from the coeliac and superior mesenteric plexuses.

SURGICAL PHYSIOLOGY

GASTRIC MOTILITY

Food is passed from the oesophagus into the stomach, where it is stored, ground and partially digested. As food enters the stomach, the muscles in the stomach walls relax and intragastric pressure rises only slightly. This effect is known as receptive relaxation, and is mediated by the vagus nerve. It is followed by muscular contractions that increase in amplitude and frequency, starting in the fundus and moving down towards the body and antrum. In the antrum, the main role is the grinding of food and propulsion of small amounts (now called chyme) into the duodenum when the pyloric sphincter relaxes.

Gastric emptying is controlled by two mechanisms: hormonal feedback and a neural reflex called the entero-gastric reflex. In the former, fat in the chyme is the main stimulus for the production of a number of hormones, the most powerful being cholecystokinin, which exerts a negative feedback effect on the stomach, decreasing its motility. The enterogastric reflex is initiated in the duodenal wall, and this further slows stomach emptying and secretion.

GASTRIC SECRETIONS

Classically, gastric secretion has been divided into three phases:

- *Cephalic (neural) phase.* Signals arise in the central cortex or appetite centres, triggered by the sight, smell, taste and thought of food, and travel down the vagus nerves to the stomach.
- *Gastric phase.* Food (in particular protein digestion products) causes the release of acid, this release controlled by a negative feedback mechanism dependent upon the pH of the stomach. The gastric phase accounts for the greatest part of daily secretion, approximately 1.5 litres.
- *Intestinal phase.* The presence of food in the duodenum triggers the release of a number of hormones, including duodenal gastrin. These exert a positive feedback effect on the stomach, causing a small increase in gastric secretion.

Mucus is produced by all regions of the stomach. It is composed mainly of glycoproteins, water and electrolytes, and serves two important functions. It acts as a lubricant, and it protects the surface of the stomach against the powerful digestive properties of acid and pepsin. Bicarbonate ions are secreted into the mucus gel layer and this creates a protective buffer zone against the effects of the low pH secretions. Alkaline mucus is produced in the duodenum and small intestine, where it has a similar function of mucosal protection.

The parietal cells in the stomach are responsible for the production of acid. Acid secretion by these cells is stimulated by two main factors: acetylcholine, released by the vagus nerve, and gastrin from the antrum. Acetylcholine and gastrin act on neuroendocrine cells located close to the parietal cells. On stimulation, these cells release histamine, which has a paracrine action on the parietal cell, stimulating acid production and secretion. Parietal cells secrete acid via an active transport mechanism, the proton pump. Somatostatin, gastric inhibitory peptide and vasoactive intestinal peptide inhibit acid secretion.

Pepsin is a proteolytic enzyme produced in its precursor form, pepsinogen, by the peptic cells found in the body and fundus of the stomach. Pepsinogen production is stimulated by acetylcholine from the vagus nerve. The precursor is then converted to its active form, pepsin, by the acid contents of the stomach.

Intrinsic factor is also produced by the parietal cells. It is a glycoprotein that binds to vitamin B_{12} present in the diet and carries it to the terminal ileum. Here specific receptors for intrinsic factor exist and the complex is taken up by the mucosa. Intrinsic factor is broken down and vitamin B_{12} is then absorbed into the blood stream.

PEPTIC ULCERATION

Peptic ulceration affects areas of mucosa exposed to acidic gastric contents. The main pathology is an imbalance between the acid–pepsin system and the mucosal ability to resist digestion. Ulceration can occur at a number of sites, including the oesophagus, stomach, duodenum, and in the jejunum following a gastrojejunostomy. Rarely, ulceration may occur in the ileum close to a Meckel's diverticulum containing ectopic acid-secreting gastric mucosa. Duodenal ulcers occur four times more commonly than gastric ulcers.

Pathology

Duodenal ulcers usually occur in the first part of the duodenum and 50% occur on the anterior wall. The majority of gastric ulcers develop on the lesser curvature in the distal half of the stomach. They may coexist with duodenal ulcers in 10% of patients.

Duodenal ulcers may be acute or chronic. Ulcers with a history of less than 3 months' duration and with no evidence of fibrosis are considered to be acute. Gastric ulcers generally run a chronic course.

Gastric ulcers may be benign or malignant. Malignancy was once thought to be a complicating factor of benign gastric ulceration. It is now realized that malignant change in a benign ulcer is rare, and that such ulcers are in fact probably malignant from the outset. Duodenal ulcers are very rarely malignant.

Aetiology

Helicobacter pylori

H. pylori is present in around 50% of the world's population, its prevalence increasing with age. It is more prevalent in developing countries, where poor and crowded living conditions are commonplace, and here the infection is probably acquired in early life via the faecal–oral or oral–oral route. Once an individual is infected, the *H. pylori* persists; in the majority of patients, there are no symptoms.

H. pylori is detected in 95% of patients with duodenal ulceration. It infects the mucosa of the antrum of the stomach, where it causes an inflammatory response. This gastritis stimulates the gastrin-producing (G) cells of the antrum to increase gastrin production. The subsequent hypersecretion of acid provides an ideal environment for gastric metaplasia of the duodenal mucosa to occur. The colonization of the metaplastic areas by *H. pylori* further damages the mucosa, and ultimately duodenal ulceration occurs.

H. pylori is found in approximately 75% of cases of gastric ulcers, although its role here is less well defined. It may be that the gastritis facilitates the access of acid and pepsin to the stomach mucosa. It seems that the key factor is decreased mucosal resistance, with excess acid having less of a role. Indeed, most patients with gastric ulceration have a normal or decreased secretory capacity.

Non-steroidal anti-inflammatory drugs (NSAIDs)

This group of drugs includes aspirin, ibuprofen and diclofenac. Their role as anti-inflammatory agents centres on their inhibition of prostaglandin synthesis by inhibiting the action of cyclo-oxygenase. In the stomach, prostaglandins are responsible for the production of mucus and bicarbonate. These both help to protect the stomach mucosa from acid by maintaining an alkaline buffer zone. By inhibiting prostaglandin synthesis, NSAIDs damage the gastric mucosa and are implicated in 30% of gastric ulcers. They may also be responsible for the small number of *H. pylori*-negative duodenal ulcers.

Smoking

This is an aetiological factor in both duodenal and gastric ulceration, but is more important in gastric ulceration. Smoking also delays ulcer healing, and there is an increased likelihood of complications (e.g. bleeding or perforation) developing in smokers.

Genetic factors

First-degree relatives of patients with a duodenal ulcer are at increased risk of developing a duodenal ulcer themselves. This risk is further increased if ulcers develop in patients under 20 years of age. First-degree relatives of patients with gastric ulcers are also at increased risk of developing gastric ulcers.

Zollinger–Ellison syndrome

This is a rare syndrome caused by a gastrin-secreting tumour (gastrinoma), which is normally found in the pancreas but may occasionally be found in the duodenum or stomach. Approximately 30% of patients have features consistent with multiple endocrine neoplasia syndrome (MEN I). Hypergastrinaemia results in a greatly increased risk of peptic ulceration. Diarrhoea may be a prominent feature, owing to large volumes of acid being secreted into the small intestine. Inactivation of the pancreatic lipase causes steatorrhoea. Complications of ulceration (pain, bleeding and stenosis) are common.

The diagnosis of Zollinger–Ellison is problematic, but ulceration in unusual sites, at an early age, or ulcers persisting despite medical treatment should be reviewed with a high index of suspicion and serum gastrin measured. Computed tomography (CT) or magnetic resonance imaging (MRI) and selective angiography may be used to localize the tumour and its metastases, if present.

Cure is effected by removal of the tumour wherever possible, although this may be made more difficult by the presence of metastatic disease, a very small tumour or multifocal disease. Removal is often supplemented with control of acid secretion using proton pump inhibitors.

Other factors

Other patients at risk of peptic ulceration include those with blood group O and those with hyperparathyroidism. Hyperparathyroidism causes elevated calcium levels, thus stimulating acid secretion. With resolution of the condition, spontaneous ulcer healing usually occurs.

Clinical features

Recurrent well-localized epigastric pain is typical of peptic ulcer disease. Classically, the pain of a gastric ulcer occurs during eating and is relieved by vomiting. Patients with duodenal ulceration characteristically describe pain when they are hungry. This pain is relieved by food, antacids, milk and vomiting. Often, however, these well-defined features are not present, and it is usually impossible to differentiate between the pain of gastric ulceration and that of duodenal ulceration. Other symptoms associated with peptic ulcer disease include heartburn, anorexia, waterbrash (a sudden flow of saliva into the mouth) and intolerance of certain foods. Intermittent vomiting may occur. Where persistent vomiting is troublesome, the possibility of gastric outlet obstruction should be considered. Such vomiting tends to be projectile and may contain recognizable food eaten many hours previously.

Differential diagnosis

Epigastric pain, with or without the other symptoms described above, may present in a variety of other conditions, both surgical and medical (Table 17.1).

The diagnosis of peptic ulcer disease may not be straight-forward. This is particularly true in the elderly patient on NSAIDs. In such patients, pain may be absent and they may present for the first time with complications of ulceration, such as bleeding or perforation.

Diagnosis

The full blood count may indicate iron-deficiency anaemia in the patient with a chronically bleeding ulcer. The bio-

17

Table 17.1	CAUSES OF EPIGASTRIC PAIN

Surgical
- Biliary colic or acute cholecystitis
- Pancreatitis
- Mesenteric ischaemia
- Perforation of a viscus
- Acute appendicitis
- Gastro-oesophageal malignancy

Medical
- Gastro-oesophageal reflux disease
- Myocardial infarction
- Pulmonary embolism
- Lower lobe pneumonia
- Irritable bowel syndrome

chemical screen may reveal dehydration and hypokalaemia from vomiting. Where hypergastrinaemia is suspected (e.g. Zollinger–Ellison syndrome), serum gastrin should be estimated. Calcium may be elevated in patients with hyperparathyroidism.

Endoscopy is now preferred to contrast studies in the investigation of peptic ulcer disease. It allows good visualization (Fig. 17.2) and biopsy of lesions, and the detection of *H. pylori* using the CLO test. In the latter, a biopsy specimen taken from the antrum is placed in a gel containing urea. Ammonia released by the action of the *H. pylori*-derived urease is detected and causes a colour change—in most kits, from yellow to pink/red. Biopsy of gastric ulcers is particularly important, as malignancy needs to be excluded.

Contrast studies are still used where endoscopy is con-traindicated, e.g. the use of Gastromiro studies in suspected perforation. They have no role as a first-line investigation for uncomplicated disease.

Ultrasound may be useful to exclude coexistent patholo-gy. Cholelithiasis and peptic ulcer disease share similar symptoms and often coexist. In addition to identifying gall-stones, ultrasound is useful for assessing the pancreas, and provides information regarding the texture of the liver and

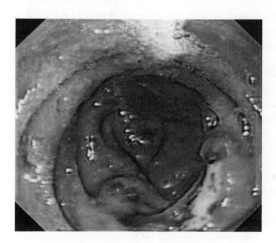

Fig. 17.2   Endoscopic appearance of a duodenal ulcer.

the presence of intraperitoneal fluid or gas in the acute setting.

SPECIAL FORMS OF ULCERATION

Stress ulceration refers to erosions or ulceration of the stomach or duodenum occurring in certain circumstances. These include severe illness, trauma, prolonged mechanical ventilation, multiple organ failure, sepsis and major surgery. The aetiology is not fully defined, although acid and mucosal ischaemia appear to be key elements. Medical prophylaxis using proton pump inhibitors may be useful in such circumstances.

Cushing's and Curling's ulcers are special forms of stress ulceration that occur following central nervous injury and burns, respectively. Hypersecretion of acid is not always essential for stress ulceration to occur, but does appear to be important in both of these conditions. In neurosurgical injury, raised intracranial pressure may be responsible for an increase in vagal activity and hence the increase in gastric secretion. The ulcers resulting from hypersecretion are usually single and, in common with other forms of peptic ulceration, may be complicated by perforation and bleeding.

MANAGEMENT OF UNCOMPLICATED PEPTIC ULCER DISEASE

Since the discovery of the link between *H. pylori* and peptic ulceration, the management of uncomplicated ulcer disease has changed greatly. Surgery has become outdated, its use now being limited to patients in whom malignancy has been proven, and those in whom complications, e.g. bleeding, perforation or stenosis, have developed.

The aims of medical treatment are symptomatic relief, accelerated ulcer healing and the prevention of ulcer relapse.

Medical management
General measures helpful in the management of peptic ulcers include the avoidance of NSAIDs, smoking and excessive alcohol. In *H. pylori*-negative patients on NSAIDs, in whom the use of these drugs cannot be avoided altogether, the least damaging agents should be used, e.g. ibuprofen. The protective role of selective cyclo-oxygenase inhibitors (so-called COX-2 inhibitors) in minimizing peptic ulceration is not fully established. These should be pre-scribed with an antisecretory agent. Antisecretory agents include selective histamine receptor antagonists and proton pump inhibitors (PPIs). H_2 antagonists competitively inhibit histamine at the target cell receptor and can decrease acid secretion by up to 80%. They have been largely replaced by the PPIs (e.g. omeprazole or lansoprazole). These agents act by irreversibly inhibiting H^+/K^+ ATPase and thus are powerful inhibitors of acid secretion.

Other agents that may be used to supplement anti-secretory agents include bismuth compounds, sucralfate, prostaglandin analogues and antacids.

Eradication of H. pylori

- *Duodenal ulcers.* Eradication of the *H. pylori* has become the mainstay of management in patients with

---

EBM 17.1   THE ROLE OF *HELICOBACTER PYLORI* ERADICATION IN THE TREATMENT OF PEPTIC ULCERATION

'RCTs have found that Helicobacter eradication is superior to acid-lowering drugs in duodenal ulcer healing, and both are superior to no treatment. In preventing duodenal ulcer recurrence, eradication therapy was similar to maintenance acid-lowering drugs, but eradication therapy was superior to no treatment. In gastric ulcer healing, eradication therapy was similar to acid-lowering drugs. In preventing gastric ulcer recurrence, eradication therapy was superior to no treatment.'

Ford A, et al. Cochrane Database of Systematic Reviews 2004; CD003840.

EBM 17.2   PEPTIC ULCER RECURRENCE IN PATIENTS ON NSAIDS OR ASPIRIN

'In an RCT in patients with healed gastric ulcer and successful eradication therapy, misoprostol or a proton pump inhibitor was superior to placebo in preventing ulcer recurrence. An RCT in Helicobacter-positive patients taking NSAIDs showed that eradication therapy did not prevent duodenal ulcer formation.'

Goldstein JL, et al. Clin Ther 2004; 26:1637–1643.
Lai KC, et al. Aliment Pharmacol Ther 2003; 17:799–805.

---

a duodenal ulcer (EBM 17.1). Eradication therapies comprise an antisecretory agent, typically a PPI, together with one or more antibiotics. The course is usually given for 1–2 weeks. Eradication rates of greater than 90% occur with good compliance, although reinfection following successful eradication is possible. Without eradication therapy, approximately 80% of ulcers will recur within 1 year (EBM 17.2). Complete resolution of symptoms is a good indicator of successful eradication. However, where symptoms persist, it is advisable to recheck the *H. pylori* status. This may be done using the *H. pylori* breath test. Like the CLO test, this relies on the hydrolysis of urea by *H. pylori*. Urea is labelled with ^{13}C which, when hydrolysed, is expired as $^{13}CO_2$. The test should be undertaken at least 4 weeks after finishing the course of eradication therapy. Earlier testing may give rise to false negative results owing to suppression of the bacterium rather than true eradication. True persisting infection should be treated with an alternative eradication course.

- *Gastric ulcers.* Malignancy should be excluded by endoscopic biopsy before a diagnosis of benign gastric ulcer is made. Where a patient is found to be *H. pylori*-positive at endoscopy, eradication therapy should be instituted. Without eradication, the relapse rate is in the region of 50%, but this falls to less than 10% with successful eradication therapy. Endoscopic surveillance of a treated ulcer should continue until healing is complete. Failure to heal warrants further biopsies.

Surgical management

- *Duodenal ulceration.* Surgery for uncomplicated duodenal ulceration is now extremely rare. Operations such as a truncal vagotomy, highly selective vagotomy, or gastric resectional surgery have had little role since the introduction of eradication therapy.
- *Gastric ulceration.* Failure of conservative therapy to heal a gastric ulcer is an indication for surgical intervention. Where malignancy cannot be excluded or is suspected, resection of the ulcer is the treatment of choice. The extent and type of resection will be determined by the position of the ulcer within the stomach and its suspected malignant potential. Benign distal ulcers may be treated by a Billroth I gastrectomy, whereby the distal part of the stomach is removed and the proximal stump anastomosed to the duodenum (Fig. 17.3A). More proximal ulcers usually necessitate a Polya-type reconstruction involving anastomosis of the gastric remnant to the jejunum (Fig. 17.3B).

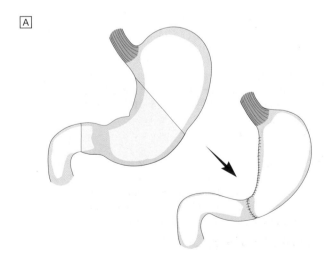
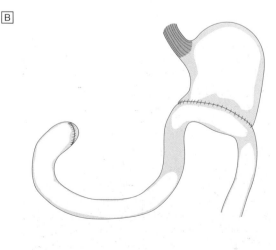

Fig. 17.3   Gastrectomy for peptic ulceration.
A Billroth I after partial gastrectomy. B Polya or Billroth II reconstruction.

A number of patients are still alive who have had anti-ulcer surgery. A number of them will be suffering long-term effects of such surgery.

Dumping

This arises in up to 20% of patients following gastric resection and encompasses a range of vasomotor symptoms, including light-headedness, tachycardia, flushing, sweats and palpitations. Occasionally, these are accompanied by diarrhoea and vomiting.

Early dumping (or dumping syndrome proper) occurs 15–30 minutes after eating. The rapid emptying of hyperosmolar (mainly carbohydrate) gastric contents into the small intestine leads to the influx of fluid down an osmotic gradient into the bowel lumen. The symptoms associated with the syndrome are due to both the sudden contraction of the extracellular fluid compartment and intestinal distension causing increased peristalsis. The patient often needs to lie down until the symptoms pass. In the majority of patients, symptoms improve spontaneously with conservative measures, which include taking smaller, dry and frequent meals, avoiding excessive carbohydrate intake, and avoiding liquids at mealtimes.

Late dumping is much less common than early dumping. It is a reactive hypoglycaemia caused by more rapid absorption of glucose from the upper small intestine. This causes hyperglycaemia, which in turn leads to increased insulin production and rebound hypoglycaemia. The symptoms are of a similar nature to those of the dumping syndrome proper (or early dumping), but may include hunger and confusion and occur 1–3 hours after eating. Late dumping is symptomatically controlled with sugar.

Diarrhoea

Rapid influx of gastric contents into the small intestine and an interruption of vagal fibres to abdominal viscera are thought to be responsible. The diarrhoea may be associated with mild steatorrhoea. Codeine-related compounds or loperamide may be used to treat the diarrhoea, although they are not always helpful. Eating small, dry meals lacking in refined carbohydrates can help. Surgical methods to slow bowel transit have not proved to be successful.

General nutritional effects

Up to 40% of patients lose weight following surgery for peptic ulcers. For the most part, decreased oral intake is responsible, and this may be due to vomiting or dumping. Early satiety following surgery (e.g. due to a small gastric remnant) may also contribute. Malabsorption may also play a role, as there is generally accelerated emptying of gastric contents into the small intestine following surgery. Bacterial overgrowth may also contribute to malabsorption.

Anaemia

This may occur some time after any form of gastric surgery and is particularly common following complete gastrectomy. The picture may be one of iron, B_{12} or folate deficiency, or a mixture of the three. Iron deficiency is the most common and may be part of a generalized poor intake, as described above. It may also result from depressed acid-dependent reduction of iron salts, this process being necessary for the body's utilization of iron. B_{12} deficiency

---

> **BOX 17.1 PEPTIC ULCERATION**
>
> - Peptic ulceration results from an imbalance between acid–pepsin secretion and the ability of the mucosal defences (mucosa, mucus and trapped bicarbonate) of the gastrointestinal tract to withstand acid and pepsin injury
> - Three factors known to cause peptic ulceration are infection with *Helicobacter pylori*, the use of non-steroidal anti-inflammatory drugs and the rare Zollinger–Ellison syndrome
> - Duodenal ulceration is more common than gastric ulceration; other sites that may be affected are the oesophagus, jejunum and Meckel's diverticulum
> - The incidence of peptic ulceration is declining and the need for elective surgery has fallen dramatically with the availability of antisecretory drugs, such as the H_2-receptor antagonists and the proton pump inhibitors, in combination with antibiotics (eradication therapy)
> - Despite the falling incidence, complications of peptic ulceration (bleeding and perforation) are still major causes of death in elderly patients

occurs when insufficient intrinsic factor is available for its absorption. This usually only arises after extensive gastric resection, as the stomach generally produces far more intrinsic factor than is actually needed for B_{12} absorption. Folate deficiency may result from poor oral intake.

Osteoporosis and osteomalacia

These conditions are associated with partial gastrectomy owing to decreased absorption of calcium and vitamin D. Such bone disease may manifest itself many years postoperatively as pathological fractures. Vitamin D and calcium supplementation is indicated on a long-term basis, especially in women.

Carcinoma

Following partial gastric resection, there is an increased risk of the long-term development of gastric cancer. The aetiology is not clear, but the reflux of bile into the stomach, relative hypochlorhydria and *H. pylori* infection are likely to play a role.

Cholelithiasis

Current evidence suggests that there is an increased risk of developing gallstones following surgery for peptic ulcers. The mechanisms involved have not been fully established.

COMPLICATIONS OF PEPTIC ULCERATION REQUIRING OPERATIVE INTERVENTION

PERFORATION

- *Duodenal ulcers.* Up to 50% of patients will have had no previous ulcer symptoms. The incidence of duodenal ulcer perforation is decreasing, probably due in part to improvements in the medical management of duodenal ulcers. Perforation usually occurs in acute ulcers on the anterior wall of the duodenum.
- *Gastric ulcers.* Gastric ulcer perforation is less common than duodenal ulcer perforation. It has a peak incidence in the elderly, and consequently the associated

morbidity and mortality are higher. Gastric perforation has a strong association with NSAID use.

Clinical features

The acute onset of severe unremitting epigastric pain is strongly suggestive of the possibility of perforation. Thereafter, the range of symptoms depends on the intra-abdominal course. The patient may be pale, shocked and peripherally shut down secondary to generalized peritonitis. Irritant stomach contents in the peritoneal cavity may give rise to shoulder-tip pain, resulting from irritation of the diaphragm. Vomiting may occur. The abdomen does not move freely with respiration, and marked tenderness, guarding, fear of movement and board-like rigidity may be found on examination. Respiration is shallow and bowel sounds are usually absent.

Generalized peritonitis does not occur in some patients because the perforation seals over with omentum. In others, the fluid tracks down the right paracolic gutter, simulating acute appendicitis. Silent perforations may also occur, and are only found incidentally on a chest X-ray.

Diagnosis

In 60% of cases of perforation, an erect chest X-ray will demonstrate free air under the diaphragm, although the absence of free air does not exclude a perforation (Fig. 17.4). A lateral decubitus film can be useful where an erect chest X-ray is not feasible, e.g. because of shock or disability.

A moderate hyperamylasaemia may be found with a perforated duodenal ulcer. High amylase levels are more suggestive of pancreatitis. Where there is still doubt over the diagnosis, an emergency water-soluble contrast meal or an abdominal CT scan may be indicated.

Management

The initial management, as for other causes of peritonitis, consists of resuscitation, oxygen, intravenous fluids and antibiotics (e.g. cefuroxime and metronidazole), and the passage of a nasogastric tube. Adequate analgesia and antiemetics should be given as necessary. A urinary catheter enables close monitoring of urine output.

Operative management is indicated in most patients, but rapid operative intervention should not be substituted for thorough resuscitation. Although a laparoscopic approach to treatment is favoured by some, its superiority over open surgery is yet to be established:

- *Duodenal ulcers.* Surgery usually involves simple closure, whereby the ulcer is under-run with sutures or plugged using an omental patch (Fig. 17.5), coupled with a thorough peritoneal lavage. All patients should be given eradication therapy. In some cases, there may be a place for the non-operative management of perforated ulcers. This may be appropriate in patients with silent perforations and those too ill to undergo

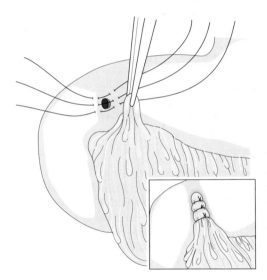

Fig. 17.5 Closure of duodenal perforation.

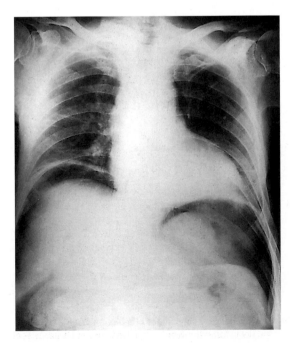

Fig. 17.4 Chest X-ray showing air under the diaphragm.

BOX 17.2 PERFORATED PEPTIC ULCER

- Perforated duodenal ulcer is more common than perforated gastric ulcer
- Ulcer perforation still carries a significant mortality (10%), particularly in the elderly and those with intercurrent disease
- Free gas beneath the diaphragm on an erect abdominal or chest film confirms the diagnosis in two-thirds of cases; a Gastromiro meal may be helpful if free gas is not present
- Perforated duodenal ulcers can be dealt with by simple closure and the application of an omental patch, followed by eradication therapy
- Patients who present late or who are deemed too ill for operation can be managed by conservative means (nasogastric aspiration and intravenous fluids, antibiotics and antisecretory drugs)
- Perforated 'gastric ulcers' frequently prove to be perforated gastric tumours (15% of cases), but simple closure and omental patch is the treatment of choice following biopsy of the ulcer wall

17

laparotomy (e.g. due to severe cardiorespiratory disease). Where the decision has been made not to operate, management consists of supportive treatment with nasogastric suction, *H. pylori* eradication therapy, intravenous fluids and antisecretory agents. Close supervision of the patient is necessary, as evidence of clinical deterioration suggests failure of conservative treatment.

- *Gastric ulcers.* Approximately 15% of perforated gastric ulcers prove ultimately to be malignant. However, current practice suggests biopsy of the ulcer wall, followed by simple closure or local excision of the ulcer, is best. If the ulcer turns out to be malignant, a minority will progress to gastric resection following tumour staging (see below).

ACUTE HAEMORRHAGE

The differential diagnosis of upper gastrointestinal bleeding is summarized in Table 17.2. Upper gastrointestinal bleeding presents with haematemesis (vomiting blood) and/or melaena (the passage of black tarry stool that has a very characteristic smell). Melaena results from the digestion of blood by enzymes and bacteria. Less commonly, melaena may be the result of a bleed from the right colon. Very rarely, if bleeding is very brisk, upper gastrointestinal bleeding may present as fresh rectal bleeding, in which case signs of cardiovascular instability are present. Slow chronic blood loss may be asymptomatic and detected on rectal examination by a positive faecal occult blood test.

Diagnosis

History and examination

A full history and examination are essential in determining the cause of the bleeding. Pointers to the diagnosis include the past medical history (peptic ulcer disease, previous bleeding, liver disease, previous surgery, coagulopathies), drug history (most importantly, NSAIDs and anticoagulants) and social history (alcohol abuse).

Specific features to be looked for include those suggestive of acute substantial blood loss and shock (hypotension, tachycardia, tachypnoea and pallor), and

signs of liver disease and portal hypertension (spider naevi, portosystemic shunting and bruising). The latter are particularly important, as variceal haemorrhage necessitates specific treatment.

Blood tests

The full blood count may be normal immediately after an acute bleed but will fall once haemodilution has occurred. The test may show anaemia, suggestive of more chronic blood loss. Urea is often high following a gastrointestinal bleed, due to the absorption of blood and its subsequent metabolism by the liver. Coagulation derangement occurs in the presence of significant liver disease.

Management

Resuscitation

Bleeding is now the most common cause of death from peptic ulcer disease and resuscitation is vital. Following the administration of high-flow oxygen, intravenous access is obtained and blood taken for the investigations noted above. A sample is also taken for blood cross-matching and intravenous fluids started.

A nasogastric tube is passed to monitor the bleeding and prevent aspiration. A urinary catheter is inserted. A central or arterial line may aid resuscitation. Volume replacement is gauged against pulse, blood pressure, urine output and central venous pressure. Over-transfusion or rapid transfusion in those with compromised cardiac function can lead to pulmonary oedema.

Detection and endoscopic treatment

The aims of management of bleeding peptic ulcers are to identify the bleeding point, arrest the bleeding (bleeding ceases spontaneously in 90% of patients) and prevent recurrence. Once resuscitation has stabilized the patient, endoscopy is used to detect the site of bleeding (Fig. 17.6), doing so in 80–90% of cases. Endoscopy may also be

Table 17.2 CAUSES OF UPPER GASTROINTESTINAL BLEEDING	
• Peptic ulceration	50%
• Mucosal lesions including gastritis Duodenitis and erosions	30%
• Mallory–Weiss tear	5–10%
• Varices	5–10%
• Reflux oesophagitis	5%
• Angiodysplasia	2%
• Carcinoma	Uncommon
• Aortoduodenal fistula	Uncommon
• Dieulafoy syndrome (rupture of a large tortuous submucosal artery normally found in the body of the stomach)	Rare
• Coagulopathies	Uncommon

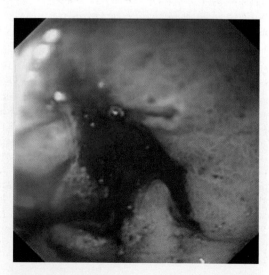

Fig. 17.6 Endoscopy appearance of a bleeding duodenal ulcer. Note the clot in the ulcer crater—a sign indicating a significant risk of rebleeding.

BOX 17.3 BLEEDING FROM PEPTIC ULCERATION

- Bleeding affects some 20% of peptic ulcer patients and remains a major source of mortality in patients older than 55 years
- Bleeding from peptic ulceration is the most common cause of upper gastrointestinal bleeding, but bleeding from gastritis, duodenitis and erosions is almost as common (each responsible for 30–40% of cases)
- The three priorities are to prevent exsanguination (prompt resuscitation), define the source of bleeding (endoscopy) and institute appropriate therapy
- Almost 90% of patients stop bleeding on conservative management. Factors associated with further bleeding include old age, shock on admission, endoscopic stigmata (arterial spurting, visible vessel, fresh clot), and gastric rather than duodenal ulcer
- The conventional operation in those who continue to bleed from duodenal ulceration consists of opening the duodenum and under-running the bleeding point. Bleeding gastric ulcer can be treated using similar principles or by excision of the ulcer. Very rarely, partial gastrectomy may be necessary
- Surgery can now be avoided in many cases by using endoscopic means (injection, laser or heat coagulation) to arrest continued bleeding

---

Table 17.3 CAUSES OF GASTRIC OUTLET OBSTRUCTION

- Peptic ulcer disease
- Malignancy
  Stomach antrum
  Pancreas
  Lymphomas
- Crohn's disease of duodenum
- Adult hypertrophic pyloric stenosis
- Inflammation of adjacent organs
- Gastroparesis

17

used to stop or prevent further bleeding. This is appropriate when stigmata of recent haemorrhage are present. These include active bleeding from the ulcer base, the presence of a visible vessel, and adherent clot overlying the ulcer. These features are associated with a significantly increased risk of further bleeding from the ulcer. Injection sclerotherapy (e.g. with adrenaline (epinephrine) 1:10 000 or sclerosants) is commonly used, but other methods include the use of heat probes and clips. Therapeutic endoscopy can also be used in the management of oesophageal and gastric varices and vascular malformations.

In patients in whom endoscopy does not identify the bleeding point, angiography may be used, but the limitation of this investigation is that it can only detect active bleeding of greater than 1 ml/min. In these patients, selective embolization can be used to stop the bleeding and thus avoid the need for surgery. The main drawback of this is that in some cases it may lead to mesenteric ischaemia.

Surgical management

Emergency surgery may be indicated if endoscopy reveals bleeding from a major artery and where attempted injection sclerotherapy is unable to control the bleeding directly; 50% of patients with active arterial bleeding and 30% with a visible vessel at the ulcer base are ultimately likely to require surgery. When bleeding recurs after therapeutic endoscopy, a further endoscopy may be able to control the bleeding. Recurrent bleeding is associated with significant morbidity and mortality, particularly in the elderly. Continuing bleeding is particularly common in those with a chronic ulcer and is more common in gastric ulceration. The type of operation used depends on the site of the bleeding ulcer and the comorbidity of the patient:

- *Duodenal ulcers.* A bleeding duodenal ulcer may simply be under-run with sutures, through a duodenotomy (opening of the anterior wall of the duodenum) to gain access to the ulcer. Once tolerating oral fluids, the patient should be started on *H. pylori* eradication therapy empirically.
- *Gastric ulcers.* With a bleeding gastric ulcer, the possibility of malignancy must be considered. The ulcer must be biopsied in all cases to determine its nature. In young fit patients, the ulcer should be excised completely by taking a small wedge resection. In elderly patients or those with significant comorbidity, under-running of the ulcer may be preferable, at least in the first instance. If the pathology result confirms malignancy, then the patient should have accurate staging and further treatment as indicated. If the ulcer proves to be benign, *H. pylori* eradication is indicated. NSAIDs should be avoided.

PYLORIC STENOSIS

Pyloric stenosis consists of narrowing of the pyloric channel, leading to gastric outlet obstruction. The obstruction may be anywhere in the region of the pylorus, but most commonly occurs in the first part of the duodenum. The most common cause in adults is peptic ulceration but other causes are shown in Table 17.3.

Clinical features

Gastric outlet obstruction presents with symptoms of fullness and often a constant dull pain in the epigastrium. Projectile vomiting of large volumes of undigested and partially digested food matter is characteristic. This is more common later in the day and when lying down, and usually relieves the sensation of fullness. There may be associated weight loss.

On examination there is commonly epigastric fullness associated with signs of dehydration and weight loss. Visible gastric peristalsis may be seen and is diagnostic of gastric outlet obstruction. A succussion splash (i.e. an audible splashing noise when the patient is gently rocked from side to side) is often elicited.

Management

When gastric outlet obstruction is suspected, a large-bore nasogastric tube is passed. Often, large volumes of non-bilious gastric contents can be aspirated and undigested food may be recognized. Intravenous access is obtained and bloods sent for full blood count, urea and electrolytes.

Biochemical analysis usually reflects dehydration, with a low sodium, potassium and chloride and a high urea and bicarbonate. The further obligatory loss of potassium by the kidneys results in a hypokalaemic metabolic alkalosis. As the alkalosis worsens, potassium stores become so depleted that hydrogen ions are excreted instead of potassium by the kidney, and the result is aciduria—the so-called paradoxical aciduria of gastric outlet obstruction. If the history of outlet obstruction is chronic, biochemistry may also reflect a degree of starvation (i.e. hypoalbuminaemia).

Gastric outlet obstruction is further investigated using radiological contrast studies (e.g. barium meal) or endoscopy. Endoscopy is the investigation of choice, as biopsies can establish the nature of the obstruction.

In most patients there is no indication for urgent laparotomy and their fluid and electrolyte balance should be corrected prior to any surgery. In long-standing cases, there may also be some benefit from intravenous feeding prior to surgery to improve the patient's overall nutritional status. Surgery is not always necessary and, assuming the pathology is benign, a course of PPIs may be sufficient to heal the ulceration and relieve the obstruction. Where surgery is necessary and where the pathology is benign, a pyloroplasty or gastrojejunostomy may suffice, but antrectomy is a more reliable operation to minimize the risk of ulcer recurrence. Where malignancy is identified, more radical surgery may be necessary.

INFANTILE HYPERTROPHIC PYLORIC STENOSIS

Infantile hypertrophic pyloric stenosis is a common cause of vomiting in the first 8 weeks of life. Male, first-born infants are most frequently affected and there is a higher incidence in the presence of an affected male relative. Infants present with vomiting of increasing amounts of milk feed, until they vomit after every meal. The vomiting is classically described as 'projectile', but the fact that the vomiting occurs after every feed is a much more important observation. The child will cry with hunger after vomiting the feed, but further attempts to satisfy this hunger will result in further vomiting. Continuing vomiting will result in dehydration, loss of gastric acid, and the classic picture of a hypokalaemic, hypochloraemic, metabolic alkalosis. The child may have paradoxical aciduria.

The diagnosis can be made clinically. Visible gastric peristalsis and palpation of the hypertrophied pylorus during feeding clinch the diagnosis. This is possible in 60–75% of cases. In the remainder, ultrasound scanning will reveal thickening and lengthening of the pyloric canal. After a period of careful rehydration to correct the biochemical imbalances, a pyloromyotomy is performed using an open or, in a few centres, a laparoscopic technique. The serosa of the pylorus is cut and the thick, hypertrophied muscle tumour is split down to the mucosa.

Complications following this operation are rare, but include haemorrhage, inadequate myotomy, wound infection and wound dehiscence.

GASTRIC NEOPLASIA

BENIGN GASTRIC NEOPLASMS

Benign tumours of the stomach may arise from epithelial or mesenchymal tissue. Adenomatous polyps may be single or multiple and are the most common benign epithelial neoplasm. Gastrointestinal stromal tumours are likely to be benign if measuring less than 5 cm in maximum dimension. Such benign lesions may be an incidental finding during investigation, but can give rise to bleeding or intermittent pyloric obstruction with vomiting. The benign nature of these lesions is confirmed by endoscopic biopsy. Small lesions may be removed at endoscopy by diathermy wire, but large polyps should be resected surgically in view of the risk of malignancy.

MALIGNANT GASTRIC NEOPLASMS

Gastric carcinoma

Epidemiology
Adenocarcinoma is the most common malignancy affecting the stomach. It accounts for 90% of malignant tumours found within the stomach, lymphomas, carcinoids and gastrointestinal stromal tumours making up the rest. The incidence of gastric cancer has decreased substantially in the last 50 years. Gastric cancer principally affects those in the 60–80-year age group, but is not infrequently seen in younger patients. Where once the tumour was more commonly noted in the gastric antrum, its incidence in this region has diminished and a corresponding increase in incidence in the proximal stomach has occurred. The male:female ratio is 2:1. Gastric cancer has the fifth poorest 5-year survival rate after cancer of the pancreas, liver, oesophagus and lung.

Aetiology
No definitive aetiological agents have been recognized but the environment is thought to have considerable influence. Environmental factors include diet and socioeconomic status. In addition, several conditions have been described that are associated with the development of malignant change within the stomach:

- *Diet.* Gastric cancer is noted more commonly where malnutrition is prevalent. It has also been associated with the use of certain preservatives in food; nitrates, nitrites and nitrosamines have been implicated. Where soils are rich in nitrates or dietary intake is high, gastric carcinoma is more common. A high vitamin intake is thought to be protective against the development of cancer of the stomach. Diets rich in carotene and vitamins C and E have been shown to reduce the incidence of intestinal metaplasia in the stomach, a condition thought to be associated with malignant change.
- *H. pylori infection.* Recent epidemiological studies have suggested that *H. pylori* may be associated with an increased incidence of malignant change within

17

EBM 17.3   THE ROLE OF *HELICOBACTER PYLORI* ERADICATION IN THE PREVENTION OF GASTRIC CANCER

'RCTs have found that Helicobacter *eradication reduces the risk of developing gastric cancer as long as pre-malignant lesions do not pre-exist at the time of eradication.*'

Ley C, et al. Cancer Epidemiol Biomarkers Prev 2004; 13:4–10.
Wong BC, et al. JAMA 2004; 291:187–194.

the stomach (EBM 17.3). At the present time, it is thought that its ability to produce ammonia as well as other mutagenic chemicals may play a part in neoplastic transformation of the gastric mucosa. Such changes are thought to be enhanced by lack of vitamin C.

- *Gastric polyps.* Hyperplastic and adenomatous polyps are the most frequently found, but only the latter have significant malignant potential. Studies have shown that over one-quarter of adenomatous polyps may show malignant changes within them. Furthermore, gastric carcinoma is frequently encountered in stomachs affected by polyps. This suggests that conditions necessary for the development of polyps may also enhance the development of malignancy.
- *Gastroenterostomy.* Where there has been a previous gastric resection or duodenal bypass for benign disease and the remaining stomach has been anastomosed to the bile-containing upper gastrointestinal tract, the stomach remnant is more vulnerable to malignant change than the intact stomach. The risk of malignant change increases with the time elapsed since surgery. Patients who have had gastric resections with gastroenterostomy may be 4–5 times more liable to develop gastric carcinoma in the stomach remnant than the normal population.
- *Chronic gastric ulcer disease.* It is thought that chronic peptic ulceration in the stomach increases the risk of malignant change within the ulcer. It has been extremely difficult to assess the true level of risk with such ulcers, but it is thought to be low. Such chronic ulcers, however, deserve close observation by endoscopy and biopsy at frequent intervals until they have healed.
- *Chronic atrophic gastritis.* This condition is associated with a loss of the gastric glands from the stomach mucosa. It has been noted to be more frequent in patients at increased risk of developing stomach cancer. Chronic atrophic gastritis is associated with pernicious anaemia, which is linked to an increased risk of gastric cancer. Such patients have a fourfold increased risk compared to the normal population.
- *Intestinal metaplasia.* This condition arises when the gastric mucosa is replaced by mucosa containing glands that have features more in common with those found in the small intestine. Such changes are usually found in the distal part of the stomach and are associated with an increased risk of development of gastric carcinoma.
- *Gastric dysplasia.* When the gastric mucosal cells become less uniform in size, shape and organization, dysplastic changes may result and may be low- or high-grade. Patients with high-grade dysplasia often have associated malignant change.
- *Host factors.* Blood group A is associated with an increased risk of developing gastric cancer. A variety of oncogenes have been associated with stomach cancer.

Early gastric cancer

Early gastric cancer results when neoplastic cells are limited to the mucosa or submucosal layers of the stomach wall. By definition, this type of cancer is confined to the most superficial layers of the stomach wall but it can be associated in a small minority of patients with lymph node metastases. Such tumours, if adequately treated surgically, are associated with 5-year survival rates in excess of 90%. The survival rate will depend upon the depth of invasion of the tumour and the presence or absence of lymph node metastases at the time of surgical excision. Early gastric cancer in the UK accounts for approximately 10% of all resected cases of gastric adenocarcinoma.

Advanced gastric cancer

The vast majority of malignant tumours found in the stomach are of the advanced gastric adenocarcinoma type. These tumours have penetrated more deeply into the stomach wall than those of early gastric cancers, and many will have transgressed the stomach wall to invade adjacent structures. Lymphatics are more frequently involved than in early gastric cancer. Should the entire thickness of the stomach wall have been penetrated, transperitoneal spread and invasion of surrounding structures by tumour is frequent. Haematogenous spread also occurs via the portal system and may lead to metastases in the liver. Advanced gastric cancer is therefore frequently associated with a variety of distant manifestations that preclude surgical resection for cure. Another feature may be linitis plastica, a diffuse thickening of the stomach wall, making it rigid and non-distensible (Fig. 17.7).

Factors affecting survival in advanced gastric cancer

The survival of patients with advanced gastric cancer depends upon their state of fitness at the time of diagnosis, and on the stage of the cancer when it is discovered and treated. Treatment usually implies surgical resection, as this is the only effective means of possible cure available at present. For surgery to be curative, excision must be adequate, with margins clear of the tumour and with satisfactory en bloc resection of all possible involved lymph nodes (EBMs 17.4 and 17.5). Such surgery will offer the best chance of cure or a prolonged disease-free interval before recurrence. Less than half of patients diagnosed with gastric cancer will be suitable for gastric resection.

Poor survival has been correlated with depth of tumour invasion through the stomach wall, involvement of tumour resection margins and the presence of lymph node metastases. Transgression of the tumour through the stomach wall is associated with very poor survival, as the tumour is able to spread transperitoneally and therefore seed the peritoneum with malignant cells, making complete surgical excision impossible.

17

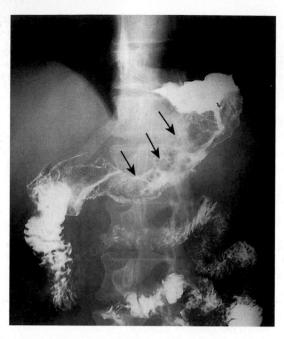

Fig. 17.7 Barium meal examination showing extensive gastric carcinoma causing narrowing of the gastric lumen (arrowed).

EBM 17.4 THE ROLE OF THE SENTINEL LYMPH NODE IN GASTRIC CANCER

'The use of sentinel node mapping and biopsy in planning the need for and radicality of lymph node dissection in gastric cancer is controversial. Two papers, one from Europe and one from China, suggest opposing views regarding tumour spread to the sentinel node.'

Moenig SP, et al. Anticancer Res 2005; 25:1349–1352.
Cheng LY, et al. World J Gastroenterol 2004;
10:3053–3055.

EBM 17.5 D1 VERSUS D2 (RADICAL) LYMPH NODE DISSECTION IN GASTRIC CANCER

'Systematic reviews have failed to show a benefit for more radical resection because of the increased morbidity and mortality of more radical lymphadenectomy, which rises further if a splenectomy or pancreatectomy is performed. Subgroup analysis suggests a survival benefit for T_3 and T_4 tumours with more radical surgery. Learning curves of surgeons and centres performing low-volume cancer surgery may confound any benefit of more radical surgery.'

McCulloch P, et al. Cochrane Database of Systemic Reviews 2004; CD001964.

A comprehensive pathological classification of tumours has enabled the prognosis of a particular stage of cancer to be estimated. Such staging is usually classified according to the tumour size (T), the node status (N), and the presence or absence of distant metastases (M) (Table 17.4).

Table 17.4 TNM CLASSIFICATION OF GASTRIC CARCINOMA*	
T (Tumour)	
• T_1	Tumour invades lamina propria or submucosa
• T_2	Tumour invades muscularis propria or subserosa
• T_3	Tumour invades serosa
• T_4	Tumour invades adjacent structures
N (Node)	
• N_0	No lymph node involvement
• N_1	Fewer than 7 lymph nodes involved by tumour
• N_2	7–15 lymph nodes involved by tumour
• N_3	More than 15 lymph nodes involved by tumour
M (Metastases)	
• M_0	No metastases
• M_1	Metastases present

* Greene FL, Page DL, Fleming ID, et al, eds. AJCC cancer staging manual. 6th edn. Springer-Verlag: New York; 2002.

Clinical features of gastric malignancy

The symptomatology of gastric carcinoma may be subtle, and mild symptoms of indigestion, flatulence or dyspepsia may be the early signs of malignancy. Such symptoms should not be overlooked and should not be treated without further investigation, particularly in patients in a vulnerable age group (> 40 years).

The severity of symptoms is not invariably associated with the stage of disease. More advanced gastric cancer tends to be associated with weight loss, anaemia, dysphagia, vomiting, epigastric or back pain, or the presence of an epigastric mass. The patient may also manifest signs of more widespread distant metastases, such as jaundice (liver secondaries or compression of the biliary tree by enlarged lymph nodes), ascites, spurious diarrhoea (secondary to pelvic infiltration), and signs and symptoms of intestinal obstruction secondary to malignant deposits on the bowel.

Diagnosis

Diagnosis is made on the basis of a thorough medical history and clinical examination. Weight loss may be evident. An epigastric mass may be palpable and ascites may be present. The liver and supraclavicular lymph nodes should be palpated for metastatic disease. A digital rectal examination may detect transcolonic spread to the pelvis. Thereafter, general tests assessing the patient's nutritional status and renal and hepatic function, as well as a full blood count, should be carried out. The diagnosis is confirmed by upper gastrointestinal endoscopy and biopsy of any suspicious lesions. Following histological diagnosis, the patient needs to have the tumour staged, and an assessment of comorbidity should also be made.

Staging of gastric carcinoma

CT of the chest and abdomen should be carried out to visualize the lungs, liver, peritoneal cavity, and perigastric and retroperitoneal lymph nodes (Fig. 17.8). Laparoscopy with laparoscopic ultrasound may help to detect small metastases within the liver, and laparoscopy alone may detect small-volume ascites and very small tumour nodules on the peritoneal surface not detected by CT. Endoscopic

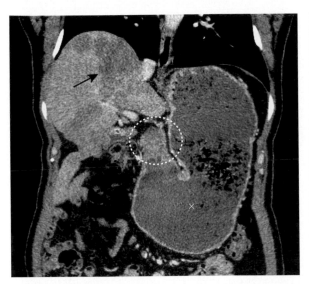

Fig. 17.8   Coronal reconstruction of a distal gastric cancer (dashed circle), with gross dilatation (cross) of the more proximal stomach (by fluid and air).
The liver is enlarged by bulky metastases (arrowed).

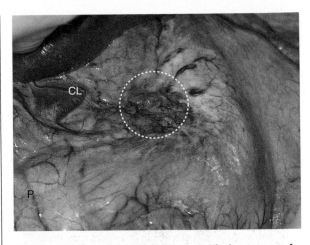

Fig. 17.9   Operative view of gastric cancer on the lesser curve of the stomach, with obvious nodes (dashed circle) close to the tumour in the lesser omentum.
The left lobe of the liver is being retracted upwards and the caudate lobe (CL) of the liver is visible through the lesser omentum. The pylorus (P) is evident in the bottom left of the picture.

ultrasound has little role in the staging of gastric cancer at present.

Where the disease is thought to be resectable (T_1–T_3 and no evidence of distant metastases) and the patient is sufficiently fit, surgical resection with the associated lymphatic drainage is indicated. Occasionally, when there has been direct invasion of other structures from the stomach tumour (T_4), wide resection for cure involving the resection of adjacent organs can be considered. This radical resection of the stomach along with its draining lymph nodes is termed a D2 resection, as opposed to a more limited nodal dissection close to the stomach wall and the tumour, termed a D1 resection. When neighbouring organs such as the pancreas are included in the en bloc resection, this is termed a D3 resection.

Resection with curative intent—radical total gastrectomy

This procedure involves the removal of the entire stomach, together with the distal part of the abdominal oesophagus and the proximal part of the duodenum. In such a radical procedure, attention is also paid to the removal of surrounding structures in which metastases may occur. These include the greater and lesser omenta and related lymph nodes (Fig. 17.9). For more proximal gastric cancers, splenectomy may be necessary for tumour clearance.

Reconstruction involves refashioning the small bowel, allowing bile to enter lower down the gastrointestinal tract, thereby preventing regurgitation of corrosive bile into the lower oesophagus. The most common form of reconstruction is Roux-en-Y (Fig. 17.10).

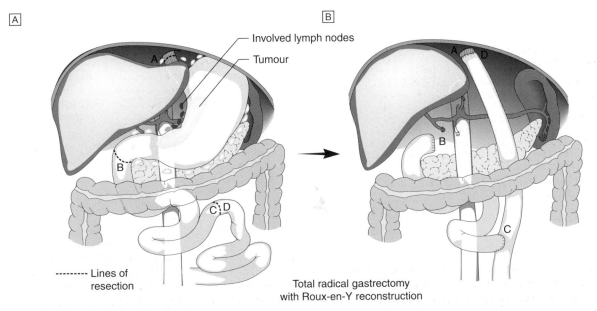

A Before surgery.

Involved lymph nodes
Tumour

Total radical gastrectomy with Roux-en-Y reconstruction

-------- Lines of resection

Fig. 17.10   Resection with curative intent.
A Before surgery. B Total radical gastrectomy with Roux-en-Y reconstruction.

17

BOX 17.4   GASTRIC CARCINOMA

- Gastric cancer is the second most common cause of death from gastrointestinal malignancy (i.e. after colorectal cancer)
- The disease is particularly common in Japan, Chile, Iceland and Eastern Europe, but its incidence in many Western countries has declined markedly throughout the last century, for reasons that are not clear
- Aetiological factors include pernicious anaemia, atrophic gastritis and achlorhydria, and previous partial gastrectomy. Dietary factors (smoked foods, low intake of fresh fruit and vegetables), the formation of carcinogenic nitrosamines (from dietary nitrate) and occupational factors (mining, rubber, asbestos) are also implicated
- Many patients have incurable and unresectable disease at presentation, and overall 5-year survival rates in Western countries are less than 15%
- Lymph node involvement is a major determinant of survival in patients undergoing gastric resection; the 5-year survival rate in patients with uninvolved nodes is 50%, whereas with involved nodes it is only 10%
- Five-year survival rates of 90% have been achieved in Japan following resection of screening-detected cancers confined to the mucosa/submucosa

---

On occasion, it may be possible to carry out radical sub-total gastrectomy, in which 90% of the stomach is removed and a small proximal cuff is left close to the cardia, thereby allowing a small gastric reservoir to remain. This is thought to allow better digestive functioning post-operatively, but such gastric preservation can only take place if appropriate clearance of the tumour has been achieved.

Such radical procedures should carry a mortality of less than 5%.

Palliative bypass

This type of operation is designed principally for advanced distal gastric tumours that are unresectable for cure and fixed to vital structures such as the common bile duct or major vessels or pancreas. Bypass is achieved by anastomosing the small bowel (jejunum) to the stomach proximal to the obstructing lesion (Fig. 17.11).

Palliative care

With advanced disease or if the patient is unfit, palliative measures such as stenting or laser therapy may be required to control the worst symptoms of the tumour. Chemotherapy and radiotherapy have only a limited role in the palliation of disease in a small proportion of patients. Recent trials have suggested that combinations of drugs, including epirubicin, cisplatin and 5-fluorouracil, may cause shrinkage of some gastric carcinomas and may in some circumstances render previously inoperable tumours operable (EBM 17.6).

EBM 17.6   THE ROLE OF PALLIATIVE CHEMOTHERAPY IN GASTRIC CANCER

'Systematic reviews show a modest survival benefit for palliative chemotherapy in gastric cancer, with ECF (epirubicin, cisplatin and 5-fluorouracil) regimens currently amongst the more effective. Newer combinations with irinotecan- or taxane-based regimens show promising results.'

Wohrer SS, et al. Ann Oncol 2004; 15:1585–1595.

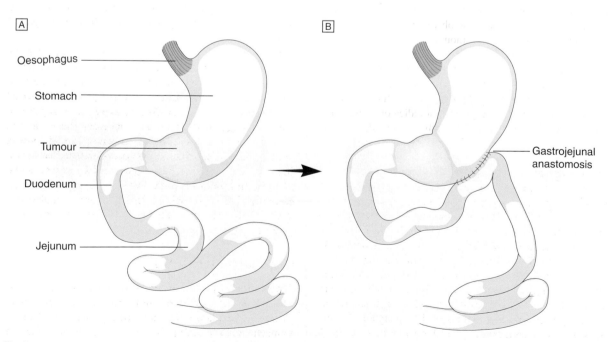

Fig. 17.11   Palliative bypass procedure for gastric carcinoma.
[A] Obstructing antral gastric carcinoma. [B] Jejunum anastomosed to stomach proximal to obstructing tumour.

Table 17.5 **EXAMPLES OF STAGES OF GASTRIC CANCER AND THEIR PROGNOSIS**	
Stage	5-year survival (%)
$T_1N_0M_0$	95+
$T_1N_1M_0$	70–80
$T_2N_1M_0$	45–50
$T_3N_2M_0$	15–25
M_1	0–10

Prognosis

When the tumour is confined to the mucosa or submucosa without lymph node or distant metastases, a 5-year survival of the order of 95–100% can be achieved. With increasing penetration of the tumour through the stomach wall and increasing numbers of nodes involved, the 5-year survival decreases. A further deterioration occurs when distant metastases are present, in which case 5-year survival is unusual (Table 17.5).

OTHER GASTRIC TUMOURS

Gastrointestinal stromal tumours (GIST)

These were previously described as leiomyomas or leiomyosarcomas, according to their malignant potential as judged by the pathologist. They are now known to be a different kind of cancer, with a specific treatment that controls the growth. They account for less than 1% of all gastric malignancies. Such tumours are more commonly found in resected or postmortem specimens as incidental findings. Only infrequently do they contribute to clinical problems such as bleeding or obstruction. GIST are now considered to be stromal tumours, as it is believed that they may arise from stromal fibroblasts, whereas previously they were thought to have arisen from smooth muscle cells. It is difficult to ascertain the malignant potential of these tumours, but histological features (mitotic figure counts) as well as size are significant indicators. Metastatic tumour in lymph nodes or other organs confirms malignancy.

Lymphomas

The stomach represents the most common site for gastrointestinal lymphomas, which are malignant aggregations of lymphatic tissue. Many lymphomas are thought to arise from mucosa-associated lymphoid tissue and are therefore frequently referred to as MALT lymphomas. In such cases, there is a frequent association with the presence of *H. pylori* infection, which, it is thought, may bring about a lymphomatous change. Such lymphomas are usually low-grade and may respond to eradication of the *H. pylori* infection. Occasionally, lymphomas may transform to a high-grade type of tumour that carries a poorer prognosis. Such tumours are more likely to require more aggressive treatment with chemotherapy. Surgery

is reserved for specific indications such as perforation or bleeding.

Carcinoid tumours

These are tumours of neuroendocrine origin that vary enormously in their malignant potential. The majority encountered are benign, but occasionally malignant carcinoids can be extremely aggressive. When associated with liver metastases, they can result in the carcinoid syndrome, which is related to the over-production of 5-hydroxytryptamine.

MISCELLANEOUS DISORDERS OF THE STOMACH

MÉNÉTRIER'S DISEASE

This is a condition of gastric mucosal hypertrophy, in which the mucosal rugal folds are grossly enlarged in the fundus and body of the stomach; the antrum is usually spared. Mucosal hypertrophy may lead to abnormally large secretions of mucus or acid. Over-secretion of acid and protein-rich mucus may contribute to symptoms of epigastric pain and hypoproteinaemia.

Ménétrier's disease is associated with a high incidence of malignancy in the stomach; once it has been diagnosed, total gastrectomy is indicated in the otherwise fit patient.

GASTRITIS

This common condition is due to inflammation of the gastric mucosal lining. It may be caused by a variety of injurious agents, both chemical and bacteriological. It is frequently associated with over-indulgence in alcohol. Biliary gastritis is seen in the presence of bile in the stomach (frequently seen after Polya-type partial gastrectomy).

Gastritis may arise as a consequence of extreme stress resulting from shock, and this form is therefore more frequently encountered in the intensive care situation. Such gastritis is thought to be a consequence of mucosal hypoperfusion and acidosis secondary to a shock-like state. This combination leads to mucosal ischaemia and resulting stress gastritis, which can cause loss of mucosa resulting in erosions that may on occasion bleed profusely. Gastritis may be lessened or prevented by resuscitation, administering mucosal protective agents, and neutralizing or minimizing gastric acid secretion. Surgery is undertaken rarely to control massive haemorrhage resulting from gastritis.

DIEULAFOY'S LESION

A condition of profuse bleeding from an abnormal vessel situated in the gastric mucosa and not associated with ulceration, Dieulafoy's lesion is usually found in the upper stomach. Such bleeding is treated initially by injection sclerotherapy, but may require open gastrotomy and oversewing of the bleeding point.

17

GASTRIC VOLVULUS

Volvulus results from twisting of the stomach about its long axis between the two relative fixed points of the oesophageal hiatus and the duodenum. The volvulus often takes place into a hiatus hernia. Complications of this include obstruction and strangulation, both of which necessitate emergency surgery. The diagnosis is confirmed by chest X-ray and contrast studies. Immediate laparotomy is advised to reduce the hernia, repair the diaphragmatic defect and anchor the stomach in the abdomen to prevent recurrence.

BEZOARS

Accumulations of hair (trichobezoars) or vegetable matter (phytobezoars) or combinations of the two (trichophyto-bezoars), these may on occasion form a complete cast of the stomach, and the ensuing reduced nutritional intake contributes to malnourishment. The diagnosis is made by barium examination and surgical removal is advisable.

MISCELLANEOUS CONDITIONS OF THE DUODENUM

DUODENAL OBSTRUCTION

Common causes of duodenal obstruction are pyloric stenosis and carcinoma of the pancreas. Rarer causes include blockage by mesenteric lymph nodes, duodenal diverticulum, duodenal atresia, annular pancreas and chronic duodenal ileus. If surgical treatment is required, bypass by duodenojejunal or gastrojejunal anastomosis is often appropriate. Symptomatic diverticula may have to be excised. Chronic duodenal ileus is an ill-defined entity that may affect visceroptotic females and rapidly growing, thin children. It has been suggested that the duodenum is obstructed by the superior mesenteric vessels as they cross its third part, but most surgeons are sceptical about this explanation. The condition is usually self-limiting in children, but in adults surgical bypass may have to be considered.

DUODENAL DIVERTICULA

The duodenum is the second most common site for diverticulum formation in the gastrointestinal tract. The diverticula rarely develop before the age of 40 years, and are often found at the point of entry of the common bile duct. They are frequently discovered incidentally at endoscopy or on barium meal examination, but can cause obstruction, bleeding and inflammation (diverticulitis). Symptomatic diverticula should be excised if it is certain that they are the cause of problems.

DUODENAL TRAUMA

Duodenal damage may follow severe crush injury of the upper abdomen (Ch. 9).

SURGERY FOR OBESITY

Obesity is an increasing problem world-wide. It is defined as a body mass index (BMI) greater than 32; morbid obesity represents a BMI greater than 38. (Until recently, the cut-offs were 30 and 35 respectively.) The effect of obesity on the respiratory, cardiovascular, locomotor and metabolic systems, as well as on mental health, can be severe. Patients with morbid obesity have a significantly reduced life expectancy; for example, a person with a BMI of 45 at the age of 25 will have a reduction in life expectancy of 11 years.

Prevention is better than cure and indeed there is no current 'cure' for obesity. Weight reduction programmes combining reduced calorie intake with increased exercise have variable results. Weight loss is slow and the programme often requires to be followed for many, many months. Furthermore, a change in eating and exercising behaviour is necessary if the weight loss is to be maintained long-term.

Patients who are morbidly obese can benefit from obesity or bariatric surgery. Such patients need to be assessed very carefully, taking account of their mental state, physical fitness, and the presence of medical conditions that lead to obesity but can be corrected by treatment (e.g. hypothyroidism). The careful selection of patients involves a multidisciplinary team approach.

A number of operations have been performed for obesity in the past. Many of the intestinal bypass operations and jaw wiring procedures are relegated to history. Current obesity surgery is designed to be restrictive or malabsorptive:

- *Restrictive*—decreases food intake, as the patient suffers early satiety even after small meals. Overeating causes upper abdominal pain, and vomiting may be required to relieve it.
- *Malabsorptive*—alters digestion, leading to food intake being poorly absorbed and eliminated in the stool. Overeating typically leads to excessive diarrhoea and flatulence.

OPERATIONS FOR OBESITY

Current options include gastric banding, vertical banded gastroplasty, gastric bypass and duodenal switch. All these operations can be performed laparosopically. However, the technical difficulty of such surgery increases in the order that these operations are listed above. The more complex operations are more likely to lead to better excess weight loss in the short term. However, there is increasing evidence to show that the percentage of excess weight loss at 3 years is similar for gastric banding and gastric bypass. The procedures can be combined; for example, gastric banding is technically easier to perform in the very obese patient who has a BMI greater than 55. Once excess weight loss has plateaued, removing the band and performing a gastric bypass may allow further excess weight loss.

The gastric band is a ring with an inflatable inner cuff, which is placed laparoscopically a short distance below the

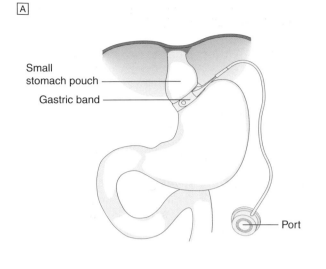

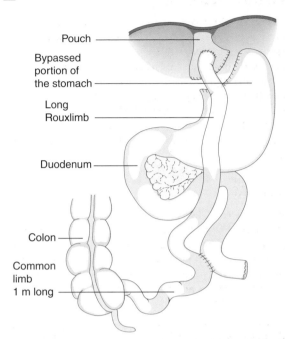

Fig. 17.12   Surgery for obesity.
A Gastric banding. B Gastric bypass.

oesophagogastric junction, creating a small (approximately 50 ml) gastric pouch (Fig. 17.12A). The cuff can be inflated or deflated via injections into a port site located in the subcutaneous tissues, in order to tighten or relax the cuff around the stomach. The tighter the cuff, the longer food-stuffs entering the gastric pouch will take to exit through the ring into the remainder of the stomach and intestinal tract, prolonging the feeling of satiety.

Gastric bypass involves stapling the stomach closed a short distance below the oesophagogastric junction (Fig. 17.12B). A Roux limb is then brought up and anas-tamosed to the small proximal gastric remnant. Depending on the size of the pouch and calibre of the anastomosis, there will be a degree of restrictive activity, as well as a

major malabsorptive element, as food will enter the distal jejunum and proximal ileum without exposure to bile or pancreatic and other digestive enzymes.

Vertical banded gastroplasty is now rarely performed. Duodenal switch is a complex operation reserved for a minority of obese patients.

Most patients with restrictive-type surgery find that they can eat more with time as the gastric remnant dilates. Hopefully, however, the target weight loss will have been achieved and improved eating habits established to allow maintenance of a healthier weight.

COMPLICATIONS OF OBESITY SURGERY

Obesity per se increases the risk of all types of surgery: in particular, chest infection, deep venous thrombosis and wound infection.

Careful follow-up of patients by the multidisciplinary team is necessary, not only to monitor weight loss, but also to ensure that malnutrition of vitamins, trace elements, essential fatty acids and other important constituents of the diet does not occur. Patients who continue to eat chocolate and ice-cream to excess may not lose weight with the restrictive-type operations.

Most patients who lose significant weight will develop gallstones and, in some, cholecystectomy may be indicated at the same time as obesity surgery.

Following significant weight loss, plastic surgery procedures may be necessary to remove excess skin, especially from the abdomen, thighs and arms.

BOX 17.5   SURGERY FOR OBESITY

- Obesity is an increasing problem in the developed world, both as a cause of disease and as a factor reducing life expectancy
- Many diseases in the morbidly obese, such as diabetes mellitus and hypertension, can be 'cured' following weight loss
- Surgery in the morbidly obese is, in general, associated with significantly increased morbidity and mortality
- Surgery to reduce oral intake (restrictive) or reduce absorption of eaten foodstuffs (malabsorptive) can lead to long-term maintenance of excess weight loss
- The current operation of first choice is the laparoscopic gastric band, in view of its relative ease of insertion, complication rate and excess weight loss maintenance over subsequent years

18

O.J. GARDEN

The liver and biliary tract

THE LIVER

ANATOMY

The liver is the largest abdominal organ, weighing approximately 1500 g. It extends from the fifth intercostal space to the right costal margin. It is triangular in shape, its apex reaching the left midclavicular line in the fifth intercostal space. In the recumbent position, the liver is impalpable under cover of the ribs. The liver is attached to the undersurface of the diaphragm by suspensory ligaments that enclose a 'bare area', the only part of its surface without a peritoneal covering. Its inferior or visceral surface lies on the right kidney, duodenum, colon and stomach.

Topographically, the liver is divided by the attachment of the falciform ligament into right and left lobes; fissures on its visceral surface demarcate two further lobes, the quadrate and caudate (Fig. 18.1). From a practical standpoint, it is the segmental anatomy of the liver, as defined by the distribution of its blood supply, that is important to the surgeon.

SEGMENTAL ANATOMY

The portal vein and hepatic artery divide into right and left branches in the porta hepatis. Occluding either branch at surgery produces an easily visible line of demarcation that runs from the gallbladder bed behind and to the left of the inferior vena cava, thus separating the two hemilivers. Each hemiliver is further divided into four segments corresponding to the main branches of the hepatic artery and portal vein. In the left hemiliver, segment I corresponds to the caudate lobe, segments II and III to the left lobe, and segment IV to the quadrate lobe. The remaining segments (V–VIII) comprise the right hemiliver (Fig. 18.2).

BLOOD SUPPLY AND FUNCTION

The liver normally receives 1500 ml of blood per minute and has a dual blood supply, 65% coming from the portal vein and 35% from the hepatic artery, which supplies 50% of the oxygen requirements.

The principal venous drainage of the liver is by the right, middle and left hepatic veins, which enter the vena cava (Fig. 18.2). In 25% of individuals, there is an inferior right hepatic vein, and numerous small veins drain direct into the vena cava from the caudate lobe (segment I). The functional unit of the liver is the hepatic acinus. Sheets of liver cells (hepatocytes) one cell thick are separated by interlacing sinusoids through which blood flows from the peripheral portal tract into the hepatic acinus to the central branch of the hepatic venous system. Bile is secreted by the liver cells and passes in the opposite direction along the small canaliculi into interlobular bile ducts located in the portal tracts (Fig. 18.3).

The liver has an important role in nutrient metabolism and is responsible for storing glucose in the form of glycogen, or converts it to lactate for release into the systemic circulation. Amino acids are utilized for hepatic and plasma protein synthesis or catabolized to urea. The liver has a central role in the metabolism of bilirubin and bile salts, drugs and alcohol. It is the principal organ for storage of a number of minerals and vitamins, and is responsible for the production of the vitamin K-dependent factors II, VII, IX and X. The liver is also the largest reticuloendothelial organ in the body and its Kupffer cells play a role in the removal of damaged red blood cells, bacteria, viruses and endotoxin, much of which enter the body from the gut.

18

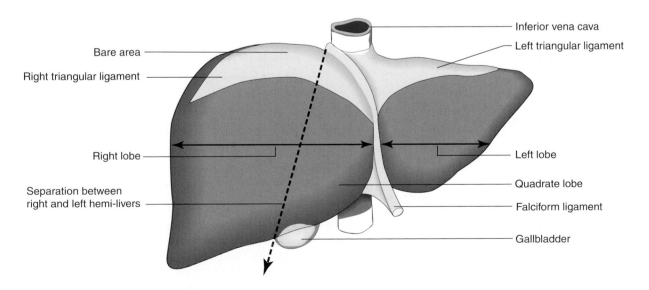

Fig. 18.1 Surgical anatomy of the liver.
The broken line represents the separation between right and left hemilivers.

18

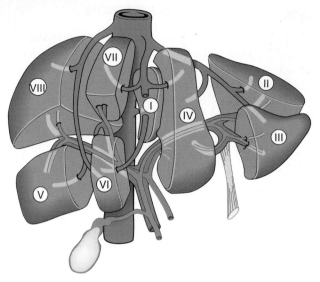

Fig. 18.2   Segmental anatomy and venous drainage.

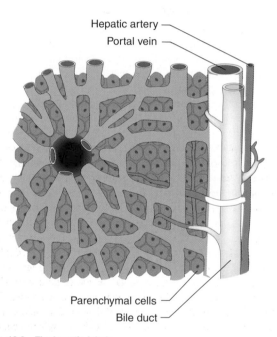

Hepatic artery

Portal vein

Parenchymal cells

Bile duct

Fig. 18.3   The hepatic lobule.
Sinusoids drain into the central hepatic vein.

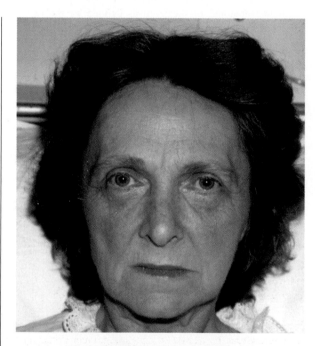

Fig. 18.4   Patient demonstrating the features of jaundiced skin and sclera.

BOX 18.1   SURGICAL ANATOMY

- The liver is divisible into right and left hemilivers (each having four segments) using a line running from the gallbladder fossa to the inferior vena cava
- Each hemiliver receives a branch of the hepatic artery and portal vein; 65% of liver blood flow and 50% of its oxygen supply are provided by the portal vein
- The hepatocytes are arranged in lobules, each of which has a central branch of the hepatic vein and peripheral portal tracts (containing a branch of the hepatic artery, portal vein and bile duct)
- Liver anatomy allows the surgeon to perform right hepatectomy, left hepatectomy and extended right hepatectomy (i.e. resecting all of the liver to the right of the falciform ligament). Resection of individual segments is also possible

---

JAUNDICE

Jaundice is caused by an increase in the level of circulating bilirubin and becomes obvious in the skin and sclera when levels exceed 50 μmol/l (Fig. 18.4). It may result from excessive destruction of red cells (haemolytic jaundice), from failure to remove bilirubin from the blood stream (hepatocellular jaundice), or from obstruction to the flow of bile from the liver (cholestatic jaundice) (Fig. 18.5). Congenital non-haemolytic hyperbilirubinaemia (Gilbert's syndrome) is a relatively rare cause of jaundice due to defective bilirubin transport; the jaundice is usually mild and transient, and the prognosis is excellent.

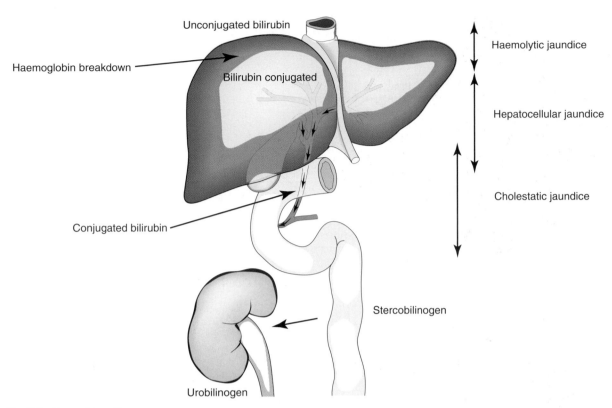

Unconjugated bilirubin

Haemoglobin breakdown

Bilirubin conjugated

Haemolytic jaundice

Hepatocellular jaundice

Cholestatic jaundice

18

Conjugated bilirubin

Stercobilinogen

Urobilinogen

Fig. 18.5   Types of jaundice.

To the surgeon, the most important type of haemolytic jaundice is that caused by hereditary spherocytosis, in which splenectomy may be necessary (Ch. 19). Haemolytic jaundice may also occur after blood transfusion and after operative or accidental trauma, when haematoma formation produces a pigment load that exceeds hepatic excretory capacity.

Hepatocellular jaundice is usually a medical rather than a surgical condition, although its recognition in patients presenting with abdominal pain is important, as surgical intervention may aggravate the hepatocellular injury.

Cholestatic jaundice due to intrahepatic obstruction of bile canaliculi may be a feature of acute and chronic liver disease and can be caused by drugs (e.g. chlorpromazine). This form of jaundice must be differentiated from that due to extrahepatic obstruction, the cause of which has most surgical relevance. Extrahepatic obstruction most commonly results from gallstones or cancer of the head of the pancreas. Other causes include cancer of the periampullary region or major bile ducts, extrinsic compression of the bile ducts by metastatic tumour, iatrogenic biliary stricture and choledochal cyst.

DIAGNOSIS

History and clinical examination

An accurate diagnosis of the cause of jaundice must be made as quickly as possible to allow prompt institution of appropriate treatment (Fig. 18.6). The age, sex, occupation, social habits, drug and alcohol intake, history of injections or infusions, and general demeanour of the patient must be considered. A history of intermittent pain, fluctuant jaundice and dyspepsia suggests calculous obstruction of the common bile duct, whereas a history of weight loss and relentless progressive jaundice favours a diagnosis of neoplasia. Obstructive jaundice is likely if there is a history of passage of dark urine and pale stools, and if the patient complains of pruritus (owing to an inability to secrete bile salts into the obstructed biliary system). Hepatocellular jaundice is likely if there are stigmata of chronic liver disease, such as liver palms, spider naevi, testicular atrophy and gynaecomastia. The abdomen must be examined for evidence of hepatomegaly or gallbladder distension, and for signs of portal hypertension such as splenomegaly, ascites and large collateral veins (caput medusae) in the abdominal wall.

Biochemical and haematological investigations

Haemolytic jaundice is suggested if there are high circulating levels of unconjugated bilirubin but no bilirubin in the urine. Serum concentrations of liver enzymes are normal in these circumstances and the appropriate haematological investigations should be set in train.

In jaundice due to biliary obstruction, the circulating bilirubin is conjugated by the liver and rendered water-soluble; it can then be excreted in the urine and gives it a dark colour. As bile cannot pass into the gastrointestinal tract, the stool becomes pale and urobilinogen is absent from the urine. Obstruction increases the formation of alkaline phosphatase from the cells lining the biliary canaliculi, producing raised serum levels. This rise in serum

18

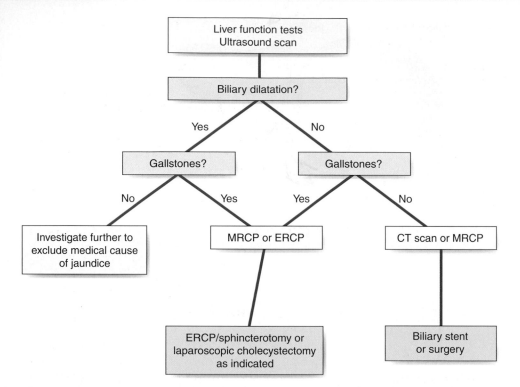

Fig. 18.6 Investigation of the jaundiced patient.

alkaline phosphatase precedes that of bilirubin and its fall is more gradual once obstruction is relieved. Serum transaminase and lactic dehydrogenase levels may rise in obstruction. Conversely, swelling of the parenchyma in hepatocellular jaundice frequently produces an element of intrahepatic biliary obstruction and a modest rise in serum alkaline phosphatase concentration.

A full blood count and coagulation screen should be undertaken as a matter of routine and viral status should be determined, if appropriate. The presence of anaemia may signify occult blood loss, and a low white cell or platelet count may indicate hypersplenism due to portal hypertension. Prolongation of the prothrombin time may be present in both hepatocellular and cholestatic jaundice, but should readily correct within 36 hours with the administration of parenteral vitamin K when jaundice is cholestatic.

Radiological investigations

If the clinical picture and biochemical investigations suggest that jaundice is obstructive, radiological techniques can be used to define the site and nature of the obstruction.

Ultrasonography

In skilled hands, this key investigation is safe, non-invasive and reliable. In the present context, it is used to define whether the patient has duct dilatation or gallbladder distension due to obstruction, and to confirm the need for more invasive investigations. Ultrasonography will also detect gallstones and space-occupying lesions in the liver and pancreas, although overlying bowel gas may prevent a clear view of the pancreas.

Magnetic resonance cholangiopancreatography (MRCP)

This non-invasive investigation is likely to replace other forms of invasive radiological imaging of the bile duct and pancreas. Magnetic resonance imaging (MRI) has the advantage that it does not introduce infection into an obstructed biliary system or the pancreatic duct; it also enables assessment of the vascular anatomy and the parenchyma of the liver and pancreas. This is important in patients presenting with symptoms suggestive of malignant obstructive jaundice.

Endoscopic retrograde cholangiopancreatography (ERCP)

This examination outlines the biliary and pancreatic systems by injecting dye through a cannula inserted into the papilla of Vater by means of an endoscope passed into the duodenum. It gives more detailed information than ultrasonography and, as will be discussed later, also allows endoscopic treatment of gallstones, biopsy of periampullary tumours, and relief of obstructive jaundice by the insertion of stents. The investigation may be complicated by acute pancreatitis, and prophylactic antibiotics should be administered to reduce the risk of cholangitis. Haemorrhage and perforation are less frequent complications.

Percutaneous transhepatic cholangiography (PTC)

Used less often than formerly, this is useful in assessing obstruction of the upper biliary tree. It provides a clear outline of the biliary system by the injection of contrast through a slim flexible needle passed percutaneously into the liver. The technique may cause bleeding or bile leakage and can be complicated by bacteraemia and septicaemia; coagulation status must be checked and antibiotic cover should be given.

Computed tomography (CT)
This can be used to identify hepatic, bile duct and pancreatic tumours in jaundiced patients. It often demonstrates the dilated biliary tree to the level of the obstruction, and may show dissemination to adjacent lymph nodes.

Other radiological investigations
These are seldom needed. Isotopic liver scanning has been superseded by ultrasonography and CT. Selective angiography is not used to diagnose the cause of jaundice, but is used by some to assess resectability if there is neoplastic obstruction; it also identifies vascular anomalies.

Liver biopsy
Liver biopsy is valuable in patients with unexplained jaundice, in whom an obstructing lesion has been excluded by ultrasonography. If lesions have been identified, a 'targeted' liver biopsy can be conducted under ultrasound or CT control. It may be preferable and safer to undertake biopsy at laparoscopy. Prothrombin time, platelet count and hepatitis B surface antigen (HBsAg) status must always be determined, and clotting abnormalities should be corrected before biopsy is undertaken.

Laparoscopy
Laparoscopy is used increasingly in the evaluation of liver disease and obstructive jaundice. It is best undertaken under general anaesthesia. In patients with malignant obstruction of the biliary tree, it may have a vital role in the staging of the tumour, as peritoneal dissemination and small hepatic metastases may be apparent.

Laparotomy
Laparotomy is no longer necessary to establish the cause of jaundice and is only undertaken to remove the causal lesion or relieve biliary obstruction. Intra-operative ultrasonography and operative cholangiography may give useful additional information in patients with neoplasia and biliary obstruction. Appropriate pre-operative preparation is particularly important in jaundiced patients.

CONGENITAL ABNORMALITIES

Simple cysts within the liver are common; they are lined by biliary epithelium and contain serous fluid, but never communicate with the biliary tree. They rarely produce symptoms, are associated with normal liver function, and on ultrasound or CT scan have no discernible wall (Fig. 18.7). In the few patients who develop symptoms, cysts tend to recur following aspiration, and sclerosis by alcohol injection is of little value for large symptomatic cysts. Surgical management consists of deroofing and may be undertaken by laparoscopic means. Polycystic disease is a rare cause of liver enlargement and may be associated with polycystic kidneys as an autosomal dominant trait. In symptomatic patients, it may be necessary to combine a deroofing procedure with hepatic resection.

Cavernous haemangiomas are one of the most common benign tumours of the liver and may be congenital. Women are affected six times more frequently than men. Most haemangiomas are small solitary subcapsular growths found incidentally at laparotomy or autopsy, but they are sometimes detected on ultrasound examination as densely hyperechoic lesions that mimic hepatic tumours. These lesions rarely give rise to pain. Resection may be considered for symptomatic lesions exceeding 5 cm in diameter.

LIVER TRAUMA

After the spleen, the liver is the solid organ most commonly damaged in abdominal trauma, particularly following road traffic accidents. Stab injuries and gunshot wounds of the liver are also increasing in incidence. These are considered in Chapter 9.

BOX 18.2 JAUNDICE

- Jaundice is a yellowish discoloration of the tissues that becomes clinically apparent when serum bilirubin levels exceed 50 µmol/l (normal < 20 µmol/l)
- It may be due to excessive haemolysis, hepatic insufficiency or cholestasis; cholestatic (obstructive) jaundice is the type encountered in surgical practice
- The two most common causes of surgical obstructive jaundice are cancer of the head of the pancreas and stones in the common bile duct (choledocholithiasis)
- In cholestatic jaundice, the bilirubin has been conjugated by the hepatocytes and is therefore soluble in water and can be excreted in the urine; patients with obstructive jaundice typically have dark urine and pale stools and may have pruritus (thought to be due to the accumulation of bile salts)
- Obstructive jaundice is characterized by elevated serum alkaline phosphatase levels in addition to hyperbilirubinaemia, and may be accompanied by modest elevations in transaminase (aminotransferase) levels, reflecting liver damage

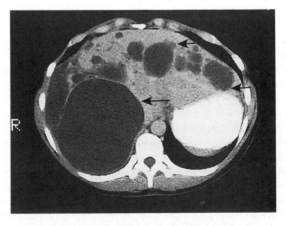
Fig. 18.7 CT scan demonstrating multiple biliary cysts appearing as hypodense areas within both lobes of the liver (arrowed).

HEPATIC INFECTIONS AND INFESTATIONS

Liver abscesses can be classified as bacterial, parasitic or fungal. Bacterial abscess is the most common type in Western medicine, but parasitic infestation is an important cause world-wide. Fungal abscesses are found in patients receiving long-term broad-spectrum antibiotic treatment or immunosuppressive therapy, and may complicate actinomycosis.

PYOGENIC LIVER ABSCESS

Infection from the biliary system is now more common due to the increasing use of radiological and endoscopic intervention. Infection may spread through the portal vein from abdominal sepsis (e.g. appendicitis, diverticulitis), via the hepatic artery from a septic focus anywhere in the body, or by direct spread from a contiguous organ (e.g. empyema of the gallbladder). Abscess formation may follow blunt or penetrating injury, and in one-third of patients the source of infection is indeterminate (cryptogenic). Common organisms are:

- *Streptococcus milleri*
- *Escherichia coli*
- *Streptococcus faecalis*
- *Staphylococcus aureus*
- anaerobes (*Bacteroides* spp).

Clinical features
The onset of symptoms is often insidious and the patient may present with a pyrexia of unknown origin. There is sometimes a history of sepsis elsewhere, particularly within the abdomen, and pain in the right hypochondrium. Other patients present with swinging pyrexia, rigors, marked toxicity and jaundice. The liver is often enlarged and tender.

Investigations
Plain radiographs may show elevation of the diaphragm, pleural effusion and basal lobe collapse. Leucocytosis is usually present and liver function tests (LFTs) are deranged. Ultrasonography or CT is used to define the abscess (which is often irregular and thick-walled) and to facilitate percutaneous aspiration for culture. ERCP may be useful if biliary obstruction is thought to be responsible.

Management
Untreated abscesses often prove fatal because of spread within the liver to multiple sites, and because of septicaemia and debility. The principles of treatment are percutaneous drainage of accessible abscesses under ultrasound guidance, and antibiotic therapy selected on the basis of culture of blood or pus. It is unusual to have to resort to formal surgical drainage. Percutaneously or surgically placed drainage tubes are left in place and the size of the cavity is monitored by serial X-rays following the injection of contrast material. Multiple small abscesses may require prolonged treatment with antibiotics for up to 8 weeks.

AMOEBIC LIVER ABSCESS

Entamoeba histolytica is a protozoal parasite that infests the large intestine and is endemic in many tropical regions. Trophozoites released by the cyst in the intestine may penetrate the mucosa to gain access to the portal venous system and so spread to the liver. The abscess is large and thin-walled, is usually solitary and in the right lobe, and contains brown sterile pus resembling anchovy sauce.

Clinical features
Right upper quadrant pain may be accompanied by anorexia, nausea, weight loss and night sweats. Tender enlargement of the liver is invariable, although jaundice is uncommon. Other signs include basal pulmonary collapse, pleural effusion and leucocytosis.

Investigations
Ultrasound and CT liver scans are used to demonstrate the site and size of the abscess, which often has poorly defined margins. The stools should be examined for amoebae or cysts. Direct and indirect serological tests to detect amoebic protein are available.

Management
Early diagnosis is important, and treatment may be commenced empirically in areas where the problem is endemic. Treatment consists of the administration of metronidazole (800 mg 8-hourly for 5 days) and usually results in rapid resolution. The abscess should be aspirated by needle puncture, if there is no clinical response within 72 hours. If untreated, an amoebic abscess may rupture into the peritoneal cavity or into a bronchus.

HYDATID DISEASE

This less common infestation is caused in humans by one of two forms of tapeworm, *Echinococcus granulosus* and *E. multilocularis*. The adult tapeworm lives in the intestine of the dog, from which ova are passed in the stool; sheep or humans serve as the intermediate host by ingesting the ova (Fig. 18.8). The condition is most common in sheep-rearing areas. Ingested ova hatch in the duodenum and the embryos pass to the liver through the portal venous system. The wall of the resulting hydatid cyst is surrounded by an adventitial layer of fibrous tissue and consists of a laminated membrane lined by germinal epithelium, on which brood capsules containing scolices develop.

Clinical features
The disease may be symptomless, but chronic right upper quadrant pain with enlargement of the liver is the common presentation. The cyst may rupture into the biliary tree or peritoneal cavity, the latter sometimes causing an acute anaphylactic reaction due to absorption of foreign hydatid protein. Other complications include secondary infection and biliary obstruction with jaundice.

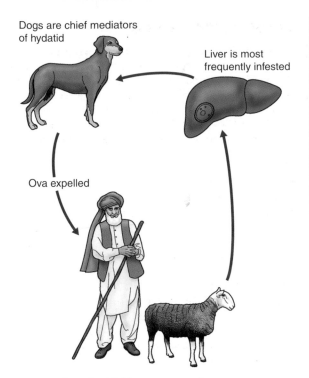

Fig. 18.8   Life cycle of *Echinococcus granulosus.*

Table 18.1   CAUSES OF PORTAL HYPERTENSION
Obstruction to portal flow
Pre-hepatic
• Congenital atresia of the portal vein
• Portal vein thrombosis
Neonatal sepsis
Pyelophlebitis
Trauma
Tumour
• Extrinsic compression of the portal vein
Pancreatic disease
Lymphadenopathy
Biliary tract tumours
Intrahepatic
• Cirrhosis
• Schistosomiasis
Post-hepatic
• Budd–Chiari syndrome
• Constrictive pericarditis
Increased blood flow (rare)
• Arteriovenous fistula
• Increased splenic blood flow in hypersplenism

18

Investigations

Eosinophilia is common and serological tests, such as complement fixation, are available to detect the foreign protein. Hydatid cysts commonly calcify and may be seen on a plain film of the abdomen. Alternatively, they can be detected by ultrasound or CT scan of the liver and are recognizable by their thick wall, which may contain multiple daughter cysts.

Management

In asymptomatic patients, small calcified cysts may require no treatment. Patients can be treated successfully with albendazole or mebendazole but this may be prolonged. Large symptomatic cysts are best managed by complete excision, together with the parasites contained within.

PORTAL HYPERTENSION

Portal hypertension is caused by increased resistance to portal venous blood flow, the obstruction being pre-hepatic, hepatic or post-hepatic. Rarely, it results primarily from an increase in portal blood flow. The normal pressure of 5–15 cmH$_2$O in the portal vein is consistently exceeded (above 25 cmH$_2$O). The causes of portal hypertension are shown in Table 18.1. Portal vein thrombosis is a rare cause and is most commonly due to neonatal umbilical sepsis. By far the most common cause of portal hypertension is cirrhosis of the liver. This results from chronic liver disease and is characterized by liver cell damage, fibrosis and nodular regeneration. The fibrosis obstructs portal venous return and portal hypertension

develops. Arteriovenous shunts within the liver also contribute to the hypertension.

Alcohol is the most common aetiological factor in developed countries, whereas in North Africa, the Middle East and China, schistosomiasis due to *Schistosoma mansonii* is a common cause. Chronic active hepatitis and primary and secondary biliary cirrhosis may result in portal hypertension, but in a large number of patients the cause remains obscure (cryptogenic cirrhosis).

Post-hepatic portal hypertension is rare. It is most frequently due to spontaneous thrombosis of the hepatic veins and this has been associated with neoplasia, oral contraceptive agents, polycythaemia and the presence of abnormal coagulants in the blood. The resulting Budd–Chiari syndrome is characterized by portal hypertension, liver failure and gross ascites.

EFFECTS OF PORTAL HYPERTENSION

As a result of gradual chronic occlusion of the portal venous system, collateral pathways develop between the portal and systemic venous circulations. Portosystemic shunting occurs at three principal sites (Fig. 18.9).

The most important consequence of shunting is the development of varices in the submucosal plexus of veins in the lower oesophagus and gastric fundus. Oesophageal varices may rupture, to cause acute massive gastrointestinal bleeding. Such bleeding occurs in about 40% of patients with cirrhosis. The initial episode of variceal haemorrhage is fatal in about one-third of patients, and the great majority of those who survive the initial haemorrhage bleed again. Bleeding from retroperitoneal and periumbilical collaterals

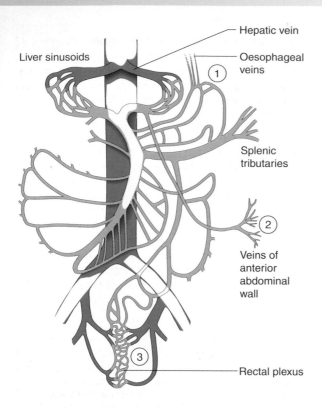

- Hepatic vein
- Oesophageal veins ①
Liver sinusoids

Splenic tributaries

② Veins of anterior abdominal wall

③ Rectal plexus

Fig. 18.9 The portal venous system.
Sites of portosystemic shunting are marked 1–3.
Retroperitoneal communications also exist.

is troublesome during abdominal surgery, and collaterals may develop and cause bleeding at the site of stomas. Anorectal varices are not uncommonly found at proctoscopy but rarely cause bleeding.

Progressive enlargement of the spleen occurs as a result of vascular engorgement and associated hypertrophy. Haematological consequences are anaemia, thrombocytopenia and leucopenia (with the resulting syndrome of hypersplenism). Ascites may develop and is due to increased formation of hepatic and splanchnic lymph, hypoalbuminaemia, and retention of salt and water. Increased aldosterone and antidiuretic hormone levels may contribute.

Portosystemic encephalopathy is due to an increased level of toxins such as ammonia in the systemic circulation. This is particularly likely to develop where there are large spontaneous or surgically created portosystemic shunts. Gastrointestinal haemorrhage increases the absorption of nitrogenous products and may precipitate encephalopathy.

CLINICAL FEATURES

Patients with cirrhosis frequently develop anorexia, generalized malaise and weight loss. Clinical manifestations of liver disease may be present, such as hepatosplenomegaly, ascites, jaundice and spider naevi. The serum bilirubin may be elevated and the serum albumin depressed. Anaemia may be present and the leucocyte count raised (or depressed if there is hypersplenism). The prothrombin time and other indices of clotting may be abnormal. Clinical and biochemical parameters are used as the basis of the modified Child's classification (Table 18.2). Patients allocated to grade A have a good prognosis, whereas those in grade C have the worst prognosis.

Table 18.2 ASSESSMENT OF PATIENTS WITH PORTAL HYPERTENSION USING A MODIFICATION OF CHILD'S GRADING SYSTEM

	Points scored		
Criterion	1	2	3
Encephalopathy	None	Minimal	Marked
Ascites	None	Slight	Moderate
Bilirubin (μmol/l)	< 35	35–50	> 50
Albumin (g/l)	> 35	28–35	< 28
Prothrombin ratio	< 1.4	1.4–2.0	> 2.0

Grade A = 5–6 points; grade B = 7–8 points; grade C = 10–15 points.

EBM 18.1 VARICEAL BLEEDING IN CIRRHOSIS: ASSESSMENT AND PROPHYLAXIS

'Severity of cirrhosis is best described using the Child–Pugh score. If grade 3 varices are diagnosed, patients should have primary prophylaxis, irrespective of the severity of the liver disease. Pharmacological therapy with propranolol is the best available modality for primary prophylaxis, with variceal band ligation recommended in cases of intolerance or contraindication to propranolol.'

Jalan R, Hayes PC, British Society of Gastroenterology. Gut 2000; 46 suppl 3–4:III 1–III 15.

Patients with portal hypertension usually present to a surgeon because of active uncontrolled bleeding from oesophageal varices, or for consideration of elective surgery for varices that have been resistant to non-surgical management.

ACUTE VARICEAL BLEEDING

Patients presenting with acute upper gastrointestinal bleeding are carefully examined for evidence of chronic liver disease (EBM 18.1). Distended collateral veins may be visible, particularly around the umbilicus, where they give rise to a 'caput medusae'. Slurring of speech, a flapping tremor or dysarthria may point to encephalopathy, and this may be precipitated or intensified by the accumulation of blood in the gastrointestinal tract.

The key investigation during an episode of active bleeding is endoscopy. This allows the detection of varices and defines whether they are or have been the site of bleeding. It is important to remember that peptic ulcer and gastritis are common complaints that occur in 20% of patients with varices. Even though a patient is known to have chronic liver disease and varices, bleeding cannot be assumed to be due to the varices.

Management

The priorities in the management of bleeding oesophageal varices are summarized in Table 18.3.

Active resuscitation

Large volumes of blood may be lost rapidly and the aim is to replace blood loss quickly with a view to urgent endoscopy. Many patients have coagulation defects from the outset, and thrombocytopenia is a common manifestation of hypersplenism. Fresh blood is preferred for transfusion purposes and the advice of the haematologist is sought regarding the use of fresh-frozen plasma (FFP) or platelet transfusion.

Endoscopy

This is performed at the earliest opportunity. The tortuous varices are usually in three columns and most prominent in the lower third of the oesophagus. Haemorrhage usually occurs from varices at the lowest few centimetres of the oesophagus. Rarely, bleeding occurs from varices in the gastric fundus.

Control of bleeding

Of the medical agents used to lower portal venous pressure and arrest bleeding, the synthetic form of somatostatin, octreotide, is most commonly employed. If variceal haemorrhage is apparent at the initial endoscopy, the injection of a sclerosant such as ethanolamine, or the application of bands is now used to arrest the bleeding (EBM 18.2). If haemorrhage is torrential and prevents direct injection, balloon tamponade may be used to stop the bleeding.

The four-lumen Minnesota tube (Fig. 18.10) has largely replaced the three-lumen Sengstaken–Blakemore tube. The four lumina allow:

EBM 18.2   CONTROL OF VARICEAL BLEEDING

'Variceal band ligation is the method of choice for control of variceal haemorrhage, with endoscopic variceal sclerotherapy as second choice. If endoscopy is unavailable, vasoconstrictors such as octreotide or glypressin, or a modified Sengstaken tube may be used while more definitive therapy is arranged. In case of bleeding that is difficult to control, a modified Sengstaken tube should be inserted until further endoscopic treatment, transjugular intrahepatic portosystemic stent shunting (TIPSS) or surgical treatment, with the mode of treatment (surgical intervention such as oesophageal transection or TIPSS) determined by the specialist centre.'

Jalan R, Hayes PC, British Society of Gastroenterology. Gut 2000; 46 suppl 3–4:III 1–III 15.

Table 18.3   PRIORITIES IN THE MANAGEMENT OF BLEEDING OESOPHAGEAL VARICES

Active resuscitation
- Group and cross-match blood
- Establish i.v. infusion line(s)
- Monitor
  - Pulse
  - Blood pressure
  - Hourly urine output
  - Central venous pressure

Assessment of coagulation status
- Prothrombin time
- Platelet count

Urgent endoscopy

Control of bleeding
- Endoscopic banding or sclerotherapy
- Tamponade (Minnesota tube) if bleeding uncontrolled
- Pharmacological measures (e.g. vasopressin/octreotide)

Treatment of hepatocellular decompensation

Treatment/prevention of portosystemic encephalopathy

Prevention of further bleeding from varices
- Injection sclerotherapy
- Stapled oesophago-gastric junction
- Portosystemic shunting/transjugular intrahepatic portosystemic stent shunting (TIPSS)
- Liver transplantation

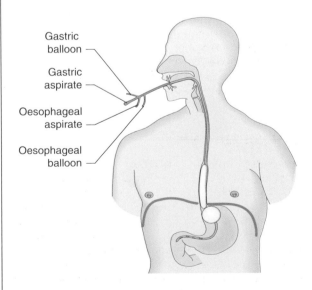

Fig. 18.10   Oesophageal tamponade using a Minnesota tube.

Gastric balloon
Gastric aspirate
Oesophageal aspirate
Oesophageal balloon

18

- aspiration of gastric contents
- compression of the oesophago-gastric varices by the inflated gastric balloon
- compression of the oesophageal varices by the inflated oesophageal balloon
- aspiration of the oesophagus and pharynx to reduce pneumonic aspiration.

Balloon tamponade arrests bleeding from varices in over 90% of patients, but the tube is not left in place for more than 24–36 hours for fear of causing oesophageal necrosis. Tamponade should be regarded as a holding measure that allows further resuscitation and treatment of hepatic decompensation before more definitive measures are used.

Prevention of further bleeding

A number of methods are now available to reduce the risk of further variceal bleeding (EBM 18.3).

EBM 18.3 PREVENTION OF FURTHER VARICEAL BLEEDING AND INFECTION

'Following control of active variceal bleeding, the varices should be eradicated using variceal band ligation. TIPSS may be used in certain centres with particular expertise; it is more effective than endoscopic treatment in reducing variceal rebleeding but does not improve survival and is associated with more encephalopathy.'

'Infection is common after upper gastrointestinal bleeding in cirrhotic patients and is a major cause of morbidity and mortality. All patients presenting with an episode of variceal bleed should have antibiotic prophylaxis with ciprofloxacin 1 g/day for 7 days.'

Jalan R, Hayes PC, British Society of Gastroenterology. Gut 2000; 46 suppl 3–4:III 1–III 15.

Injection sclerotherapy

Although originally undertaken by means of a rigid oesophagoscope under general anaesthesia, this is now carried out by fibreoptic endoscopy. Injection is repeated at weekly or fortnightly intervals until the varices are completely sclerosed. Excessive or too frequent injection may be complicated by ulceration and necrosis, sometimes with a fatal result.

Endoscopic banding

Just as haemorrhoids can be managed by the application of elastic bands, endoscopic applicators are now available that can be used to occlude varices at the oesophago-gastric junction. The reduced risk of oesophageal ulceration and perforation has resulted in this technique being favoured over sclerotherapy in many centres.

Surgical disconnection

This is rarely used in the management of variceal haemorrhage. The gastric vein and short gastric veins are ligated, and the distal oesophagus is transected and reanastomosed just above the cardia using a stapling gun (Fig. 18.11). Stapled oesophageal transection occludes flow into the varices, but carries considerable morbidity and mortality when employed as a last resort in the emergency situation.

Emergency portosystemic shunting

This has a high mortality and has been abandoned in most centres. Elective portosystemic shunting is still used occasionally to decompress the portal system and reduce the risk of further variceal haemorrhage, but portosystemic encephalopathy can be troublesome. Rarely, operation is considered in patients with severe liver disease and when there is a clear indication for liver transplantation.

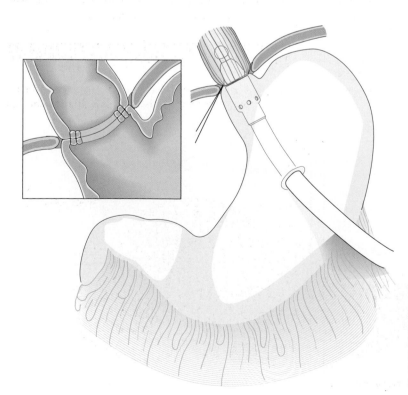

Fig. 18.11 Oesophageal stapling.
The gun is inserted through an anterior gastrostomy. A ligature is tied just above the cardia, invaginating a flange of oesophageal wall between the two parts of the gun. Inset: the gun has been fired, simultaneously resecting a full-thickness ring of oesophageal wall and anastomosing the cut ends with staples.

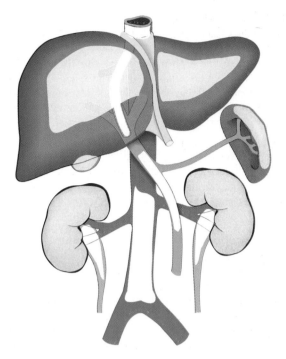

Fig. 18.12 Transjugular intrahepatic portosystemic stent shunting (TIPSS).

BOX 18.3 PORTAL HYPERTENSION

- Portal hypertension is almost always due to obstruction to portal flow (rather than increased inflow), and may be pre-hepatic, hepatic or post-hepatic
- Cirrhosis of the liver is the most common cause of portal hypertension in developed countries, and alcoholic cirrhosis is most often responsible
- Portosystemic shunts develop between gastric and oesophageal veins, in the retroperitoneum and periumbilical area, and occasionally in the anorectum. Varices in the submucosa of the lower oesophagus are a common source of major bleeding, but gastritis (portal gastropathy) can be responsible
- Child's grading (A, B or C) is based on encephalopathy, ascites, bilirubin and albumin levels, and prothrombin time, and is a valuable prognostic index
- Variceal bleeding may be controlled by injection sclerotherapy or endoscopic banding, although balloon tamponade (four-lumen Minnesota tube) may sometimes be needed
- Surgical portosystemic shunts effectively decompress oesophageal varices and reduce rebleeding, but can cause encephalopathy and have been largely replaced by transjugular intrahepatic portosystemic stent shunting (TIPSS)
- Although injection sclerotherapy (or banding) reduces the risk of rebleeding and may improve survival rates, long-term outcome is determined by the nature and severity of the underlying liver disease

Types of shunt procedure

There are several anatomical sites at which portosystemic shunts can be performed but most of these operations have been replaced by non-surgical approaches to treatment. In transjugular intrahepatic portosystemic stent shunting (TIPSS, Fig. 18.12), a metal stent is inserted via the transjugular route using a guidewire passed through the hepatic vein to the intrahepatic branches of the portal vein. The technique is a relatively safe means of decompressing the portal system as general anaesthesia and laparotomy are avoided. The risk of encephalopathy is similar to that of a surgical portosystemic shunt, but the procedure is now considered routinely before surgical intervention in both the acute and the elective settings.

ASCITES

Ascites can be controlled by bed rest, salt and water restriction, and a diuretic such as the aldosterone inhibitor, spironolactone. If refractory, ascites can be treated by inserting a peritoneojugular (LeVeen) shunt, which allows one-way flow between the peritoneum and the jugular vein (Fig. 18.13). It is unusual for the shunt to remain patent for more than 12 months, but this may suffice for patients with refractory ascites and advanced liver disease who are not candidates for liver transplantation.

TUMOURS OF THE LIVER

Hepatic tumours can be benign or malignant, and primary or secondary. Primary tumours may arise from the

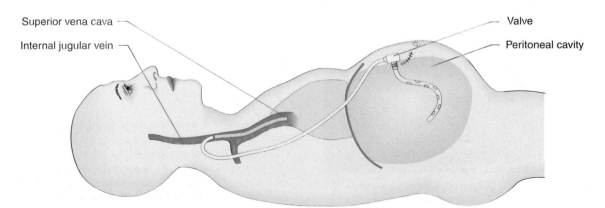

Fig. 18.13 Peritoneovenous (Le Veen) shunt to relieve ascites.

parenchymal cells, the epithelium of the bile ducts, or the supporting tissues.

BENIGN HEPATIC TUMOURS

Cavernous haemangioma

This is the most common benign liver tumour. Most cavernous haemangiomas are asymptomatic and are detected on ultrasonography as a dense hyperechoic lesion, or are found incidentally at laparotomy. These lesions rarely reach a sufficient size to produce pain, abdominal swelling or haemorrhage. Heart failure occasionally develops, if there is a large arteriovenous communication. Lesions discovered incidentally at laparotomy should be left alone; needle biopsy can be hazardous. Large symptomatic lesions should normally be resected only by an experienced surgeon.

Biliary hamartomas

These are small fibrous lesions that are often situated beneath the capsule of the liver. They can be mistaken for a small metastatic tumour unless a biopsy is obtained.

Liver cell adenomas

These are relatively uncommon and are found almost exclusively in women. They may be associated with the use of contraceptives containing high levels of oestrogen. The majority present as solitary, well-encapsulated lesions, but malignant transformation has been reported. They may be asymptomatic but generally present with right hypochondrial pain as a result of haemorrhage within the tumour. Superficial tumours may bleed spontaneously and present with symptoms of haemoperitoneum. Adenomas may be detected by ultrasonography or CT. LFTs and serum α-fetoprotein levels are usually normal. Percutaneous biopsy should be avoided because of the risk of haemorrhage.

Treatment consists of formal hepatic resection because of the difficulties of distinguishing adenoma from a well-differentiated hepatoma, concerns that lesions may undergo

malignant transformation, and the known risk of spontaneous haemorrhage.

Focal nodular hyperplasia of the liver

This is more common in females. The lesion is generally asymptomatic and may regress with time or on withdrawal of the contraceptive pill. Hyperplasia can be differentiated from adenoma by the central fibrous scar, which is often visible on ultrasound or CT (Fig. 18.14). Such lesions do not undergo malignant transformation and do not require excision unless symptomatic.

PRIMARY MALIGNANT TUMOURS OF THE LIVER

Hepatocellular carcinoma (hepatoma)

Hepatocellular carcinoma (hepatoma) is relatively uncommon in the developed world but is common in Africa and the Far East. In the West, about two-thirds of patients have pre-existing cirrhosis and many others have evidence of hepatitis B or C infection. In Africa and the East, 'aflatoxin' (derived from the fungus, *Aspergillus flavus*, which contaminates maize and nuts) is an important hepatocarcinogen.

Clinical features

The diagnosis is usually made late in the course of the disease. In non-cirrhotic patients, the tumour may have grown to a considerable size before giving rise to abdominal pain or swelling. In cirrhotic patients, hepatoma may become manifest as sudden deterioration in liver function, often associated with extension of the tumour into the portal venous system. Common presenting features include abdominal pain, weight loss, abdominal distension, fever and spontaneous intraperitoneal haemorrhage. Jaundice is uncommon unless there is advanced cirrhosis. Examination may reveal features of established liver disease and hepatomegaly is invariable.

Investigations

LFTs are generally deranged. Although early detection of hepatocellular carcinoma in susceptible individuals can be pursued by a policy of serial measurement of α-fetoprotein (an oncofetal antigen) and ultrasound scanning, this tumour marker is present in only one-third of the white population with hepatocellular carcinoma, compared to 80% of African patients with this disease.

The lesion may be detected and characterized by abnormal ultrasound scanning. Percutaneous needle aspiration cytology and needle biopsy for histological confirmation should be reserved for patients who are not being considered for hepatic resection, as these investigations carry a small but significant risk of tumour dissemination and haemorrhage.

Abdominal CT or MRI is valuable in planning resection and excluding the presence of nodal involvement. Pulmonary metastases may not be evident on chest X-ray and their presence should be excluded by a CT scan of the thorax, if resection is contemplated. Peritoneal dissemination of the tumour may only be excluded by laparoscopy. Hepatocellular carcinoma is seen as an extremely vascular lesion on arteriography, and propagation

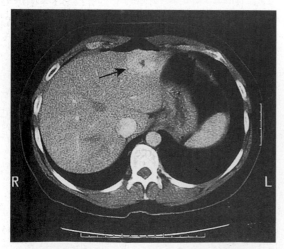

Fig. 18.14 Intravenous enhanced CT scan demonstrating a hypervascular lesion in the left lobe of the liver (arrowed). This symptomatic focal nodular hyperplastic lesion was removed by left lobectomy.

of tumour thrombus along the portal vein or its branches may be demonstrated.

Management

In non-cirrhotic patients, large tumours (particularly those of the fibrolamellar type) may be amenable to liver resection. Cirrhotic patients have less hepatic functional reserve, and even those with well-preserved liver function may only tolerate limited segmental resection. In cirrhotic patients, multicentricity is common and satellite lesions often surround the primary tumour, so that cure is uncommon.

For advanced tumours, systemic chemotherapy with doxorubicin (adriamycin), methotrexate or 5-fluorouracil may have palliative value, although response rates of less than 20% are the norm. More encouraging results have been reported following local embolization of these agents plus lipiodol by selective arteriography (chemo-embolization).

The disease is usually advanced at presentation and the 5-year survival rate is less than 10%. Liver transplantation has been used in the treatment of this tumour, but the best results are reported in cirrhotic patients in whom an incidental hepatoma has been found on examination of the resected specimen following the transplant.

Cholangiocarcinoma

This adenocarcinoma may arise anywhere in the biliary tree, including its intrahepatic radicles. It accounts for less than 10% of malignant primary neoplasms of the liver in Western medicine, although its incidence is rising. Risk factors include chronic parasitic infestation of the biliary tree in the Far East, and choledochal cysts (see below).

Jaundice, pain and an enlarged liver are the common presenting features, although there may be coexisting biliary infection causing the tumour to masquerade as a hepatic abscess. Resection offers the only prospect of cure but is seldom feasible when cholangiocarcinoma arises in the liver substance. Cholangiocarcinoma arising from the extrahepatic bile ducts is considered later.

Other primary malignant tumours

- *Angiosarcoma* (Fig. 18.15). This rare tumour of the liver may arise after industrial exposure to vinyl chloride or exposure to the previously used radiological contrast medium, Thorotrast.
- *Haemangioendothelioma*. This presents as a diffuse multifocal tumour and is rarely resectable at presentation.
- *Biliary cystadenoma*. This rare condition of the liver, with a marked female predominance, has a 1:4 risk of malignant transformation and should be resected.

METASTATIC TUMOURS

The liver is a common site for metastatic disease; secondary liver tumours are 20 times more common than primary ones. In 50% of cases, the primary tumour is in the gastrointestinal tract; other common sites are the breast, ovaries, bronchus and kidney. Almost 90% of patients with hepatic metastases have tumour deposits in other sites.

Hepatomegaly and tenderness are distinctive features, and individual deposits may be palpable. The patient is often cachectic, and ascites or jaundice may be present. Pyrexia occurs in up to 10% of patients. The alkaline phosphatase and γ-glutamyl transpeptidase are often raised. Ultrasound and CT scans may demonstrate multiple filling defects. The diagnosis can be confirmed by aspiration cytology or needle biopsy undertaken under ultrasound control. Such invasive investigation may be unnecessary when resection is being considered.

18

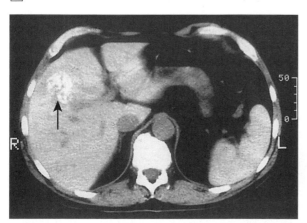

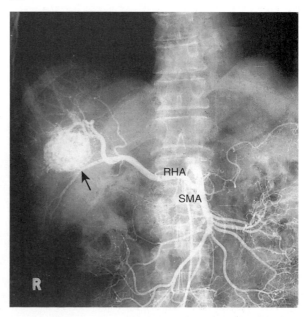

Fig. 18.15 Angiosarcoma.
A CT scan demonstrating a lesion in segment V (arrowed). B Angiography shows an extremely vascular lesion (arrowed) taking its blood supply mainly from an aberrant right hepatic artery (RHA) arising from the superior mesenteric artery (SMA).

18

There is no effective treatment for most patients with hepatic metastases. Both lobes of the liver are usually involved, making surgical resection impossible. In some tumours, notably those arising from the colon and rectum, apparently solitary metastases or metastases confined to one or other lobe may be resected. A careful search for other metastases is required, including local recurrence of the original primary tumour (e.g. colonoscopy) and dissemination elsewhere (e.g. CT of the thorax). In well-selected patients, 5-year survival rates of 30–40% have been reported following resection. Non-curative resection may be considered as a means of palliation in patients with symptomatic hepatic metastases from a carcinoid tumour.

LIVER RESECTION

Resection involves mobilization of the liver from its peritoneal attachments. Following isolation, ligature and division of the appropriate vessels, the devascularized lobe or segment is separated by careful dissection, which may be facilitated by the use of an ultrasonic dissector. Intervening biliary and vascular channels can be defined and divided between ligatures. The hepatic veins or tributaries are controlled by suture ligation following removal of the resected specimen.

Modern techniques of hepatic resection have greatly reduced operative blood loss, with a subsequent reduction in morbidity and mortality. Adequate drainage of the operating field following resection may minimize the consequences of post-operative bile leakage or bleeding. Post-operative monitoring should include blood gas, glucose and lactate measurement. Hepatic dysfunction may be evident from prolongation of the prothrombin time in major liver resectional surgery.

LIVER TRANSPLANTATION

This is considered in Chapter 29.

THE GALLBLADDER AND BILE DUCTS

ANATOMY OF THE BILIARY SYSTEM

The biliary tree consists of fine intrahepatic biliary radicles that drain individual liver segments before forming the right and left hepatic ducts. The left hepatic duct runs a mainly extrahepatic course and joins the right hepatic duct to form the common hepatic duct. This is joined at a variable position by the cystic duct to form the common bile duct, which ends at the papilla of Vater, usually in the second part of the duodenum (Fig. 18.16).

The common bile duct is approximately 8 cm long and up to 10 mm in diameter. It lies in the free edge of the lesser omentum before passing behind the first part of the duodenum and through the head of the pancreas. It is usually joined by the pancreatic duct just before entering the duodenum.

The gallbladder lies in a bed on the undersurface of the liver between its right and left halves. It is a muscular structure with a fundus, body and neck. Hartmann's pouch is a dilatation of the gallbladder outlet adjacent to the origin of the cystic duct, in which gallstones frequently become impacted. The gallbladder is supplied by the cystic artery, a branch of the right hepatic artery.

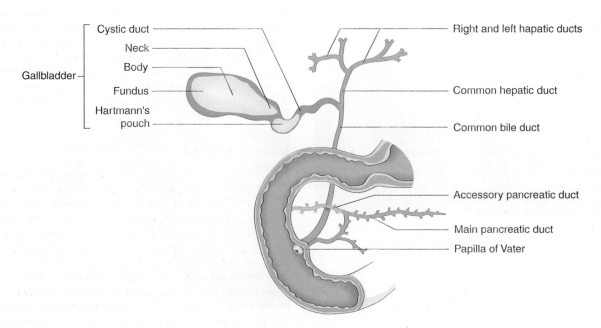

Fig. 18.16 Anatomy of the biliary tree.

PHYSIOLOGY

BILE SALTS AND THE ENTEROHEPATIC CIRCULATION

Bile acids are synthesized by the liver from cholesterol. The primary bile acids, chenodeoxycholic and cholic acid, are conjugated with glycine or taurine to increase their solubility in water, and the conjugates (e.g. glycocholic and taurocholic acid) form sodium and potassium bile salts. In the intestine, bacterial action produces the secondary bile salts, deoxycholic and lithocholic acid.

Bile salts can combine with lipids to form water-soluble complexes called micelles, within which lecithin and cholesterol can be transported from the liver. Bile salts are also detergents and a reduction in surface tension allows fat to be emulsified in the intestine, thus facilitating its digestion and absorption. On reaching the distal ileum, 95% of the bile salts are reabsorbed, transported back to the liver and passed once again into the biliary system. This enterohepatic circulation (Fig. 18.17) allows a relatively small bile salt pool (2–4 g) to circulate through the intestine some 6–12 times a day. The daily faecal loss equals that of hepatic synthesis (0.2–0.6 g/24 hrs). When bile is excluded from the intestine, 25% of ingested fat may appear in the

> **BOX 18.4   BILE SALTS**
>
> - The primary bile acids, chenodeoxycholic and cholic acid, are conjugated with glycine or taurine and form sodium or potassium bile salts (e.g. sodium taurocholate)
> - Bile salts are vital for the excretion of cholesterol in bile; cholesterol is insoluble in water and must be transported in water-soluble complexes (micelles) with bile salts and lecithin
> - Bile salts are detergents, and on reaching the intestine they emulsify fat and facilitate the digestion and absorption of fat and fat-soluble vitamins
> - Bile salts must not be confused with bile pigments (e.g. bilirubin), which are waste products and excreted in bile. The small bile salt pool (2–4 g) is conserved by reabsorption of bile salts from the terminal ileum
> - Disease or resection of the terminal ileum prevents the enterohepatic circulation of bile salts and is associated with a high incidence of cholesterol gallstones and diarrhoea (owing to the cathartic action of bile salts on the colon)

faeces and there is marked malabsorption of fat-soluble vitamins, including vitamin K.

The gallbladder has a capacity of 50 ml and can concentrate bile by a factor of 10. It contracts in response to cholecystokinin (CCK), which is released from the duodenal mucosa by the presence of food, notably fatty acids. Gallbladder contraction is accompanied by reciprocal relaxation of the sphincter of Oddi. The secretion of bile is promoted by the hormone secretin. The vagus nerve also stimulates bile secretion and gallbladder contraction. Some 1–2 litres of bile are produced by the liver.

CONGENITAL ABNORMALITIES

Congenital abnormalities of the gallbladder and bile ducts are common. The gallbladder may be absent (agenesis), double, intrahepatic, partitioned with a fold in the fundus (Phrygian cap), or multiseptate. The cystic duct may be absent or join the right hepatic duct rather than the common hepatic duct, and accessory ducts may be present. The cystic artery may be duplicated or may arise from the common hepatic or left hepatic artery. These anomalies are important in that great care must be taken to avoid the inappropriate division of major ducts and arteries in the course of cholecystectomy.

BILIARY ATRESIA

Failure of development of the duct system occurs once in every 20 000–30 000 births and is the most common cause of prolonged jaundice in infancy. Jaundice usually becomes apparent in the first 2–3 weeks of life and the liver and spleen usually enlarge. LFTs show an obstructive pattern. Liver biopsy reveals cholestatic jaundice, but differentiation from neonatal hepatitis is often surprisingly difficult.

In extrahepatic biliary atresia, a Roux loop of jejunum is anastomosed to the intrahepatic duct system in the hilum of the liver (Kasai operation). A delay in treatment will result in jaundice and cholangitis, allowing cirrhosis to develop, with portal hypertension and ascites.

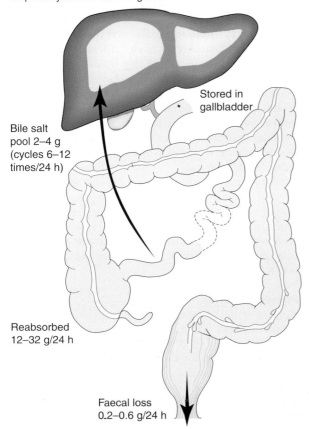

Hepatic synthesis 0.2–0.6 g/24 h

Stored in gallbladder

Bile salt pool 2–4 g (cycles 6–12 times/24 h)

Reabsorbed 12–32 g/24 h

Faecal loss 0.2–0.6 g/24 h

Fig. 18.17   The enterohepatic circulation.

CHOLEDOCHAL CYSTS

Cystic transformation of the biliary tree (choledochal cyst) is rare. The most common type results in a saccular dilatation of the common bile duct, which often has an abnormal termination that enters the pancreatic duct within the head of the pancreas. This may allow reflux into the biliary system, resulting in pain, inflammation, calculus formation and malignant transformation. The abnormalities are probably congenital, although diagnosis may be delayed until adult life.

In the neonate, the cyst may present with jaundice or spontaneous perforation. The adult patient usually presents with intermittent pain and jaundice, and may have attacks of pancreatitis. LFTs show a cholestatic pattern, and ultrasonography and cholangiography (MRCP or ERCP) establish the diagnosis (Fig. 18.18). In view of the significant risk of malignant transformation, excision of the cyst is indicated.

Caroli's disease consists of cystic biliary dilatation that is more marked in the peripheral intrahepatic ducts. Recurring infection may progress to cirrhosis and liver failure. When Caroli's disease is found in association with congenital hepatic fibrosis, portal hypertension is often present. Endoscopic, percutaneous and surgical manipulation of the biliary tree is best avoided, and liver transplantation may have a valuable role in management.

GALLSTONES

PATHOGENESIS

Gallstones are common in Europe and North America but less so in Asia and Africa. Their incidence increases with age. In developed countries, they occur in at least 20% of women over the age of 40; the incidence in males is about one-third of that in females. The disease has increased markedly in frequency and cholecystectomy is the most common elective abdominal operation in many Western countries.

Gallstones are formed from the constituents of bile. The great majority result from failure to keep cholesterol in micellar form in the gallbladder, and pigment stones are less common. Most cholesterol stones become mixed with bile pigments as they increase in size; such 'mixed' stones are much more common than pure cholesterol stones.

Cholesterol stones

Cholesterol stones are particularly common in middle-aged obese multiparous women. Stone formation is encouraged if bile becomes supersaturated with cholesterol (i.e. lithogenic), either by excessive cholesterol excretion or by a reduction in the amount of bile salt and lecithin available for micelle formation. Supersaturation is most likely to occur while the bile is concentrated in the gallbladder, and is favoured by stasis or decreased gallbladder contractility. The formation of cholesterol crystals is the key event, and this 'nucleation' may be due to coalescence of cholesterol molecules or their precipitation around particles of mucus, bacteria, calcium bilirubinate or mucosal cells. Pure cholesterol stones are yellowish-green with a regular shape but rough surface. They are usually solitary, whereas mixed stones are darker and are usually multiple.

Cholesterol stones are particularly common in some tribes of North American Indians, where more than 75% of women over 40 are affected. Such individuals have a small bile salt pool. Conversely, the high incidence of stones in Chilean women reflects high levels of cholesterol excretion. Obesity and high-calorie or high-cholesterol diets favour cholesterol stone formation by producing highly supersaturated gallbladder bile. Drastic weight reduction and diets designed to lower serum cholesterol levels may also promote stone formation by mobilizing cholesterol and increasing its excretion.

Disease or resection of the terminal ileum and drugs such as colestyramine favour cholesterol nucleation by reducing the bile salt pool. Hormonal influences are reflected in an increased incidence of stone formation in women taking oral contraceptives or post-menopausal oestrogen replacement. Pregnancy may also have an effect by increasing stasis within the gallbladder.

Pigment stones

Pigment stones consist of calcium bilirubinate and are usually multiple and small. They are more prevalent in those areas of the world where haemolytic blood disorders are most common: for example, Mediterranean countries and malarial regions. Stones found in Western patients are usually composed of black pigment, whereas brown pigment stones are common in people from the Far East. Pigment stones account for 25% of all gallstones in Western patients, but for 60% of those in some Far Eastern countries such as Japan.

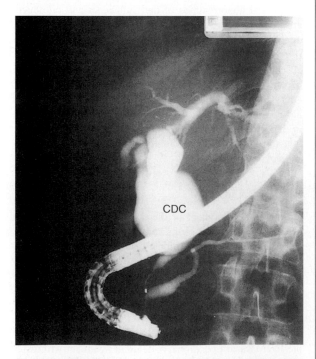

Fig. 18.18 ERCP demonstrating the common type of choledochal cyst (CDC) involving the common bile duct.

18

Chronic haemolysis favours pigment stone formation by increasing pigment excretion, and stone formation is common in congenital spherocytosis, haemoglobinopathy and malaria. Cirrhosis and biliary stasis are also important associations. Some patients with brown pigment stones have increased amounts of unconjugated bilirubin in the bile. In Far Eastern patients, this may be due to the action of β-glucuronidase produced by *E. coli*, an organism that invades duct systems infested with *Clonorchis sinensis* or *Ascaris lumbricoides*.

PATHOLOGICAL EFFECTS OF GALLSTONES

Acute cholecystitis and its complications

This is usually produced by obstruction of the neck of the gallbladder or cystic duct by a stone. Bacteria are cultured from the bile in approximately one-half of patients with gallstones, and unrelieved obstruction in the presence of this infected bile may produce an empyema. The thickened gallbladder becomes intensely inflamed, oedematous and occasionally gangrenous. The fundus of the distended, inflamed gallbladder may perforate, giving rise to localized abscess formation and occasionally to biliary peritonitis. The common organisms implicated in inflammation of the gallbladder are *E. coli*, *Klebsiella aerogenes* and *Strep. faecalis*. Staphylococci, clostridia and salmonella are occasionally present. These organisms may be cultured from the blood if there is bacteraemia.

Chronic cholecystitis

Repeated bouts of biliary colic or acute cholecystitis culminate in fibrosis, contraction of the gallbladder and chronic inflammatory change with marked thickening of the wall. The gallbladder ceases to function. Chronic inflammatory change may be present in the absence of gallstones, as is the case in the gallbladders of typhoid carriers.

Mucocoele

A mucocoele develops when the outlet of the gallbladder becomes obstructed in the absence of infection. The imprisoned bile is absorbed, but clear mucus continues to be secreted into the distended gallbladder.

Choledocholithiasis

When gallstones enter the common bile duct, they may pass spontaneously or give rise to obstructive jaundice, cholangitis or acute pancreatitis. Gallstone pancreatitis most commonly occurs when a small stone becomes temporarily arrested at the ampulla of Vater.

Gallstone ileus

This uncommon form of intestinal obstruction occurs when a large gallstone becomes impacted in the intestine. Stones large enough to block the gut generally gain access by eroding through the wall of the gallbladder into the duodenum.

Carcinoma

The incidence of carcinoma of the gallbladder is increased in patients with long-standing gallstones.

BOX 18.5 GALLSTONES

- Most gallstones form because of failure to keep cholesterol in solution. This can result in pure cholesterol stones, but more commonly the stones also acquire a content of bile pigment as they enlarge, forming 'mixed' stones
- Pigment stones are the most common type of stone in some Far Eastern countries, but are less common in Western society, where they are associated with chronic haemolysis, biliary stasis and cirrhosis
- Only 15% of stones contain enough calcium to be seen on a plain film
- The majority of individuals with gallstones are asymptomatic and remain so; the presence of gallstones is not in itself an indication for cholecystectomy
- Gallbladder stones may cause flatulent dyspepsia, biliary colic, acute cholecystitis and gallbladder cancer (although the latter is so rare that this consideration does not affect the decision not to treat asymptomatic stones)
- Gallstones that migrate into the bile duct can cause obstructive jaundice, cholangitis and acute pancreatitis, although they often remain asymptomatic
- Gallstone ileus is a rare form of intestinal obstruction; stones large enough to obstruct the gut are usually too large to pass through the ampulla of Vater and have gained access to the gut by an internal fistula involving the gallbladder

---

COMMON CLINICAL SYNDROMES ASSOCIATED WITH GALLSTONES

The majority of individuals with gallstones are asymptomatic or have only vague symptoms of distension and flatulence. Fewer than half of such patients develop symptoms or complications from their gallstones within 10 years.

Biliary colic

Biliary colic is due to transient obstruction of the gallbladder from an impacted stone. There is severe gripping pain, often developing after meals or in the evening, which is maximal in the epigastrium and right hypochondrium with radiation to the back. Despite being continuous, the pain may wax and wane in intensity over several hours, and vomiting and retching are common. Resolution occurs when the stone falls back into the gallbladder lumen or passes onwards into the common bile duct. The patient then recovers rapidly, but repeated bouts of colic are common. In some cases, the obstruction does not resolve and the patient develops acute cholecystitis.

Acute cholecystitis

Acute cholecystitis is a more prolonged and severe illness. It usually begins with an attack of biliary colic, although its onset may be more gradual. There is severe right hypochondrial pain radiating to the right subscapular region, and occasionally to the right shoulder, together with tachycardia, pyrexia, nausea, vomiting and leucocytosis. Abdominal tenderness and rigidity may be generalized but are most marked over the gallbladder. Murphy's sign (a catching of the breath at the height of inspiration while the gallbladder area is palpated) is usually present. A right hypochondrial

18

18

BOX 18.6 ACUTE CHOLECYSTITIS

- In the great majority of cases acute cholecystitis is associated with gallstones and results from obstruction of gallbladder outflow
- In contrast to biliary colic, which results from obstruction alone, acute cholecystitis is associated with infection and is a systemic illness
- The patient appears unwell, has pyrexia and tachycardia, and is tender in the right hypochondrium; Murphy's sign is almost always positive
- In 90% of cases, acute cholecystitis will settle with conservative treatment (nil by mouth, intravenous fluids, antibiotics, nasogastric suction if appropriate)
- In 10% of cases, disease progression leads to life-threatening complications: notably, empyema, gangrene and perforation
- Given that the gallbladder is permanently diseased and that complications may supervene, most surgeons now advocate early cholecystectomy (i.e. within 5 days) for acute cholecystitis

---

mass may be felt. This is due to omentum 'wrapped' around the inflamed gallbladder.

In 85–90% of cases, the attack settles within 4–5 days. In the remainder, tenderness may spread and pyrexia and tachycardia persist or worsen. The development of a tender mass, associated with rigors and marked pyrexia, signals empyema formation. The gallbladder may become gangrenous and perforate, giving rise to biliary peritonitis. Jaundice can develop during the acute attack. Usually, this is associated with stones in the common bile duct, but compression of the bile ducts by the gallbladder may be responsible.

Acute cholecystitis must be differentiated from perforated peptic ulcer, high retrocaecal appendicitis, acute pancreatitis, myocardial infarction and basal pneumonia. Acute cholecystitis can develop in the absence of gallstones (acalculous cholecystitis), although this is rare.

Chronic cholecystitis

Chronic cholecystitis is the most common cause of symptomatic gallbladder disease. The patient gives a history of recurrent flatulence, fatty food intolerance and right upper quadrant pain. The pain is worse after meals and is often associated with a feeling of distension and heartburn. The differential diagnosis includes duodenal ulcer, hiatus hernia, myocardial ischaemia, chronic pancreatitis and gastrointestinal neoplasia.

Mucocoele

In this condition, the patient often presents with a history of biliary colic and a non-tender piriform swelling in the right hypochondrium. There is little systemic upset and no pyrexia.

Choledocholithiasis

Stones may be present in the common bile duct of some 5–10% of patients with gallstones. There is little muscle in the wall of the bile duct, and pain is not a symptom unless the stone impedes flow through the sphincter of Oddi. The vast majority of stones in the common bile duct originate in the gallbladder. 'Primary' duct stones are extremely rare.

Impaction of a stone at the sphincter obstructs the flow of bile, producing jaundice, pale stools and dark urine. Obstruction commonly persists for several days but may clear spontaneously, as a result either of passage of the stone or of its disimpaction. Small stones may pass through the common bile duct without causing symptoms. In longstanding obstruction the bile ducts become markedly dilated and the diameter of the common bile duct may exceed its upper limit of 10 mm. A totally obstructed duct system becomes filled with clear 'white bile', as back pressure on the hepatocytes prevents clearance of bilirubin and mucus secretion is increased.

Infection of an obstructed biliary tract causes cholangitis, which is characterized by attacks of pain, pyrexia and jaundice (the so-called triad of Charcot), frequently in association with rigors. Long-standing intermittent biliary obstruction may lead to secondary biliary cirrhosis.

Acute pancreatitis may be associated with a stone in the common bile duct (Ch. 19).

Obstructive jaundice due to stones in the common bile duct has to be distinguished from other causes of obstructive jaundice, notably malignant obstruction and cholestatic jaundice. Acute viral or alcoholic hepatitis may occasionally be confused with obstructive jaundice.

Courvoisier's law

Fibrosed gallbladders that contain stones cannot distend when pressure increases in the obstructed biliary tree. Courvoisier's law states that if the gallbladder is palpable in the presence of jaundice, the jaundice is unlikely to be due to stone. This law is not inviolate. Distended gallbladders are not always easy to feel but can be detected readily by ultrasound.

OTHER BENIGN CONDITIONS OF THE GALLBLADDER

Cholesterosis

Cholesterosis or 'strawberry gallbladder' is a condition in which the mucous membrane of the gallbladder is infiltrated with lipid and cholesterol. It affects middle-aged and elderly patients of either sex.

Cholesterol stones are found in the gallbladders of half of these patients. Macroscopically, the mucosa is brick-red and speckled with bright yellow nodules. Symptoms of acute and chronic cholecystitis may be produced, and cholecystectomy is required in the symptomatic patient.

Adenomyomatosis

This rare condition is characterized by mucosal diverticula (Rokitansky–Aschoff sinuses) that particularly affect the fundus and penetrate the muscular layers to the serosa. Muscular hypertrophy and inflammatory cell infiltrates are present. The diagnosis is often only made following cholecystectomy, as the gallbladder frequently contains stones or biliary gravel.

Acute acalculous cholecystitis

About 5% patients with acute cholecystitis have acalculous inflammation. The condition may be precipitated by major surgery, bacteraemia, trauma, pancreatitis or other serious illness, and may complicate parenteral nutrition. The inflammatory reaction in the gallbladder wall may be intense and severe, leading to gangrene and perforation. In ill patients, percutaneous drainage (cholecystostomy) under ultrasound guidance may be considered, but urgent cholecystectomy is often advisable.

INVESTIGATION OF PATIENTS WITH SUSPECTED GALLSTONES

Blood tests
A full blood count may reveal a neutrophilia in acute cholecystitis or its complications. An elevated serum bilirubin or alkaline phosphatase may signify the presence of common duct stones.

Plain abdominal X-ray
As only 15% of gallstones contain enough calcium to be seen on a plain radiograph, this investigation is seldom used in diagnosis. Gas is occasionally seen outlining the biliary tree if there is a fistula between the biliary tract and the gut, as in gallstone ileus or following choledochoduodenostomy. Previous endoscopic sphincterotomy also allows gas to enter the biliary tree.

Ultrasonography
Ultrasonography permits inspection of the gallbladder, its wall and its contents, and demonstrates dilatation of the intrahepatic and extrahepatic biliary tree. Stones reflect the ultrasonic wave and are thrown into prominence by the acoustic shadow they produce (Fig. 18.19). The technique is extremely accurate in skilled hands. As it does not depend on hepatic excretion of contrast, it can be used in both jaundiced and non-jaundiced patients, and therefore has supplanted oral cholecystography.

Cholangiography
Intravenous cholangiography is rarely used since intravenous injection of an iodine-containing contrast agent carries a small but definite risk of severe (and even fatal) anaphylactoid reaction. MRCP is used increasingly to assess the biliary tree non-invasively and ERCP is reserved for removing stones detected in the common bile duct following endoscopic sphincterotomy. Complications include cholangitis and pancreatitis. PTC is more likely to be used in the evaluation of biliary malignancy.

SURGICAL TREATMENT OF GALLSTONES

Patients with symptomatic gallstones are usually advised to undergo cholecystectomy to relieve symptoms and avoid complications (EBM 18.4). Patients with asymptomatic gallstones are treated expectantly, particularly if they are elderly or suffering from medical conditions likely to increase the risk of surgery. In younger patients, there may be a stronger case for surgery despite the absence of symptoms, particularly if the stones are multiple and likely to cause complications, such as acute pancreatitis.

The principles of surgical treatment involve removal of the gallbladder and the stones it contains, while ensuring that no stones remain within the ductal system. 'Open' cholecystectomy may be required if the equipment and expertise for laparoscopic cholecystectomy are not available, but is now undertaken in less than 5% of patients with symptomatic gallstones. A laparoscopic procedure may not be possible in the patient who has previously undergone multiple abdominal operations or who is grossly obese. Pregnancy is considered a relative contraindication to laparoscopy in the first trimester because of the risk of anaesthetic agents to the developing fetus, and also because of the risk of spontaneous abortion.

Conversion from a laparoscopic procedure to open cholecystectomy should be seen as a limitation of the minimally invasive technique and not as a failure of the surgeon. Laparotomy is mandatory when the anatomy in the area of the cystic duct and artery cannot be defined readily, if uncontrolled bleeding occurs, or if the bile duct is injured (EBM 18.5).

Open cholecystectomy
The gallbladder is usually approached through a right subcostal incision. Following careful inspection and palpa-

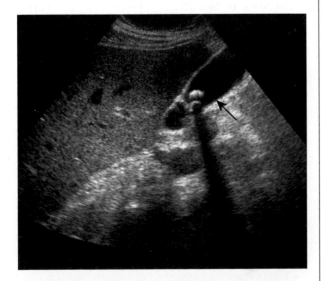

Fig. 18.19 Ultrasound scan of the gallbladder demonstrating the hyperechoic features of a solitary gallstone (arrowed) along with the typical acoustic shadow.

EBM 18.4 SURGICAL TREATMENT OF GALLSTONES
'Asymptomatic gallstones do not require treatment by laparoscopic cholecystectomy unless there is a high risk of gallbladder cancer. Once a patient with gallstones becomes symptomatic, elective cholecystectomy is indicated. Laparoscopic cholecystectomy is associated with less pain, shorter hospital stay, faster return to normal activity and less abdominal scarring than open cholecystectomy. These advantages are also evident when the procedure is used in acute cholecystitis.'   *NIH Consensus Statement 1992 Sep 14–16; 10(3):1–20. Kiviluoto T, et al. Lancet 1998; 351:321–325.*

18

18

tion of the abdominal contents to exclude other pathology, the cystic duct and artery are identified. Intra-operative cholangiography is performed under image intensification by cannulating the cystic duct and following the injection of contrast. The cholangiogram displays the anatomy of the duct system, identifies ductal stones, and confirms that dye passes freely into the duodenum (Fig. 18.20). Once the films have been inspected, the cystic duct and artery are ligated and divided and the gallbladder is removed. A retrograde approach, in which the gallbladder is mobilized 'fundus first', can be used when inflammation makes visualization of the biliary anatomy difficult, and in difficult cases a subtotal cholecystectomy may avoid damage of vital structures.

Some surgeons pursue a policy of selective cholangiography, obtaining a cholangiogram only in patients at high risk of having ductal stones. The presence of such stones may be suspected if there is a history of jaundice or pancreatitis, if pre-operative LFTs are abnormal, or if dilatation of the common bile duct or the presence of multiple gall-

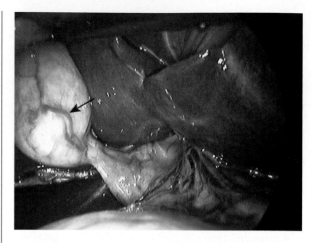

Fig. 18.21   Laparoscopic view of the gallbladder attached to the main bile duct beneath the liver and showing the branches of the cystic artery (arrow) on the gallbladder surface.

bladder stones has been detected on ultrasound. At surgery, a stone may be palpable in the duct system.

Following removal of the gallbladder, haemostasis is secured and the wound is closed. Many surgeons leave a drain in the subhepatic space to prevent the development of a collection and to identify leakage of bile, although the value of this approach has been questioned.

Laparoscopic cholecystectomy

Access to the peritoneal cavity is obtained through three or four cannulae inserted through the anterior abdominal wall and following insufflation of the peritoneal cavity with CO_2. The gallbladder is retracted by grasping forceps inserted through the most lateral cannula in order to display the structures at the porta hepatis. An excellent view of the operating field is obtained with the laparoscope (Fig. 18.21), and the cystic duct and artery are isolated by dissection with instruments passed through the remaining cannulae.

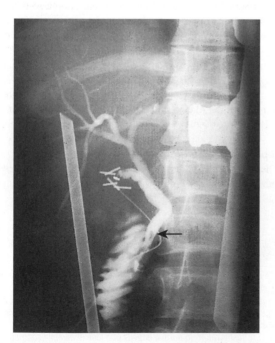

Fig. 18.20   Operative cholangiogram undertaken at laparoscopic cholecystectomy (note the radio-opaque ports).
The extrahepatic ducts are seen and there is flow of contrast into the duodenum. A small radiolucent calculus is present at the lower end of the common bile duct (arrow).

BOX 18.7   CHOLECYSTECTOMY

- Cholecystectomy is the standard treatment for symptomatic gallbladder stones; alternatives (stone dissolution, extracorporeal lithotripsy) are now seldom used
- Open cholecystectomy has been largely superseded by laparoscopic cholecystectomy, but conversion to open operation is still sometimes needed
- Cholecystectomy now has a low operative mortality (0.2%); inadvertent injury to the bile duct (0.2% incidence) remains the main source of major morbidity
- Some 5–10% of patients undergoing cholecystectomy have ductal stones, many of which are unsuspected. Opinions vary as to whether intra-operative cholangiography should be undertaken routinely to detect such stones
- In the era of laparoscopic cholecystectomy, there is a growing tendency not to perform routine operative cholangiography, and to extract symptomatic duct stones by non-operative means (i.e. at endoscopic papillotomy)
- If ductal stones cause symptoms, they frequently give rise to cholangitis and Charcot's triad of pain, jaundice and fever (often with rigors)

EBM 18.6   EXPLORATION OF THE COMMON BILE DUCT

'Patients undergoing cholecystectomy do not require ERCP pre-operatively if there is a low probability of choledocholithiasis. Laparoscopic common bile duct exploration and post-operative ERCP are both safe and reliable in clearing common bile duct stones.'

Nathanson L, et al. Ann Surg 2005; 242:912–188.

Some surgeons have found it difficult to undertake operative cholangiography routinely with this approach, and have either abandoned its use or relied upon intravenous cholangiography, MRCP or ERCP in the pre- or post-operative period to exclude the presence of common bile duct stones.

The cystic duct and artery are divided between metal clips and the gallbladder is dissected from the liver using diathermy. Extraction of the gallbladder through a cannula site may require extension of the incision or the tedious removal of individual stones from the gallbladder. Care must be taken to secure haemostasis, and many surgeons leave a drain in the subhepatic space.

Exploration of the common bile duct

This is undertaken much less often with the free availability of ERCP and sphincterotomy (EBM 18.6). At open surgery, if stones are present in the duct system, the common bile duct is opened longitudinally between stay sutures (choledochotomy) and the stones are extracted with forceps (Desjardins forceps) or a Fogarty balloon catheter. Following exploration, further check cholangiogram films are obtained, or the interior of the duct can be inspected with a rigid or fibreoptic choledochoscope.

The opening in the common bile duct is closed around a T-tube, the long limb of which is brought out through a stab incision in the abdominal wall (Fig. 18.22). This serves as a safety valve to allow the escape of bile if there is a temporary obstruction to flow into the duodenum following duct exploration. It also facilitates the installation of iodine-containing dye to obtain a T-tube cholangiogram some 7–10 days following surgery. If this shows free flow of dye into the duodenum and no residual duct stones, the T-tube can be clamped before removal.

If, at operation, a stone is firmly impacted at the lower end of the common bile duct, it may have to be removed through the duodenum. Transduodenal sphincterotomy and sphincteroplasty increase the risk of post-operative morbidity and mortality, and are undertaken rarely.

With the reluctance of some surgeons to perform operative cholangiography during laparoscopic cholecystectomy, increasing reliance has been placed on removing common bile duct stones at ERCP. Other surgeons continue to adhere to the principles employed at open cholecystectomy and explore the common bile duct by means of a choledochotomy or through the dilated cystic duct. Retained stones can be removed with the aid of a small-diameter fibreoptic choledochoscope under direct vision, or by means of a wire basket or an inflatable balloon catheter using the image intensifier. The surgeon can suture

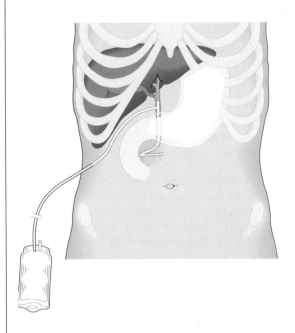

Fig. 18.22   T-tube drainage of the common bile duct.

or leave a drain in the cystic duct, or can oversew the choledochotomy over a T-tube or stent.

COMPLICATIONS OF CHOLECYSTECTOMY

The post-operative stay of patients undergoing open cholecystectomy may exceed 7 days. Respiratory complications are not uncommon and there is a significant risk of wound infection (see below). Operative mortality following elective open cholecystectomy is low (0.2%), but is increased tenfold if there is obstructive jaundice or if the common bile duct has to be explored.

Post-operative stay is reduced greatly with laparoscopic cholecystectomy, which in some centres is undertaken as a day-case procedure. Complications resulting from a major abdominal wound are undoubtedly avoided, but there is concern regarding the apparent increased incidence of injury to the bile duct. Failure of the patient to recover quickly following the procedure, the development of abdominal pain or the need for additional analgesia in the immediate post-operative period should cause the surgeon to consider the complications of haemorrhage or bile leakage, and mandates further assessment by LFTs and abdominal imaging. Mortality and morbidity related to the laparoscopic procedure have also been reported. Nevertheless, the advantages to the patient of this minimally invasive technique have led to its widespread adoption by surgeons.

Haemorrhage

This may originate from the cystic artery or the gallbladder bed. Significant intra-abdominal bleeding may not be readily apparent, but should be suspected from the development of pain or if the patient exhibits early features of

18

hypovolaemic shock. Blood may issue from the drain, if one is present, and re-exploration is mandatory.

Infective complications

Wound infection from organisms present in the bile (notably *E. coli, Klebsiella aerogenes* and *Strep. faecalis*) can be reduced following cholecystectomy by the intravenous administration of a cephalosporin at the time of induction of anaesthesia, although the routine use of this group of drugs at laparoscopic cholecystectomy has recently been questioned (EBM 18.7). A longer course of antibiotics may be prescribed when operating on patients with obstructive jaundice, cholangitis, or complications such as acute chole-cystitis or empyema when significant bile contamination of the peritoneal cavity has occurred. Collections of bile and/or blood readily become infected after cholecystectomy. Formal drainage may be needed if this progresses to the formation of a subhepatic or subphrenic abscess.

Bile leakage

This may be due to a ligature or clip slipping off the cystic duct, the accidental division of an unrecognized accessory duct, damage to the common bile duct, or retention of a duct stone after exploration. Bile leakage may be evidenced by the development of abnormal LFTs and localized or gener-alized abdominal pain. It may be contained if a drain is in place. In the absence of biliary peritonitis, a persistent leak requires investigation by means of endoscopic cholan-giography. Surgery may be needed if biliary peritonitis develops.

Retained stones

Following bile duct exploration, the post-operative T-tube cholangiogram (see above) may reveal a retained stone in the bile duct. Small stones can sometimes be flushed into the duodenum by irrigating the T-tube with saline, and their passage may be facilitated if glucagon is given to relax the sphincter of Oddi. If the duct cannot be cleared by irrigation, delayed extraction of the stones may be undertaken under radiological control. The patient is discharged with the T-tube in place. This is removed 4–6 weeks later and a steerable catheter passed along its track into the bile duct. A wire (Dormia) basket can be passed along the catheter to catch and withdraw the retained calculus (Fig. 18.23).

In some patients, unsuspected stones may be left in the bile duct at cholecystectomy. Such stones usually give rise to complications such as jaundice, cholangitis and pan-creatitis in the months and years following cholecystectomy. ERCP can be used to confirm the presence of such retained stones (Fig. 18.24) and endoscopic papillotomy is performed to recover them (Fig. 18.25). In this technique,

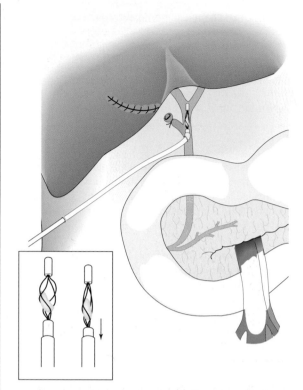

Fig. 18.23 Removal of a retained common bile duct stone.

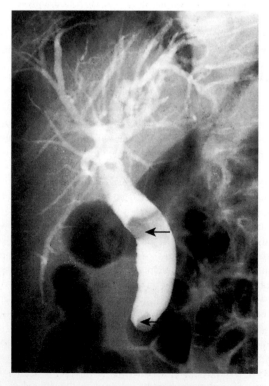

Fig. 18.24 Endoscopic retrograde cholangiography demonstrating multiple stones (arrows) within the biliary tree.
These calculi were removed from the dilated bile duct by balloon extraction following sphincterotomy.

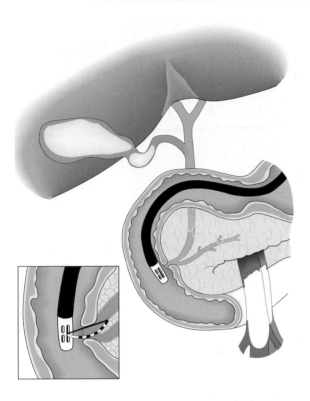

Fig. 18.25 Endoscopic papillotomy to remove retained stones.

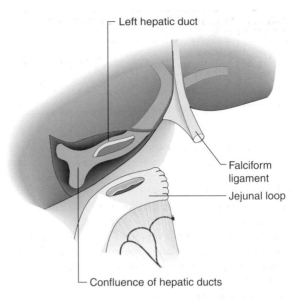

Fig. 18.26 Relief of bile duct stricture by anastomosis of a loop of jejunum to the distended biliary tree above the stricture (hepaticojejunostomy Roux en Y).

18

a diathermy wire attached to a cannula is passed through the duodenoscope and used to divide the sphincter of Oddi. The stones can then be extracted with a Dormia basket or balloon catheter. The same method can be used to extract stones detected in the immediate post-operative period. If the stones are too large to be withdrawn or the patient is unwell, a stent or a catheter can be left in the biliary system (nasobiliary catheter). The stones can be crushed (lithotripsy) and removed at a later date by means of a repeat endoscopic examination. It is uncommon to have to operate to retrieve retained bile duct stones.

Bile duct stricture

About 90% of benign duct strictures result from damage during cholecystectomy, in which the duct is divided, ligated or devascularized. This last mechanism appears to be a common cause of injury at laparoscopic cholecystectomy. Other causes of injury include division of a ligated common bile duct that has been mistaken for the cystic duct, division of the right hepatic duct below the point of anomalous insertion of the cystic duct, and encirclement of the common bile duct by the ligature or clip used to close off the cystic duct. Strictures only occasionally result from abdominal trauma or erosion of the bile duct by a gallstone (Mirizzi's syndrome).

If the common bile duct is completely occluded, progressive obstructive jaundice develops in the post-operative period. If there is a partial stricture, attacks of pain, fever and obstructive jaundice signal the development of cholangitis. The serum alkaline phosphatase and transaminase concentrations are usually elevated, and blood cultures may be positive during attacks of fever. If left untreated, persistent cholangitis and obstruction progress to secondary biliary cirrhosis, hepatic abscess formation, portal hypertension and liver failure.

The site and extent of the stricture must be defined radiologically. After ultrasonography has been performed, MRCP, ERCP and/or PTC are undertaken. Reconstructive surgery is carried out in a specialist centre and usually necessitates bringing up a Roux loop of jejunum and anastomosing this to the distended biliary system above the stricture (Fig. 18.26).

Post-cholecystectomy syndrome

This term is used to embrace a group of complaints such as post-prandial flatulence, fat intolerance, epigastric and right hypochondrial discomfort, and heartburn, which may follow cholecystectomy. The complaints tend to be more trouble-some when cholecystectomy has been performed in the absence of gallstones. Investigations are usually negative, but some patients prove to have retained stones or other alimentary disorders such as peptic ulceration, gastritis and chronic pancreatitis. It is possible that some patients develop pain because of functional abnormalities of the sphincter of Oddi (see below).

MANAGEMENT OF ACUTE CHOLECYSTITIS

Patients with acute cholecystitis are admitted to hospital. The pulse, blood pressure and temperature are monitored,

265

18

EBM 18.8   TIMING OF CHOLECYSTECTOMY

'Early cholecystectomy for acute cholecystitis is associated with a better outcome than delayed cholecystectomy.'

Papi C, et al. Am J Gastroenterol 2004; 99(1):147–155.
Shikata S, et al. Surgery 2005; 35:553–560.

and analgesics, intravenous fluid and a broad-spectrum antibiotic such as a cephalosporin are prescribed. Patients are given nothing by mouth and a nasogastric tube is passed if they are vomiting. The majority of patients settle within a few days on this regimen. Failure to settle suggests the presence of an empyema.

Some surgeons delay operation for 2–3 months after the attack in the expectation that the acute inflammatory reaction will have resolved by then, but most now prefer to perform cholecystectomy during the same admission and within 72 hours of the onset of the attack (EBM 18.8). Provided the operation is carried out by an experienced surgeon and under antibiotic cover, 'early' cholecystectomy is not associated with an increased incidence of complications. The duration of the illness and hospitalization is reduced, and further attacks of acute cholecystitis during the waiting period for elective surgery are averted. It should be noted that this is a planned procedure carried out after appropriate investigation (ultrasonography) and with all facilities, on a routine elective list. Laparoscopic cholecystectomy is more difficult to perform in the acute setting, but is the method preferred by most surgeons.

If surrounding inflammation makes identification of the relevant anatomical structures difficult, drainage of the gallbladder with removal of stones (cholecystostomy) may be performed as an interim measure. Elective cholecystectomy is usually performed approximately 2 months later.

ATYPICAL 'BILIARY' PAIN

More difficulty arises with patients who have attacks of pain consistent with biliary colic but in whom investigations such as ultrasonography, oral cholecystography and ERCP reveal no abnormality. Some of these patients with 'acalculous biliary pain' may eventually prove to have non-biliary disease, such as peptic ulceration, chronic pancreatitis or 'irritable' colon. In the majority, no explanation for the symptoms can be found, although recent evidence suggests that some may be suffering from a functional disorder of the sphincter of Oddi (Fig. 18.27). Endoscopic manometry may be useful in identifying patients who may benefit from endoscopic sphincterotomy.

NON-SURGICAL TREATMENT OF GALLSTONES

Dissolution therapy with bile salts is no longer popular in the management of gallstone disease. Percutaneous extraction or dissolution of gallstones is possible, but the efficacy and complications of this approach have been questioned. Destruction of stones by extracorporeal shock-wave

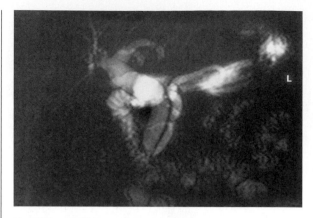

Fig. 18.27   MRCP in a patient who underwent laparoscopic cholecystectomy 5 years before the development of recurrent right upper quadrant pain.
The bile and pancreatic ducts are dilated secondary to biliary dyskinesia.

lithotripsy has been used in selected patients but, like the previous treatments, has largely been made redundant with the advent of laparoscopic cholecystectomy.

MANAGEMENT OF ACUTE CHOLANGITIS

This condition is caused by incomplete obstruction of the biliary tree and is more often due to common bile duct stones. It is not frequently observed as a presenting feature of malignancy, but may result from instrumentation of the biliary tree during the investigation or treatment of malignant obstructive jaundice.

The patient is often extremely unwell, with evidence of septic shock. Treatment involves resuscitation, the administration of appropriate antibiotics, and decompression of the biliary tree. Given the high associated morbidity and mortality of surgical intervention, decompression is normally achieved by endoscopic means. When common bile duct stones are responsible, it may be necessary to drain the biliary tree temporarily by means of a stent, even if sphincterotomy and stone extraction have apparently been successful.

OTHER BENIGN BILIARY DISORDERS

ASIATIC CHOLANGIOHEPATITIS

There has been a decline in the incidence of this condition, which occurs in the Far East and is particularly common in coastal Chinese communities. Suppurative cholangitis develops and pigment stones form in the intrahepatic and extrahepatic biliary tree. Deconjugation of bilirubin glucuronide by bacteria may be implicated in stone formation, and *E. coli* and *Strep. faecalis* can often be isolated from the bile and portal blood.

The clinical features are those of obstructive jaundice, pain and fever, and liver abscesses may form. Cholangitis is treated with antibiotics, and stones in the duct can be removed by percutaneous, endoscopic and operative means. Ductal obstruction may be treated by choledochoduodenostomy or hepaticojejunostomy. A limb of the Roux loop of jejunum may be left in a subcutaneous position to facilitate subsequent percutaneous manoeuvres to treat residual or recurrent calculi. Hepatic resection may be indicated if suppuration and obstruction have led to regional destruction of liver tissue.

PRIMARY SCLEROSING CHOLANGITIS

In this condition, both intrahepatic and extrahepatic bile ducts may become indurated and irregularly thickened. There is a marked chronic inflammatory cell infiltrate and fibrous narrowing of the biliary tree. The aetiology of the condition is unknown, but it may have an immunological basis. Over three-quarters of patients also suffer from ulcerative colitis; other associated conditions include retroperitoneal fibrosis, immunodeficiency syndromes and pancreatitis. Bile duct carcinoma can develop, and obstruction can give rise to bacterial cholangitis and secondary biliary cirrhosis.

The condition frequently affects young adults and gives rise to intermittent attacks of obstructive jaundice, pruritus and pain. ERCP and liver biopsy are the mainstays of diagnosis. Medical treatment is generally unsatisfactory, and the outlook is extremely variable. Duct strictures can sometimes by treated by surgical bypass or the insertion of stents, but such manoeuvres may compromise the ability to undertake successful liver transplantation, which offers the only prospect of cure.

TUMOURS OF THE BILIARY TRACT

CARCINOMA OF THE GALLBLADDER

Carcinoma of the gallbladder is rare and almost invariably associated with the presence of gallstones. The condition is four times as common in females as in males. About 90%

of lesions are adenocarcinomas; the remainder are squamous carcinomas.

Direct invasion commonly obstructs the bile duct or porta hepatis, and early lymphatic and haematogenous dissemination is common. Initial symptoms are indistinguishable from those of gallstones but jaundice, if present, is unremitting. A mass may be palpable. Many tumours are detected incidentally at cholecystectomy for the treatment of gallstones. Some surgeons recommend an aggressive approach of segmental resection, involving segments IV, V and VI of the liver and dissection of the regional lymph nodes. Tumours presenting with jaundice cannot be cured by resection, and palliation by endoscopic or percutaneous insertion of a stent or surgical bypass is required. The 5-year survival rate is less than 5%.

CARCINOMA OF THE BILE DUCTS

Cholangiocarcinoma is a relatively uncommon cancer that affects the elderly and which is increasing in frequency. The tumour may arise at any site within the biliary tree and can be multifocal. Tumours can be classified based on the level of involvement of the biliary tree (Fig. 18.28). Polypoidal tumours are uncommon but carry a more favourable outlook. Sclerotic lesions involving the confluence of the hepatic ducts (Klatskin tumour) pose considerable problems in management. The lesions are said to be slow-growing, but this has been over-emphasized. Cholangiocarcinoma may develop in patients with underlying primary sclerosing cholangitis or choledochal cyst.

Clinical features
Progressive obstructive jaundice, often preceded by vague dyspeptic pain, is the usual presenting feature. The gallbladder may become obstructed because of cystic duct involvement, and mucocoele or empyema can develop, but generally it is impalpable. Anorexia and weight loss are common. Pruritus is often particularly distressing.

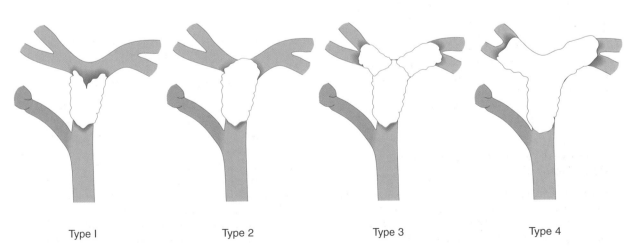

Type I   Type 2   Type 3   Type 4

Fig. 18.28 **Classification of cholangiocarcinoma.**

18

Management

The diagnosis of malignant obstruction may be made on the history and clinical findings. The presence of intrahepatic duct dilatation and a collapsed gallbladder on ultrasound scan are highly suggestive of a tumour involving the common hepatic duct. Resectability is best assessed by CT or MRI to exclude the presence of hepatic metastases and nodal involvement and to assess vascular invasion.

Carcinoma of the common bile duct is treated by the Whipple operation (p. 281) if the tumour is localized and the patient is fit for radical resection. Long-term survival following this procedure is better in patients with cholangiocarcinoma than in those with carcinoma of the head of the pancreas.

Carcinoma of the upper biliary tract is resectable in only 10% of patients, some of whom may require hepatic resection to achieve satisfactory clearance of the tumour. Following resection, the remaining biliary tree is anastomosed to a Roux loop of jejunum. In the majority of patients not submitted to resection, palliation can be achieved by insertion of a stent by endoscopic or percutaneous transhepatic techniques (Fig. 18.29). Most stents are liable to occlusion, exposing the patient to repeated attacks of cholangitis and/or jaundice. Some surgeons prefer surgical palliation, which can be effected by intrahepatic anastomosis of a Roux loop of jejunum to the segment III duct in the left lobe of the liver. Although decompression of only one-half of the biliary tree is achieved, this operation provides effective palliation in the short term. Few patients with cholangiocarcinoma survive for more than 18 months. The role of systemic chemotherapy and/or radiotherapy has yet to be established.

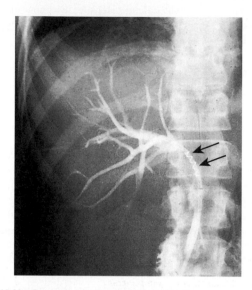

Fig. 18.29 Percutaneous transhepatic cholangiogram demonstrating a stricture at the confluence of the hepatic ducts. This lesion has the typical appearance of a cholangiocarcinoma and has been managed by percutaneous insertion of a stent (arrowed).

19

O.J. GARDEN

The pancreas and spleen

THE PANCREAS

SURGICAL ANATOMY

The pancreas develops from separate ventral and dorsal buds of endoderm that appear during the fourth week of fetal life. The ventral pancreas develops in association with the biliary tree, and its duct joins the common bile duct before emptying into the duodenum through the papilla of Vater (Fig. 19.1). During gestation, the duodenum rotates clockwise on its long axis, and the bile duct and ventral pancreas pass round behind it to fuse with the dorsal pancreas. Most of the duct that drains the dorsal pancreas joins the duct draining the ventral pancreas to form the main pancreatic duct (of Wirsung); the rest of the dorsal duct becomes the accessory pancreatic duct (of Santorini) and enters the duodenum 2.5 cm proximal to the main duct. In fetal life, the common bile duct and main pancreatic duct are dilated at their junction to form the ampulla of Vater. In extra-uterine life, only 10% of individuals retain this ampulla, although the great majority still have a short common channel between the two duct systems.

The pancreas lies retroperitoneally, behind the lesser sac and stomach. The head of the gland lies within the C-loop of the duodenum, with which it shares a blood supply from the coeliac and superior mesenteric arteries (Fig. 19.2). The superior mesenteric vein runs upwards to the left of the

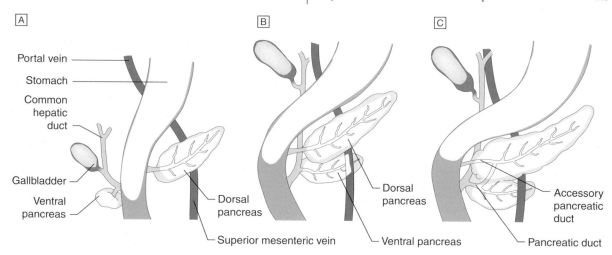

Fig. 19.1 The development of the pancreas.

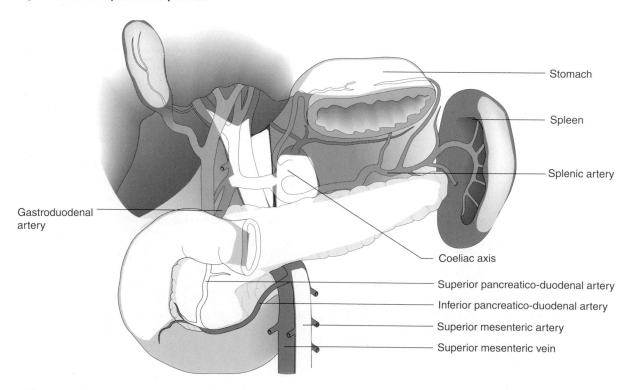

Fig. 19.2 Anatomical relationships of the pancreas.

uncinate process, and joins the splenic vein behind the neck of the pancreas to form the portal vein. The body and tail of the pancreas lie in front of the splenic vein as far as the splenic hilum, and receive arterial blood from the splenic artery as it runs along the upper border of the gland. The intimate relationship of the friable pancreas to these major blood vessels is the reason that bleeding is problematic after pancreatic trauma. The close association between the common bile duct and the head of pancreas explains why obstructive jaundice is so common in cancer of the head of the pancreas, and why gallstones frequently give rise to acute pancreatitis.

SURGICAL PHYSIOLOGY

EXOCRINE FUNCTION

The exocrine pancreas is essential for the digestion of fat, protein and carbohydrate. The pancreas secretes 1–2 litres of alkaline (pH 7.5–8.8) enzyme-rich juice each day. The enzymes are synthesized by the acinar cells and stored there as zymogen granules. Trypsin is the key proteolytic enzyme; it is released in an inactive form (trypsinogen) and is normally only activated within the duodenum by the brush border enzyme, enterokinase. Once trypsin has been activated, a cascade is established whereby the other proteolytic enzymes become activated in turn. Lipase and amylase are secreted as active enzymes. The alkaline medium required for the activity of pancreatic enzymes is provided by the bicarbonate secreted by the ductal epithelium.

Pancreatic secretion is stimulated by eating. Hormonal and neural (vagal) mechanisms are involved. Food entering the duodenum (notably fat and protein digestion products) releases cholecystokinin (CCK), which stimulates pancreatic enzyme secretion, while at the same time causing the gallbladder to contract and increase bile flow into the intestine. Acid in the duodenum releases the hormone secretin, which stimulates the pancreas to secrete watery alkaline juice.

ENDOCRINE FUNCTION

The islets of Langerhans are distributed throughout the pancreas. Although they account for only 2% of the weight of the gland, they receive 10% of its blood supply. Interaction between the endocrine and the exocrine pancreas is facilitated by the close proximity of islets and acini, and by a local 'portal' system in which blood draining from the islets enters a capillary network around neighbouring acinar cells before entering the tributaries of the portal vein. Four types of islet cell are recognized: A cells produce glucagons; B cells, insulin; D cells, somatostatin; and PP cells, pancreatic polypeptide. Glucagon and insulin have well-established physiological roles; the function of the other islet products is uncertain, but somatostatin and pancreatic polypeptide may serve as local (paracrine) regulators, rather than as circulating (endocrine) messengers. Gastrin-producing (G) cells are not normally found in the pancreas, except in the rare Zollinger–Ellison syndrome (Ch. 17).

PANCREATIC PAIN

The parasympathetic nervous system has no role in the perception of pancreatic pain. Painful stimuli from the pancreas are transmitted by sympathetic fibres that travel along the arteries of supply to the coeliac ganglion, and from there to segments 5–10 of the thoracic spinal cord via the greater (and lesser) splanchnic nerves.

CONGENITAL DISORDERS OF THE PANCREAS

Annular pancreas is a rare cause of duodenal obstruction, resulting from failure of rotation of the ventral pancreas.

In approximately 5% of individuals, the ducts draining the dorsal and ventral pancreas fail to fuse, giving rise to pancreas divisum. This means that the secretions of the larger dorsal pancreas have to drain to the duodenum through the smaller accessory duct. There is no evidence to suggest a strong association between pancreas divisum and acute or chronic pancreatitis.

Rests of pancreatic tissue may be found at a variety of sites within the gut wall, but are most common in the duodenum, stomach and proximal small bowel. Such heterotopic tissue remains asymptomatic, but can cause ulceration, bleeding and obstruction.

Cystic fibrosis affects the sweat glands, pancreas and bronchial mucous glands. Meconium ileus can produce surgical problems by giving rise to intestinal obstruction in neonates.

PANCREATITIS

Pancreatitis may be acute or chronic. After an attack of acute pancreatitis, the gland usually returns to anatomical and functional normality, whereas chronic pancreatitis is associated with a permanent derangement of structure and function. Some patients suffer from recurrent acute pancreatitis but enjoy relatively normal health between attacks.

ACUTE PANCREATITIS

Acute pancreatitis is a common cause of emergency admission to hospital. Britain has 100–200 new cases per million of the population each year and the incidence continues to rise, possibly as a result of increasing alcohol consumption. The disease is relatively rare in children, but all adult age groups may be affected. Roughly 1 in 4 patients proves to have severe disease, and of these 1 in 4 will die.

Aetiology

Conditions associated with the development of acute pancreatitis are listed in Table 19.1; gallstones and alcohol are of overriding importance.

19

Table 19.1   CAUSES OF ACUTE PANCREATITIS
Non-traumatic (75%) **Major factors** • Biliary tract disease (50%) • Alcohol (20–30%)
Minor factors • Viral infection (mumps, Coxsackie) • Drugs (e.g. steroids) • Hyperparathyroidism • Hyperlipidaemia • Scorpion bites (Trinidad) • Hypothermia • Pancreatic cancer • Polyarteritis nodosa • Previous Polya gastrectomy
Traumatic (5%) • Operative trauma • Blunt or penetrating injury • Investigation (ERCP or angiography) **Idiopathic (20%)**

Gallstone pancreatitis

Gallstones are present in some 40% of patients in the UK who develop acute pancreatitis. Most of these have many small stones in the gallbladder, a wide cystic duct, and a common channel between the common bile duct and the main pancreatic duct (Fig. 19.3). It is now believed that stones or biliary sand may impact transiently in the common channel and so promote the reflux of bile into the pancreatic duct and/or impair the normal flow of pancreatic juice. It has also become apparent that many patients with 'idiopathic acute pancreatitis' are actually suffering from pancreatitis caused not by stones per se, but by debris containing microcrystals of cholesterol and calcium bilirubinate granules (so-called biliary sludge). The causal significance of gallstones and biliary sludge in acute pancreatitis is underlined by the fact that further attacks are exceptional once biliary tract disease has been eradicated.

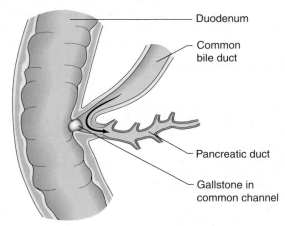

Duodenum

Common bile duct

Pancreatic duct

Gallstone in common channel

Fig. 19.3   A common channel shared by the bile duct and the pancreatic duct may allow gallstone pancreatitis.

Alcohol-associated pancreatitis

The proportion of cases of acute pancreatitis linked to alcohol varies in different parts of the world. In Scotland the figure is around 30%, whereas in some parts of France and North America it may be as high as 50–90%. The mechanism responsible is uncertain. Alcohol consumption normally exceeds 80 g day immediately prior to an attack, but genetic vulnerability is likely. Alcohol may cause the secretion of unduly viscid juice, with the formation of protein plugs and impairment of flow, and may also generate toxic free radicals that directly damage the gland. Alcohol-associated pancreatitis frequently causes permanent damage to the gland, with progression to chronic pancreatitis.

Other causes

Of the other rarer causes, pancreatitis following ERCP has assumed a greater importance because of the increasing number of such diagnostic procedures being undertaken, and owing to the particularly severe form of disease following over-injection of contrast into the pancreatic duct. A small number of patients may have a family history of acute pancreatitis. There is a high incidence of pancreatic cancer when familial pancreatitis proceeds to its chronic form. The most common causes in children are the mumps virus, trauma (particularly from the ends of bicycle handlebars impacting on the epigastrium) and multi-organ failure.

Pathophysiology

Pancreatic inflammation ranges in severity from mild oedema to severe necrosis and haemorrhage. In general, oedematous pancreatitis is usually mild and settles on conservative treatment, whereas necrotizing pancreatitis is frequently severe, often leading to complications, the need for operation and death.

Local effects

The exact mechanism responsible for acute pancreatitis remains uncertain. Reflux of duodenal juice and/or bile into the pancreatic duct and obstruction to the flow of pancreatic juice may trigger premature activation of pancreatic enzymes within the duct system. Intraduct activation of trypsin, chymotrypsin, phospholipase, catalase and elastase may then unleash a chain reaction of cell necrosis, further enzyme release and changes in the microcirculation. Rupture of the duct system permits autodigestion of the gland. The continued release of activated proteolytic enzymes is responsible for increased capillary permeability, protein exudation, retroperitoneal oedema and peritoneal exudation. Vasoactive kinins such as kallikrein are also released, and activated macrophages may release cytokines. Alcohol induces spasm of the sphincter of Oddi and increases the sensitivity of acinar cells to CCK hyperstimulation, resulting in enhanced intracellular protease activation.

General effects

The majority of patients who develop severe pancreatitis have evidence of early organ dysfunction at the time of admission or soon thereafter. Worsening organ failure is associated with a poor outcome. Profound hypovolaemic shock may follow the fluid, protein and electrolyte loss that results from altered capillary permeability, and metabolic upsets result from cytokine release. Endotoxin can be detected in the systemic circulation in many patients, indicating that bacteria and their products may also be implicated in the circulatory upset. Other factors that contribute to the systemic upset include acute renal failure (possibly due to a combination of hypovolaemia, endo-toxaemia and local intravascular coagulation), acute respira-tory distress syndrome (ARDS, due to altered permeability in pulmonary capillaries), consumptive coagulopathy, and altered liver function (due to hepatocyte depression and/or obstruction of the common bile duct by a gallstone or pancreatic oedema).

Clinical features

Constant severe or agonizing pain in the epigastrium, with radiation through to the back, is usually prominent. Pain can also be experienced in either hypochondrium. Nausea, vomiting and retching are often marked.

Clinical examination often reveals much less tenderness, guarding and rigidity than might have been expected from the patient's history. Shock is often present in severe pancreatitis. Bruising around the umbilicus (Cullen's sign) or brawny discoloration of the flanks (Grey–Turner's sign) is an uncommon, relatively late sign of severe pancreatitis but is indicative of a poor prognosis. Obstructive jaundice may be apparent in patients with pancreatitis due to an impacted gallstone, but is usually transient. A pleural effusion may be detected in about 20% of cases, and is almost always left-sided; it probably represents the effect of inflammation tracking retroperitoneally to involve the pleura.

Diagnosis

The key to the diagnosis of acute pancreatitis is a high index of suspicion and measurement of the serum amylase concentration (EBM 19.1). Previous attacks of flatulent dyspepsia, biliary colic or jaundice may suggest biliary pancreatitis. Alcohol intake should be documented.

EBM 19.1 DIAGNOSIS AND PROGNOSIS OF ACUTE PANCREATITIS

'Although amylase is widely available and provides acceptable accuracy of diagnosis, where lipase estimation is available it is preferred for the diagnosis of acute pancreatitis.'
'Available prognostic features which predict complications in acute pancreatitis are clinical impression of severity, obesity or APACHE II.8 in the first 24 hours of admission, and C-reactive protein > 150 mg/l, Glasgow score 3 or more or persisting organ failure after 48 hours in hospital. Patients with persisting organ failure, signs of sepsis or deterioration in clinical status 6–10 days after admission will require computed tomography.'

Working Party of the British Society of Gastroenterology; Association of Surgeons of Great Britain and Ireland; Pancreatic Society of Great Britain and Ireland; Association of Upper Gastrointestinal Surgeons of Great Britain and Ireland. Gut 2005; 54 suppl 3:iii 1–9.

Biochemistry

The diagnosis is usually supported by a raised total serum amylase of at least three times the upper limit of normal (generally > 1000 U/l). Hyperamylasaemia reflects the rupture of acinar cells and parts of the ductal system, with the release of amylase into the circulation. The serum amylase levels usually rise rapidly (within 6 hours) but are often raised only transiently, returning to normal within 48 hours. Serum lipase levels also rise in acute pancreatitis, the rise being slower but more sustained, but this test is not generally undertaken routinely by most laboratories.

As shown in Table 19.2, a number of other conditions can produce hyperamylasaemia, although the rise is seldom as high as 1000 U/l. Most conditions causing such 'false positive' rises in serum amylase demand prompt surgical intervention, whereas surgery is usually avoided whenever possible in the early stages of acute pancreatitis. Approximately 30% of fatal attacks of pancreatitis are diagnosed at post-mortem. If there is significant diagnostic doubt, urgent ultrasonography or computed tomography (CT) may reveal the true diagnosis. False negative results occur in 5–10% of cases of acute pancreatitis, in that the patient is seen before (exceptionally) or after the hyperamylasaemia has occurred. There is no correlation between the height of the serum amylase level and the severity of the attack.

Radiology

A left-sided pleural effusion or features of ARDS may be seen on chest X-ray. A bowel empty of gas except for a 'sentinel loop' of jejunum may reflect local ileus, and in some cases gas is seen in the hepatic and splenic flexures but not the transverse colon—the 'colon cut-off' sign. Radio-opaque gallstones may be seen in some patients with gallstone pancreatitis.

Ultrasonography may reveal swelling of the pancreas with peripancreatic fluid collections and oedema, and may detect gallstones. CT is not usually performed as part of the initial diagnostic assessment but may also reveal pancreatic and peripancreatic swelling, the development of necrosis (see below) and the presence of gallstones. Although there is considerable interest in magnetic resonance imaging (MRI), it is not suitable for patients requiring significant intensive care support. Gastrografin studies are not normally indicated, unless ulcer perforation cannot be excluded.

Table 19.2 NON-PANCREATIC DISORDERS CAPABLE OF CAUSING HYPERAMYLASAEMIA

- Acute cholecystitis
- Perforated duodenal ulcer
- High intestinal obstruction
- Mesenteric vascular occlusion
- Bowel strangulation
- Dissecting aortic aneurysm
- Ruptured aortic aneurysm
- Ruptured ectopic pregnancy

19

Differentiation between gallstone- and alcohol-associated pancreatitis

It may not be evident from the history and presentation whether the attack of pancreatitis is due to gallstone disease or to alcohol. On the one hand, there may be a history of alcohol abuse in a patient with known gallstone disease, whereas on the other, it should be remembered that some patients with no obvious predisposing factors may be shown to have gallstones during a subsequent readmission for an attack of idiopathic pancreatitis. Table 19.3 lists some of the ways in which alcohol and gallstones can be differentiated as potential causes of an attack of acute pancreatitis.

Assessment of severity

Most patients with severe attacks have some evidence of systemic organ dysfunction at presentation. This may be obvious clinically from the shocked state of the patient, or formal 'prognostic factor scores', such as the Glasgow system, can be used (Table 19.4). Urea and electrolyte measurements reflect the state of hydration and are helpful in managing fluid and electrolyte balance. Liver function tests (LFTs) may show hyperbilirubinaemia and elevation of liver enzymes, particularly in patients with gallstone pancreatitis. Hyperglycaemia and glycosuria can occur transiently in severe disease. Arterial blood gas analysis may reveal severe hypoxia. Moderate polymorphonuclear leucocytosis is common. Serum calcium levels may fall in severe disease. At one time, it was believed that this reflected the formation of calcium soaps following fat necrosis within the abdomen, but it is now recognized that much of the fall reflects the drop in serum albumin levels caused by protein exudation. A marked reduction in the level of ionized calcium is unusual and frank tetany is exceptional.

It should be appreciated that predictive systems require 48 hours for full evaluation, by which time clinical assessment is almost as accurate. Progress can be monitored by regular clinical evaluation, and a rising APACHE II score or a rising level of C-reactive protein (see below) may help to identify patients in need of urgent investigation and surgical intervention. Serum levels of interleukin-6 (IL-6), trypsinogen activation peptide and leucocyte elastase have been shown to be excellent markers of disease severity but are not generally available. If deterioration occurs, contrast-enhanced CT may detect pancreatic necrosis.

Management

There is no specific treatment for acute pancreatitis and most attacks settle with conservative management. All patients with suspected severe disease should be managed in a high-dependency or intensive care environment.

Conservative treatment

- *Pain relief.* Severe pain requires the administration of opiates; pethidine is frequently prescribed.
- *Treatment of shock.* Large volumes of crystalloid solution, plasma or dextran may be needed to maintain circulating blood volume and to correct intravascular hypovolaemia. Oxygen is essential in shocked patients, in whom pulse, blood pressure, urine output and central venous pressure should be monitored (Ch. 3).
- *Suppression of pancreatic function.* Oral fluids and diet are withheld. A nasogastric tube may relieve vomiting but there is no evidence that routine nasogastric intubation is beneficial.
- *Inhibition of pancreatic secretion or enzymes.* There is no evidence to support the use of the somatostatin analogue, octreotide. Similarly, several trials have shown no advantage to the use of the antiprotease, aprotinin (Trasylol), and gabexate mesylate in the treatment of pancreatitis.
- *Prevention of infection.* Antibiotic prophylaxis has been advocated by some as a means of reducing the risk of secondary infection. Others have been concerned that the more widespread use of antibiotics will result in an increased incidence of severe fungal infection. Consensus supports the use of a prophylactic antibiotic such as an intravenous cephalosporin for predicted severe disease.
- *Inhibition of inflammatory response.* There is currently no evidence to support the use of agents such as the platelet-activating factor (PAF) antagonist, lexipafant, as a means of reducing the inflammatory response in acute pancreatitis.
- *Nutritional support.* A reduction in acute-phase response and septic complications may result from enteral support rather than intravenous nutrition, although this requires the passage of a nasojejunal tube. There remains doubt as to whether outcome is affected, but enteral nutrition should be favoured where possible in patients with severe pancreatitis and its complications (EBM 19.2).

Table 19.3 DIAGNOSIS OF ALCOHOL- OR GALLSTONE-ASSOCIATED PANCREATITIS

	Alcohol	Gallstones
Female patient	+/–	+
History of alcohol abuse	+++	+/–
History of gallstone disease	+/–	+++
Family history of gallstones	+/–	++
High serum amylase level	+	++
Abnormal liver function tests	+	+++
Radiological evidence of gallstones	+/–	+++

Table 19.4 GLASGOW SYSTEM USED TO PREDICT SEVERITY OF ACUTE PANCREATITIS*

Criterion	Measurement
Age	> 55 years
White cell count	> 15 x 10^9/l
Blood glucose (no diabetic history)	> 10 mmol/l
Serum urea (no response to i.v. fluids)	> 16 mmol/l
PaO_2	< 8 kPa (60 mmHg)
Serum calcium	< 2.0 mmol/l
Serum albumin	< 32 g/l
Serum lactate dehydrogenase	> 600 U/l
Serum aspartate aminotransferase	> 100 U/l

* Factors are assessed within 48 hours of admission; three or more positive criteria indicate the presence of severe disease.

EBM 19.2   NUTRITIONAL SUPPORT IN ACUTE PANCREATITIS

'The evidence is not conclusive to support the use of enteral nutrition in all patients with severe acute pancreatitis. However, if nutritional support is required, the enteral route should be used if that can be tolerated.'

Working Party of the British Society of Gastroenterology; Association of Surgeons of Great Britain and Ireland; Pancreatic Society of Great Britain and Ireland; Association of Upper Gastrointestinal Surgeons of Great Britain and Ireland. Gut 2005; 54 suppl 3:iii1–9.

- *Other measures.* Peritoneal lavage with isotonic crystalloid solutions was once advocated as a means of removing enzymes and vasoactive substances from the peritoneal cavity and so preventing their absorption. However, recent trials have shown no reduction in mortality or morbidity in patients with severe acute pancreatitis.

Endoscopic treatment

When gallstones are suspected to be the cause of acute pancreatitis, consideration may be given to the endoscopic retrieval of such stones from the biliary tree using a basket or balloon following endoscopic sphincterotomy. When patients are admitted with a mild attack of pancreatitis, there is no need to institute such active therapy, as in most cases the offending gallstone will pass on into the duodenum spontaneously. In patients with severe disease that does not settle promptly on conservative management, endoscopic stone retrieval may abort the attack and reduce morbidity and mortality. All patients with predicted severe disease and any patient with suspected cholangitis should therefore undergo urgent endoscopic retrograde cholangiopancreatography (ERCP) and sphincterotomy.

Surgical treatment

Acute pancreatitis is managed conservatively whenever possible, but surgery is indicated under the following circumstances:

1. *When the diagnosis is uncertain.* If alternative causes of hyperamylasaemia are suspected, laparotomy is occasionally needed to confirm the diagnosis. It is accepted, however, that unnecessary laparotomy increases morbidity in patients with acute pancreatitis. If acute pancreatitis is present, no further action is usually needed, although when gallstones are found, consideration should be given to cholecystectomy.
2. *When the patient fails to improve on conservative management or deteriorates.* If the general condition and other indices (e.g. APACHE II score or C-reactive protein level) are deteriorating, the presence of pancreatic and peripancreatic necrosis must be suspected. A dynamic CT scan is obtained urgently, the term dynamic reflecting the fact that contrast is injected into the circulation so that it can be seen whether all of the pancreas enhances (and therefore has a blood supply and is not necrotic). If there is extensive infected necrosis (gas visible radiologically or a positive culture on

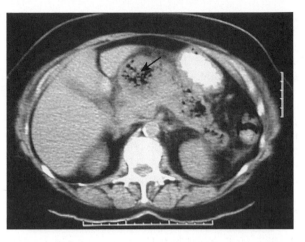

Fig. 19.4   CT scan showing a fluid collection with gas in an area of infected necrosis.

needle aspiration), urgent laparotomy is usually needed (Fig. 19.4).

3. *When gallstones are present.* Modern practice favours the 'early' eradication of gallstones in the course of the first admission with pancreatitis, and surgery is undertaken once the attack of acute pancreatitis has settled and following the diagnosis of gallstones. In patients with severe disease who fail to settle promptly, ERCP may both confirm the presence of stones and allow their removal following endoscopic sphincterotomy, thus permitting resolution of the attack. It cannot be overemphasized that patients who have had an attack of gallstone pancreatitis should not be allowed to have another because of failure to eradicate gallstones. Biliary surgery consists of cholecystectomy with operative cholangiography to ensure that there are no stones in the duct system that also require removal. A laparoscopic approach is normally possible in patients with mild disease during the same admission.
4. *When complications develop* (see below).

Complications

Pancreatic pseudocyst

A pancreatic pseudocyst is a collection of pancreatic secretions and inflammatory exudate enclosed in a wall of fibrous or granulation tissue. It differs from a true cyst in that the collection has no epithelial lining and is surrounded by inflammatory tissue. Pseudocysts form most commonly in the lesser sac or in the adjacent retroperitoneum, and differ from acute collections in that they persist for 4 or more weeks from the onset of acute pancreatitis. Small pseudocysts are usually asymptomatic and resolve spontaneously. In about 10% of patients, larger collections persist and can pose problems.

Pseudocysts typically do not declare themselves for some weeks after the episode of pancreatitis. Persistent or intermittent abdominal discomfort and mild to moderate hyperamylasaemia usually signal their presence, and larger collections may compress neighbouring structures to cause

19

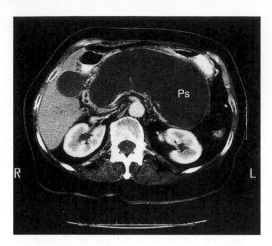

Fig. 19.5   CT scan showing a massive pseudocyst (PS) displacing the stomach and duodenum.

vomiting and obstructive jaundice. Ultrasonography is of great value in monitoring the progress of inflammation and in detecting pseudocyst formation, although a CT scan may better assist in determining the appropriate approach to treatment (Fig. 19.5). Some cysts become so large that they are palpable and, in some cases, visible.

The presence of a pseudocyst is not in itself an indication for surgical treatment. Approximately 50% of asymptomatic pseudocysts will resolve up to 12 weeks following the onset of acute pancreatitis. Treatment is indicated only if the pseudocyst is enlarging, and aims to avoid infection of the contents, haemorrhage or rupture. It normally consists of drainage of the pseudocyst into a Roux loop of jejunum (pseudocyst–jejunostomy), the stomach (pseudocyst–gastrostomy) or duodenum (pseudocyst–duodenostomy), whichever appears most appropriate (Fig. 19.6). As the tissues holding the sutures must be firm, it is desirable to avoid surgery within 6 weeks of the onset of the acute attack to allow the pseudocyst to 'mature', if possible. In the absence of necrosis, endoscopic cystogastrostomy may offer an alternative to surgery, but the relative roles of surgical and endoscopic drainage are yet to be determined.

Pancreatic abscess

A pancreatic abscess is a circumscribed intra-abdominal collection of pus, usually in proximity to the pancreas, containing little or no pancreatic necrosis. The presentation often resembles that of pancreatic pseudocyst, but the patient is usually more ill, and has pyrexia and leucocytosis. The presence of an abscess is confirmed by ultrasonography or CT (Fig. 19.4). Treatment consists of adequate external drainage under antibiotic cover and is achieved by laparotomy or endoscopic drainage combined with lavage, which allows the debridement of any associated necrosis.

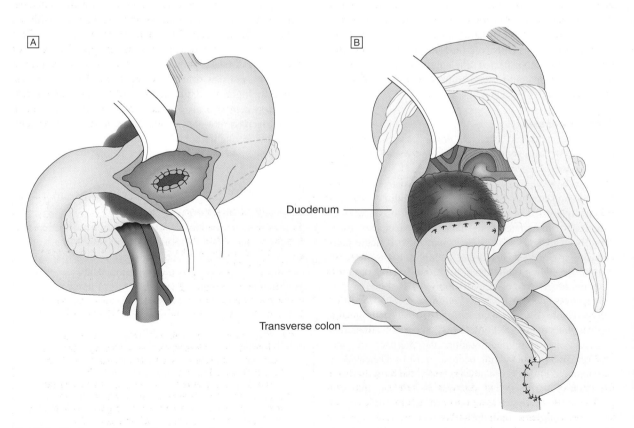

Duodenum

Transverse colon

Fig. 19.6   Treatment of pancreatic pseudocyst.
A Transgastric cystogastrostomy. B Cystojejunostomy Roux-en-Y. (Note that the loop is usually brought retrocolic and not antecolic, as shown here.)

EBM 19.3   COMPLICATIONS OF ACUTE PANCREATITIS

'*Patients with signs of cholangitis require urgent ERCP and endoscopic sphincterotomy or duct drainage by stenting to ensure relief of biliary obstruction. All patients with persistent symptoms and greater than 30% pancreatic necrosis, and those with smaller areas of necrosis and clinical suspicion of sepsis, should undergo image-guided fine-needle aspiration to obtain material for culture 7–14 days after the onset of pancreatitis.*'

Working Party of the British Society of Gastroenterology; Association of Surgeons of Great Britain and Ireland; Pancreatic Society of Great Britain and Ireland; Association of Upper Gastrointestinal Surgeons of Great Britain and Ireland. Gut 2005; 54 suppl 3:iii1–9.

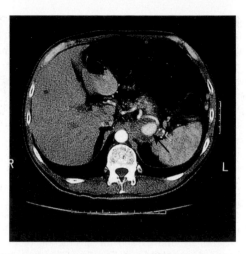

Fig. 19.7   Intravenous contrast-enhanced CT scan showing a splenic artery aneurysm (arrow) secondary to pancreatic necrosis.

Pancreatic necrosis

The development of retroperitoneal necrosis is not in itself an indication for surgery. In patients with a secondary deterioration in organ failure scores or systemic signs of infection, CT- or ultrasound-guided fine-needle aspiration of the pancreatic or peripancreatic tissue is required (EBM 19.3). If the presence of infection is confirmed, surgery is needed. Blunt finger debridement can be undertaken, and multiple retroperitoneal drains are placed before abdominal closure and post-operative lavage. Open packing of the debrided abdomen has been described; others have favoured a minimally invasive technique employing a rigid endoscope. A feeding jejunostomy may be inserted so that feeding can continue without reliance on intravenous nutrition. As might be expected, the mortality of necrotizing pancreatitis is higher (10% or more) than that of oedematous pancreatitis (2% or less). Percutaneous approaches to necrosectomy have shown considerable promise and may reduce the need for prolonged high-dependency care.

Progressive jaundice

Persistent or progressively deepening jaundice suggests that a gallstone is impacted at the lower end of the biliary tree, or that the bile duct is compressed by pancreatic inflammation or pseudocyst formation. ERCP can be used to remove any impacted stones following endoscopic sphincterotomy.

Persistent duodenal ileus

Protracted ileus usually reflects continuing pancreatic inflammation. In the absence of an indication for operation (e.g. pancreatic necrosis, pseudocyst formation), conservative management is instituted and nutritional status maintained by tube feeding (nasoenteric fine-bore tube) or parenteral nutrition while the pancreatitis is resolving.

Gastrointestinal bleeding

Severe acute pancreatitis may be complicated by bleeding from gastritis, erosions or duodenal ulceration, and prophylactic H_2-receptor antagonists are advisable in all such cases. Splenic vein thrombosis is evident in up to 15% of patients dying from acute pancreatitis, and may contribute to blood loss as a result of gastropathy in the early stages and, rarely, gastric varices in the late stages. If bleeding develops, the guidelines for investigation and management are as outlined in Chapter 18. On rare occasions, laparotomy (preceded, if possible, by angiography) is urgently required for massive intraperitoneal bleeding due to erosion of blood vessels by the inflammatory process (Fig. 19.7).

Pancreatic ascites

Rarely, amylase-rich fluid accumulates within the abdomen. This complication is increasingly associated with an alcohol-related attack in a malnourished patient. This may result from rupture of an immature pseudocyst, or of the pancreatic duct or one of its tributaries. A pleural effusion may be evident. Treatment consists of gut rest and intravenous nutritional support. ERCP may demonstrate the leak or distal obstruction of the pancreatic duct. A pancreatic stent may avoid the need for pancreatic surgery.

BOX 19.1   ACUTE PANCREATITIS

- Acute pancreatitis is defined as an attack of pancreatic inflammation, after which the gland returns to anatomical and functional normality
- Gallstones (50% of cases) and alcohol (30% of cases) are the outstanding causes of acute pancreatitis
- In 1 in 4 cases, the attack is severe, as assessed by prognostic factor scoring; in 1 in 4 patients with severe pancreatitis, the attack proves fatal
- In most cases, the pancreatic inflammation is mild and oedematous, and settles on conservative management. Necrotizing pancreatitis is frequently severe and often leads to complications, the need for surgery, and death
- Severe attacks of gallstone pancreatitis can often be aborted if a stone occluding the lower end of the biliary tree can be removed by endoscopic papillotomy. Once gallstones have been eradicated, recurrent attacks of gallstone pancreatitis are exceptional

Prognosis

Following resolution of the acute attack, the prognosis depends on the aetiological factor involved. The biliary tree must be fully investigated in all cases, as gallstone pancreatitis has an excellent long-term outlook once chole-cystectomy has been carried out and gallstones have been cleared from the biliary tree.

The prognosis in alcohol-associated pancreatitis is less favourable. Many patients are unwilling or unable to abstain from drinking, and suffer further attacks of acute pancreatitis with progression to chronic pancreatitis.

CHRONIC PANCREATITIS

Chronic pancreatitis is a chronic inflammatory condition characterized by fibrosis and the destruction of exocrine pancreatic tissue.

Aetiology

Chronic pancreatitis is a relatively rare disease but its incidence may be increasing with the growing problem of alcoholism. Although alcohol is by far the most common aetiological factor, being implicated in some 70–80% of cases, the factors that predispose some patients to develop chronic pancreatitis are poorly understood. Smoking appears to be an important co-factor. In parts of equatorial Africa, the Middle East and India, adolescents and young adults may suffer from so-called tropical pancreatitis. This was once thought to be a consequence of malnutrition, but it is now thought that toxins in dietary staples such as cassava are responsible and that malnutrition is a result rather than a cause of the condition. Rare causes of chronic pancreatitis include hyperparathyroidism, traumatic duct strictures, gallstones and pancreas divisum, although the significance of the last is still uncertain.

Pathophysiology

The secretion of an unduly viscid pancreatic juice may allow protein plugs to form in the duct system, and these plugs subsequently calcify to form duct stones. Impaired flow of pancreatic juice then leads to inflammation, stricture formation in the duct system, and progressive replacement of the gland by fibrous tissue. Loss of acinar tissue is eventually reflected by steatorrhoea and, in time, loss of islet tissue may lead to diabetes mellitus.

Clinical features

Pain is the outstanding feature in most cases. It is characteristically epigastric with marked radiation through to the back, and is often eased by leaning forward or getting down on all fours. In some cases, the pain is precipitated by eating, or the patient learns to avoid certain foods, notably fatty ones. The application of heat sometimes brings relief, and permanent discoloration of the skin may reflect the continued use of heat pads or hot water bottles. The progressive use of powerful opioid analgesics can result in drug dependency.

Weight loss is usual and reflects a combination of inadequate intake, a poor diet and malabsorption. Steatorrhoea is common, the bowel motion being pale,

bulky, offensive, floating on water, and difficult to flush. Diabetes mellitus develops in about one-third of patients, but islet function is often preserved for some years following the onset of exocrine insufficiency.

Other less common manifestations of chronic pancreatitis include transient or intermittent obstructive jaundice, duodenal obstruction and splenic vein thrombosis (leading to splenomegaly, hypersplenism and gastric and oesophageal varices).

Investigations and diagnosis

Abdominal plain films and CT scans may reveal the speckled calcification typical of chronic pancreatitis. Ultrasonography and CT can be used to detect pancreatic enlargement, and may also reveal pseudocysts, dilatation of the pancreatic duct and splenomegaly. MRCP or ERCP is of great value and must always be performed to reveal the architecture of the pancreatic duct, if surgery is contemplated. When investigating these patients, it must be borne in mind that cancer of the pancreas may block the duct system and cause pancreatitis, and that the two conditions can coexist. Pancreatic endocrine function is assessed by measurement of random blood glucose levels, supplemented if necessary by a glucose tolerance test.

Exocrine function can be measured in a multitude of ways, but insufficiency may not be detectable until 90% of the pancreatic parenchyma is destroyed. Furthermore, function tests do not differentiate between chronic pancreatitis and pancreatic cancer. If necessary, faecal fat excretion can be measured over 3–5 days while the patient's fat intake is controlled at 100 g/day (normal individuals excrete less than 5 g/day), or fat absorption can be measured by isotopic labelling of dietary fat. More often, a trial of oral pancreatic supplements is attempted.

Management

The diagnosis of chronic pancreatitis is not in itself an indication for surgery. Considerable clinical judgement is needed to determine the need for, and timing of, operation. In most cases, intractable pain is the cardinal indication for surgery; operation does not restore pancreatic endocrine and exocrine function and, at best, merely slows their decline.

Conservative management

This consists of encouraging abstinence from alcohol, relief of pain, treatment of exocrine and endocrine insufficiency, and attempts to improve nutritional status. Opiates are avoided, if possible, but their use may prove essential to relieve pain. Coeliac plexus block is rarely of value and at best provides relief for a few weeks or months. Diabetes mellitus is treated by appropriate means (diet, oral hypo-glycaemic agents or insulin). Steatorrhoea is treated by pancreatic exocrine supplements, and modern position-release preparations (e.g. Creon) minimize the enzymic degradation of the supplements by acid and pepsin during their passage through the stomach. Oral pancreatic enzyme supplements in the absence of exocrine insufficiency have not been shown conclusively to reduce analgesic consumption.

19

Surgical treatment

This is indicated if pain is intractable; when neighbouring structures, such as the common bile duct, duodenum, portal or splenic vein, are sufficiently compressed to produce symptoms; when pseudocysts or abscesses develop; or when cancer cannot be excluded.

In general, the objective is to relieve pain or compression, while at the same time conserving as much pancreatic tissue and function as possible. In about one-third of cases, the pancreatic duct system is dilated sufficiently to allow these objectives to be achieved by a drainage operation. Frequently, there are multiple strictures throughout the length of the duct, which must be slit open so that a Roux loop of jejunum can be anastomosed to the entire length of the pancreatic duct as a longitudinal pancreaticojejunostomy (Fig. 19.8). Approximately 70% of patients remain pain-free or substantially improved when assessed 5 years after this operation, and the avoidance of resection often means that pancreatic function does not worsen appreciably.

If drainage is not feasible, part or all of the pancreas will have to be resected by distal pancreatectomy if the disease is confined to the distal part of the gland, and pancreaticoduodenectomy if affecting the head of the gland. This approach has recently been avoided in favour of a procedure that combines a 'coring out' of the pancreatic head with pancreaticojejunostomy. In some patients, the entire pancreas appears to be so diseased that total pancreatectomy is undertaken, but this must be regarded as a last resort, given the permanent brittle diabetes and exocrine insufficiency that follow. Approximately 70% of patients are

pain-free or substantially improved when assessed 5 years following resection. As with all aspects of chronic pancreatitis, the results of surgery are better in patients who continue to abstain from alcohol.

NEOPLASMS OF THE PANCREAS

Neoplasms of the exocrine pancreas are common and are almost always malignant, whereas neoplasms of the endocrine pancreas are rare and may be benign.

NEOPLASMS OF THE EXOCRINE PANCREAS

Benign pancreatic neoplasms such as cystadenomas frequently remain asymptomatic until their size causes pressure on surrounding structures. Such lesions are more common in females and, unlike pseudocysts, they are not associated with a preceding history of pancreatitis or

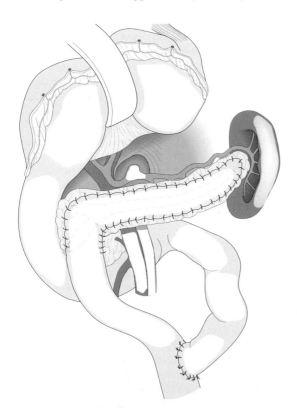

Fig. 19.8   Pancreatic duct decompression by longitudinal pancreaticojejunostomy.

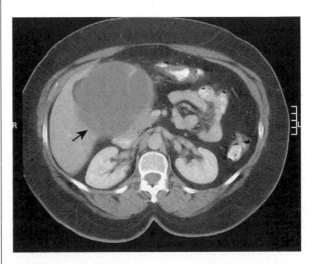

Fig. 19.9   CT scan showing a mucinous cystadenoma (arrow) in the head of the pancreas.

19

alcohol abuse. The serum amylase is usually normal. Imaging techniques may not reliably differentiate such lesions from a pseudocyst (Fig. 19.9). Resection of the affected part of the pancreas is usually needed, but the prognosis thereafter is excellent.

Malignant neoplasms of the pancreas are almost invariably ductal adenocarcinomas. Acinar cell carcinomas, cystadenocarcinomas and sarcomas are all rare.

ADENOCARCINOMA OF THE PANCREAS

Aetiology

The cause of pancreatic cancer is unknown. It is increasing in frequency and is now the fourth most common cause of cancer death in males and the sixth most common in females in many developed countries. It affects approximately 100 per million of the population in the UK and USA, and accounts for about 10% of all cancers of the alimentary system. It carries a dismal prognosis.

Men are more commonly affected than women and the peak incidence lies between 55 and 70 years of age. Factors thought to increase the risk of pancreatic cancer include tobacco smoking and a high-fat high-protein diet. The disease may occur in family clusters.

Pathology

The great majority of adenocarcinomas arise from ductal rather than acinar tissue. The head of the gland is at least two-thirds more commonly affected than the body or tail. The cancer spreads locally and disseminates to nerve bundles, to local lymphatics, and to lymph nodes around the gland. Regardless of the site of origin, spread outside the reach of surgical cure is usual by the time the disease is diagnosed. It is hardly surprising that 90% of patients are dead within a year of the diagnosis being made, and that survival beyond 5 years is truly exceptional.

Cancer arising from the ampullary region, distal common bile duct and duodenum has a much better outlook than cancer of the pancreas. It may be that biliary obstruction occurs so early that the tumour is discovered at a stage where resection is still curative.

Clinical features

Obstructive jaundice, with the passage of dark urine and pale stools, is the common presenting feature of cancer of the head of the pancreas. It is usually progressive, in contrast to the intermittent jaundice of calculous obstruction. Pruritus is frequently troublesome. In keeping with Courvoisier's law, the gallbladder is frequently palpable in patients with obstructive jaundice due to pancreatic cancer. When cancer arises in the body and tail of the pancreas, jaundice is more likely to be due to liver metastases or the involvement of nodes in the porta hepatis.

Weight loss is invariable and may be the first symptom, reflecting a combination of inadequate intake, malabsorption and depressed liver function. Pain is present in about 70% of patients at the time of diagnosis and most have ill-defined upper abdominal pain or discomfort. Neoplastic infiltration can cause severe back pain, which is an ominous symptom signalling unresectability.

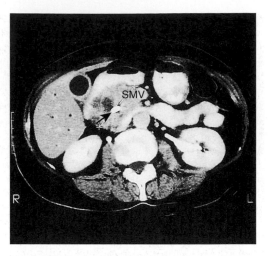

Fig. 19.10 CT scan showing a 6 cm adenocarcinoma in the head of the pancreas.
A stent (arrow) is evident within the invaded bile duct and the tumour comes into contact with the superior mesenteric vein (SMV).

Diabetes mellitus or impaired glucose tolerance is present in one-third of patients. Steatorrhoea is common, and failure to absorb the fat-soluble vitamin K may cause coagulopathy.

Trousseau's sign of thrombophlebitis migrans is a late manifestation in some patients but is not specific for this form of cancer.

Investigations and diagnosis

Many patients with pancreatic cancer are anaemic at the time of diagnosis. A stool examination revealing occult blood loss should, however, raise the possible diagnosis of an ampullary tumour. In patients with jaundice, its obstructive nature is confirmed by examination of the urine, stool and blood (Ch. 18). Ultrasonography will detect dilatation of the biliary tree, will exclude gallstones, and may show the mass lesion in the pancreas or reveal liver metastases. The more recent introduction of high-quality spiral (helical) CT with thin-cut examination of the pancreas has improved the staging of pancreatic malignancy (Fig. 19.10). However, neither CT nor ultrasonography can differentiate between neoplasia and chronic pancreatitis with absolute accuracy. If biliary obstruction is present, cholangiography is used to define the site and nature of the obstruction; MRCP is preferred to ERCP as it is less invasive and displays both pancreatic and biliary duct systems, so determining the need for therapeutic intervention such as stent insertion (see below and Fig. 19.11). A common finding in pancreatic cancer is the 'double duct sign', in which both the pancreatic duct and the common bile duct are narrowed as they pass through the neoplasm. Endoscopy also allows lesions in the gastroduodenal lumen to be biopsied, and pancreatic juice and bile can be sampled for cytological examination.

Circulating tumour markers (e.g. CA 19–9) lack sensitivity and specificity but may be useful in the follow-up of treated patients and in the detection of recurrence following resection.

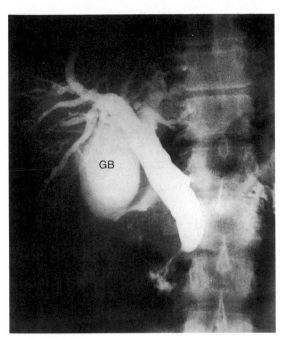

Fig. 19.11 **A cholangiogram obtained at ERCP demonstrating a dilated gallbladder (GB) and biliary tree above a pancreatic cancer obstructing the intrapancreatic portion of the common bile duct.**

Every effort should be made to obtain cytological or histological confirmation of the malignant nature of any mass lesions revealed radiologically. This is particularly important if surgery is not contemplated, as a number of benign lesions (e.g. chronic pancreatitis) can masquerade as malignancy, whereas a number of malignancies (e.g. lymphoma) that can mimic pancreatic cancer have a far better prognosis if recognized and treated appropriately. Pancreatic tissue can be safely obtained by percutaneous fine-needle aspiration under ultrasound or CT scan guidance or by endoscopic ultrasonography, although this is not generally undertaken if resection is being considered.

CT of the abdomen should be undertaken to assess local invasion of tumours considered to be resectable and to exclude distant metastases. The use of laparoscopy has been promoted in selected patients to exclude dissemination of disease (peritoneal seedlings or liver metastases) that might not be easily detected by conventional radiological imaging and that would preclude radical surgery.

Management

Surgical resection offers the only prospect of cure, but only about 10% of patients are candidates for radical surgery. In most cases, the presence of advanced disease, advanced age or intercurrent disease means that palliation is the objective of management. In jaundiced patients, coagulopathy should be corrected by the parenteral administration of vitamin K. Patients should be well hydrated to avoid post-operative renal failure, and prophylactic antibiotics should be given.

Curative treatment

The standard operation of radical pancreaticoduodenectomy (Whipple's procedure) entails block resection of the head of the pancreas, the distal half of the stomach, the duodenum, gallbladder and common bile duct. Reconstruction is achieved by anastomoses between the jejunum and the pancreatic remnant, common hepatic duct and gastric remnant, respectively (Fig. 19.12). The procedure used to carry a prohibitively high operative mortality,

A

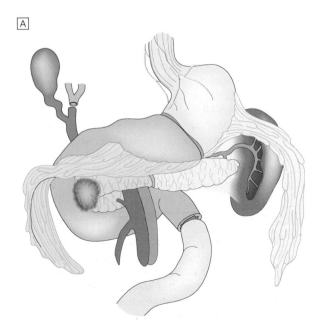

B

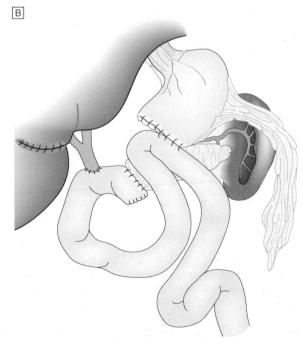

Fig. 19.12 **Whipple procedure.**
A The resected area. B The anastomoses performed. (The gallbladder is usually removed.)

but in specialist hands this should now be less than 1–2%. It has been suggested that prior drainage of the biliary tree by endoscopic or percutaneous means may introduce infection and thereby increase the risk of post-operative infection. In practice, the majority of patients have already undergone stent placement at the time of diagnostic ERCP. Although 5-year survival rates of 20% following resection have been reported in a series of selected patients, overall survival rates are little better than those obtained by palliative surgery and cure remains exceptional. Attempts to improve the radicality of resection by removing all of the pancreas have proved disappointing; total pancreatectomy offers no advantage in terms of operative mortality or long-term survival, and also confers permanent diabetes and exocrine insufficiency. Although adjuvant chemoradiation therapy is favoured in the USA following pancreatic resection, there is no strong evidence to demonstrate an additional benefit from radiotherapy compared to chemotherapy alone (EBM 19.4).

The prospects for patients with cancer of the peri-ampullary region, distal common bile duct or duodenum are less gloomy, with 5-year survival rates ranging from 20% to 40%.

Palliative treatment

The relief of jaundice, pruritus, pain and duodenal obstruction is the objective of palliative treatment (EBM 19.5).

EBM 19.4   SURGICAL RESECTION IN PANCREATIC CANCER

'Resectional surgery should be undertaken only in specialist centres, to increase resection rates and reduce hospital morbidity and mortality. Percutaneous biliary drainage prior to resection in jaundiced patients does not improve surgical outcome and may increase the risk of infective complications. Gemcitabine single-agent chemotherapy is recommended to prolong duration of survival following resection.'

Pancreatic Section, British Society of Gastroenterology; Pancreatic Society of Great Britain and Ireland; Association of Upper Gastrointestinal Surgeons of Great Britain and Ireland; Royal College of Pathologists; Special Interest Group for Gastro-Intestinal Radiology. Gut 2005; 54 suppl 5:v1–16.

EBM 19.5   PALLIATIVE TREATMENT OF PANCREATIC CANCER

'Relief of obstructive jaundice will be adequately achieved by placement of a plastic stent, but surgical bypass may be preferred in patients likely to survive more than 6 months. Endoscopic stent placement is preferable to transhepatic stenting.'
'Neurolytic coeliac plexus block should be considered at the time of palliative surgery, or undertaken by percutaneous or endoscopic approaches in non-surgical patients.'
'Pancreatic enzyme supplements should be used to maintain weight and improve quality of life.'

Pancreatic Section, British Society of Gastroenterology; Pancreatic Society of Great Britain and Ireland; Association of Upper Gastrointestinal Surgeons of Great Britain and Ireland; Royal College of Pathologists; Special Interest Group for Gastro-Intestinal Radiology. Gut 2005; 54 suppl 5:v1–16.

BOX 19.3   PANCREATIC CANCER

- Ductal adenocarcinoma of the pancreas is predominantly a disease of the ageing population and showed a threefold increase in incidence during the 20th century
- Aetiological factors include a high-fat, high-protein diet and smoking
- As the head of the pancreas is the most common site for tumour formation, obstructive jaundice is commonly the presenting complaint. Other features include weight loss, steatorrhoea and diabetes mellitus
- Late presentation is the rule and 90% of patients are dead within a year of diagnosis
- Only 10% of patients are potential candidates for curative resection (Whipple's operation) and overall 5-year survival rates are close to zero
- Endoscopic stenting now offers an alternative to palliative surgical bypass of the obstructed biliary system, but duodenal obstruction by tumour is also a problem in up to 10% of patients

---

In the past, operation was usually undertaken to bypass the obstructed biliary system (cholecyst-jejunostomy or choledochojejunostomy), and gastrojejunostomy was carried out to treat or prevent blockage of the duodenum by continued tumour growth. In many cases, operation can now be avoided by the insertion of a prosthetic stent by endoscopic or percutaneous means. Stenting suffers from the disadvantages that it cannot deal with or prevent duodenal obstruction, and that the stents frequently encrust and block after about 3 months, so that their replacement becomes necessary. Some surgeons have therefore promoted a policy of surgical bypass in selected patients with unresectable malignancy.

Mean survival following palliative intervention is only about 4 months, and few patients live for more than a year. Prolonged survival raises doubt about the diagnosis of cancer, underlining the need to have cytological or histological confirmation of the diagnosis in all cases.

Although there is evidence that survival rates can be improved by chemotherapy, the benefits obtainable with currently available regimens do not justify their use outside controlled clinical trials. Pain relief is a vital part of the management of advanced pancreatic cancer, and coeliac plexus block should be considered if pain cannot be controlled by appropriate analgesic therapy. In some patients with intractable pain, thoracoscopic splanchnicectomy has been advocated.

NEOPLASMS OF THE ENDOCRINE PANCREAS

These rare neoplasms may give rise to defined syndromes as a result of the over-secretion of peptide products, but some tumours that appear histologically to be of neuroendocrine origin neither contain identifiable products on immunohistochemistry nor give rise to circulating products. The most common islet cell tumour is the insulinoma, which has an annual incidence of 1 per million of the population. It arises from B cells and results in the over-secretion of insulin, with episodes of hypoglycaemia. Gastrinomas arise from G cells and give rise to the Zollinger–Ellison syndrome (Ch. 17). Tumours of the A cells producing glucagon are known as glucagonomas, and excessive secretion of vasoactive intestinal peptide (VIP) from vipomas produces pancreatic cholera (see below). Some tumours may produce more than one peptide, or the pattern of secretion may vary with time. A proportion of patients have tumours and/or hyperplasia of the parathyroid glands or anterior pituitary gland and are regarded as suffering from multiple endocrine neoplasia type I (MEN I; Ch. 24).

INSULINOMA

Insulinomas are usually single, small (< 2 cm in diameter) benign tumours that may affect any part of the pancreas. Multiple insulinomas are usually associated with MEN I. Less than 10% of insulinomas are malignant, but such tumours are often larger than 2 cm in diameter.

Clinical features

Hypoglycaemia may give rise to mild symptoms, but over the years there is gradual intellectual and motor impairment with insidious personality changes. More severe attacks of hypoglycaemia can produce sweating, palpitations, tremulousness, and a wide variety of transient psychoneurological symptoms with episodes of bizarre behaviour. Because of memory lapses, the patient may not recall these events, and the diagnosis only comes to light when they are found in a hypoglycaemic coma. Attacks are typically precipitated by fasting and relieved by taking glucose. Some patients are misdiagnosed as suffering from psychiatric illness, epilepsy, alcoholism or brain tumours, and it is not unusual for 2–3 years to elapse between the first symptom and establishment of the correct diagnosis.

Diagnosis

The diagnosis of insulinoma demands a high index of suspicion and rests on:

- the demonstration of hypoglycaemia after fasting (blood glucose concentration of less than 2.2 mmol/l after an overnight 12–14-hour fast)
- the confirmation that hypoglycaemia is due to inappropriate insulin secretion.

In patients with insulinoma, serial plasma insulin levels remain inappropriately high in the face of falling glucose levels. Factitious hypoglycaemia caused by insulin injection is a rare problem occasionally encountered in members of medical and nursing staff. It can be excluded by measuring C-peptide levels at the same time as insulin levels are determined. If exogenous insulin is being administered, there is no corresponding C-peptide production.

Once the presence of an insulinoma has been confirmed, a variety of methods can be used to localize the tumour(s). Ultrasonography, CT and selective angiography are successful in less than 50% of cases, owing to the small size of the tumour. Endoscopic ultrasonography offers a safe, accurate method of localization. In many centres experienced in the management of such lesions, pre-operative assessment is limited to confirmation of inappropriate secretion of insulin.

BOX 19.4 INSULINOMA

- Insulinoma is the most common endocrine tumour of the pancreas (but is still rare, having an annual incidence of 1 per million of the population)
- The diagnosis of insulinoma is often delayed, as the episodes of hypoglycaemia (usually precipitated by fasting and relieved by food) are often misinterpreted (e.g. as being due to brain tumour, psychiatric upset or epilepsy)
- The diagnosis is confirmed by demonstrating that fasting produces hypoglycaemia in association with inappropriately *high* insulin levels
- Measurement of C-peptide levels (one molecule of C-peptide is released for every molecule of insulin) excludes factitious hypoglycaemia
- Most insulinomas are small benign tumours that may be difficult to locate; they are usually treated by enucleation

---

Management

Surgical removal of the tumour is the treatment of choice, although patients can be controlled temporarily by diazoxide (a diabetogenic antihypertensive drug; 5 mg/kg daily in three divided doses, given orally). At laparotomy, the pancreas is fully exposed and carefully palpated. All but a few lesions will be evident to the surgeon's palpating hand or on intraoperative ultrasound. Most insulinomas can be enucleated, but resection of the affected part of the pancreas is occasionally necessary. If the tumour cannot be found, distal pancreatectomy used to be recommended in the mistaken belief that insulinomas were more common in the body and tail of the gland. If no tumour is found, it is better to close the abdomen, control hypoglycaemia with diazoxide, and carry out interval selective venous sampling or endoscopic ultrasonography in order to localize the lesion for re-operation.

If a malignant insulinoma is found confined to the pancreas, resection is indicated. Chemotherapy using streptozotocin may prove useful, if there is unresectable or metastatic disease, although this is often poorly tolerated because of its toxic side-effects. Symptoms of hyperinsulinism can be controlled by diazoxide, if necessary.

GLUCAGONOMA AND VIPOMA

Excessive glucagon production may give rise to a syndrome of necrotizing dermatitis, painful glossitis, stomatitis, bowel upset, weight loss, diabetes mellitus and anaemia. Plasma levels of glucagon are raised. Vipomas may be solitary and benign but half are malignant. Over-secretion of VIP causes a syndrome of profuse watery diarrhoea, hypokalaemia and achlorhydria also known as 'pancreatic cholera'. The systemic upset may be profound, with daily loss of 5 litres or more of potassium-rich stool and the production of marked metabolic alkalosis. The patient may be confused from profound dehydration and metabolic alkalosis, and ileus and abdominal distension may lead to the suspicion of intestinal obstruction. Diagnosis rests on recognition of the typical syndrome and the detection of increased levels of VIP in the circulating blood.

Both types of tumour may be defined by CT or angiography. Resection often reverses the their effects. The aim

19

is to remove the tumour, although this may necessitate total or subtotal pancreatectomy. In the case of solitary tumours, surgery may be curative. In unresectable cases and those with metastases, streptozotocin or the somatostatin analogue, octreotide, may be useful in controlling symptoms.

THE SPLEEN

SURGICAL ANATOMY

The spleen is a friable blood-filled organ lying in the left upper quadrant of the abdomen behind the 9th, 10th and 11th ribs (Fig. 19.13). It weighs about 150 g, is ellipsoid in shape and lies with its long axis along the line of the 10th rib. The convex outer surface of the spleen lies against the diaphragm and its lower pole rests on the splenic flexure of the colon below. Its concave inner surface is related to the fundus of the stomach, the tail of the pancreas and the upper pole of the right kidney. It has a fibrous capsule and, except at its hilum, is covered by peritoneum, which is reflected as ligaments running to adjacent organs. These are the lienorenal, lienogastric and lienocolic ligaments. The phrenicocolic ligament, which runs between the splenic flexure of the colon and the undersurface of the diaphragm, provides additional support.

The tortuous splenic artery arises from the coeliac axis (Fig. 19.2), which carries 40% of the splanchnic blood flow into the spleen. Venous blood drains into the portal venous system via the splenic vein. The splenic vessels are closely related to the pancreas; the artery runs within the lienorenal ligament and branches reach the splenic hilum, the only part of the spleen without a peritoneal covering. Further branches continue as the short gastric vessels that run within the lienogastric ligament to the upper part of the greater curvature of the stomach. Both the lienogastric and lienorenal ligaments and their contained vessels must be divided during splenectomy.

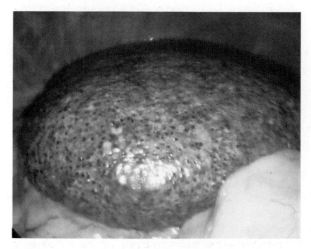

Fig. 19.13 Laparoscopic view of the spleen as a stapling device is applied to its pedicle during laparoscopic splenectomy.

Some 25% of the lymphoid tissue of the body is contained within the spleen and forms its white pulp, which consists of lymphoid follicles (Malpighian bodies) and lymphatic tissue, containing lymphocytes, macrophages and plasma cells. These cells migrate to the spleen from the bone marrow and 30–50% of them are thymus-dependent. The red pulp is a loose honeycomb of reticular tissue that contains the splenic sinusoids. The blood vessels are carried into the pulp along fibrous trabeculae, which are continuous with the capsule. Erythrocytes move in and out of the pulp tissue, so that 1% of the body's red cells and 20–30% of its platelets are sequestrated at any given moment.

The pulp of the spleen is not provided with lymphatic vessels and those present are confined to the capsule and trabeculae. Lymph nodes close to the hilum thus receive more lymph from the stomach than from the spleen, and drain to nodes along the splenic artery.

Normally, the spleen is impalpable and cannot be percussed. When enlarged, it extends downwards and medially below the costal margin. It is then best palpated bimanually, with the patient lying on the right side with the left side turned slightly forward. The distinctive notch on the antero-inferior border of the spleen may then be felt. On percussion, an enlarged spleen causes dullness over the ninth rib in the mid-axillary line. Splenomegaly is normally confirmed by abdominal ultrasound or CT scan.

SURGICAL PHYSIOLOGY

HAEMOPOIESIS

In fetal life, the spleen is a source of red blood cells and granulocytes. Extramedullary haemopoiesis occurs only in the myeloproliferative syndromes. In humans, the spleen does not act as a reservoir for blood.

FILTRATION OF BLOOD CELLS

Normal blood cells pass through the spleen unchanged, but abnormal and ageing cells are trapped. It has been estimated that 20 ml of red cells are phagocytosed daily. White cells and platelets, particularly when coated with antibodies, are also removed. Following splenectomy, there is an increased number of misshapen red cells in the peripheral blood, some containing nuclear remnants (Howell–Jolly bodies) and others containing clumps of iron (siderocytes).

IMMUNOLOGICAL FUNCTION

The spleen is an important site for effecting both cell-mediated and humoral immunity. Following splenectomy, immunological responses are impaired.

INDICATIONS FOR SPLENECTOMY

Although the recommendation to remove the spleen often comes from the haematologist, the surgeon must be aware of the indications for splenectomy and the criteria that should be fulfilled before accepting a patient for operation. The common indications are outlined below.

TRAUMA

In recent years, there has been an increasing tendency to avoid unnecessary laparotomy in trauma patients thought to have minor splenic injury. In those patients submitted to laparotomy, splenectomy is indicated only if the organ cannot be conserved by the use of haemostatic agents, local suturing or partial splenectomy. Spleens involved by pathological conditions, such as portal hypertension, polycythaemia and infective mononucleosis, are prone to rupture with minor trauma. A temporary improvement in the clinical state may precede a sudden deterioration following splenic rupture. Awareness and careful observation are critical, particularly in patients with suspected or known splenic trauma, such as subcapsular haematoma, which can lead to 'delayed rupture'.

HAEMOLYTIC ANAEMIAS

Hereditary spherocytosis

In this autosomal dominant disorder, the red blood cells are spherical rather than biconcave, are unduly fragile, and are destroyed almost exclusively in the spleen. Excess haemolysis results in anaemia, jaundice and splenic enlargement. It is a disease of remissions and relapses, with 'haemolytic crises' requiring transfusion. Pigment gallstones occur in 30–60% of cases.

Splenectomy is indicated in all cases when health is impaired, when severe haemolytic crises have occurred and when gallbladder disease is present. However, it should be avoided before the age of 3–4 years. If gallstones are present, cholecystectomy is carried out simultaneously. Both procedures can be performed by laparoscopic means.

Acquired haemolytic anaemias

Excess haemolysis may occur following exposure to agents such as chemicals, drugs or infection, and with extensive burns, or it may be an immune phenomenon. In the latter, the red cells are coated with an autoantibody, which can be detected by agglutination when antihuman globulin is added to a suspension of the patient's erythrocytes (positive Coombs' test).

Autoimmune haemolytic anaemia predominantly affects middle-aged women and causes severe haemolytic crises superimposed on a background of mild anaemia. Treatment consists of steroid therapy. Splenectomy is indicated if treatment fails from the outset or if there is a fall in the haemoglobin following the reduction or cessation of steroids.

THE PURPURAS

Idiopathic thrombocytopenic purpura (ITP)

In this disease, the presence of autoantibodies causes the premature removal of platelets. The low platelet count is associated with plentiful megakaryocytes in the bone marrow. Cyclical bleeding from the gastrointestinal tract and other sites is associated with petechiae and ecchymoses.

Platelet counts are below 50×10^9/l, and bleeding time is prolonged but clotting time is normal. The spleen is palpably enlarged in only 2–3% of patients, and dense adhesions may form around it.

Clinical course

The disease may be chronic or acute. The acute form often presents in children and there is usually a short history of a preceding viral illness. Spontaneous remission is common and the response to steroids or splenectomy is excellent. The chronic form is characterized by a course of remissions and relapses, which may last several years. Its response to steroids is poor and the outcome after splenectomy less satisfactory.

Choice of treatment

The acute form of the disease is treated initially with steroids. A rapid increase in the platelet count is associated with a good prospect of complete and lasting remission when therapy is stopped. If steroid therapy does not result in rapid remission, splenectomy is advised, except for acute ITP in children, as spontaneous remission is likely. Splenectomy is curative in about 70% of patients with the chronic form of the disease, and is usually recommended if a patient has two relapses on steroid therapy. Patients may remain asymptomatic despite a low platelet count of $20–30 \times 10^9$/l following splenectomy.

Secondary thrombocytopenia

Splenectomy is contraindicated in secondary haemorrhagic purpuras, although it may be advised if hypersplenism is associated with symptomatic secondary thrombocytopenia.

HYPERSPLENISM

This syndrome consists of splenomegaly and pancytopenia in the presence of an apparently normal bone marrow and the absence of an autoimmune disorder. There is sequestration and destruction of blood cells in the spleen, affecting predominantly white cells and platelets.

Hypersplenism may complicate a number of inflammatory conditions (e.g. rheumatoid arthritis), infections (e.g. malaria), and myeloproliferative and lymphoproliferative disorders. In portal hypertension, splenic congestion frequently leads to splenomegaly and hypersplenism.

The effects of hypersplenism include expansion of the total blood volume to fill the increased vascular spaces of the enlarged spleen and splanchnic bed. There is increased pooling of cells within the enlarged spleen and excess destruction. In the peripheral blood, there is anaemia, leucopenia and thrombocytopenia, but marrow turnover is increased, with reticulocytosis and leucoerythroblastosis. Increased amounts of urobilinogen are present in the urine.

The removal of a grossly enlarged spleen carries appreciable morbidity and mortality, and puts the patient at long-term risk from serious bacterial infection. Splenectomy must not be undertaken lightly, and the haematologist and surgeon should take into account the degree of cytopenia, the extent of splenic enlargement, the amount of discomfort caused, and the incidence of recurrent infections from leucopenia. The prognosis of the underlying cause of the

19

19

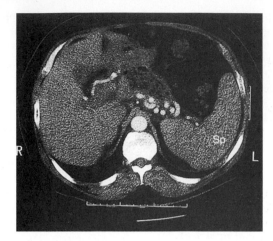

Fig. 19.14 Moderate enlargement of the spleen (Sp) in a patient with segmental portal hypertension, following an episode of acute pancreatitis.
Contrast is seen in a tortuous splenic artery.

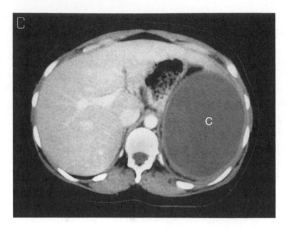

Fig. 19.15 CT scan showing the complete replacement of the upper pole of the spleen by a thick-walled cyst (C).
There was a past history of trauma.

hypersplenism and the potential difficulty of the surgical procedure should be taken into account.

Segmental portal hypertension

A localized form of portal hypertension associated with hypersplenism and oesophagogastric varices may follow occlusion of the splenic vein. Thrombosis may result from acute or chronic pancreatitis (Fig. 19.14), or the vessel may become compromised by direct invasion from a carcinoma of the pancreas. Gastric varices are particularly prominent in this condition and often communicate directly with short gastric veins. Acute variceal haemorrhage in this situation is best managed by splenectomy with ligation of the vessels on the greater curvature of the stomach, as endoscopic sclerotherapy or banding of gastric varices is difficult. Recurrent haemorrhage is unusual following surgery and the prognosis is favourable, given that there is often no associated liver disease.

PROLIFERATIVE DISORDERS

Myelofibrosis

It is recognized that this condition is due to an abnormal proliferation of mesenchymal elements in the bone marrow, spleen, liver and lymph nodes, and that extramedullary haemopoiesis occurs at many sites. Most patients present over the age of 50 years. The spleen may be grossly enlarged and splenic infarcts may occur. Splenectomy decreases transfusion requirements and, by relieving the discomfort of a grossly enlarged spleen, also improves symptoms.

Lymphomas

In non-Hodgkin's lymphoma, splenectomy is only indicated in the rare event that a primary neoplasm is confined to the spleen or, in both myelo- and lymphoproliferative conditions, to reduce transfusion requirements when hypersplenism is a problem.

Other tumours

Of the other rare tumours, haemangiomas (capillary or cavernous) may reach sufficient size to cause splenic enlargement, with a consumptive coagulopathy and haemorrhagic tendency.

MISCELLANEOUS CONDITIONS

Cysts of the spleen

Cysts of the spleen are uncommon. They are usually single (Fig. 19.15) but occasionally multiple. Single cysts may be congenital, degenerative or parasitic:

- *Congenital* cysts are due to an embryonic defect and result in a dermoid-like lesion. They are lined by flattened epithelium and contain thin blood-stained fluid or thick creamy material, sometimes with hair and teeth.
- *Degenerative* cysts result from liquefaction of an infarct or haematoma. There may be a past history of minor trauma. The wall is fibrous and often calcified, and the cyst is filled with brownish fluid or paste-like material.
- *Parasitic* cysts are due to infection with *Echinococcus granulosus* (hydatid disease).

Splenic cysts normally cause no symptoms and are often discovered fortuitously. Symptomatic cysts may present with left upper quadrant pain radiating to the back or left shoulder. The lesion may be recognized by CT or ultrasound scan, investigations that are usually sufficient to characterize the nature of the cyst. Intervention is not indicated for small congenital or degenerative cysts. Large symptomatic cysts are treated by partial or complete splenectomy.

Abscess of the spleen

A splenic abscess is rare. It should be suspected when progressive splenic enlargement is associated with

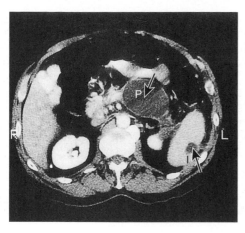

Fig. 19.16   CT scan showing a splenic infarct (arrow I) in a patient who has developed a pseudocyst (arrow P) following a severe attack of pancreatitis.

bacteraemia and abscess formation at other sites. Splenectomy, although desirable, may not prove feasible and drainage may be preferable.

Splenic infarct

Splenic infarct may present with acute onset of left upper quadrant pain in a patient with known hypersplenism. Asymptomatic infarcts may be observed in patients following a severe attack of pancreatitis (Fig. 19.16). These may resolve with the formation of a splenic cyst, but do not require surgical intervention.

Splenic artery aneurysm

This is a relatively common complication of atherosclerosis in elderly patients. The calcified wall of the aneurysm is visible on X-ray and there is obvious calcification of the tortuous splenic artery. The presence of a small, uncomplicated atherosclerotic aneurysm is not necessarily an indication for surgical treatment. The natural history of these lesions is not well known, particularly as they often affect elderly, frail patients. Bleeding can occur, however, and operation is then mandatory. A splenic aneurysm may rarely arise from a peripancreatic abscess, following an attack of acute pancreatitis. Haemorrhage in this setting is associated with a high mortality rate.

Congenital aneurysms are rare; they are more common in women and may rupture during pregnancy. An asymptomatic congenital aneurysm may be discovered on abdominal X-ray as a thin calcified ring shadow. Because of the risk of rupture, it should be treated electively. As most congenital aneurysms lie close to the splenic hilum, splenectomy is usually required, although it may occasionally be possible to conserve the spleen by relying on the collateral arterial blood supply from the short gastric arteries.

OTHER INDICATIONS FOR SPLENECTOMY

Removal of the spleen may be required as part of other surgical procedures, such as distal pancreatectomy and radical gastrectomy for carcinoma and, less frequently, for certain types of splenorenal shunt.

SPLENECTOMY

PRE-OPERATIVE PREPARATION

In the pre-operative period, particular attention must be paid to the full blood count and coagulation status. In the presence of any bleeding tendency, transfusion of blood, fresh frozen plasma or platelets may be required to bring the coagulation profiles to as near normal as possible before surgery. For thrombocytopenia, platelets should be available to cover the operation and the post-operative phase.

Accessory spleens in the splenic hilum, splenic pedicle or omentum may account for relapse of the condition for which the splenectomy was performed. Scintiscanning after the administration of ^{51}Cr-labelled red cells may be used to detect functioning accessory splenic tissue, although a careful search at operation should identify this.

Prophylactic antibiotics should be administered with the pre-medication because of the increased risk of infection. As the stomach is handled during splenectomy, a nasogastric tube should be inserted.

In cases of suspected splenic trauma, laparotomy is normally undertaken through a long vertical incision. For an elective splenectomy, access is usually gained via a left subcostal incision. Rarely, a thoraco-abdominal incision is necessary to remove a large spleen. Laparoscopic splenectomy is now favoured by some surgeons, although delivery of an enlarged spleen from the abdomen may pose difficulties.

TECHNIQUE

A normal-sized non-adherent spleen is removed after first mobilizing it medially by dividing its lateral peritoneal attachments. The splenic artery and vein are doubly ligated and divided. Finally, the lienogastric ligament, with its contained short gastric vessels, is divided between ligatures.

When the spleen is enlarged or adherent to surrounding organs or the diaphragm, preliminary mobilization may not be possible and the vascular pedicle is dissected first. Alternatively, the splenic artery may first be ligated in continuity so that the spleen shrinks in size, allowing it to be mobilized and the vessels to be ligated close to the splenic hilum.

Drainage of the abdomen is not normally required after the removal of a normal-sized spleen. After removal of an enlarged organ, oozing from adhesions and the cut edge of the peritoneum is common. This should be controlled by electrocautery or, if large collateral vessels are present, by oversewing of the peritoneal edge.

Drains are not used (as they may actually increase the incidence of subphrenic sepsis), unless there is a possibility that the tail of the pancreas has been injured or there is persistent oozing due to a coagulation defect.

19

POST-OPERATIVE COURSE AND COMPLICATIONS

Any bleeding tendency increases the likelihood of post-operative haemorrhage. Hypotension and circulatory collapse within 48 hours of surgery indicate the need to re-explore the abdomen.

Serum amylase levels should be monitored in the immediate post-operative period, since pancreatitis may result from handling and bruising of the pancreatic tail during mobilization of the spleen. Pancreatic fistula formation is uncommon, although gastric fistula (involving the greater curvature of the stomach) can follow injury to the greater curvature of the stomach when the short gastric vessels are ligated in the lienogastric ligament.

Left lower lobe collapse or atelectasis is the most frequent complication of splenectomy but usually responds to conservative measures. Subphrenic abscess may arise from pancreatic or gastric injury, inadequate haemostasis or inappropriate use of drains.

Low-dose heparin is advised in all patients undergoing splenectomy, since the transient increase in the platelet and white cell count following splenectomy may predispose to venous thrombosis. In patients with portal hypertension, splenectomy may be complicated by splenic vein thrombosis, with propagation of clot into the portal vein.

Loss of lymphoid tissue reduces immune activity and impairs the response to bacteraemia. The risk of overwhelming post-splenectomy sepsis is greatest when splenectomy is performed in childhood, but a slightly increased incidence of death from pneumonia, complicated by disseminated intravascular coagulation and adrenal failure, has also been reported in adults. As most infections occur within 3 years of splenectomy, some surgeons advise prophylactic penicillin for this period. Although this is mandatory in young children, there remains some debate regarding its benefit in adults.

Elective splenectomy should be preceded by the administration of pneumococcal, meningococcal and *Haemophilus influenzae* vaccine. These are best administered 2–3weeks prior to surgery, but are still effective if given post-operatively.

BOX 19.5   SPLENECTOMY

- The spleen is the intra-abdominal organ most frequently ruptured during blunt abdominal trauma. Rupture is particularly liable to occur if the spleen is pathologically enlarged
- Other indications for splenectomy include hereditary spherocytosis, acquired haemolytic anaemia, idiopathic thrombocytopenic purpura, hypersplenism, and myeloproliferative disorders such as myelofibrosis
- Following traumatic rupture or laceration of the spleen, there is now increased emphasis on conservation rather than splenectomy, whenever this is safe and feasible
- Splenectomy in childhood (and to a lesser extent in adult life) carries an appreciable risk of overwhelming post-splenectomy sepsis, and pneumococcal infection is frequently responsible
- If splenectomy is unavoidable, the patient should receive pneumococcal, meningococcal and *Haemophilus influenzae* vaccine (before splenectomy, if possible), and may benefit from prophylactic penicillin. The duration of penicillin therapy is uncertain but the risk of sepsis is greatest in the first few years after splenectomy

Section 4
LOWER GASTROINTESTINAL SURGERY

M.G. DUNLOP

The intestine and appendix

INTRODUCTION

Conditions affecting the small and large intestine are extremely common in the general population and so are a frequent reason for consultation with community practitioners, outpatient referral, or admission to surgical and medical gastroenterological units as well as infectious disease units. Intestinal disease can affect individuals at any time of life, with self-limiting problems such as infective diarrhoea being common in the very young, inflammatory conditions being prevalent in early and middle adulthood, and degenerative disorders such as cancer, diverticular disease and ischaemia becoming more common with progressing age. These conditions result in similar symptoms and so there can sometimes be difficulty in differentiating chronic from acute conditions. Similarly, self-resolving disorders in which watchful waiting is appropriate may be difficult to distinguish from those that require timely diagnosis and active intervention.

BOX 20.1 CLINICAL ASSESSMENT OF A PATIENT WITH GASTROINTESTINAL SYMPTOMS

- Gastrointestinal symptoms are very common
- Most symptoms are due to self-resolving illness
- Patient age is an important factor when considering the differential diagnoses
- Duration of symptoms is an important arbiter of the need for investigation
- Careful assessment of the nature and severity of symptoms is important and may indicate peritonitis, obstruction or severe inflammation
- Symptoms of self-resolving intestinal disorders that are managed conservatively are often indistinguishable from major problems
- Investigation usually requires invasive endoscopy and radiation dosage as part of imaging

---

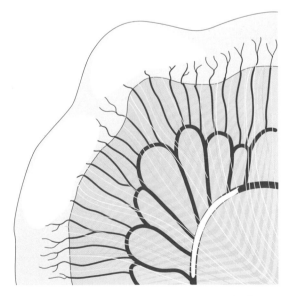

Fig. 20.1   Arterial arcades supplying the small intestine from the superior mesenteric artery.

Hence, there is a conflict between the need for prompt investigation and diagnosis of conditions that require early investigation and intervention and an approach appropriate to those conditions that can be treated conservatively. Furthermore, because of the nature of the anatomy of the large and small intestine, investigation may require invasive endoscopy and/or a significant radiation dose as a consequence of currently available imaging modalities. Thus, careful history and examination, informed by knowledge of the hierarchy of likely diagnoses for a given age group with a particular symptom constellation and clinical signs, are essential when assessing patients with intestinal problems.

APPLIED SURGICAL ANATOMY AND PHYSIOLOGY

ANATOMY AND FUNCTION OF THE SMALL INTESTINE

The small bowel extends from the pylorus to the ileocaecal valve and ranges in length from 3 to 9 metres. The jejunum, which comprises two-fifths of the small intestine, is of wider calibre than the ileum, and the diameter of the gut lumen narrows progressively from the duodenojejunal flexure to the ileocaecal valve. The small bowel mucosa comprises a single layer of columnar cells in a villiform structure that dramatically increases the absorptive area of the mucosa. Columnar glandular epithelium is interspersed with mucus-secreting cells, Paneth cells and amine precursor uptake and decarboxylation (APUD) cells derived from the neural crest. The epithelium is supported on a strong submucosa. Between the inner layer of circular muscle and the outer longitudinal layer runs Auerbach's myenteric plexus, which comprises vagus parasympathetic fibres and sympathetic fibres from the lesser and greater splanchnic nerves. This plexus controls orderly propulsive contractions of the muscular layers of the gut wall. The sympathetic nervous system mediates the sensation of visceral pain, and a submucosal plexus (Meissner's plexus) of autonomic nerves innervates the glandular cells in the epithelium.

The small intestine is supplied by the superior mesenteric artery, which runs in the root of the small bowel mesentery, supplying the bowel by a series of arterial arcades (Fig. 20.1). These midgut vessels communicate through the pancreaticoduodenal arcade with the coeliac axis. The superior mesenteric supply also communicates with that of the inferior mesenteric artery by contributing to the colonic marginal artery through the left branch of the middle colic artery, anastomosing to the ascending branch of the left colic artery. This so-called 'watershed' at the splenic flexure is often a region of limited perfusion, and so the colon is at risk of ischaemia in pathological conditions. Venous blood drains via the superior mesenteric vein to the portal vein. Lymphoid aggregates in the submucosa (Peyer's patches) are more numerous in the ileum, and lymph drains to regional nodes in the root of the mesentery before passing to the cisterna chyli.

20

The principal function of the small bowel is absorption of amino acids, short peptides, sugars and fats, as well as minerals, vitamins and other micronutrients. Its secretory and digestive functions supplement those of the upper digestive tract. The mucosa is thrown into circular folds (plicae semilunares) and carpeted by finger-like villi, giving an absorptive area of 200–500 m². Some 5–8 litres of fluid enter the jejunum each day, of which only 1–2 litres normally pass to the colon.

ANATOMY AND FUNCTION OF THE LARGE INTESTINE AND APPENDIX

The main function of the large bowel is absorption of water and also sodium, particularly on the proximal colon, whereas the left colon and rectum act as a reservoir until defaecation is appropriate. Mucus is secreted as a lubricant. The large bowel mucosa consists of columnar epithelium interspersed with mucus-secreting goblet cells. The villi are shorter than those of the small intestine, and crypts pass down to the muscularis mucosa, which is supported by a strong submucosa. The large bowel extends from the ileocaecal valve to the upper anal canal. The ileocaecal valve has relevance in the presence of colonic obstruction because, if it remains competent, increasing pressure within the colon may result in perforation. The caecum is a blind pouch in the right iliac fossa; the appendix opens from its base at the point where the taeniae coli converge. The transverse and sigmoid colons have mobility by virtue of possessing a mesentery, whereas ascending and descending colon are only partially peritonealized.

The true rectum is demarcated by coalescence of the taeniae coli of the sigmoid colon to form a continuous outer muscular tube. The upper third of the rectum has peritoneal cover on its front and sides, but the middle third is peritonealized only anteriorly as it passes downwards in the hollow of the sacrum to the anorectal junction. The lower third of rectum lies beneath the peritoneal floor of the pelvis.

The inferior and superior mesenteric arteries supply the colon and anastomose via a marginal artery (Fig. 20.2) that allows collateral supply in the event of arterial occlusion, but at the splenic flexure this arterial communication is tenuous. The superior rectal artery is the continuation of the inferior mesenteric artery; it supplies the rectum and anastomoses with the middle and inferior rectal arteries (branches of the internal iliac arteries). Blood from the inferior mesenteric vein drains into the splenic vein. Lymph drains from the colon to epicolic and paracolic nodes close to the bowel wall, and to regional nodes at the origin of the superior and inferior mesenteric vessels (Fig. 20.3). Lymph from the rectum drains upwards to superior rectal and inferior mesenteric nodes, whereas anal canal lymph drains to inguinal nodes. Knowledge of the lymphatic drainage has considerable

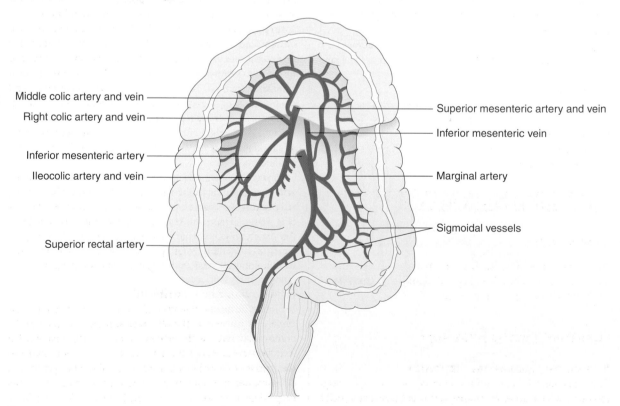

Middle colic artery and vein

Right colic artery and vein

Inferior mesenteric artery

Ileocolic artery and vein

Superior rectal artery

Superior mesenteric artery and vein

Inferior mesenteric vein

Marginal artery

Sigmoidal vessels

Fig. 20.2 **Blood supply of the large intestine from the branches of the superior and inferior mesenteric arteries.**

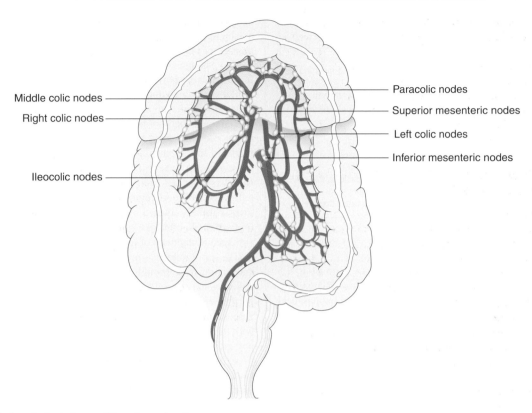

Fig. 20.3 **Lymphatic drainage of the colon and rectum.**

relevance to surgical lymphadenectomy performed as part of radical cancer clearance, as well as to radiotherapy for rectal and anal cancers.

The appendiceal lumen is lined by colonic epithelium and the submucosa contains lymphoid follicles, which are prominent in childhood but regress in adolescence. In older patients, the lumen may eventually be obliterated by fibrosis. It develops as a conical diverticulum, which projects from the medial wall of the caecum some 2 cm below the ileocaecal junction as the taeniae coli converge on the root of the appendix. The appendix has no known function in humans.

DISORDERS OF THE APPENDIX

APPENDICITIS

Acute appendicitis remains the most common acute abdominal emergency in childhood, adolescence and early adult life. Its management is addressed in Chapter 15.

TUMOURS OF THE APPENDIX

Benign tumours of the appendix

The appendix is the most common site for carcinoid tumours, which arise from argentaffin cells of the APUD system and are usually distinct yellow submucosal lesions located near the tip of the appendix. They account for 85% of all appendiceal tumours and are found in 0.5% of all appendices removed surgically. The vast majority are benign, but tumours larger than 2 cm can infiltrate the wall of the appendix and spread to the mesenteric and regional lymph glands. It is very rare for appendiceal carcinoid tumours to give rise to liver metastases and the carcinoid syndrome. Appendicectomy is sufficient treatment for most appendiceal carcinoid tumours, but right hemicolectomy is necessary if the tumour is larger than 2 cm, if it involves the caecum, or if the lymph nodes are affected.

Other benign tumours of the appendix include adenoma and cystadenoma. A mucocoele of the appendix may be confused with a tumour and arises due to chronic obstruction of the appendix base and accumulation of mucin in the lumen. Such simple mucocoeles are cured by appendicectomy. Mucin-secreting cystadenoma of the appendix is important, as it can result in pseudomyxoma peritonei.

Pseudomyxoma peritonei

This is a rare but distressing condition, with around 50 new cases per year in the UK. It results from seeding of the peritoneal cavity with mucus-secreting cells that have a low mitotic rate and can cause pressure symptoms owing to the amount of mucin produced. In a substantial proportion of cases, death results from the need for repeated excisions to palliate symptoms. Occasionally, the underlying basis of the condition is a true malignant mucus-secreting

20

BOX 20.2   TUMOURS OF THE APPENDIX

- Around 85% of all appendiceal tumours are carcinoids, the appendix being the most common site of carcinoid tumour in the gastrointestinal tract
- Carcinoid tumours are found in 0.5% of surgically removed appendices, but lymph node involvement is rare and metastases are extremely rare
- Mucin-secreting cystadenoma is important because, if ruptured, it may lead to pseudomyxoma peritonei
- Appendix adenocarcinoma is rare and may be associated with hereditary non-polyposis colorectal cancer (HNPCC)
- Pseudomyxoma peritonei is a rare, capricious condition that causes pressure symptoms on intestine and other intra-abdominal organs, and for which there is no curative therapy

---

adenocarcinoma of the appendix. Median survival is 2.5 years and few patients are alive at 5 years. The mucin-secreting cells are clonally derived from appendiceal tumour. Surgical debulking is frequently necessary but rarely curative, and the lesions respond poorly to chemotherapy and radiotherapy. Recently, there has been a move towards radical surgical debulking and excision of the entire peritoneum, combined with topical instillation of hot mitomycin C. However, there is an appreciable surgical mortality and morbidity, and long-term follow-up has tempered initial enthusiasm, as the results are not so favourable. Hence, symptom control and tailored surgical resection remain the mainstay of treatment for most patients.

Adenocarcinoma

Adenocarcinoma of the appendix is an uncommon but highly malignant neoplasm, which frequently presents with involved regional lymph nodes at diagnosis. The clinical presentation may mimic acute appendicitis or appendix mass. Right hemicolectomy is the treatment of choice, even in cases where the diagnosis is only apparent at histological assessment of an appendicectomy specimen. In cases with involved lymph nodes, adjuvant chemotherapy with standard large bowel regimens (see below) should be considered. Appendix adenocarcinoma often affects younger patients, and may arise in association with the autosomal syndrome of hereditary non-polyposis colorectal cancer (HNPCC).

CLINICAL ASSESSMENT OF THE SMALL AND LARGE INTESTINE

HISTORY AND CLINICAL EXAMINATION

Painful contraction of the midgut (small bowel, and right and transverse colon) due to obstruction or inflammation results in periumbilical colic, whereas that of the hindgut (distal large bowel) results in lower abdominal colic. Nausea and vomiting are early and predominant features of small bowel disorders, particularly high small bowel obstruction. In contrast, large bowel conditions, particularly obstruction, present with the predominant features of abdominal distension and altered bowel habit, whereas vomiting is a late feature. Normal bowel habit may range from the passage of one motion every 3 days to three per day.

The passage of blood or mucus per rectum is a common feature of large bowel disease. It is important to differentiate 'outlet-type' bleeding from sinister blood loss, when the blood is mixed with the stool and there may be associated altered bowel habit or tenesmus. Outlet bleeding is typically bright red and may be present only on toilet paper or spattered in the pan separate from the stool. There may be associated perianal pain, due to fissure or prolapsed piles. Blood originating from the distal bowel is usually bright red, whereas blood coming from the upper gastrointestinal tract is usually altered by gut bacteria and becomes black (melaena). Weight loss, malaise and anaemia are common non-specific features of intestinal disease.

The oral mucous membrane, hands, fingernails, eyes and conjunctiva should be inspected. Examination of the abdomen may reveal distension, a mass or visible peristalsis. In thin subjects, the caecum is often palpable, and the descending and sigmoid colon may be palpable when loaded with faeces. Hepatomegaly due to metastatic disease should be excluded. Abdominal auscultation determines the presence and pitch of bowel sounds and occasionally reveals an arterial bruit. Digital rectal examination is essential to detect blood and mucus. Three-quarters of rectal cancers and up to one-third of all colorectal cancers can be felt rectally. In patients with lower gastrointestinal symptoms, there is no rationale for checking the faeces for occult blood, as the sensitivity of the guaiac faecal occult blood (FOB) test is only 55% at best, on 3 consecutive days. Thus investigation should not be influenced by the lack of FOB positivity, making the test redundant in the assessment of symptomatic patients.

INVESTIGATION OF THE LUMINAL GASTROINTESTINAL TRACT

Stool culture is widely used for investigation of diarrhoeal illnesses, and should include culture and sensitivity, tests for toxin such as *Clostridium difficile*, and tests for cysts, ova and parasites. Currently available imaging modalities for investigation of the small bowel comprise plain radiography, barium follow-through, small bowel enema (a variation of the follow-through, in which barium is instilled directly into the duodenum through a tube), computed tomography (CT), magnetic resonance imaging (MRI), long fibreoptic enteroscopy, capsule video-endoscopy, labelled white cell radionuclide scanning and labelled red cell radionuclide scanning. In the investigation of suspected coeliac disease, biopsy of the small bowel was previously undertaken by orojejunal capsule biopsy (Crosby capsule), but this has been almost totally superseded by upper gastrointestinal video-endoscopy and biopsy. The terminal ileum can be inspected at colonoscopy, double-contrast barium enema frequently allows visualization of the terminal ileum, and a pneumocolon technique can also be used with barium follow-through to obtain double-contrast views of the terminal ileum. Suspected coeliac disease is now frequently diagnosed by serum antibody assays, including anti-endomysial antibodies and IgA antigliadin antibodies. Tests of absorptive capacity may involve assessment of carbohydrate absorption by a xylose absorption test, which directly tests the ability to absorb monosaccharides; a disaccharidase absorption test; disaccharide breath tests; and direct disaccharidase enzyme activity assessed directly from mucosal biopsy. The glucose tolerance test may be flat in impaired small bowel function but has poor specificity and is seldom used. The main tests of fat absorption are 2- or 5-day faecal fat tests and the ^{14}C-triolein breath test. The specific functions of the terminal ileum can be assessed by the Schilling test, and bile salt absorption by the SeHCAT test. Faecal calprotectin is a useful non-specific test of inflammation of the large and small intestine and can be used to monitor inflammatory bowel disease. Bacterial overgrowth can be assessed using the glucose breath test, ^{14}C-xylose and ^{14}C-glycocholate breath tests. Small bowel aspiration can be carried out by nasojejunal tube or at enteroscopy for bacterial culture.

Direct inspection of the large bowel includes proctoscopy, rigid sigmoidoscopy, flexible sigmoidoscopy and colonoscopy. These techniques allow biopsy and facilitate snare removal of colorectal polyps using cauterizing diathermy. Plain radiography is used extensively in the emergency situation but is seldom of value in elective investigation. Contrast radiography of the colon is undertaken routinely using double contrast (air and barium) to allow detailed inspection of the mucosa. Cross-sectional imaging using CT and MRI is also widely used in the staging of colorectal cancer and has considerable utility in the assessment of the acute abdomen. Other available investigations include tests of colonic transit using ingested radio-opaque markers. This investigation is not used routinely but is relevant to the assessment of megacolon and slow-transit constipation.

PRINCIPLES OF OPERATIVE INTESTINAL SURGERY

The crucial role of the small bowel in maintaining nutrition requires that resectional surgery should aim to retain the maximum possible length of bowel. Ileocaecal resection for Crohn's disease may result in gallstone formation and megaloblastic anaemia, owing to poor absorption of bile salts and vitamin B_{12}. Conversely, loss of the entire large bowel can be tolerated with little impact on nutritional status, but occasionally water and salt depletion can occur, especially in hot climates.

Small intestinal anastomoses heal well, owing to their excellent blood supply and rich submucosal arteriolar plexus. Small bowel content clears after 12 hours of fasting, and so apart from fasting the patient, no specific bowel preparation is required for planned small bowel resection. The large intestine microcirculation consists of a series of small end-arteries, which, combined with the presence of faeces with a high density of bacterial colonization, results in poor anastomotic healing compared to those of the small intestine. This produces a higher anastomotic leak rate for colocolic or colorectal anastomoses.

In view of the risk of anastomotic leakage, there is a lower threshold for the formation of a stoma in patients who require large bowel anastomosis, particularly in the emergency setting when the bowel lumen contains liquid faeces, as this increases the risk of peritoneal contamination. In specialist centres, every effort is made to reconstitute large bowel continuity in both elective and emergency resectional surgery. In emergency surgery for left-sided colonic obstruction or perforation, a total colectomy with anastomosis of the ileum to the rectum may be considered to avoid a colorectal anastomosis in the presence of faecal loading. Segmental left-sided resection and the formation of a colostomy (Hartmann's operation) avoid an anastomosis, but many specialist colorectal surgeons prefer left-sided resection with primary anastomosis.

In the elective setting, there is time to allow reduction in faecal content by a low-residue diet for 2 days preoperatively and a liquid diet for the day before surgery. The bowel may be cleared using mechanical bowel preparations comprising cathartic laxatives such as Picolax, or osmotic laxatives such as polyethylene glycol (KleanPrep); for right-sided resections, however, there is no requirement for bowel preparation and there is a move away from any bowel preparation because of lack of any evidence for benefit in recent meta-analyses. Prophylactic antibiotic therapy usually comprises a single dose of a broad-spectrum cephalosporin to cover coliforms, in combination with metronidazole to cover anaerobic bacteria.

INFLAMMATORY BOWEL DISEASE

In view of the similarities in clinical presentation and in management aspects of both conditions, it is useful to discuss Crohn's disease and ulcerative colitis together (Table 20.1). The key difference between the two conditions is that ulcerative colitis affects the colon and rectum exclusively, whereas Crohn's disease can affect the whole gastrointestinal tract; inflammation is restricted to the mucosa in ulcerative colitis, but transmural inflammation is a hallmark of Crohn's disease. There are also important implications for prognosis, as surgery for ulcerative colitis is curative, whereas Crohn's disease frequently follows a relapsing course, despite medical or surgical intervention.

CROHN'S DISEASE

Although originally described as a disease affecting the terminal ileum, it is now clear that any part of the gastrointestinal tract can be involved, from mouth to anus. In 50% of cases both small and large bowel are involved, whereas in 25% of cases large bowel alone is affected. The incidence is increasing in developed countries and the annual rate is currently 5–7 cases per 100 000 in the UK population. At the time of initial clinical presentation, the features of Crohn's disease may be indistinguishable from those of ulcerative colitis. Indeed, in cases of colonic Crohn's disease, it may be difficult to differentiate the two conditions, even after resection and histological assessment.

Table 20.1   CLINICAL FEATURES OF ULCERATIVE COLITIS AND CROHN'S DISEASE

	Crohn's disease	Ulcerative colitis
Incidence	5–7 per 100 000 and rising	10 per 100 000 and static
Extent	May involve entire gastrointestinal tract	Limited to large bowel
Rectal involvement	Variable	Almost invariable
Disease continuity	Discontinuous (skip lesions)	Continuous
Depth of inflammation	Transmural	Mucosal
Macroscopic appearance of mucosa	Cobblestone, discrete deep ulcers and fissures	Multiple small ulcers, pseudopolyps
Histological features	Transmural inflammation, granulomas (50%)	Crypt abscesses, submocosal chronic inflammatory cell infiltrate, crypt architectural distortion, goblet cell depletion, no granulomas
Presence of perianal disease	75% of cases with large bowel disease; 25% of cases with small bowel disease	25% of cases
Frequency of fistula	10–20% of cases	Uncommon
Colorectal cancer risk	Elevated risk (relative risk = 2.5) in colonic disease	25% risk over 30 years for pancolitis
Relationship with smoking	Increased risk, greater disease severity, increased risk of relapse and need for surgery	Protective, first attack may be preceded by smoking cessation within 6 months

Cigarette smoking is the single most important risk factor for developing the disease, and is associated with increased disease severity and frequency of relapse, as well as the need for surgical intervention. The underlying aetiology has previously been attributed to nutritional deficiency and increased intestinal permeability, and immunological factors have been postulated. However, there is now strong evidence implicating the gut bacterial flora in the pathogenesis of inflammatory bowel disease and of Crohn's disease in particular. Recently, a gene involved in host–bacteria interaction, *CARD15 (NOD2)*, has been identified. Particular genetic variants that influence protein function have been associated with risk of the disease and with disease severity and location. It seems likely that other genes in this pathway will also be involved, and this is the focus of much current research activity.

Pathology

Macroscopically, Crohn's disease produces a cobblestone appearance, in which oedematous islands of mucosa are separated by crevices or fissures; these can extend through all coats of the bowel wall. Serpiginous ulceration is common, and fibrosis produces strictures of varying number and length. Multiple areas of inflammation are common, but intervening bowel appears normal (i.e. skip lesions, Fig. 20.4). Full-thickness involvement of the bowel wall leads to serosal inflammation, adhesion to neighbouring structures, and sinus or fistula formation. Microscopically, there are deep fissuring ulcers, oedema and inflammatory cell infiltrates with foci of lymphocytes and non-caseating granulomas in 50% of cases.

Clinical features

Crohn's disease is a chronic disorder with exacerbations, remissions and a varied clinical presentation. Continuous or episodic diarrhoea is associated with recurring abdominal pain and tenderness, lassitude and fever. Declining general health, malabsorption and weight loss, with failure to thrive and to reach developmental milestones, are common in affected children.

Examination may reveal malnutrition and there may be a palpable abdominal mass. There may be features of subacute intestinal obstruction, and this may be due to active disease, stricturing of 'burnt-out' disease, or adhesions from previous surgical intervention. Fistula formation occurs in 20% of patients with small and large bowel disease, and in 10% of those with large bowel disease only. The fistula may communicate with other loops of bowel, other viscera (e.g. bladder, vagina) or the skin. External fistulae most often result from surgical intervention and commonly involve the anterior abdominal wall or perineum. Abscesses can result from subclinical bowel perforation. Free perforation is

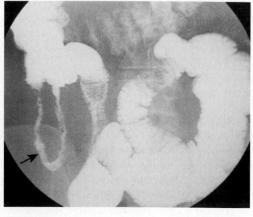

Fig. 20.4   Multiple small bowel strictures in Crohn's disease.
The arrow indicates the longest stricture.

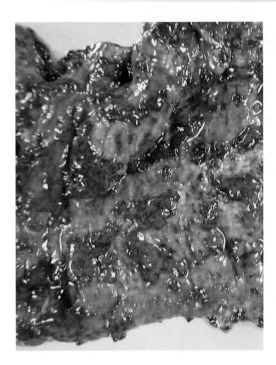

Fig. 20.5 Fulminant Crohn's colitis.

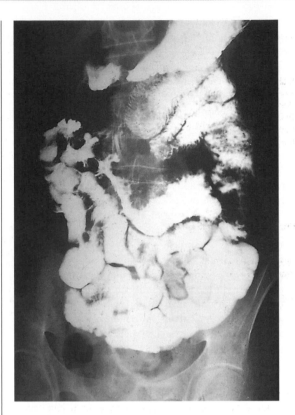

Fig. 20.6 Small bowel contrast enema in Crohn's disease, showing a long irregular stricture and typical rose-thorn ulceration.

relatively uncommon because the inflamed segment usually adheres to surrounding structures. Although less common than in ulcerative colitis, toxic dilatation can complicate colonic disease. Fulminant Crohn's colitis is shown in Figure 20.5; deep ulcers and fibrosis with mucosal oedema and inflammation can be seen.

Crohn's disease is associated with an elevated (2.5 times increased) risk of carcinoma of the colon. It is important to consider the possibility of malignancy in patients with relapsing symptoms from long-standing disease that has been relatively quiescent. There is no evidence that surveillance is beneficial, and many patients with colonic Crohn's eventually need to have their colon removed.

One-quarter of patients with small bowel Crohn's disease and three-quarters of those with large bowel disease have troublesome anal lesions, including ulceration, abscess, oedematous skin tags, fissure and fistula. Anal fissures are often multiple and indolent, and extend to involve any part of the perineum, including the vagina or scrotum. Systemic manifestations include anterior uveitis, iritis, polyarthropathy, ankylosing spondylitis, liver disease (e.g. sclerosing cholangitis) and erythema nodosum. Disease of the terminal ileum or its resection increases the incidence of gallstones.

Investigations

In the non-emergency situation, general assessment includes evaluation of nutritional status and the detection of anaemia, which may be due to iron deficiency from chronic blood loss. Normocytic anaemia of chronic disease or macrocytic anaemia due to vitamin B_{12} or folate malabsorption may result. Elevated erythrocyte sedimentation rate (ESR) and acute-phase proteins such as C-reactive protein are useful in monitoring disease, but are not specific for diagnostic

purposes. The standard diagnostic investigation is barium follow-through (or small bowel enema). A typical appearance on small bowel contrast enema is shown in Figure 20.6; rose-thorn ulcers and a long irregular stricture of the terminal ileum at the site of previous ileocaecal resection may be seen. Active disease produces radiological evidence of thickening, luminal narrowing and separation of loops, and is often associated with ulceration, spike-like fissures and a cobblestone appearance. Skip lesions and fistula formation may be apparent. Proctoscopy, sigmoidoscopy and colonoscopy are used to determine the presence and extent of large bowel disease. Biopsy of macroscopically normal rectum at sigmoidoscopy or colonoscopy may reveal occult large bowel involvement, particularly if there has been troublesome perianal involvement. Double-contrast barium enema may be useful in assessing the extent of disease and may delineate fistula formation.

Management

Medical management

Attention to nutritional state is essential and anaemia should be corrected by transfusion if life-threatening or symptomatic. Supplemental iron and/or vitamins may be appropriate if the anaemia is less severe. Malnourishment should be managed by a high-protein, low-residue or elemental diet. Hydrophilic colloid preparations and codeine phosphate may help diarrhoea, and colestyramine can be used to bind bile salts and prevent their cathartic effects on the colon in patients with small bowel disease. There is no evidence

20

that low-residue and elemental diets have real value in inducing remission of Crohn's disease.

Steroids can be used in the acute phase (prednisolone 30–60 mg daily by mouth), but every attempt should be made to avoid long-term steroid therapy in view of the risk of complications. There are no drugs that can guarantee freedom from relapse, but Crohn's disease may respond to 5-aminosalicylic acid (5-ASA) agents, such as mesalazine and olsalazine. These agents may be useful in colonic disease and, in some cases, for relapsing terminal ileal disease, and there is limited evidence that maintenance therapy may marginally reduce the risk of relapse. Immunosuppression using azathioprine (3 mg/kg daily) or 6-mercaptopurine can be used in resistant cases to induce remission and also to maintain it. However, there are concerns about complications of long-term immuno-suppression and the agents are not generally continued beyond 2 years without review; they are seldom used beyond 4 years. Monoclonal antibodies to tumour necrosis factor-α (TNF-α) are now used frequently in specialist centres and have a place in patients with fistulating Crohn's disease. Newer agents such as anti-integrins are now being tested in clinical trials.

Surgical management

Almost all patients with Crohn's disease require surgery at some stage. Surgery may have a role in the acute management of abscess or perforation, and in the chronic situation where there are frequent relapses on maximum medical management or failure to respond in subacute disease. Perianal and chronic burnt-out disease with fibrosis and stricturing may necessitate intervention for intermittent bowel obstruction. Operation is reserved for patients who are not thriving on medical management or who have complications (notably, obstruction, abscess, perforation and fistula; EBM 20.1). Uninvolved bowel should be preserved and the residual small bowel length documented. Stricturoplasty is a useful technique that involves longitudinal division of the strictured small bowel, with closure of the defect transversely to widen the intestinal lumen. Radical surgery is contraindicated, as the risk of recurrence is determined by the natural history of the disease rather than the extent of surgery. The recurrence rate following small bowel resection is around 30%, as opposed to less than 20% in colonic disease. In the initial phases of colonic Crohn's disease, segmental resection is preferred to bypass of affected segments. However, many patients eventually undergo proctocolectomy and ileostomy. In perianal Crohn's disease, loculated pus can be drained and radical surgery should be avoided, as the disease tends to recur. Fistulae should be laid open and complex reconstructions avoided.

BOX 20.3   INDICATIONS FOR SURGERY IN CROHN'S DISEASE

Elective
- Chronic subacute obstruction due to fibrotic strictures, adhesions or refractory disease
- Symptomatic disease unresponsive to or poorly controlled by medical management
- Chronic relapsing disease on discontinuation of medical management and steroid dependency
- Complications of medical management (e.g. osteoporosis)
- Concerns about long-term immunosuppression, risk of malignancy and viral/atypical infections
- Perianal sepsis and fistula
- Enterocutaneous fistula
- Onset of malignancy, including colorectal adenocarcinoma and small bowel lymphoma
- Rarely, control of debilitating extra-colonic manifestations such as iritis and sacroiliitis

Emergency
- Fulminant colitis or acute small bowel relapse unresponsive to medical management
- Acute bowel obstruction
- Life-threatening haemorrhage
- Abscess or free perforation
- Perianal abscess

ULCERATIVE COLITIS

In developed countries, the annual incidence is approxi-mately 10 new cases per 100 000 population, but the disorder is very rare in developing countries. The cause is unknown, but most interest centres on an immunological basis for the disease, interacting with dietary constituents. Ulcerative colitis affects all age groups but the peak incidence occurs in young adults. In 95% of cases, the disease is contiguous, affecting the rectum and extending proximally (Table 20.1). In 5% of cases, it is segmental and the rectum is occasionally spared. There is substantial risk of colorectal adenocarcinoma in cases with pancolitis (Table 20.1). Although ulcerative colitis is primarily a disease of the large bowel, systemic manifestations (iritis, polyarthritis, sacroiliitis, hepatitis, erythema nodosum, pyoderma gangrenosum) can occur. Primary sclerosing cholangitis (PSC) affects 2–5% of cases of ulcerative colitis; it tends to indicate severe disease and predict complications including pouchitis. Many patients with PSC will eventually develop liver failure and liver transplantation may be indicated.

Pathology

The characteristic feature of ulcerative colitis is involvement restricted to the mucosa and submucosa of the large bowel. However, with severe relapse, there may be full-thickness involvement, with inflammatory infiltrate. Abscesses form at the base of the colonic crypts, which may burst horizontally or occasionally radially to involve deeper layers of the bowel wall. The abscesses have a surrounding inflammatory infiltrate and coalesce to form crypt abscesses, which undermine the mucosa and cause ulcera-

---

EBM 20.1   CROHN'S DISEASE AND ULCERATIVE COLITIS

'Colonoscopic surveillance may reduce colorectal cancer risk.'
'Surgical resection is required in patients resistant to medical management and for complications of Crohn's disease.'

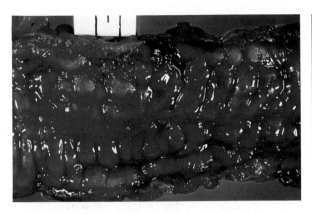

Fig. 20.7 Macroscopic appearance of fulminant ulcerative colitis.

tion of the overlying mucosa (Fig. 20.7). The intervening mucosa becomes oedematous and may form inflammatory pseudopolyps. Histologically, there is infiltration of chronic inflammatory cells, crypt architectural distortion and goblet cell depletion. Importantly, there are no granulomas. The bowel loses its haustrations and becomes thick and rigid, although strictures are uncommon. There can sometimes be difficulty in distinguishing ulcerative colitis from Crohn's colitis, and there may even be migration from one pheno-type to the other. In this instance, the term 'indeterminate colitis' is used to denote uncertainty. There are important implications for surgical treatment, since ileo-anal pouch is to be avoided in cases of Crohn's colitis.

Other rare subtypes of colitis are collagenous and lymphocytic colitis (collectively known as microscopic colitis), characterized by chronic diarrhoea, normal endoscopic and radiological findings, and typical findings on histological examination of colonic tissue. Microscopic colitis occurs more commonly in females; it can affect people of all ages but has a mean in the seventh decade. Collagenous colitis is characterized by macroscopically normal colonic mucosa overlying a typically thickened subepithelial collagen band on histological examination. Lymphocytic colitis is characterized by an increased number of lymphocytes in the submucosa but lacks the features of either ulcerative or Crohn's colitis. It can have a segmental distribution and so differentiation from Crohn's colitis is important. There may be an association with a coexistent autoimmune disorder or the use of drugs such as non-steroidal anti-inflammatory drugs (NSAIDs).

Clinical features

Ulcerative colitis characteristically runs an intermittent course of relapse and remission, although some patients may have a chronic continuous variant. In some cases, the initial attack is fulminant, and toxic dilatation with exacerbation of abdominal and systemic symptoms may occur at any time. Diarrhoea with the passage of mucus and blood is typical of relapse. Abdominal pain and tenderness may be present and intermittent pyrexia is common. Passage of 10–15 or more stools each day is not unusual. Rather than increased faecal frequency, it is the incapacitating faecal urgency that is most distressing for most patients, causing a significant degradation of quality of life.

Careful rectal examination should detect anal complications such as fissure, fistula and haemorrhoids, which are present in 25% of cases. The rectal mucosa often feels thick and boggy. Sigmoidoscopy (with biopsy) is the key investigation and reveals a red, matt granular mucosa with contact bleeding. In the early stages of disease, the only sign on sigmoidoscopy may be loss of the rectal mucosal vessels. As the disease progresses, severe ulceration leads to fulminant colitis, the complications of which include dramatic nutritional depletion, toxic dilatation, perforation and severe bleeding. During an exacerbation, the dilated colon may become paper-thin.

Investigations

Expert colonoscopy is the mainstay of diagnosis and assessment of disease severity and extent. The endoscopic features of a case of severe acute colitis are shown in Figure 20.8. Although less frequently used than colonoscopy, barium enema may also help in the assessment of the extent of disease (Fig. 20.9) but is contraindicated in patients with fulminant colitis and those with toxic dilatation because of the risk of precipitating perforation. Typical changes include loss of haustrations, fluffy granularity of the mucosa, and pseudopolyps. Undermining ulcers may create a double contour to the edge of the colon. Widening of the retrorectal space, due to perirectal inflammation and reduced distensibility of the rectum, is common. In an acute attack, plain films of the abdomen may reveal a dilated gas-filled colon in which pseudopolyps are evident. When toxic dilatation is suspected, daily plain X-rays are essential to monitor progress. So-called 'backwash ileitis' may produce a dilated and featureless terminal ileum in which the mucosa appears granular. In the acute phase, it is essential to collect stool cultures to exclude supervening bacterial infection and especially *Cl. difficile*, which is prevalent in hospital practice.

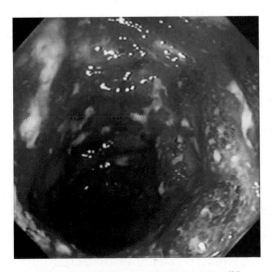

Fig. 20.8 Colonoscopic appearance of severe acute colitis.

20

20

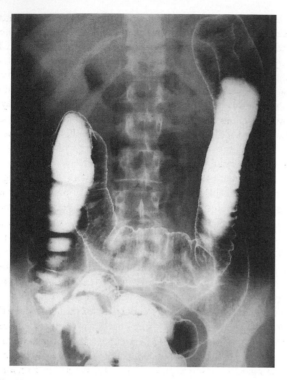

Fig. 20.9   Barium enema appearance of ulcerative colitis.

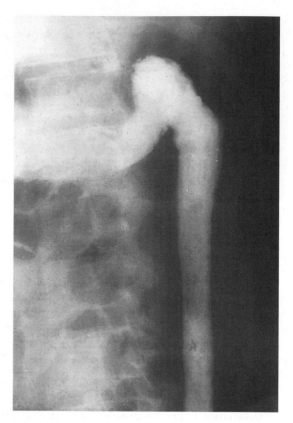

Fig. 20.11   Barium enema appearance of chronic ulcerative colitis, showing a 'lead pipe' colon.

Ultimately, over a period of years of chronic colitis, the bowel may become short and featureless, resembling a smooth tube. Figure 20.10 shows the colonoscopic appearance of chronic burnt-out colitis, and Figure 20.11 the barium enema features. Colonoscopy has an important place in the diagnosis and surveillance of colitis by detecting evidence of dysplasia.

Management

Medical management

With fluid and electrolyte replacement, correction of anaemia, adequate nutrition, steroid therapy, and timely surgical intervention when appropriate, 97% of patients survive their first attack. However, over 70% are destined to have recurrent episodes. High-dose systemic steroids (oral prednisolone, intravenous methylprednisolone or hydrocortisone) are needed during an acute relapse. Immunosuppression with either azathioprine or ciclosporin A may be helpful for those who do not respond. Topical steroids delivered by enema or suppository usually control mild attacks of proctocolitis. Long-term aminosalicylates, such as mesalazine or olsalazine, have been shown to reduce the risk of relapse when a patient is in remission, and are now preferred to sulfasalazine, which is effective but has significant side-effects. Nicotine patches have been used effectively to induce remission in view of the rationale that smoking appears to be protective for ulcerative colitis. However, side-effects are greater and such an approach is therefore used in only a very limited number of cases. Around 15% of all patients diagnosed with ulcerative colitis will eventually require surgery. The risk varies from 1 in 50 for those with mild proctitis, to 1 in 20 for moderately severe colitis, and 1 in 2 for those with extensive disease.

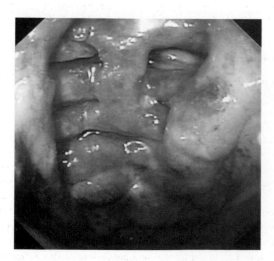

Fig. 20.10   Colonoscopic appearance of chronic burnt-out colitis.

Surgical management

Indications for surgery in the emergency and elective setting include fulminant colitis that fails to respond promptly to aggressive medical therapy, perforation, toxic dilatation and massive bleeding. Patients presenting as an emergency are catabolic, malnourished, immunosuppressed by their disease and medical interventions, bacteraemic and even septic. Hence, surgery should be limited and, in the acute setting, bowel reconstruction is inadvisable. Modern management comprises a 'first aid' operation of colectomy and ileostomy to allow the patient to recover. The rectum is closed over as a stump in the pelvis, or by bringing out the distal end as a mucous fistula. Completion proctectomy and the formation of an ileo-anal pouch are undertaken following recovery from the emergency operation, usually after 6 months. It is important that patients understand that it is essential to remove the residual rectum because of the substantial lifetime rectal cancer risk.

In the elective setting, definitive reconstructive surgery is possible because the patient is fit and well nourished, and complications are much reduced over those in the emergency situation. Indications for surgery include failure of medical management or repeated relapses on medical treatment. Failure to thrive, as reflected in retardation of growth and sexual development in children, or malnourishment and anaemia in adults, is a common indication for operation. Local complications that influence the decision to operate include those affecting the perineum and the rare instance when a stricture has formed. The onset of biopsy-proven dysplasia or early carcinoma in chronic disease and the onset of fulminant colitis unresponsive to maximal medical management necessitate surgical intervention.

Modern surgical practice aims to preserve continence following removal of the entire diseased large bowel. Restorative proctocolectomy with retention of the anal sphincters and reconstruction by formation of an ileal pouch anastomosed to the upper anal canal are now standard. This approach has the benefits of removing all but a tiny cuff of rectal mucosa in the upper anal canal, and also maintaining the ability of the patient's bowel to move normally. A temporary ileostomy may be required. Faecal urgency is eliminated and the overall quality of life is excellent, despite the passage of 4–6 liquid motions per day. A Koch's pouch may be considered following panproctocolectomy as an alternative to permanent ileostomy. Although the patient does not require a stoma bag, the pouch needs to be emptied by cannulating the stoma spout.

Cancer surveillance in ulcerative colitis

There is a substantial risk of colorectal cancer in long-standing ulcerative colitis, and this is now a major factor contributing to the decision to operate. Carcinoma is often difficult to detect in colitis, is usually poorly differentiated and has a poor prognosis. Regardless of disease extent, around 2% of all patients will develop cancer at 10 years, 8% at 20 years and 18% at 30 years. In pancolitis, the overall risk is around 25% after 30 years. Early age at first onset (especially < 15 years of age), pancolitis, a family history of colorectal cancer and associated PSC are strong predictors of cancer risk. Cancer surveillance is recommended in the long-term management of patients with chronic ulcerative colitis, and colonoscopy should be performed at 2-yearly intervals (EBM 20.1). Random biopsies are taken at surveillance colonoscopy, since dysplasia indicates a high risk of cancer occurrence. Dysplasia-associated lesion or mass (DALM) is a high-risk indicator of impending cancer development. In patients with high-grade dysplasia or DALM, restorative proctocolectomy is now recommended because the cancer risk is > 60% in the next 2 years. In many cases of DALM, there is already evidence of malignancy on pathological assessment of the resected colon. A prophylactic restorative proctocolectomy may be considered in patients with pancolitis, especially when ulcerative colitis was diagnosed before the age of 15 years, rather than accepting the uncertainties of a prolonged surveillance programme without proven benefit. Fully counselled patient involvement is essential in such decisions.

DISORDERS OF THE SMALL INTESTINE

SMALL BOWEL NEOPLASMS

Small bowel tumours account for less than 5% of all gastrointestinal neoplasms.

Benign tumours

Solitary neoplasms include adenomatous or villous polyps, hamartomas, lipomas, haemangiomas and leiomyoma (many of which may have been miscategorized as gastrointestinal stromal tumours (see below). Multiple hamartomas are found in the Peutz–Jeghers syndrome (see below). Benign tumours are rarely symptomatic and so the true incidence is unknown. Symptoms may arise as a result of intussusception or bleeding, particularly in the case of leiomyoma and the hamartomatous lesions of Peutz–Jeghers syndrome.

BOX 20.4 INDICATIONS FOR SURGERY IN ULCERATIVE COLITIS

Elective

- Symptomatic disease unresponsive to or poorly controlled by medical management
- Chronic relapsing disease on discontinuation of medical management and steroid dependency
- Complications of medical management
- Concerns about long-term immunosuppression, risk of malignancy and viral/atypical infections
- Severe dysplasia on surveillance biopsies
- Onset of colorectal adenocarcinoma
- Rarely, control of debilitating extra-colonic manifestations such as iritis and sacroiliitis

Emergency

- Fulminant colitis unresponsive to maximal medical management
- Toxic megacolon
- Free perforation
- Life-threatening haemorrhage
- Acute complications of medical management

20

20

Malignant tumours

The diagnosis of a malignant tumour of the small intestine is difficult because symptoms are ill defined and intermittent. Small bowel imaging, such as a follow-through contrast study, may not reveal a lesion because of overlying loops of unaffected small bowel. Abdominal CT or MRI may be useful. Enteroscopy may detect a lesion, but biopsy is not yet possible as a routine because the channel for many current enteroscopes does not permit passage of a biopsy wire. Video capsule endoscopy may detect a lesion.

Gastrointestinal stromal tumours (GISTs)

GISTs are an interesting group because recent integration of molecular, clinical and pathological understanding has led to a new application of a class of chemotherapeutic drugs. GISTs are the most common form of mesenchymal tumour of the intestinal tract. The lesions are derived from smooth muscle of gut tube; 50–60% are in the stomach, 20–30% in small bowel, 10% in rectum and 5% in oesophagus. It has become clear that there is a spectrum from benign to malignant and that the more malignant lesions have a poor prognosis, tending to recur locally and to metastasize. Recent findings have shown that *c-Kit* expression can help differentiate malignant from benign phenotype. The Kit protein is a transmembrane tyrosine kinase receptor and most GISTs have a mutation in either the *c-Kit* gene or the platelet-derived growth factor receptor alpha gene (PDGFRA). The mutations cause the respective oncoproteins to exhibit constitutive tyrosine kinase activity and promote cell growth due to up-regulation in tumour cells. Pathological assessment of immunohistochemical stains for Kit protein, combined with an assessment of the numbers of mitotic figures in histological fields from biopsy or resected specimens, can help predict biological behaviour. Understanding that *c-Kit* oncogene is one of the molecular lesions involved in GIST development and progression, as well as predicting behaviour, has allowed the development of new anticancer agents such as imatinib mesylate, a tyrosine kinase inhibitor that inhibits the activities of Kit and PDGFRA, and has been shown to be useful in treating malignant GIST lesions.

Adenocarcinoma

The duodenum and upper jejunum are the most common sites of this rare tumour. Adenocarcinomas, which are usually poorly differentiated and are mucin-secreting, may be associated with HNPCC. Resection of the affected segment is carried out, but palliative bypass may be all that is possible, as the disease often presents late.

Lymphoma

Coeliac disease is a predisposing factor in small bowel T-cell lymphoma, which, along with B-cell lymphoma, can cause intermittent obstruction, bleeding or perforation. The disease should be staged pre-operatively to allow further systemic or local treatment to be planned. Antigliadin and anti-endomysial antibodies should be determined and a biopsy of adjacent normal small intestine or duodenum should be assessed for villous atrophy.

Carcinoid tumour

The small bowel is the second most common site for carcinoid tumour after the appendix. Metastasis to lymph nodes is common at presentation, and obstruction and bleeding are the usual modes of presentation. There may be features of the carcinoid syndrome in the presence of liver metastasis, but blood 5-hydroxytryptamine (5-HT) levels are determined in the absence of liver metastasis. The primary tumour should be resected where possible. In many cases, the lesions are multifocal and may require multiple resections.

PEUTZ–JEGHERS SYNDROME

Peutz–Jeghers syndrome is an autosomal dominant inherited disorder with high penetrance. The gene, *LKB1/STK11*, is located on the short arm of chromosome 19 and mutations are causative in most families, although some cases are due to as yet unmapped genes. The clinical manifestations include gastrointestinal polyps and melanin pigmentation at mucocutaneous junctions, and occasionally on the dorsum of the hands and feet. Small intestinal and gastric cancers occur in around 7% of patients and the lifetime risk of colorectal cancer is around 10–20%, although these estimates may be inaccurate due to the rarity of the disorder.

Pathology

Polyps occur most commonly in the jejunum; they have a short pedicle with a lobulated surface resembling that of an adenomatous polyp or sometimes a villous tumour. On microscopy, the hamartomas consist of branches of muscularis mucosae covered by epithelium and lamina propria. Adenocarcinomatous change may occur but it is not clear whether this arises in a hamartoma or in an area of normal epithelium.

Clinical features

Most cases present in childhood or adolescence. There are usually dark brown or bluish spots on the lips and inside the mouth. The face, palms, soles, arms and perianal region can also be affected, but patients without pigmentation have been described. The usual presentation is with abdominal pain or obstruction due to intussusception of a polyp, but rectal bleeding and iron deficiency anaemia are also common. The diagnosis is usually made on clinical grounds, with the association of abdominal colic and typical pigmentation in childhood or early adulthood. Assessment of the small bowel is complicated because the radiation dose associated with repeated barium small bowel follow-through or CT examinations restricts their use. Recent advances in gastrointestinal contrast MRI technology hold promise (Fig. 20.12).

Management

Treatment is conservative wherever possible. However, laparotomy, enterotomy and polypectomy are required frequently. On-table enteroscopy can reduce the numbers of enterotomies and allows inspection of the whole length of the gastrointestinal tract from oesophagus to anus, with removal of all polyps. Upper and lower gastrointestinal surveillance endoscopy is recommended, as the cancer

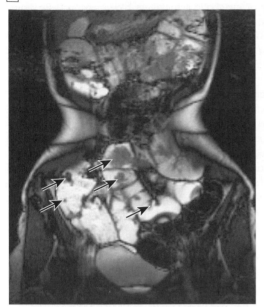

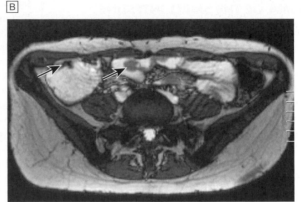

Fig. 20.12 Peutz–Jeghers syndrome.
A Abdominal MRI (coronal view) showing multiple polypoid filling defects (arrowed) due to hamartomatous polyps. B Cross-sectional MRI of a large jejunal polyp.

risk is high. However, because of the rarity of the condition, there is no strong evidence to support this approach.

DIVERTICULA OF THE SMALL INTESTINE

Meckel's diverticulum

This is the most common congenital abnormality of the gastrointestinal tract, being present in 2% of people; it comprises persistence of part of the vitello-intestinal duct. The diverticulum is around 5 cm long and arises from the antimesenteric border of the ileum some 50 cm from the ileocaecal valve. It is a true diverticulum and in 10% of cases its tip is connected to the umbilicus by a fibrous cord. Heterotopic mucosa is found in 50% of symptomatic diverticula; it is most often acid-secreting gastric mucosa but pancreatic tissue may also be present. Only 5% of Meckel's diverticula cause symptoms, most frequently in childhood or early adult life. Bleeding from peptic ulceration is the most common cause of severe gastrointestinal bleeding in childhood. Intestinal obstruction may occur due to intussusception of the diverticulum, or to a loop of bowel becoming trapped beneath or twisted around (volvulus) a band extending to the umbilicus. Acute diverticulitis produces abdominal pain and tenderness, pyrexia and leucocytosis, and may mimic acute appendicitis.

Symptomatic Meckel's diverticula should be excised. Asymptomatic diverticula found incidentally at laparotomy should be left alone, unless the neck is narrow or nodularity suggests that the diverticulum contains abnormal mucosa. In patients with unexplained gastrointestinal bleeding, heterotopic mucosa within a Meckel's diverticulum can be detected by scintiscanning after injection of ^{99m}Tc-labelled sodium pertechnetate.

Jejunal diverticulosis

Jejunal diverticula are acquired during adult life. Only one or two diverticula may be present, but often diverticulosis is very extensive, with multiple wide-mouthed sacs caused by herniation of mucosa into the mesentery at the site of vessel penetration of the gut wall. Jejunal diverticulosis may first be diagnosed at laparotomy for complicated disease, or incidentally by barium studies or at operation. The diverticula may cause bleeding, inflammation, malabsorption (due to bacterial over-colonization) and perforation. Occasionally, fish bones or even NSAID tablets can become trapped in a diverticulum and cause local perforation. In symptomatic disease, the affected segment of bowel may have to be locally resected, leaving other affected areas in situ.

RADIATION INJURY

External beam irradiation or internal irradiation using radioactive implants can cause proctocolitis and enteritis. The terminal ileum is the most commonly affected site within the small bowel. In the acute phase, oedema, inflammation and ulceration may produce diarrhoea, lower abdominal pain, tenesmus, mucus discharge and rectal bleeding. Subsequently, the bowel may thicken, with fibrosis and stricture. Topical steroids or topical aminosalicylates, such as a mesalazine enema, may give symptomatic relief of proctitis. Stricture and fistula formation usually require resection of the affected bowel. If the fistula affects the rectum and vagina, excision of the whole rectum and replacement with fresh colon from outside the irradiated field, employing a colo-anal J-pouch reconstruction, may be required. A defunctioning ileostomy has to be used with caution, as the small bowel itself often has been irradiated.

ISCHAEMIA OF THE SMALL INTESTINE

In developed countries, small intestinal ischaemia is usually due to atheromatous occlusion with superadded thrombosis of the superior mesenteric artery. Factors predisposing to mesenteric thrombosis include hypovolaemia or hypoperfusion of the gut resulting from trauma, cardiogenic shock, cardiac arrhythmia and septic shock. Arterial embolism can result from atrial fibrillation or recent myocardial infarction. In a third of patients dying from acute ischaemic necrosis of the midgut, there is no demonstrable occlusion of a major vessel, and in these cases low perfusion is responsible. Other causes include polycythaemia, sickle cell disease and disseminated intravascular coagulation. Arteritis should be suspected where there are other stigmata or a history of disseminated arteritis, such as pre-existing renal failure. Impaired venous return from the gut can be due to hyperviscosity syndromes and prothrombotic tendency, but are also seen in the presence of malignancy and portal hypertension. Ischaemic necrosis may progress to necrosis of all bowel layers with gangrene and perforation, but recovery may ensue if flow is restored within 6 hours. Slow resolution of a short segment of ischaemia may result in fibrosis and stricture formation in the longer term.

ACUTE SMALL BOWEL INFARCTION

Acute occlusion of the superior mesenteric artery (SMA) is predominantly a disease of the elderly and leads to complete necrosis and gangrene of most of the midgut. Massive resection is inevitable unless flow can be restored within 6 hours. Even if the patient survives, the resulting nutritional problems may prove overwhelming.

Clinical features

The diagnosis should be considered in all patients with acute abdominal pain who have no signs of other underlying disease. Early diagnosis is often difficult as the symptoms and signs are non-specific. There may be a preceding history of chronic or episodic abdominal pain associated with meals, diarrhoea and weight loss. Cardiac arrhythmias, notably atrial fibrillation, are often present on initial presentation. Abdominal pain is a predominant symptom and may be associated with vomiting. In a third of cases, there is watery or bloody diarrhoea. The pain varies in its location but is generally central, severe and constant in nature. Abdominal tenderness, guarding and rigidity are late signs denoting gangrene and perforation, and cardiovascular collapse signifies hypovolaemia and sepsis.

Investigations and diagnosis

In almost all cases, the diagnosis is made on the basis of clinical suspicion. As many affected patients are old and frail, with multiple comorbidities, a decision must be taken early as to whether active management is indicated. Plain abdominal films may reveal calcified atheroma in the mesenteric arteries and aorta, and there may be dilated thickened gas-filled small bowel loops. Gas in the bowel wall or in the peritoneal cavity is a grave sign. Marked leucocytosis and hyperamylasaemia are common, but the finding of metabolic acidosis on blood gas analysis should raise strong suspicion of bowel ischaemia. Arteriography is seldom helpful in practice because of the late presentation of most cases. The decision to undertake laparotomy should be taken on clinical grounds.

Management

Following vigorous resuscitation, gangrenous bowel requires resection, but this may be futile in elderly patients with extensive midgut involvement. In some instances of acute occlusion, arterial flow can be restored by embolectomy or thrombectomy. A 'second-look' laparotomy 24 hours later may be useful. The prognosis is poor, with an overall mortality of 70–90%. Survival is restricted almost exclusively to patients in whom a defined vascular occlusion is treated early. Mesenteric venous occlusion has an equally bad prognosis, and treatment is usually confined to resection of the gangrenous bowel and anticoagulation.

CHRONIC MESENTERIC ISCHAEMIA

Chronic mesenteric ischaemia results in repeated bouts of ill-defined colicky central abdominal pain, typically commencing 20–30 minutes after eating. Weight loss is almost universal due to a 'fear of food', brought about by pain after the patient eats. Diagnosis is often elusive and is usually preceded by extensive investigation to exclude other conditions of the small or large bowel, such as Crohn's disease and malignancy. Mesenteric arteriography may be diagnostic but must be taken in the context of symptoms because atheromatous change in mesenteric vessels is common.

PARALYTIC ILEUS

Paralytic ileus is a term that refers to lack of propulsive contractions of the small intestine, affecting both jejunum and ileum, although the ileus can be localized in some instances. Treatment is usually focused on the underlying cause. Ileus is common after surgery owing to handling of the bowel and in the presence of peritonitis due to any cause, such as perforated duodenal ulcer, pancreatitis, appendicitis and mesenteric ischaemia. Metabolic and electrolyte abnormalities, such as hypokalaemia, hyponatraemia, uraemia and diabetic ketoacidosis, can result in ileus. Drugs such as tricyclic antidepressants and lithium may be implicated in some cases.

MECHANICAL OBSTRUCTION

Both large and small bowel obstruction can be classified as intraluminal, intramural and extramural (Table 20.2), but the most common causes of small intestinal obstruction in developed countries are adhesions and obstructed hernia. The most common cause of large bowel obstruction is colorectal cancer. Treatment usually requires operation and should be focused on the underlying cause of obstruction.

Table 20.2 AETIOLOGY OF INTESTINAL OBSTRUCTION

	Small intestine	Large intestine
Intraluminal	Food bolus obstruction Gallstone ileus Trichobezoar/hairball (rare and restricted to patients with intellectual impairment or with psychiatric illness)	Concreted bowel motion (usually associated with stricture due to other disorder such as diverticular disease)
Intramural	Crohn's disease Radiation stricture Tumour Ischaemic stricture (Caecal cancer)	Large bowel malignancy Diverticular stricture Volvulus (sigmoid colon or caecum) Crohn's disease Ischaemic stricture Ulcerative colitis (rare)
Extramural	Adhesions Incarcerated hernia Extrinsic compression by tumour Intussusception (usually predisposing cause in adults, e.g. caecal tumour)	Adhesions very rare Incarcerated large hernia incorporating sigmoid or intraperitoneal caecum Extrinsic compression by tumour

20

NON-NEOPLASTIC DISORDERS OF THE COLON AND RECTUM

COLONIC DIVERTICULAR DISEASE

Colonic diverticular disease is an acquired condition that is extremely common in developed countries, being present to some extent in more than 60% of people over the age of 70 years but rare before the age of 35. Hence, the term diverticular *disease* is almost a misnomer in these countries. The condition is linked with a low-fibre diet and is rare in populations whose staple diet is high in fibre. Although the whole colon can be affected, the segment most commonly involved is the sigmoid colon, probably related to the high intraluminal pressure generated at this site when a low-residue diet is consumed. Muscular hypertrophy can be detected radiologically before diverticulae develop. The pulsion diverticulae emerge between the mesenteric and antimesenteric taeniae and result from herniation of mucosa through the circular muscle at the sites of penetration of blood vessels. The true rectum is never affected by diverticular disease because of differences in the arrangement of the blood supply and also because the outer longitudinal smooth muscle tube encompasses the full circumference of the rectum, unlike the arrangement of the taeniae in the colon. In addition to the common acquired colonic diverticular disease that may affect the caecum, there is a rare congenital solitary diverticulum of the caecum that can arise from the medial wall close to the ileocaecal valve and can extend upwards retroperitoneally. Caecal diverticulum may become obstructed by a faecolith and inflamed, producing a clinical picture indistinguishable from appendicitis.

Colonic diverticular disease is frequently asymptomatic and often picked up incidentally on investigation of the gastrointestinal tract for symptoms that are not actually due to the disease itself. However, it may give rise to intermittent lower abdominal and left iliac fossa pain and altered bowel habit (usually constipation), although urgency of defaecation may be a feature in a minority and occasional minor rectal bleeding can occur. The sigmoid colon may be tender. Barium enema reveals muscle thickening and multiple diverticula (Fig. 20.13).

Patients should be advised to take a high-fibre diet, supplemented if necessary by bran or a bulk laxative such as methylcellulose. Stimulant laxatives and purgatives are to be avoided. Antispasmodics, such as propantheline or mebeverine, may be useful if there is smooth muscle spasm and colicky pain. There is evidence that NSAIDs increase the risk of complications and advice should be given to avoid these agents wherever possible. Surgical

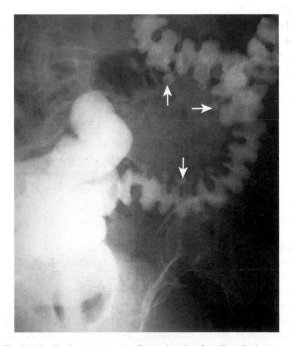

Fig. 20.13 Barium contrast radiography showing diverticular disease (arrowed).

EBM 20.2   DIVERTICULAR DISEASE

'Surgery is required for complicated diverticular disease and acute cases failing to respond to antibiotics.'

Table 20.3   COMPLICATIONS OF COLONIC DIVERTICULAR DISEASE

Inflammation
- Peridiverticulitis
- Pericolic abscess

Intestinal obstruction
- Colonic fibrous stricture
- Stricture and inflammatory mass
- Adherent small bowel loops

Perforation
- Purulent peritonitis
- Faecal peritonitis

Fistula formation
- Colovesical
- Colovaginal
- Enterocolic
- Cutaneous (rare in modern practice)

Bleeding
- Chronic intermittent blood loss
- Massive lower gastrointestinal haemorrhage

---

resection of the affected segment may be indicated if there are persistent symptoms, or when carcinoma cannot be excluded by radiology or colonoscopy (EBM 20.2).

Complicated diverticular disease

Although most diverticular disease is asymptomatic, serious complications are a frequent cause for emergency admission to surgical wards and are life-threatening and debilitating. Complications of diverticular disease are causally linked to inflammation (Table 20.3). Faeces inspissated in a diverticulum may produce stasis and a local inflammatory response. Infection spreads locally and results in peridiverticulitis, producing a low-grade pyrexia and left iliac fossa pain. Persistent infection may cause necrosis and the formation of a peridiverticular abscess. Patients presenting with established diverticular abscess are usually toxic and may not respond to antibiotics. Free perforation of the peridiverticular abscess may result. Diverticulitis is also the underlying cause of diverticular bleeding.

Diverticulitis

Peridiverticulitis presents with pyrexia, leucocytosis, nausea and vomiting, and there is often a history of altered bowel habit. Pain and tenderness in the left iliac fossa are almost universal and a mass may be palpable. The diagnosis is primarily a clinical one, with the typical presentation being sufficient to treat the patient expectantly. The diagnosis may be secured by gentle colonoscopy or flexible sigmoidoscopy and biopsy of inflamed segments. However,

peridiverticulitis may not be apparent from within the bowel lumen itself. Barium enema is a useful test to make the diagnosis of diverticular disease, with the assumption that inflammation was present previously, but this is best avoided for 4–6 weeks to allow the infection to settle.

Treatment comprises fasting or clear fluids by mouth, bed rest, intravenous fluids and broad-spectrum antibiotics, such as a cephalosporin and metronidazole. Failure to settle suggests the development of pericolic abscess, and surgical resection and peritoneal toilet combined with abscess drainage may be required. In the absence of rapid improvement within 36–48 hours, intravenous and oral contrast-enhanced CT should be undertaken. The presence of an abscess indicates the need for surgical resection. Such patients have a very high chance of ongoing sepsis and future surgery is almost certain due to chronic symptoms, even if the acute bout settles with antibiotics. Approximately one-third of all patients admitted with acute diverticular disease undergo surgery during the index admission, while the remainder settle and have no further attacks. Around 10% of these patients will eventually require surgery comprising sigmoid colectomy with primary anastomosis.

Perforation

Rupture of a pericolic abscess gives rise to purulent peritonitis, whereas free perforation of the bowel produces faecal peritonitis. The patient is usually profoundly ill, with septic shock, dehydration, marked abdominal pain, tenderness and distension. Intravenous broad-spectrum antibiotics and vigorous pre-operative resuscitation are essential, followed by resection of the affected bowel and peritoneal lavage. Specialist colorectal surgeons may elect to perform an anastomosis in view of the fact that only 30% of colostomies are ever closed, and so the risk of a second laparotomy may be avoided. If peritoneal contamination is severe and there is poor bowel perfusion of the gut, a colostomy may be preferable. The most common approach is to bring the proximal end on to the surface and oversew the rectum (Hartmann's procedure), although the distal end may be exteriorized as a mucous fistula. Continuity can be restored after bowel preparation, but this should not be for at least 3 months. The mortality of perforated diverticular disease is 10–20% but may be as high as 50% in the elderly with faecal peritonitis.

Stricture formation and obstruction

Long-standing diverticular disease may cause stricture formation and subacute intestinal obstruction. Such strictures are often very difficult to distinguish from malignant strictures, particularly as diverticular disease coexisting with a cancer is very common. In many instances, a resection is undertaken without a firm diagnosis of cancer being established.

Fistula

Diverticular disease can give rise to fistulae to other viscera, in particular the bladder. The small bowel and vagina may also be affected but cutaneous fistulae are very rare in modern surgical practice. Colovesical fistula is less common in women because the uterus is interposed between bladder and sigmoid colon. The patient usually complains of dysuria and the passage of cloudy urine, with bubbling on micturition (pneumaturia). The diagnosis may be confirmed by barium enema but may not reveal the fistula in every case, because it is often intermittent. Cystoscopy is not infrequently undertaken because many patients present to the urology service with chronic bladder instability and infections. A CT scan may reveal air in the bladder and show the fistulous tract itself. Treatment consists of resection of the affected segment, usually a sigmoid colectomy, with synchronous repair of the bladder.

Bleeding

Diverticular disease may present with persistent fresh rectal bleeding or massive haemorrhage, which should be differentiated from angiodysplasia, haemorrhoids, polypoid colorectal tumours and, very occasionally, fulminant inflammatory bowel disease. Colonoscopy seldom allows the bleeding site to be identified. Angiography may be helpful but the bleeding must be at the rate of 1 ml/min to be visible. It may be possible to embolize the bleeding vessel using gel foam. In some cases of unremitting torrential haemorrhage, operation has to be undertaken when a source of bleeding has not been localized. On-table lavage and colonoscopy may be helpful in allowing a segmental resection of the affected bowel. However, in some cases, a blind total colectomy and ileorectal anastomosis may be required.

ISCHAEMIA OF THE LARGE INTESTINE

The aetiology of ischaemia of the large bowel is similar to that of the small intestine. Atheroma at the origin of the inferior mesenteric artery results in relative insufficiency of the arterial supply from the marginal artery (Fig. 20.2). In rare cases where the inferior mesenteric artery is patent and an abdominal aortic aneurysm is present, colonic infarction may complicate aortic surgery if the inferior mesenteric artery is ligated. Untreated colonic ischaemia often progresses to gangrene and perforation. Some cases present with an acute bloody diarrhoeal illness known as ischaemic colitis, but others may declare symptoms from a chronic stricture.

Ischaemic colitis

In almost 50% of cases, ischaemia of the large intestine is transient and necrosis is confined to the mucosa and submucosa. The patient presents with lower abdominal pain, nausea, vomiting and bloody diarrhoea. Coexisting cardiovascular disease should raise suspicion of the diagnosis. Examination reveals tenderness and guarding, often maximal in the lower left abdomen. There is usually a leucocytosis and pyrexia. Plain abdominal radiography may reveal a thickened segment of colon and thumb printing due to submucosal oedema, which may be evident on barium enema (Fig. 20.14). Contrast studies should be carried out with water-soluble contrast such as gastrografin, because of the risk of perforation. The splenic flexure and sigmoid colon are most often affected. Ischaemic

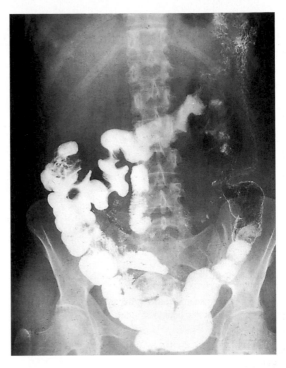

Fig. 20.14 Barium enema showing typical features of ischaemic colitis, with mucosal oedema and 'thumb printing'.

colitis is treated conservatively in the first instance unless abdominal signs reveal peritonitis, but symptoms should resolve after a few days of supportive therapy. A barium enema is indicated once the acute episode has settled, to exclude diverticular disease.

Gangrenous ischaemic colitis

The clinical presentation is localized or even generalized peritonitis. Surgery is advisable if the patient is fit and it is deemed appropriate, following consultation with the patient wherever possible, or with the family. Without surgery, death is virtually certain but the surgical mortality is around 50%. Resection of the infarcted segment with colostomy formation is the rule, as poor blood supply militates against a primary anastomosis.

Ischaemic stricture of the colon

Colicky abdominal pain, constipation and abdominal distension, following a history of an attack of bloody diarrhoea or a documented episode of ischaemic colitis, may suggest the diagnosis of ischaemic stricture. Barium enema reveals a smooth narrowing of a segment of bowel, with a funnelled appearance at either end but lacking the shouldered appearance of a malignant stricture (Fig. 20.15). Colonoscopy reveals a smooth narrowed stricture with unremarkable biopsies, or occasionally histology may reveal evidence of chronic fibrosis. Resection is usually required, but some cases never come to medical attention and are revealed by chance during a barium study at a later date.

20

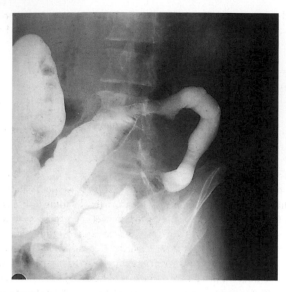

Fig. 20.15 Barium enema showing the smooth tapered appearance of a chronic benign stricture.

OTHER BENIGN CONDITIONS OF LARGE BOWEL

Irritable bowel syndrome

Irritable bowel disease is a functional bowel disease that is highly relevant to surgical practice because it presents with symptoms that are indistinguishable from structural bowel disease, such as inflammatory bowel disease and cancer. Because of the lack of discriminatory clinical features, the diagnosis is largely one of exclusion, once appropriate investigation has ruled out other disorders.

Volvulus

Volvulus of the colon most commonly affects the sigmoid colon, and rarely the caecum, and is an important differential diagnosis of any cause of large bowel obstruction, such as cancer and diverticular disease. Sigmoid volvulus is due to a twist around a narrow origin in the sigmoid mesentery. It is an acquired condition and is the most common cause of large bowel obstruction in countries with a high level of dietary fibre. In the UK, patients are usually elderly and chronic constipation is associated. The clinical presentation is of a bowel obstruction with lower abdominal pain, abdominal distension, nausea, vomiting and absolute constipation. Occasionally, the patient may present with sepsis owing to an established visceral perforation. Plain radiography reveals a characteristic Y-shaped shadow surrounded by a grossly distended colon arising out of the pelvis on a plain radiograph ('coffee bean' sign). Water-soluble contrast radiography may help and show a characteristic 'beaking' at the site of the twist. CT may be useful in atypical cases.

Sigmoid volvulus can be treated conservatively in the emergency situation by reduction and deflation, using rigid sigmoidoscopy and the placement of a large-bore tube into the sigmoid. Elective sigmoid colectomy following full bowel preparation is curative in the fit patient. In frail and demented patients or those with significant cardiac or other comorbidity, a conservative approach may be taken, but a relapse of the twist is very likely and frequent readmission is the rule. Hence, surgery is the preferred option wherever possible.

Caecal volvulus is a misnomer because it involves both the caecum and the small intestine, with the twist occurring around the superior mesenteric artery. The presence of a congenital intraperitoneal caecum predisposes to the volvulus. It is usually suggested by plain radiography showing anticlockwise rotation of dilated small bowel loops around a grossly distended caecum. Caecal volvulus usually requires emergency laparotomy because of the danger of compromise to the arterial supply of substantial lengths of the small bowel. Any infarcted bowel should be resected and this often requires right hemicolectomy. If viable, the posterior peritoneum in the right iliac fossa should be excised and the caecum sutured to the posterior abdominal wall. The narrow root of the small intestinal mesentery can be corrected by anchoring sutures.

Angiodysplasia

Angiodysplasia is an important cause of massive lower gastrointestinal haemorrhage, and may coexist with diverticular disease. The acquired submucosal arteriovenous malformations commonly affect the caecum and sigmoid colon, but any part of the large bowel can be involved. The diagnosis may be secured by visualization of a bleeding point at colonoscopy. Bleeding angiodysplastic lesions can be treated by angiographic embolization, by laser treatment or injection sclerotherapy at colonoscopy, or by resection at emergency laparotomy.

Pseudo-obstruction

Pseudo-obstruction, also known as Ogilvie's syndrome, is of particular importance as part of the differential diagnosis of mechanical large bowel obstruction, since patients typically present with abdominal distension, pain and altered bowel habit, usually constipation. In all, 25–30% of patients presenting with symptoms, signs and radiological features consistent with obstruction actually have a pseudo-obstruction. Therefore, contrast radiography is essential in all cases of suspected mechanical large bowel obstruction. Operative mortality from pseudo-obstruction is at least 15% and so surgery should be avoided wherever possible. Pseudo-obstruction is a functional disorder of the large bowel and usually arises in the elderly and frail. The underlying mechanism is not fully understood but the pathogenesis seems to involve autonomic imbalance resulting from decreased parasympathetic tone or excessive sympathetic output. There is frequently comorbidity or active disease such as chest infection. Other specific associated aetiological factors include hypokalaemia, hypocalcaemia, lithium therapy for manic depression, retroperitoneal haematoma or tumour, and diabetes.

Management is conservative and involves stimulant enemas. Colonoscopic deflation may be required in cases where caecal distension causes concern about impending caecal perforation. Intravenous erythromycin has been shown to bind to the motilin receptors in the colon and can be effective in non-resolving cases. Intravenous neostigmine has been shown to be effective when other measures fail to resolve the pseudo-obstruction. Progression of disease can lead to colonic perforation and so, in a minority of cases, colectomy and ileorectal anastomosis may be required.

Pseudomembranous colitis

Pseudomembranous colitis is associated with the use of oral broad-spectrum antibiotics in particular. *Cl. difficile* is the organism responsible in almost all cases, and can be diagnosed by stool culture or by assays for the presence of *Cl. difficile* toxin in stool or blood. Necrosis of the colorectal mucosa causes watery diarrhoea, toxaemia, shock and collapse. The stools are watery, green, foul-smelling and blood-stained, and often contain fragments of mucosal slough. A pseudomembrane is often visible on sigmoidoscopy and a biopsy confirms the diagnosis. Patients may be profoundly unwell, with dehydration and sepsis, and may require intensive resuscitation with intravenous fluid replacement. Treatment consists of oral metronidazole or vancomycin for 10 days. It is becoming more commonplace for severe cases to develop toxic megacolon that is indistinguishable from that associated with inflammatory bowel disease. This surgical emergency requires colectomy and ileostomy. An ileorectal anastomosis can be performed at a later date when the patient is fully recovered.

Hirschsprung's disease

Hirschsprung's disease affects 1 in 5000 live births and is due to the absence of ganglion cells in Auerbach's and Meissner's plexuses. It is an inherited disorder showing incomplete penetrance and variable expressivity. In some cases, there is a strong familial component, and mutations of the *RET* oncogene on chromosome 10 are responsible for most of these. *RET* gene mutations are also associated with multiple endocrine neoplasia (MEN) type II. In most cases, 5–20 cm of the distal large bowel is affected. The disease usually presents in childhood, but late presentation in adult life is not unknown. Loss of peristalsis in the affected segment leads to large bowel obstruction with gross distension of the colon proximal to the aganglionic segment. The differential diagnosis in the neonate includes imperforate anus and meconium ileus, and in older children, megacolon acquired as a result of chronic constipation. Ischaemic colitis and, in children, necrotizing enterocolitis have been reported due to super-infection with *Staphylococcus aureus*.

Barium enema reveals dilated bowel above the narrowed aganglionic segment, and lack of ganglia can be confirmed by full-thickness biopsy of the abnormal area. In neonates, treatment consists of irrigation of the bowel with saline, followed by operation at about 6 weeks to bring ganglionated bowel down to the anal verge. In older children, a preliminary colostomy may be needed to allow bowel decompression. In the rare instance where the disease is not diagnosed until adulthood, the proximal colon is usually

dysfunctional due to chronic megacolon and procto-colectomy, and ileo-anal pouch reconstruction may be preferable to anterior resection.

Acquired megacolon and idiopathic slow-transit constipation

In some children, chronic constipation may result in megacolon and is associated with behavioural problems and difficulty with toilet training. The initial complaint is often faecal soiling, but a vicious cycle of constipation and anal fissure may ensue. In adults, defaecatory problems ranging from idiopathic slow-transit constipation to adult megacolon and megarectum may arise. Electrophysiological studies have shown changes reminiscent of Hirschsprung's disease affecting the whole of the large bowel, and there may be associated gastric motility dysfunction. Examination reveals gross faecal loading of the colon and rectum. Barium studies reveal a capacious and poorly contracting bowel with huge redundant loops. Transit studies with radio-opaque markers or with radiolabelled enema typically show delayed transit.

Initial conservative management with aperients, bulk laxatives and regular enemas is successful in many cases, but faecal disimpaction under general anaesthesia may be required. Colectomy may be indicated in resistant cases but specialist advice should be sought, as severe cases are often due to neuropathy of the whole gut and surgery may not be curative.

INTESTINAL STOMA AND FISTULA

STOMA

Intestinal stomas have an important place in the management of small and large intestinal disease. An ileostomy is formed by bringing out the ileum through the abdominal wall and usually the right rectus muscle in the right iliac fossa. Ileal bowel content is irritant to skin and a spout is fashioned to allow appliances to be fitted and so prevent skin contact with bowel content (Fig. 20.16). Ileostomy comprises either an 'end' stoma, or a 'loop' or 'defunctioning' stoma. It may be employed as an adjunct

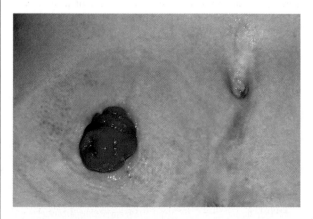

Fig. 20.16 Ileostomy sited in the right iliac fossa and showing a spout.

to resectional surgery when the disease process prevents re-anastomosis, or as a temporary stoma to allow a distal anastomosis to heal, such as for a low colorectal or ileo-anal anastomosis. End-ileostomy is used when the colon has been removed, and occasionally when small intestine distal to the stoma has been removed, as in extensive Crohn's disease.

The colon can be brought out as an end or a loop colostomy, usually in the left iliac fossa, although a transverse colostomy is brought out in the right upper quadrant. A colostomy does not require a spout, as faeces are not usually irritant to the skin. End-colostomy is used as part of a Hartmann's procedure and is an integral part of an abdominoperineal resection for rectal cancer (see below). A loop colostomy of the sigmoid colon is used to divert faeces from a diseased anorectum, such as during the management of complex perianal fistula or faecal incontinence surgery. It may also be used as palliation for pelvic cancer or during radical radiotherapy for rectal cancer. A transverse colostomy is seldom used in modern colorectal surgical practice.

INTESTINAL FISTULA

A fistula is an abnormal communication between two epithelialized surfaces, and can manifest as a communication between intestine and other parts of the gastrointestinal tract, skin, urinary tract or vagina. Intestinal fistulae may arise as part of a disease process or as an iatrogenic complication, such as leak from a surgical anastomosis or after radiotherapy. Anastomotic leak usually results in a cutaneous fistula, with bowel content appearing through the wound several days after intestinal surgery. The overall leak rate from colorectal surgery is around 5%, but 10% for rectal anastomoses. Occasionally, post-surgical leak can present as a rectovaginal fistula, in which case management is usually conservative. Peritonitis requires laparotomy and the anastomosis may have to be taken down, with the formation of a stoma. Radiation fistula typically presents several months or years after the primary treatment, owing to the late development of endarteritis obliterans and chronic microvascular ischaemia. Radiation-induced rectovaginal fistula in patients cured of the original malignancy is best treated by rectal excision and colo-anal anastomosis, to allow healing to occur in healthy non-irradiated bowel.

Disease processes resulting in fistula formation include Crohn's disease. As discussed above, complicated diverticular disease may manifest as a fistula, usually colovesical, owing to the proximity of the sigmoid colon and the dome of the bladder. Malignant tumours of the upper and lower intestine can result in any combination of fistulation. Actinomycosis and tuberculosis are rare causes of cutaneous fistula. Treatment of disease-related fistula usually requires management of the primary problem.

POLYPS AND POLYPOSIS SYNDROMES OF THE LARGE INTESTINE

The terms 'polyp' and 'tumour' are not synonymous. A polyp is an excrescence of the mucosa and so implies no pathological definition. The histological classification of colorectal polyps into four groups has clinical relevance (Table 20.4).

COLORECTAL ADENOMA

True neoplastic epithelial polyps are classified as tubular, tubulovillous and villous adenomas, depending on their histological architecture, and such classification has clinical relevance with respect to cancer risk. Adenomas affect 70% of people aged 65–69 years and 40% of asymptomatic individuals over 50 years of age. Tubular adenomas are usually pedunculated but occasionally are sessile. Tubular adenomas account for 75% of all adenomas, villous adenomas for 10%, and tubulovillous types for 15%. However, villous adenomas account for 60% of lesions larger than 2 cm. Villous tumours are most common in the rectum and some may carpet the rectum. Around 50% of such tumours have a focus of carcinoma at presentation. Villous adenomas greater than 1 cm in diameter have an approximately 30% chance of malignancy, whereas the risk in a similar-sized tubular adenoma is around 10%. Multiple adenomas are common, with 24% of patients having two tumours.

Table 20.4 CLASSIFICATION OF BENIGN INTESTINAL POLYPS

Type	Solitary	Multiple
Neoplastic	Adenoma (tubular, tubulovillous, villous)	Familial adenomatous polyposis (FAP)
Hamartomatous	Juvenile polyp	Juvenile polyposis syndrome (JPS)
	Peutz–Jeghers polyp	Peutz–Jeghers syndrome (PJS)
		Cronkhite–Canada syndrome
		Cowden's disease
Inflammatory	Benign lymphoid polyp	Benign lymphoid polyposis
		Pseudopolyposis in ulcerative colitis
Metaplastic	Metaplastic (hyperplastic)	*MYH*-associated polyposis (MAP)
	Serrated adenoma	Multiple metaplastic polyps

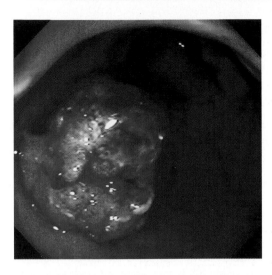

Fig. 20.17 Endoscopic appearance of a rectal adenomatous polyp.

Clinical features

The majority of polyps are asymptomatic. They may induce rectal bleeding or large bowel colic, especially when a large polyp has caused intussusception. Occasionally, a rectal polyp may prolapse through the anus. Patients with rectal villous adenomas can present with severe watery diarrhoea, and water and electrolyte depletion due to excessive mucus loss. Rectal adenomas may be palpable, but villous tumors are soft and may be missed. Distal polyps are detected readily by sigmoidoscopy, but there is a need for full colonoscopy in view of the risk of synchronous lesions. The colonoscopic appearance of a rectal adenoma is shown in Figure 20.17. Colonoscopy is superior to barium enema as it affords the opportunity for polypectomy.

Management

Colonoscopic removal of asymptomatic polyps has been shown to reduce future risk of malignant conversion. Colonoscopy with polypectomy enables histological assessment of the polyp, and advanced colonoscopic techniques such as lasering or submucosal resection are now well established for difficult cases. Smaller adenomas can be biopsied and a current applied to destroy the polyp site ('hot' biopsy). However, polypectomy using an electrocautery snare may be the only treatment required. Polyps demonstrating malignant change may be managed in this way if there are no features of poor differentiation, stalk invasion at the resection margin or invasion of submucosal lymphatics (Fig. 20.18). It may be necessary to perform surgical excision of larger polyps per-anally or by bowel resection. Transanal endoscopic microsurgery (TEM) allows resection of large rectal villous adenomas and suture of the rectum using an operating microscope.

Follow-up colonoscopy is recommended after 6–12 months and 2–3 years. The current view is not in favour of long-term follow-up once the colon has been shown to be clear of any further polyps, unless the polyps fulfilled high-risk criteria or there were recurrent lesions at the 3-year screen.

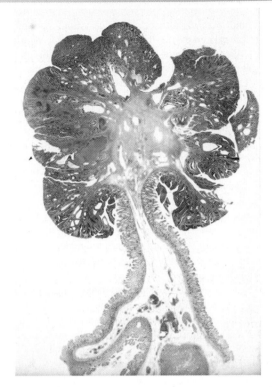

Fig. 20.18 Histological appearance of an adenomatous polyp, with malignant degeneration and early stalk invasion.

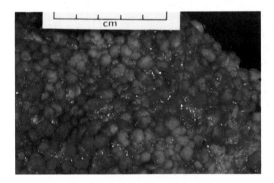

Fig. 20.19 Macroscopic features of dense polyposis due to familial adenomatous polyposis.

FAMILIAL ADENOMATOUS POLYPOSIS (FAP)

FAP is one of the most common single-gene disorders predisposing to cancer and is inherited as an autosomal dominant trait. The gene responsible is *APC*, which is located on the long arm of chromosome 5. In addition to germline changes resulting in FAP, almost every sporadic colorectal cancer has a somatic defect in the *APC* gene or in other components of the Wnt signalling pathway. The annual incidence of FAP is 1 in 6670 live births and the population prevalence is 1 in 13 528. Around 25% of affected individuals have no family history of FAP, the disease arising in these sporadic cases as the result of a new germline mutation. Direct testing from the *APC* gene is now routine. Clinicopathological diagnosis requires the presence of > 100 adenomatous polyps of the large bowel (Fig. 20.19). Polyps usually develop during the teenage

20

years and early adulthood, with a virtual certainty of colorectal cancer by the third or fourth decade if prophylactic colectomy is not undertaken. Because of effective surgical prophylaxis, FAP now accounts for less than 0.2% of all cases of colorectal cancer in the UK. Furthermore, the prevalence of colorectal cancer at diagnosis is 65% for symptomatic 'sporadic' cases and only 5% for screened family members.

Extra-colonic features

Most of the gastric polyps detected in 70% of FAP patients show cystic enlargement of the fundic glands rather than adenomatous change. Duodenal adenomas are almost universal and malignant degeneration of peri-ampullary adenoma is now the major cause of death, with 7% of patients eventually developing peri-ampullary cancer. Ileal adenomas also occur in FAP, but the risk of progression to malignancy appears to be very low. Craniofacial and long bone osteomas, when associated with epidermoid cysts, give rise to Gardner's syndrome.

Intra-abdominal desmoid tumours arise in around 10% of FAP cases. Although benign, these lesions expand and compress adjacent structures. Intra-abdominal and retro-peritoneal disease may be amenable only to surgical palliation. Treatment with toremifene, tamoxifen, sulindac, indometacin, chemotherapy and radiotherapy provides benefit in a few cases.

An epidermoid cyst arising in a prepubescent child should raise suspicion of FAP. Pigmented lesions of the retina, known as congenital hypertrophy of the retinal pigment epithelium (CHRPE), are well described in association with FAP. The lesions are asymptomatic but frequently affect both eyes. Women aged < 35 years with FAP are at 160 times greater risk of papillary thyroid carcinoma than non-FAP counterparts, but there is no excess risk in men. Other rare associations with FAP include hepatoblastoma, carcinoma of the gallbladder, bile duct and pancreas, and an increased risk of brain tumours.

Diagnosis and management

The diagnosis can be established by sigmoidoscopy and biopsy. Screening of affected individuals by direct *APC* gene mutation analysis is used to define the optimal timing of prophylactic surgery. All FAP patients should be referred to a regional genetics service for registration and gene analysis. Pre-symptomatic detection of FAP allows prophylactic colectomy before malignancy supervenes (EBM 20.3). There is no general consensus on the preferred surgical strategy, as both restorative procto-colectomy with ileo-anal pouch formation and total colectomy with ileorectal anastomosis have particular advantages. Proctocolectomy with ileostomy is seldom used in modern practice. The upper gastrointestinal tract should be screened for duodenal adenoma or carcinoma.

EBM 20.3   COLORECTAL ADENOMAS

'Prophylactic surgery is indicated for familial adenomatous polyposis.'

PEUTZ–JEGHERS SYNDROME (PJS)

This is discussed above in the section on small intestinal disorders.

JUVENILE POLYPOSIS SYNDROME (JPS)

Juvenile polyps are usually classified as hamartomas, although some regard them as inflammatory, with blockage of crypts resulting in retention cysts. Single juvenile polyps occur in around 1% of populations in developed countries, and multiple juvenile polyposis is uncommon. JPS is characterized by the development of multiple hamar-tomatous polyps throughout the gastrointestinal tract, usually when the child is aged < 10 years. Affected patients have a high risk of developing gastrointestinal cancer that ranges from 9% to 68% but is probably in the region of 50%. Because JPS is rare, there are no reliable estimates of its frequency in the general population; around 1:50 000 is a reasonable estimate, based on population registry data. JPS is associated with incomplete penetrance for both polyposis and also colorectal cancer, and less than 0.1% of all cases of colorectal cancer are attributable to JPS. The disorder exhibits genetic heterogeneity, with mutations in *SMAD4, BMPR1A/ALK3* and *PTEN* having been identified. Estimates of cancer risk are inaccurate but the lifetime risk is around 50%. Hence, surveillance has a place, and consideration should be given to prophylactic colectomy, much in the same way as in FAP. Large bowel surveillance for at-risk individuals is recommended 1–2-yearly from the age of 15–18 years; surveillance intervals can be extended after the age of 35 years. Documented gene carriers or affected cases should, however, be kept under surveillance until the age of 70 years and prophylactic surgery should be discussed.

METAPLASTIC (HYPERPLASTIC) POLYPOSIS AND *MYH*-ASSOCIATED POLYPOSIS (MAP)

Metaplastic (sometimes referred to as hyperplastic) polyps are usually less than 5 mm in diameter and occur in increasing numbers with age, being present in some 75% of the population over the age of 40 years. They tend to be pale, flat-topped, sessile plaques, found mainly in the rectum and often on the crest of mucosal folds. It is becoming recognized that at least a subset of patients with multiple metaplastic polyps early in life has a substantially elevated cancer risk. A gene involved in DNA base excision repair (*MYH*) has been shown to be associated with colorectal metaplastic polyposis with an autosomal dominant mode of inheritance. Through demonstration of an association between the gene and colorectal cancer, it appears by inference that metaplastic polyps might actually have pre-malignant potential. Histologically, the crypts are elongated, dilated and lined by columnar epithelium that has a sawtooth pattern. These polyps are often indistinguishable from adenomatous polyps, and are frequently removed because of the difficulties in differentiating them from adenomas. Some of the larger metaplastic polyps take on the features of a serrated adenoma and principally affect the caecum, where they are highly likely to progress to cancer.

OTHER RARE POLYPOSIS SYNDROMES

Turcot's syndrome

This comprises adenomatous colorectal polyposis in association with astrocytoma (also medulloblastoma or glioblastoma) of the brain or spinal cord. It is a clinical constellation and has been shown to be due to mutations in HNPCC-related genes (DNA mismatch repair genes) or in the gene that codes for FAP (*APC*). In some families, there is an autosomal recessive pattern of inheritance, suggesting a possible relationship with *MYH*-associated polyposis.

Cowden's disease

This is a rare disseminated form of gastrointestinal hamartomatous polyposis with an autosomal dominant pattern of inheritance, but most cases are due to mutations. There is a greater risk for benign and malignant disease of the breast and thyroid. All patients have warty tricholemmomas around the eyes, and these lesions are diagnostic when present in association with oral fibromas and keratoses of the hands and feet.

Cronkhite–Canada syndrome

This rare syndrome comprises intestinal polyposis with alopecia, atrophy of the nails and brown macular hyperpigmentation. Histological examination shows cystic dilatation of the crypts, similar to that seen in juvenile polyposis. The condition does not seem to be inherited.

OTHER COLORECTAL POLYPS

Benign lymphoid polyps are round, smooth, sessile tumours, usually found in the lower rectum; they vary in diameter from a few millimetres to 3 cm. They consist of an aggregate of normal lymphoid tissue covered by attenuated epithelium. They are most common in the third and fourth decades, and usually present with rectal bleeding, anal pain and tenderness, or with prolapse of the polyp. Treatment consists of local excision. Other polypoid conditions include pseudopolyps in chronic ulcerative colitis, submucosal lipoma, lymphosarcoma, carcinoid tumour and leiomyoma. Neurofibromatosis rarely results in colonic polyps. Mucosal ganglioneuromatosis has been described in association with multiple adenomatous or juvenile polyps and MEN type IIb.

MALIGNANT TUMOURS OF THE LARGE INTESTINE

COLORECTAL ADENOCARCINOMA

Large bowel adenocarcinoma is the most common gastrointestinal malignancy and is second only to lung cancer as a cause of cancer death in developed countries. There are few cancers with such dramatic environmental effects, as shown by comparing incidence between populations and by migration studies that demonstrate how a migrant population takes on the risk of the host population within a generation. In the UK, colorectal cancer accounts

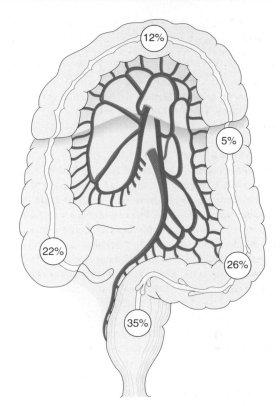

Fig. 20.20   Distribution of colorectal cancer in the large bowel in the UK.

for 14% and 12% of all cancer registration in males and females respectively, and is third-ranked cancer overall after lung and prostate in males and breast and lung in females. The lifetime risk is 5%, resulting in 32 000 cases each year. The male:female ratio for colon cancer is close to unity, whereas that for rectal cancer is 1.7:1 in high-incidence populations. The highest incidence rates are in the oldest population. The rectum and sigmoid are particularly common sites for tumours (Fig. 20.20), but in low-incidence countries, tumours are more evenly distributed. Around 3% of patients present with synchronous tumours, and another 3% develop a metachronous tumour at a later date.

Aetiology

A number of contributing factors are associated with colorectal cancer. These include male gender (males' lifetime risk 1.5 times that of females), increasing age, a strong family history of the disease and consuming a 'Westernized' diet.

Diet

Diet is a major environmental risk factor but no consistent dietary component is clearly the single factor imparting that risk. Recently, dietary fibre has again gained favour as a protective factor. A diet high in fibre is associated with lower cancer rates in certain populations and within the UK population, whereas the consumption of a diet high in fat and red meat is associated with higher cancer rates. A high-energy diet is an associated risk factor. A low-fibre,

20

EBM 20.4   PREVENTION AND DETECTION OF COLORECTAL ADENOCARCINOMA

'Aspirin and non-steroidal anti-inflammatory drugs protect from colorectal neoplasia and are associated with reduced cancer mortality.'
'Population screening by faecal occult blood test reduces mortality by 18% in those accepting screening.'

---

high-fat diet appears to increase faecal pH, and this may enhance bile acid toxicity. Brassica vegetables, such as broccoli, contain antioxidants and other potential anti-neoplastic compounds. A deficiency of dietary calcium and vitamin D is associated with increased colorectal cancer risk. Randomized trials using adenoma formation as a surrogate end-point have found no intervention that reduces risk, and so it seems likely that a combination of all the elements that make up a 'Western' diet is involved.

Protective factors

Dietary calcium and aspirin have been shown in randomized trials to reduce colorectal adenoma formation. Aspirin and other NSAIDs have been shown to be associated with a substantial reduced risk in population studies (RR 0.53), while hormone replacement therapy also seems to be protective (EBM 20.4). Despite epidemiological evidence, intervention studies do not indicate that dietary fibre protects from adenoma formation.

Smoking, alcohol and exercise

Smoking and alcohol excess are risk factors for men but women appear not to be subject to the excess risk. An association between lack of physical exercise and colorectal cancer has been observed. Colonic transit time may be reduced by exercise, but alterations in the levels of prostaglandins and antioxidant enzymes may also occur.

Inflammatory bowel disease

The risk of colorectal cancer in ulcerative colitis and Crohn's disease is discussed above.

Genetics

Genetic susceptibility has been shown to contribute 35% to the overall incidence of colorectal cancer. This genetic component ranges from an ill-defined increased risk in individuals with a positive family history, to well-defined autosomal dominant genetic traits in which the responsible genes have been identified and mutations characterized. Three broad categories of genetic susceptibility trait have been defined at the clinical and molecular level: HNPCC, dominant polyposis syndromes (FAP, PJS and JPS, discussed in the section on colorectal adenomas) and recessive inheritance (MAP, discussed above).

HNPCC is the most common autosomal dominant syndrome, accounting for 3–5% of all colorectal cancer cases. It is associated with only small numbers of adenomas, but the risk of colorectal cancer is very high, with 70% of males and 35% of females developing the disease over a lifetime. There is also an elevated risk of other malignancies, including endometrial (35% risk in females), gastric (15%), ovarian (9%), upper urinary tract (~2%) and small intestinal (~2%). Empirical HNPCC criteria comprise:

- three or more relatives with histologically proven colorectal cancer, one being a first-degree relative of the other two
- two or more generations affected
- at least one family member affected before the age of 50 years.

One case may be endometrial cancer rather than colorectal cancer. HNPCC is of major interest because it is a relatively common definable genetic cause of colorectal cancer and thus lends itself to identification of gene carriers by DNA analysis of blood samples. Mutation analysis allows targeting of those at risk for colonoscopic screening and adenoma removal, and this has been shown to be an effective cancer control measure in HNPCC.

HNPCC is due to mutation of one of the genes that participate in DNA mismatch repair. Mutations are most common in *MSH2* on chromosome 2p, *MLH1* on chromosome 2q and *MSH6* on chromosome 2p. Around 90% of large dominant HNPCC families from research studies have identifiable mutations. In clinical genetics practice, however, only 30% of selected families have mutations in one of the genes responsible. Overall, causative mutations have been identified in 2.8% of all colorectal cancer cases, but patients who develop colorectal cancer at an early age are more likely to have developed the disease because of an underlying DNA mismatch repair gene defect; 1 in 4 of patients aged < 40 years and 1 in 20 aged < 55 years at diagnosis of colorectal cancer carry a mutation, irrespective of family history.

Clinical features of established disease

Intestinal symptoms are extremely common in the general population but there are no specific symptoms that discriminate cancer from benign intestinal diseases or from symptoms common in healthy individuals. Presentation may include intermittent rectal bleeding, blood mixed with mucus, altered bowel habit, iron deficiency anaemia and colicky lower abdominal pain. Tenesmus occurs in over 50% of patients with low rectal cancers. Massive lower gastrointestinal haemorrhage is rare and so is more likely to represent underlying benign disorders rather than colorectal cancer. Abdominal wall invasion may manifest as parietal pain and occasionally leads to abscess formation. Perianal or sciatic-type pain is an ominous sign suggesting locally advanced rectal cancer. Sinister symptoms are often ignored by young patients, but 3% of presenting patients are under the age of 35. Around 15% of all patients present with obstruction and 3% have a perforation at presentation. Such complications significantly worsen the prognosis for a given tumour stage and increase the likelihood of the patient requiring a colostomy.

A full history is essential, as clinical examination is often negative. There may be signs of anaemia, and abdominal examination may reveal hepatomegaly or an abdominal mass, especially in right-sided colon cancer. There may be signs of bowel obstruction. Digital rectal

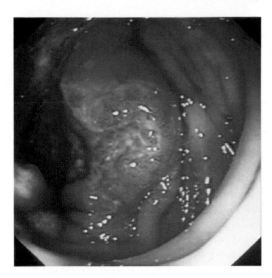

Fig. 20.21 Typical colonoscopic features of colorectal cancer.

examination is mandatory to detect low cancers and to assess fixity and sphincter involvement. An FOB test will not alter the decision to investigate the symptomatic patient and so is a superfluous investigation.

Population screening for colorectal cancer

Early detection of colorectal cancer by population screening in asymptomatic individuals has been shown to result in a 20% or so improved survival benefit in screened populations aged 50–75 years. The most extensively studied screening test is the faecal occult blood test (FOBT) using guaiac-impregnated paper—Haemoccult—but sensitivity is only 50–60%. The predictive value is around 10% for cancer and 50% for adenomas > 1 cm. Specificity is the main problem with the test, as it generates large numbers of people with positive slides but no cancer. Population screening using colonoscopy is widespread for those that can afford it in the USA, but it seems unlikely to be implemented in other countries in view of the massive cost implications. However, there is a move to offer once-only flexible sigmoidoscopy at age 50–55 years in the UK as a means of detecting adenoma formers, as well as those with early rectosigmoid cancers. This has the potential benefit of increasing cost efficiency and is currently under evaluation in a large randomized trial. Newer screening modalities are also under assessment, including cancer-specific stool DNA testing, but these approaches are many years away from formal clinical evaluation.

Investigations

Colonoscopy is the investigation of choice and is effective in identifying tumours throughout the colon and rectum (Fig. 20.21). Barium enema (Fig. 20.22) has similar diagnostic accuracy but colonoscopy has the advantage of allowing diagnostic biopsy and snaring of any adenomas proximal to the cancer. In most instances with typical features of shouldering and mucosal destruction, it is not necessary to visualize the tumour before operation. Sigmoidoscopy or colonoscopy allows visualization and

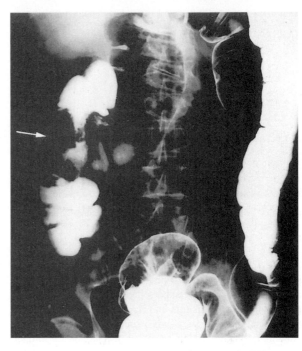

Fig. 20.22 Barium enema showing a malignant 'applecore' appearance (arrow) in the right colon, due to stenosing colorectal cancer.

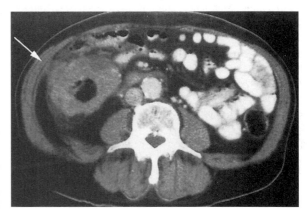

Fig. 20.23 CT scan features of colorectal cancer in a frail elderly patient.

biopsy of the tumour, particularly when the barium enema is inconclusive. Polypoidal tumours (see below) are easily visualized and snare polypectomy should be considered. In some very elderly patients, colonoscopy or barium enema may not be tolerated and oral contrast-enhanced CT scans of the abdomen may be useful (Fig. 20.23).

Pre-operative staging

Staging is a central component of pre-operative work-up, as it provides important information on prognosis, helps inform surgical strategy and indicates the need or otherwise for adjuvant pre-operative radiotherapy for rectal cancer and adjuvant post-operative chemotherapy for colorectal cancer. All patients with colon or rectal cancer should be

20

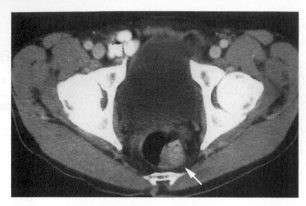

Fig. 20.24   CT scan features of early T$_1$ rectal cancer (arrowed), restricted to the bowel wall.

fully staged by CT scan of the chest, abdomen and pelvis (Fig. 20.24). Liver ultrasound and chest X-ray have now been almost totally superseded by CT scan. For rectal cancer, digital examination and rigid sigmoidoscopy should be undertaken in every case (perhaps as examination under anaesthetic, EUA) to assess the degree of tumour fixity. In addition to CT, MRI of the pelvis is now standard practice to assess the degree of local invasion. Endo-anal ultrasound may also be useful for local staging of rectal cancer, but is somewhat operator-dependent and requires considerable experience and interpretational skill on the part of the surgeon or ultrasonographer. In some cases being considered for major debilitating surgery with a view to cure, positron emission tomography (PET) has a place; it can detect tumour elsewhere in the body, and that could tip the balance of benefit away from such surgery.

MANAGEMENT OF COLORECTAL ADENOCARCINOMA

Surgery

Elective colorectal resection with curative intent

The mainstay of treatment comprises en bloc resection of the primary tumour and excision of locoregional nodes. This achieves cure in 75% of cases undergoing intended 'curative' resections. Excision of the colonic mesentery, ligation of the arterial supply at its origin, and excision of all accompanying lymph nodes achieve locoregional lymphadenectomy for the respective segment of bowel (Fig. 20.25). Resection offers cure for patients with localized disease; even for patients with lymph node metastases but no distant metastases, cure can be expected in 50% of cases with surgery alone. For rectal cancer, excision of the entire mesorectum reduces local recurrence rates to 5%. Wherever possible, bowel continuity should be restored. In specialist hands, low rectal cancer should be treated by low anterior resection and colo-anal anastomosis, and this can be combined with a small colonic J-pouch to improve defaecatory function. However, for low rectal cancer involving the sphincter muscle, it may be necessary to remove the anal sphincter as part of an abdominoperineal resection and fashion a permanent end-

colostomy. Laparoscopic colectomy is currently being evaluated in a number of randomized trials and survival outcomes are awaited. However, there are short-term benefits, with less pain and shorter hospital stay, and the approach is gaining widespread acceptance and introduction, even without evidence from RCTs of survival equivalence.

Rectal cancer can be excised per-anally under direct vision or with a resectoscope. TEM is particularly applicable to small low-lying cancers (< 3 cm). Per-anal excision has a place for T$_1$ or T$_2$ tumours and avoids major abdominal surgery. However, careful staging is essential because the recurrence rate is 25–30% if there are incomplete excision margins or if the lesion was staged inaccurately. Pathology assessment may indicate the need to proceed to formal resection and mesorectal excision.

Early polyp cancers removed at colonoscopic snare polypectomy may be treated without the need for formal transabdominal resection. However, where the pathology specimen of the snared polyp cancer shows poor differentiation or submucosal lymphatic invasion, or where the diathermized margin is involved, formal resection and regional lymphadenectomy are indicated. With the introduction of population colorectal cancer screening by FOBT, this is becoming a more common scenario.

In the elective setting, the patient should be fasted and have undergone full pre-operative work-up to assess cardiac, respiratory and any other comorbidity; reversible risk factors for major surgery should have been addressed. Bowel preparation has been radically reshaped in recent years, comprising free fluids for 48 hours prior to surgery and no mechanical bowel preparation for right-sided or total colectomy. Some centres still prefer mechanical bowel preparation (e.g. polyethylene glycol, sodium picosulfate or phospho-soda), but recent meta-analysis indicates that there is no benefit to bowel preparation, even for left-sided resections, and it may even be harmful. Hence, there is a move away from any preparation prior to colorectal surgery, apart from a phosphate enema 2 hours prior to surgery. The operation should be covered with perioperative broad-spectrum antibiotics (e.g. a third-generation cephalosporin and metronidazole) and chemical prophylaxis for deep venous thrombosis (low molecular weight fractionated heparin or calcium heparin), along with compression stockings and intra-operative intermittent pneumatic calf compression (EBM 20.5).

Emergency colorectal resection

In cases of perforation or obstruction of colorectal cancer, there is a substantially increased risk of perioperative mortality. The patient should be resuscitated before laparotomy is undertaken. For obstructed right-sided colon cancer, right hemicolectomy is the operation of choice. An ileotransverse anastomosis can be safely performed, as the ileum has an excellent blood supply and the distal colon is not obstructed. Treatment of obstructed left colon cancer is best achieved by a one-stage resection with anastomosis whenever possible. Measures that may be employed to reduce the risk of anastomotic leakage in such cases include on-table colonic lavage to remove faecal residue. Resection

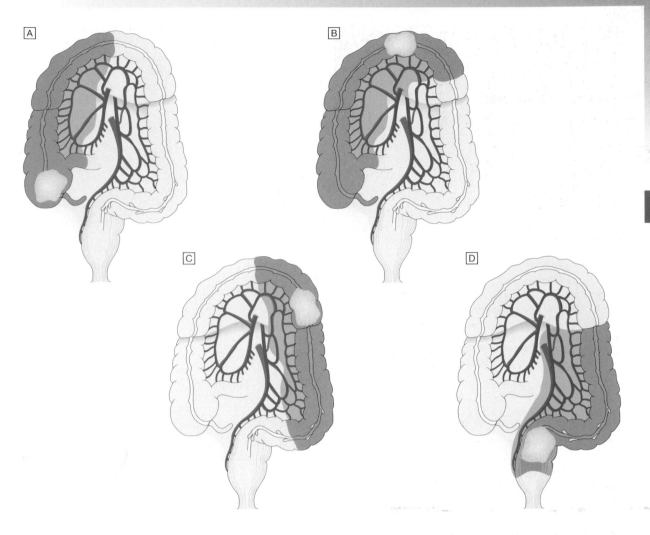

Fig. 20.25   Surgical resection for colorectal cancer in various locations.
Radical tumour resection requires clearance of the primary tumour and also the arteries supplying that part of the colon. Lymphatic drainage follows the path of arterial supply, allowing a regional lymphadenectomy. [A] Excision of a right-sided tumour and the ileocaecal, right colic and right branch of middle colic arteries. [B] Tumours of transverse colon are usually treated by extended right hemicolectomy, again taking the feeding vessels at their origin from the superior mesenteric artery. [C] For left colonic lesions, the feeding vessels are taken. [D] Anterior resection is treated by high ligation of the inferior mesenteric artery.

EBM 20.5   PREPARATION FOR SURGERY IN PATIENTS WITH COLORECTAL ADENOCARCINOMA

'Pre-operative staging is required to guide surgery and pre-operative adjuvant radiotherapy.'
'Bowel preparation is not required for colorectal resection.'
'Compression stockings and heparin are required thromboprophylaxis for patients undergoing colorectal surgery.'

---

of the entire colon and ileorectal anastomosis avoid a colocolic anastomosis and also remove any synchronous tumour (occurs in 3% of cases). Patients with gross faecal peritonitis secondary to perforation of left colon cancer usually require resection, with the creation of an end-colostomy (Hartmann's procedure). If contamination is minimal, a specialist surgeon may elect to carry out primary resection and anastomosis. As in the elective

setting, surgery should be covered with perioperative antibiotics and DVT prophylaxis.

Pathology and staging

Macroscopically, colorectal cancer may be polypoidal, ulcerating or stenosing (Fig. 20.26). Two-thirds are ulcerating and a typical lesion has raised everted edges, a slough-covered floor and indurated base. Tumours of the caecum tend to be large exophytic growths. Tumour differentiation may be classified as good, moderate or poor. Around 10–20% of tumours have mucinous histology and this tumour type has a poor prognosis. There is an increasing proportion of proximal tumours in the UK, as right colonic cancer is more common in the elderly and the UK population is ageing.

Colorectal cancer spreads by lymphatic invasion and via the portal blood to the liver. Once the peritoneum is breached, dissemination throughout the abdominal cavity

20

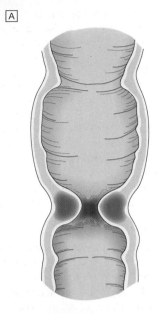 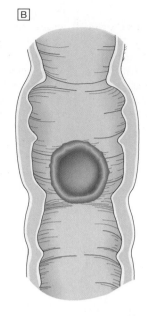 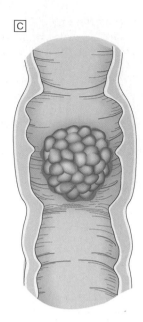

Fig. 20.26 **Macroscopic characteristics of colorectal cancer.**
[A] Stenosing. [B] Ulcerating. [C] Polypoidal.

Table 20.5	DUKES' STAGING FOR COLORECTAL CANCER	
Dukes' stage	**Description**	**Proportion of colorectal cancers (%)**
A	Spread into, but not beyond, muscularis propria	10
B	Spread through full thickness of bowel wall	30
C	Spread to involve lymph nodes	30
D*	Distant metastases	20

* There is formally no D stage in Dukes' staging; this is a misnomer, as Dukes' staging refers only to degree of local invasion and to lymphatic spread. However, the term is widely used in clinical practice.

is likely. Invasion of lymphatics results in regional lymph node involvement. Very low rectal tumours may also involve the inguinal nodes. Systemic metastases are unusual but do occur in the later stages of the disease. There are a number of tumour staging systems; in the UK, Dukes' and TNM staging systems are used exclusively (Tables 20.5 and 20.6), while the TNM stages are often grouped using the American Joint Committee on Cancer (AJCC) system (Table 20.7), which allows alignment between Dukes' and TNM staging. Pathological staging has important implications for prognosis and also for directing clinical management (EBM 20.5). Thus a decision on whether or not to offer patients adjuvant chemotherapy is guided by staging information.

Adjuvant therapy

Radiotherapy

Adjuvant pre-operative radiotherapy has an important place in the management of rectal cancer, and so pre-operative staging of rectal cancer is essential in order to plan optimal management. Radiotherapy has been shown to reduce local recurrence rates and improve survival (EBM 20.6). Most specialist centres in the UK offer selective pre-operative radiotherapy for those at increased risk of local recurrence, because there is significant morbidity associated with pelvic irradiation and many patients will be cured by surgery alone. Risk factors include a low tumour, bulky fixed lesion, anterior lesion, evidence of T_3 or T_4 stage and/or involved lymph nodes on pelvic CT or MRI. Either a 5-day short-course regimen of 45 Gy daily or a long-course regimen of 52 Gy given weekly over 3 months is administered. The former is reserved for patients with operable but tethered tumours or very low or anterior tumours, or if extra-rectal spread is evident. Fixed, inoperable tumours are best dealt with by radical radiotherapy over 3 months, and this may be combined with 5-fluorouracil (5-FU)-based chemotherapy. Post-operative radiotherapy results in poor bowel function and may damage the small intestine, and so should be avoided whenever possible.

Adjuvant chemotherapy

Systemic adjuvant chemotherapy using 5-FU alone or in combination has been shown to improve survival for Dukes' C colorectal cancer after surgical resection (EBM 20.6). There is an overall 30% improvement in survival for patients with Dukes' C tumours who receive chemotherapy, equating with an 11% absolute improvement in survival for that group and a 6% overall improvement in survival for patients with colorectal cancer of all stages. In the UK, it is now routine practice to offer chemotherapy based on 5-FU to all patients with stage C cancers who do not have significant comorbidity. Recently, it has been shown that Dukes' B tumours also gain survival benefit but this is only a 2% or so increased survival overall. Hence, adjuvant chemotherapy for Dukes' B tumours is restricted to poor-prognosis lesions, such as those that are poorly differentiated or show venous or lymphatic invasion in tumour sections. Chemotherapy based on 5-FU is considered a conventional 'first-line' chemotherapeutic regimen for colorectal cancer. An alternative approach to targeting the same pathway by use of fluorinated thymidine analogues is through inhibition of thymidylate synthase using chemical inhibitors such as capecitabine. Capecitabine has considerable benefits because it is less toxic and can be administered orally; it is now being widely introduced, replacing intravenous regimens based on 5-FU. Other newer agents, such as oxaliplatin and irinotecan (CPT-11), have been shown to be valuable additions for patients who relapse after first-line chemotherapy. Other agents such as temozolomide, used either alone or in combination with 5-FU, are showing promise in clinical trials.

Palliative therapy

In addition to resection with curative intent, surgery provides valuable, good-quality palliation for many patients with hepatic or other distant metastases. This is achieved through ameliorating symptoms or by averting distressing features of advanced local disease. In some instances, diversion of the faecal stream through a defunctioning colostomy or ileostomy may be all that is feasible, but

---

Table 20.6 TNM STAGING OF COLORECTAL CANCER

T (Tumour)

- T_x Primary tumour cannot be assessed
- T_{is} Carcinoma in situ
- T_1 Cancer invades submucosa
- T_2 Cancer invades into muscularis propria
- T_3 Cancer invades through muscularis propria and into subserosa or adjacent non-peritonealized tissues
- T_4 Cancer perforates the visceral peritoneum or directly invades adjacent organs

N (Node)

- N_x The regional lymph nodes cannot be assessed
- N_0 No regional lymph nodes involved
- N_1 Metastases in 1–3 pericolic or perirectal lymph nodes
- N_2 Metastases in 4 or more pericolic or perirectal lymph nodes
- N_3 Metastases in lymph node along the course of a major named blood vessel

M (Metastases)

- M_x The presence of distant metastases cannot be assessed
- M_0 No distant metastases
- M_1 Distant metastases

Table 20.7 AMERICAN JOINT COMMITTEE ON CANCER (AJCC) STAGE GROUPINGS AND EQUIVALENCE WITH DUKES' STAGING

AJCC	TNM	Dukes
I	$T_1N_0M_0$ or $T_2N_0M_0$ Spread into submucosa or just into muscularis propria No lymph node or distant spread	A
IIA	$T_3N_0M_0$ Spread through bowel wall into outermost layers No lymph node or distant spread	B
IIB	$T_4N_0M_0$ Spread through bowel wall into other tissues or organs No lymph node or distant spread	B
IIIA	$T_{1-2}N_1M_0$ Spread into submucosa or just into muscularis propria Spread to $\leq$ 3 nearby lymph nodes but no distant spread	C
IIIB	$T_{3-4}N_1M_0$ Spread through bowel wall into other tissues or organs Spread to $\leq$ 3 nearby lymph nodes but no distant spread	C
IIIC	Any T N_2M_0 Any T stage and spread $\geq$ 4 lymph nodes but no distant spread	C
IV	Any T Any N M_1 Any T and N stage but distant spread (e.g. liver, lung, peritoneum)	D*

* There is formally no D stage in Dukes' staging; this is a misnomer, as Dukes' staging refers only to degree of local invasion and to lymphatic spread. However, the term is widely used in clinical practice.

20

EBM 20.6 IMPROVING POST-OPERATIVE SURVIVAL RATES IN COLORECTAL ADENOCARCINOMA

'Post-operative intensive follow-up is associated with a 9% survival improvement. Adjuvant radiotherapy reduces local recurrence and improves survival. Adjuvant chemotherapy improves survival by 30% for stage III tumours and 2% for stage II tumours.'

BOX 20.5 COLORECTAL ADENOCARCINOMA

- Colorectal adenocarcinoma is the most common gastrointestinal malignancy, with 32 000 cases per annum in the UK
- It is second only to lung cancer as a cause of cancer death in developed countries, accounting for 14% of all cancers in males and 12% in females, with a 5% lifetime risk
- Around 3% of patients present with synchronous tumours, and another 3% develop metachronous tumours
- Aetiological factors include male gender, increasing age, family history, 'Westernized' diet, inflammatory bowel disease and pre-existing adenomatous polyps
- Genes have been identified for a number of genetic predisposition syndromes, accounting for ~3% of all cases. The molecular basis of the remainder of the 35% genetically determined colorectal cancer is being unravelled, offering future potential for genetic screening
- Two-thirds of all large bowel cancers occur in the rectum and sigmoid colon, and the most common clinical features are alteration in bowel habit and the passage of blood per rectum
- Diagnosis involves colonoscopy and biopsy or barium enema. Pre-operative staging is important and involves CT and MRI
- Surgery is the mainstay of treatment, involving radical local clearance combined with regional lymphadenectomy in most cases
- Adjuvant therapy options include pre-operative radiotherapy for rectal cancer and post-operative chemotherapy
- Pre-symptomatic diagnosis may be achieved by faecal occult blood testing or by surveillance colonoscopy in high-risk groups
- Overall 5-year survival is 51%. Staging systems provide useful prognosis to guide therapy and inform patients of expected outcome

---

wherever possible it is preferable to resect the tumour and involved bowel in a formal way. Hence, almost all patients will undergo some form of surgical resection, whether it be curative or palliative. In a small number of cases with poor functional status and/or extensive metastatic load and in whom surgical resection is relatively contraindicated, combined radiological and colonoscopic placement of an intraluminal expanding stent will palliate an obstructing colonic cancer.

Radiotherapy has an important role in palliation of locally advanced irresectable rectal cancer and can control pain, mucus discharge, disordered bowel habit, bleeding and faecal incontinence. It also has a value in palliation of rectal cancer recurrence and in alleviating bone pain from metastases. It may rarely be used to palliate locally invasive colonic cancer invading the abdominal wall, but this approach is restricted because the fields are difficult to define and damage to adjacent bowel is likely.

Palliative chemotherapy is now used extensively both to treat symptoms of disseminated disease, and to control disease progression and extend survival. This is especially the case with the introduction of oral capecitabine. Median life expectancy from diagnosis of hepatic metastases is now around 12–14 months.

Prognosis

Systematic population data from cancer registry show that overall 1-year and 5-year survival is 73% and 51% respectively, having improved by 20% in both males and females in the 10 years between 1992 and 2002. The marked improvement in survival from colorectal cancer is due to a combination of earlier diagnosis across all stages, improved perioperative anaesthetic and surgical management, and improved adjuvant therapies, especially chemotherapy. However, overall prognosis is even better for patients who have no evidence of metastases on pre-operative staging tests and who have undergone a resection with curative intent, with predicted survival being 75% at 5 years. This underscores the importance of pre-operative staging in informing radical surgery. The 5-year survival by Dukes' stage is 90–95% for Dukes' stage A, 65–75% for Dukes' stage B and 40–50% for Dukes' stage C. Few patients with liver or lung metastases will survive to 5 years and most die within 2 years of diagnosis. Operative mortality is low (~4%) for elective resections but rises to 25% in patients with complications such as obstruction and perforation who require emergency surgery, emphasizing the importance of early detection and surgery prior to the development of complications. Some patients with isolated hepatic metastases may be candidates for hepatic resection with a view to cure, and there is some evidence for long-term survival benefit in selected series.

OTHER MALIGNANT TUMOURS OF THE LARGE INTESTINE

Colorectal adenocarcinoma dominates the incidence of large bowel cancer and all other malignant tumours are very rare in comparison.

Squamous cancer of the large bowel

Such tumours are not simply metastatic anal carcinomas, but may arise in the caecum and proximal colon from an area of squamous metaplasia in long-standing ulcerative colitis. In the absence of chronic inflammation, an adenosquamous pattern may be seen and the prognosis is poor.

Carcinoid tumour of the large bowel

Large bowel carcinoid tumours are rare, but benign lesions may be found incidentally during rectal examination as solitary, spherical, hard, sessile, yellowish submucosal nodules. Malignant carcinoid tumors of the colon may give rise to the carcinoid syndrome, and 60% have metastasized by the time of diagnosis.

Lymphoma of the large intestine

Primary lymphomas usually arise in the rectum or caecum but are occasionally multicentric. Secondary involvement of the large bowel in generalized disease is more common. Barium enema shows a long rigid segment with intramural thickening. The diagnosis is established by endoscopic or operative biopsy. Primary lymphomas are treated by resection, followed by chemotherapy and radiotherapy. Secondary malignant lymphoma and malignant lymphomatous polyposis are treated by systemic chemotherapy and targeted radiotherapy.

Gastrointestinal stromal tumours (including leiomyosarcoma)

These tumours are rare in the large bowel and are discussed above. They arise from the muscle of the bowel wall, most usually the rectum, and are usually diagnosed by digital examination or by sigmoidoscopy. As discussed, there is a spectrum from benign to malignant and the tumours are often impossible to distinguish clinically; resection is therefore advisable. Metastasis occurs via the blood stream to the liver and lungs.

BOX 20.6   PRINCIPAL SYMPTOMS ASSOCIATED WITH DISORDERS OF APPENDIX AND INTESTINE

Appendix
- Midgut colicky pain
- Parietal right iliac fossa pain
- Nausea, vomiting
- Abdominal mass
- Systemic toxicity

Small intestine
- Nausea, vomiting
- Midgut colicky pain
- Parietal abdominal pain
- Anorexia and weight loss
- Abdominal distension
- Abdominal mass (late feature)

Large intestine
- Fresh rectal bleeding
- Altered blood per rectum (melaena)
- Passage of mucus or pus per rectum
- Altered bowel habit
- Abdominal distension
- Faecal incontinence and defaecatory urgency
- Perianal and perineal pain

BOX 20.7   PRINCIPAL DISORDERS OF APPENDIX AND INTESTINE RELEVANT TO SURGICAL PRACTICE

Appendix
- Appendicitis
- Tumours, benign or malignant

Small intestine
- Crohn's disease
- Paralytic ileus
- Mechanical obstruction
- Mesenteric ischaemia
- Tumours, benign or malignant
- Radiation damage
- Meckel's diverticulum
- Jejunal diverticulosis

Colon and rectum
- Diverticular disease
- Tumours, benign or malignant
- Mesenteric ischaemia
- Inflammatory bowel disease
    Crohn's disease
    Ulcerative colitis
    Pseudomembranous colitis
    Infective
- Volvulus
- Irritable bowel syndrome
- Angiodysplasia
- Pseudo-obstruction
- Megacolon and slow-transit constipation

ANORECTAL CONDITIONS

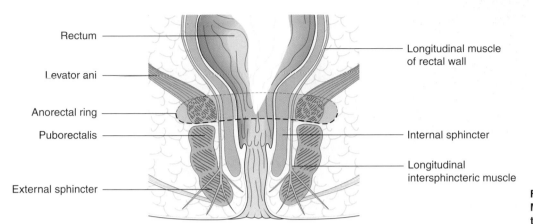

Rectum

Levator ani

Anorectal ring

Puborectalis

External sphincter

Longitudinal muscle of rectal wall

Internal sphincter

Longitudinal intersphincteric muscle

Fig. 21.1 Musculature of the anorectum.

21

INTRODUCTION

Anorectal complaints are extremely common; approximately 2–3% of the population have anorectal symptoms at any given time. A basic understanding of the principles of applied anatomy and pathophysiology helps to differentiate patients who merit specialist assessment from those who can be treated symptomatically in the first instance. There remains a great deal of social taboo, and so the symptoms associated with anorectal disorders are often ignored or hidden from relatives and doctors alike. It is important that the perianal symptoms are elicited without embarrassment to the patient or clinician. The more common disorders of the anus and rectum that are encountered in clinical practice in the UK are described in this chapter. Symptoms due to anorectal conditions overlap with those due to conditions affecting the large bowel, and so documentation of a full gastrointestinal history is essential.

APPLIED SURGICAL ANATOMY

The anus is a remarkable structure that is capable of allowing (when socially convenient) the passage of stool but is also capable of maintaining continence to gas, fluid and solid at almost all other times.

ANAL MUSCULATURE AND INNERVATION

The anal canal is 3–4 cm long in males and slightly shorter in females. It consists of two muscle layers (Fig. 21.1), known as the internal and the external sphincters. The internal sphincter is a condensation of the circular smooth muscle of the rectum and is continuous with the circular muscle of the whole of the gastrointestinal tract. It is controlled by the autonomic nervous system with fibres from the pelvic sympathetic nerves, the lower lumbar ganglia and the pre-aortic/inferior mesenteric plexus. The parasympathetic fibres arise from the sacral plexus. The smooth muscle of the internal sphincter maintains tone and contributes to resting pressure within the anal canal, so playing an important role in maintaining anal continence.

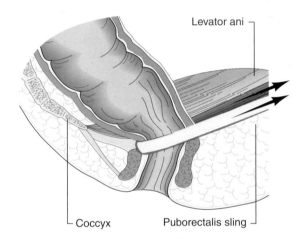

Levator ani

Coccyx

Puborectalis sling

Fig. 21.2   The puborectalis sling establishing the anorectal angle.

The longitudinal muscle of the gut ends at the anus as a series of fibrous bands that radiate to the perianal skin, and so is of little consequence in perianal disease. The striated muscle of the external sphincter is under voluntary control, being innervated bilaterally by the internal pudendal nerves and the fourth branch of the sacral plexus. The circular muscle tube of the external sphincter blends with the lower part of the levator ani, known as the puborectalis sling (Fig. 21.2). The puborectalis fibres of the levator ani originate from the posterior aspect of the pubic symphysis and pass backwards to join with the external sphincter. The levator ani muscles themselves are also important in maintaining the relationship of the anus and rectum during defaecation.

THE LINING OF THE ANAL CANAL

The cell type of the anal canal epithelium determines why certain diseases, such as tumours and viral infections, affect only particular levels of the canal. The epithelium of the anal canal is specialized and contains three distinct zones. The external zone (from the dentate line to the anal verge) is keratinized, stratified squamous epithelium.

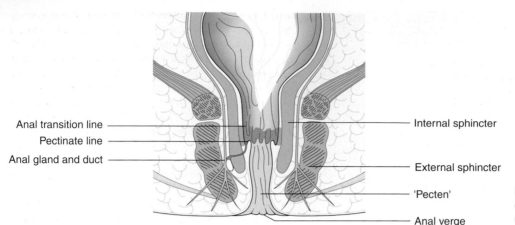

Anal transition line — Internal sphincter
Pectinate line
Anal gland and duct — External sphincter

'Pecten'

Anal verge

Fig. 21.3 The lining of the anorectal canal.

There is a short, modified, anal transitional zone of non-keratinized squamous epithelium, which lies above the dentate line, separated from the columnar epithelial of the anal canal but continuous with the rectal epithelium. The anal valves are crescentic mucosal folds that form a serrated or dentate line on the luminal aspect of the mid-anal canal (Fig. 21.3). The dentate line represents the line of fusion between the endoderm of the embryonic hindgut and the ectoderm of the anal pit. Thus, the epithelium is innervated by the autonomic nervous system and is insensate with respect to somatic sensation. The canal lining below the dentate line is innervated by the peripheral nervous system and so conditions affecting this region, such as abscess, anal fissure or tumour, result in anal pain.

The composition of the epithelium of the anorectum determines the type of tumour that affects the region. Thus, squamous cell carcinoma of the anal canal arises from the epithelium *below* the dentate line or in the transitional zone of non-keratinized squamous epithelium. Because the canal above the anal transition zone contains columnar glandular epithelium, tumours of the upper anal canal are adenocarcinoma; they are best considered as a low rectal cancer and treated accordingly.

There are 4–8 specialized anal glands located within the substance of the internal sphincter or in the space between the internal and external sphincters at the level of the mid-anal canal; these glands have ducts that open directly on to the dentate line (Fig. 21.4). They are involved in the aetiology of perianal abscess and fistula-in-ano. The precise function of the anal glands is unclear, but they secrete mucus and probably lubricate and protect the delicate epithelium of the anal transition zone. The ducts from these glands open into the folds of mucosa at the dentate line. The relevance of these glands lies in the fact that they are the source of most perianal abscesses. When an anal gland duct becomes occluded, the obstructed gland may become infected with gut organisms such as coliforms, and anaerobic bacteria such as *Bacteroides*.

THE ANAL (HAEMORRHOIDAL) CUSHIONS

Although the internal and external sphincters, the puborectalis sling and the anorectal angle play important roles in maintaining anal continence, fine control is aided by the anal 'cushions' that lie in the submucosa within the anal canal, above the dentate line. The anal cushions are

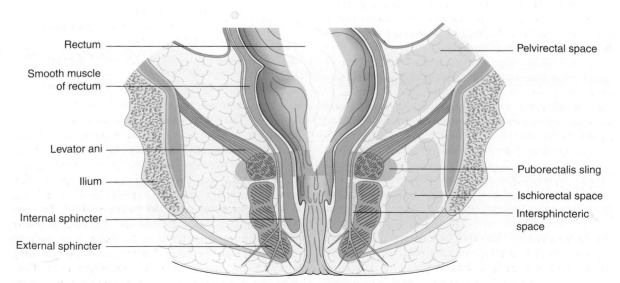

Rectum — Pelvirectal space
Smooth muscle of rectum
Levator ani
Ilium — Puborectalis sling
Internal sphincter — Ischiorectal space
External sphincter — Intersphincteric space

Fig. 21.4 Principal anorectal spaces in relation to the anal sphincters and rectum.

BOX 21.1 ANAL CONTINENCE

Anal continence is dependent on:
- intact anorectal and pelvic floor sensation
- intact anal sphincters and levator ani
- preservation of the anorectal angle
- the bulk provided by the anal 'cushions'

BOX 21.2 SEVERE ACUTE ANAL PAIN

- Severe acute anal pain may be due to intersphincteric abscess, anal fissure, perianal haematoma and, rarely, anal cancer

---

specialized vascular structures comprised of fibroconnective tissue containing arteriovenous communications, fed by the terminal branches of the superior rectal artery with inconstant anastomoses to the middle and inferior rectal arteries. There are usually three anal cushions because there are three terminal branches of the artery (left, right posterior and right anterior, corresponding with the 3, 7 and 11 o'clock positions when the patient is in the lithotomy position). These positions determine the position of haemorrhoids, which are caused by distension and prolapse of the anal cushions. Haemorrhoids are not 'varicose veins' of the anal canal, but prolapse of the specialized anal cushions; indeed, haemorrhoids are uncommon in patients with portal hypertension, despite the fact that the anal canal represents a potential portosystemic anastomosis.

LYMPHATIC DRAINAGE OF THE ANAL CANAL

The majority of the lymphatic drainage of the rectum passes superiorly through the mesorectum to follow the superior rectal artery and on to the inferior mesenteric and aortic chains. There are also some lymphatic channels that follow the course of the middle rectal arteries to drain to the nodes around the internal iliac arteries. Lymphatic drainage of the anus below the dentate line is to the inguinal lymph nodes. This anatomical distinction between the anus and the rectum has important implications for the management of tumours of the rectum and anus because anal cancer frequently metastasizes to inguinal lymph nodes, whereas rectal cancer metastasizes upwards to the mesorectum and onwards to the para-aortic chain. Thus, radiotherapy fields for anal squamous cancer normally incorporate the inguinal nodes.

ANORECTAL DISORDERS

HAEMORRHOIDS

Despite haemorrhoids (colloquially known as piles) being very common, the aetiology remains obscure. Almost all haemorrhoids are primary, with only a tiny proportion due to other factors, such as a cancer in the distal rectum. Haemorrhoids are enlarged, prolapsed anal cushions and

the pathophysiology involves degeneration of the supporting fibroelastic tissue and smooth muscle, with enlargement and protrusion of the cushions at the 3, 7 and 11 o'clock position. As the cushions prolapse, there is keratinization and hypertrophy of the overlying anal transitional zone and eventually prolapse of the columnar epithelial component in advanced stages. However, the underlying cause of the stretching of the fibroelastic support is unknown. Constipation and straining at stool are common features. These may be aggravated by a high anal sphincter pressure, with further entrapment of prolapsed piles. Haemorrhoids during pregnancy are very common and are probably due to hormonal effects inducing connective tissue laxity, combined with constipation and pressure from the baby's head. Sitting on the toilet for long periods, such as when reading, is also held to be an associated aetiological factor. However, as with other putative aetiological factors, there is no real evidence for cause and effect.

Clinical features

Bleeding and prolapse are the cardinal features and may occur in isolation or together. The bleeding is typically intermittent 'outlet-type' bleeding, separate from the stool and evident in the pan or only on wiping. There may also be aching or dragging discomfort on defaecation, and patients may self-reduce their piles to obtain relief after each bowel motion. Severe constant pain is unusual and in such cases other pathology should be suspected. In the later stages, haemorrhoids remain prolapsed at all times and there is staining of the underwear with mucus and faecal fluid. However, it is very unusual for patients to present with incontinence of solid faeces and a sphincter defect should be suspected in such cases. In cases of constant prolapse, there is often pruritus due to the discharge, with irritation of the perianal skin.

Haemorrhoids can be staged according to the degree of prolapse, but it is important to note that this classification does not necessarily relate to the amount of trouble that symptoms cause the patient:

- *First-degree* piles are those that bleed, are visible on proctoscopy but do not prolapse.
- *Second-degree* piles are those that prolapse during defaecation but reduce spontaneously.
- *Third-degree* piles are prolapsed constantly but can be reduced manually (Fig. 21.5).
- *Fourth-degree* piles are chronically and irreducibly prolapsed.

Patients may present as an emergency with a complication of haemorrhoids, such as thrombosed prolapsed piles or torrential haemorrhage. Prolapsing haemorrhoids may acutely thrombose and there is associated marked sphincter spasm. The thrombosed piles are large, swollen, irreducible haemorrhoids, which are dark blue or even black owing to necrosis and submucosal haemorrhage. They are acutely painful and tender and the diagnosis is easily made on inspection, but a rectal examination will be impossible because of pain. Major haemorrhage, resulting in significant hypovolaemia and anaemia, is unusual but should be excluded in any patient presenting with a major fresh rectal bleed.

21

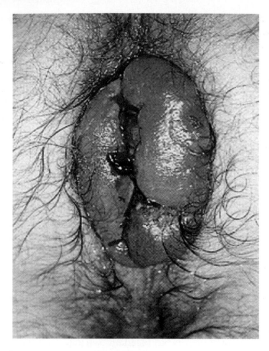

Fig. 21.5   Third-degree haemorrhoids.

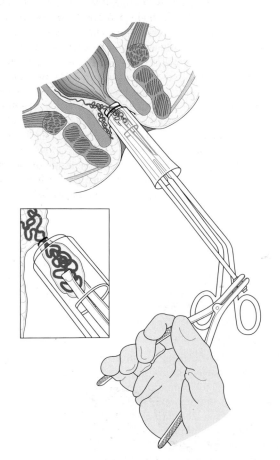

Fig. 21.6   Application of Barron's rubber band to haemorrhoids.

Examination

Assessment of suspected piles must always include consideration of other potential differential diagnoses, as the symptoms of piles and colorectal cancer can be very similar. However, piles are so common that it is important to take a sensible approach to the investigation of rectal bleeding. Indiscriminate large bowel investigation for a common complaint such as rectal bleeding, due most commonly to haemorrhoids and not to cancer, is inappropriate. Careful history is essential to guide further clinical assessment and investigation. If the bleeding is of the outlet type, there is no alteration in bowel habit and the patient is under 50 years of age, then the chance of rectal cancer is extremely remote. In such cases, digital rectal examination, combined with proctoscopy and rigid sigmoidoscopy, should secure the diagnosis. If piles are confirmed, then treatment can be instigated without recourse to imaging the rest of the colon by barium enema or colonoscopy. If the patient is older, if there is a change of bowel habit, or if there is no evidence of piles on proctoscopy, then further colonic investigation is indicated.

Examination of the perianal region should be carried out in the left lateral position. Prolapsed piles will be apparent at this stage and evidence of associated anal skin tags should be noted. Digital rectal examination is essential to assess sphincter tone and to exclude other anal conditions. First- or second-degree piles are rarely palpable, as they compress on pressure, and diagnosis is made by proctoscopy. The proctoscope should be gently inserted to the hilt and withdrawn, when bulging haemorrhoids will be visible at right anterior, right posterior and left lateral positions. Rigid sigmoidoscopy should be performed to exclude other rectal pathology.

Management

In many cases, reassurance after appropriate evaluation is all that many patients require. Specific treatment is not required for most cases, as symptoms are minor and intermittent. A high-fibre diet with plenty of vegetables is commonly recommended, although there is no good evidence that this actually provides any benefit at all. However, if constipation is a feature, it does seem reasonable advice; in some cases, bulk laxatives or stool softeners may be indicated. Patients often self-medicate with proprietary ointments and creams. There is no good evidence from controlled trials that these are effective, but if patients find that they help, then it seems reasonable to advise their intermittent use.

Non-operative approaches

There are many non-operative approaches to the treatment of haemorrhoids, the aim of which is to cause fibrosis and shrinkage of the protruding haemorrhoidal cushion in order to prevent bleeding and prolapse. Current outpatient clinic treatment approaches include application of small rubber bands to strangulate the pile (using a special Barron's bander); submucosal injection of sclerosant; and the application of heat by infrared photocoagulation. There is no strong evidence that any of these approaches is much better than doing nothing at all. In the long term, the symptoms of *untreated* piles tend to wax and wane, and the recurrence of symptoms after any of these procedures is much the same as without any treatment. However, of all the non-operative treatments, rubber band ligation (Fig. 21.6) may be the most effective in the short term. Where there is a significant

---

EBM 21.1 HAEMORRHOIDS

*'Open haemorrhoidectomy and stapled haemorrhoidectomy are
equally effective for second- and third-degree piles; rubber band
ligation has similar efficacy to haemorrhoidectomy.'*

---

cutaneous component to the piles, any of the outpatient
treatments is likely to be painful because of the cutaneous
nerve supply, and is also unlikely to succeed. In these
circumstances, the decision should be to do nothing but
reassure the patient, or to offer an operation.

Operative approaches

The principle of haemorrhoidectomy involves total removal
of the haemorrhoidal mass and the securing of haemostasis

BOX 21.3 HAEMORRHOIDS

- Haemorrhoids are common and are best treated conservatively
- Classification:
  First-degree: visible in the lumen on proctoscopy but do not prolapse
  Second-degree: prolapse on defaecation but return spontaneously
  Third-degree: remain prolapsed but can be replaced digitally
  Fourth-degree: long-standing prolapse and cannot be replaced in the anal canal
- Symptoms are outlet-type bleeding, prolapse, mucus discharge, discomfort and thrombosis
- Treatment:
  First-degree: advice on avoiding constipation and straining
  Second-degree: conservative management is best but, if they are symptomatic, banding, injection sclerotherapy or haemorrhoidectomy
  Third-degree: if symptomatic, haemorrhoidectomy
  Fourth-degree: thrombosed piles are usually treated conservatively in the first instance; interval haemorrhoidectomy is seldom required

---

of the feeding vessel. The wound can be left open or can be
closed, but there are rarely problems with healing or
infection. In some cases, there are secondary haemorrhoids
between the main right anterior, right posterior and left
lateral positions, and these are also removed as part of
the operation. Recently, a different surgical approach using
a circular stapler has been developed (EBM 21.1). This
technique aims to divide the mucosa and haemorrhoidal
cushions above the dentate line in order to transect the
feeding vessels and hitch up the stretched supporting fibroelastic tissue, rather than removing the whole haemorrhoidal
mass as in the standard haemorrhoidectomy. This 'stapled
haemorrhoidectomy' is currently undergoing clinical trials
in the UK and may have a place for the treatment of
symptomatic first- and second-degree piles. With all surgical
approaches to treating piles, it is important to consider that
the haemorrhoidal cushions contribute to fine control of
continence. Hence, an element of anal incontinence can be
one of the long-term sequelae of any haemorrhoidectomy.
Surgery should not be considered lightly.

FISSURE-IN-ANO

Fissure-in-ano is a common condition characterized by a
linear anal ulcer, often with the internal sphincter visible
in the base, affecting the anal canal below the dentate line
from the anal transition zone to the anal verge (Fig. 21.7).
There is often little in the way of granulation tissue in
the ulcer base. Owing to failed attempts at healing, there
may be a tag of skin at the lowermost extent of the fissure,
known as a 'sentinel pile'. At the proximal extent of the
fissure there may be a hypertrophied anal papilla.
Sometimes fissures will heal incompletely and mucosa
will bridge the edges of the fissure. This results in a low
perianal fistula and may present years later. Fissures are
most frequently observed in the posterior midline of the
anal canal, although anterior fissures may occur in women
following childbirth; they are rarely seen in males.

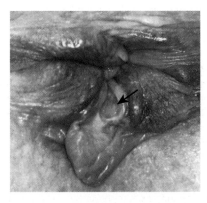

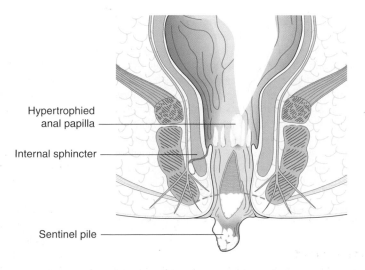

Hypertrophied
anal papilla

Internal sphincter

Sentinel pile

Fig. 21.7 Perianal fistula.
A Fistula (arrow) at the typical 6 o'clock position. B Explanatory diagram.

21

The condition most commonly affects people in their twenties and thirties, with a slight male preponderance. Most fissures are idiopathic, but it is clear that the pathophysiology involves ischaemia in the base of the ulcer, associated with marked anal spasm and a significantly raised resting anal pressure. Successive bowel motions provoke further trauma, pain and anal spasm, resulting in a vicious circle of anal pain and sphincter spasm that causes further trauma to the anal mucosa during defaecation. Fissures may be acute and settle spontaneously, but chronic anal fissure is defined as an ulcer that has been present for at least 6 weeks. Recurrent multiple or unusually extensive fissures affecting areas other than the midline should raise the suspicion of Crohn's disease, which can occasionally present with anal fissure as the sole initial complaint. Occasionally, anal fissure may be associated with ulcerative colitis. Fissure is an uncommon complication of haemorrhoidectomy and results from a non-healing wound combined with anal spasm.

Fissure-in-ano is one of the most common causes of constipation in infants and children. The pain associated with the fissure leads to a pattern of behaviour in which the child tries to avoid defaecation. This results in stool retention and rectal stool bolus formation. The rectum becomes overdistended and the child becomes unaware of the need to pass stool. Overflow incontinence and soiling result.

Clinical features and diagnosis

The most common symptoms are pain on defaecation in a young patient. There is often associated rectal bleeding of the outlet type, with blood on the paper or dripping into the pan after passing the motion. The amount of bleeding is usually minor and there may be some staining or mucous discharge in the underwear. Patients often report that it is painful to wipe the anus after moving the bowels. Pain is the predominant symptom and may be burning, tearing or sharp in nature. It may last a few hours after defaecation. There may be a history of constipation, which could be aetiologically responsible for the tear, but is more likely a response to the pain.

The diagnosis should be suspected from the history alone and is confirmed by gently parting the superficial part of the anal sphincter with the gloved fingers to reveal the characteristic linear ulcer. There may be an associated 'sentinel pile', which consists of heaped-up skin at the lowermost extent of the linear ulcer (Fig. 21.7). It is often too painful to perform a digital rectal examination or a proctoscopy, and so this is best left until after treatment is instigated. However, it is important to complete clinical assessment with rigid sigmoidoscopy at a later date. A full history is important to exclude previous perianal surgery, perianal abscess, trauma during childbirth or symptoms consistent with Crohn's disease.

Management

Many acute fissures resolve spontaneously and so treatment should be reserved for chronic symptoms of 6 weeks' or more duration. Having established that the fissure is primary, treatment is aimed at alleviating pain and anal spasm in order to break out of the vicious circle. It is important

---

EBM 21.2   ANAL FISSURE

'Internal sphincterotomy is more effective than anal stretch. The latter should not be performed because of the significant excess risk of faecal incontinence.'

---

to document reproductive history for females, as surgery may have implications for future anal continence.

The optimal approach is conservative in the first instance. Stool softeners may help, but rarely effect a cure as the sole treatment. Chemical sphincterotomy is the first-line treatment of choice, using topical nitrates (glyceryl trinitrate 0.2–0.5% or 0.5% diltiazem) as a cream applied 12-hourly to the anal canal. Unfortunately, headaches can be a dose-limiting side-effect, especially with topical nitrates, but healing can be achieved in 50–70% of chronic fissures. Other means of reduction in sphincter tone include direct injection of the sphincter with botulinum toxin, which temporarily paralyses the sphincter.

Until the relatively recent advent of chemical sphincterotomy as first-line treatment, surgery was the only option. Surgery still has a major role in the management of patients who have fissures resistant to medical treatment, or who have recurrence. Anal stretching has been abandoned, as it is associated with significant sphincter damage and the risk of incontinence (EBM 21.2). Lateral sphincterotomy is the most common operation for anal fissure and involves controlled division of the lower half of the internal sphincter at the lateral position (3 o'clock or 9 o'clock with the patient in the lithotomy position). There is a small but appreciable risk of late anal incontinence following lateral sphincterotomy. This is usually only to gas, but occasionally faecal incontinence to liquid or solid can occur, particularly in women who have had birth-related anal sphincter damage. In women, it may therefore be more appropriate to avoid further division of any sphincter muscle, and this can be achieved using an anal advancement flap or a rotation flap to cover the ulcerated base of the fissure and allow new, well-vascularized skin to heal the ulcer and reduce the associated anal spasm.

In children, treatment includes stool softeners, aperient medication and, rarely, manual disimpaction under anaesthetic. Anal stretch, while having fallen into disrepute in adult practice, is still a widely used and successful treatment for resistant cases. Topical nitrate preparations are currently the subject of controlled trials in children and are not yet in widespread use.

BOX 21.4   ANAL FISSURE

- Anal fissure is treated medically in the first instance and damage to sphincter should be avoided
- Pain on defaecation and bleeding are the outstanding symptoms
- Chemical sphincterotomy is the treatment of first choice; operative approaches are reserved for failed cases

---

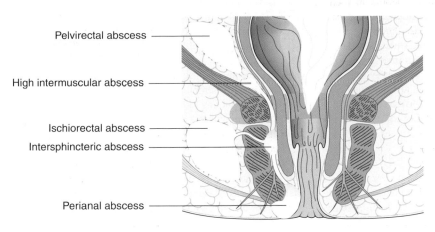

Pelvirectal abscess

High intermuscular abscess

Ischiorectal abscess

Intersphincteric abscess

Perianal abscess

Fig. 21.8 Spread of infection from the anal gland to the anorectal spaces and resultant abscess formation.

21

PERIANAL ABSCESS

Perianal abscess is a generic term encompassing the collection of pus and the formation of an abscess in the perianal, intersphincteric, ischiorectal or pelvirectal spaces (Fig. 21.8). Perianal suppuration is common, affecting men three times more frequently than women. Conditions that predispose to perianal abscess include ulcerative colitis and Crohn's disease, as well as any cause of immunosuppression such as haematological disease, diabetes mellitus, chemotherapy and human immunodeficiency virus (HIV) infection. Occasionally, patients with established sepsis elsewhere may develop metastatic suppuration in the perianal region. However, most patients who present with perianal abscess have no predisposing factors and most abscesses are cryptoglandular, initiated by blockage of the anal gland ducts (Fig. 21.3). The obstructed anal gland becomes secondarily infected with large bowel organisms such as *Bacteroides*, *Streptococcus faecalis* and coliforms. The fact that the anal glands are situated in the intersphincteric space (Fig. 21.4) explains the routes that the infection may take as pus tracks along the line of least resistance through the tissue spaces.

Clinical features

In cases where the abscess remains localized within the intersphincteric space, the patient presents with acute anal pain and tenderness. There is usually no evidence of suppuration on inspection of the perianal region. Pain often prevents digital examination, and so an anaesthetic is required. The main differential diagnosis is acute anal fissure. The diagnosis is confirmed by demonstration of a localized pea-sized lump in the intersphincteric space. True perianal abscess is the most common type, in which pus tracks inferiorly to appear at the perianal margin between the internal and external sphincters (Fig. 21.8). Symptoms are usually of 2–3 days' duration and the abscess may have discharged spontaneously. Systemic upset is minimal and anal pain is the predominant presenting complaint.

Infection tracking through the external sphincter results in an ischiorectal abscess. Ischiorectal abscess is a relatively uncommon but serious problem; it may be associated with uncontrolled diabetes and so diabetes should be excluded in all cases. As the ischiorectal space is horseshoe-shaped and there are no fascial barriers within it, infection can track posteriorly around the anus to affect the contralateral space. In such cases, the patient is toxic and pyrexial with a large, painful, fluctuant, brawny swelling affecting both buttocks, due to large volumes of pus. There is a history of perianal pain for several days, associated with difficulty in sitting.

Infection tracking upwards from the infected anal gland through the upper part of the intersphincteric space may result in a high intersphincteric (high intermuscular) abscess or a pelvirectal abscess. As these spaces encircle the anorectum above the levator muscles, abscesses can be bilateral and often present with a major systemic upset. These are complex problems meriting specialist management. With high abscesses, it is also important to consider intra-abdominal sepsis from Crohn's or diverticular abscess.

Management

An established abscess will not respond to antibiotics alone and requires surgical drainage. Treatment of perianal abscess is usually straightforward and involves drainage of the pus under general anaesthetic. Most cases are adequately dealt with by incising and deroofing the abscess at the point of maximal fluctuance. However, anatomical considerations are important, as inappropriate incision of sphincter muscle can result in incontinence in the long term. Furthermore, drainage of pus through the wrong space will create a perianal fistula (see below). At operation, pus should be sent for bacteriological assessment to determine the causative organism(s). In uncomplicated

---

BOX 21.5 ANORECTAL SEPSIS

- Most anorectal sepsis is cryptoglandular
- Perianal and ischiorectal abscesses are the most common forms of abscess in the anorectal region
- Recurrent abscess should raise suspicion of fistula and Crohn's disease
- Abscess requires incision and drainage

cases, antibiotics have no place after incision and drainage. Where there is extensive cellulitis, as is often the case with ischiorectal abscess, parenteral antibiotics, such as broad-spectrum cephalosporins and metronidazole, should be administered. Parenteral antibiotics are mandatory for diabetic patients with perianal sepsis. Unusually complex perianal sepsis or recurrent abscess should raise suspicion of underlying Crohn's disease. Sigmoidoscopy and rectal biopsy should be performed and the roof of the abscess sent for histology.

FISTULA-IN-ANO

Obstruction of the duct and infection of the anal glands constitute the underlying pathogenesis of both perianal abscess and fistula. Frank abscess precedes some cases of fistula, and inappropriate surgical drainage of perianal abscess is responsible for a small but significant proportion of fistulae. Figure 21.9 is a simplified diagram showing the classification of fistula-in-ano. In patients with recurrent perianal abscesses, a fistula tract may be identified. However, there is no need to search routinely for a fistula when draining straightforward perianal abscesses because probing may actually cause a fistula inadvertently. It is important to allow acute perianal abscesses to settle after incision and drainage before attempting to delineate a fistula. Some fistulae develop without any known perianal abscess, in which case the patient may present with a small abscess that intermittently points and discharges pus on to the perianal skin.

Perianal fistula may complicate Crohn's disease. Around 10% of patients with Crohn's disease of the small intestine, without colorectal involvement, also have perianal recurrent fistula or fissures. Hence, it is important to consider Crohn's disease in all patients with perianal fistula or sepsis that is resistant to treatment. Other rare causes of perianal fistula include ulcerative colitis, carcinoma of the anus or rectum, HIV infection, trauma and tuberculosis.

Clinical features and assessment

In most cases, the patient presents with a chronically discharging opening in the perianal skin, associated with pruritus and perianal discomfort. A careful clinical history is essential to ensure that there are no predisposing factors and also to determine whether there has been any previous surgery. Investigation requires examination under anaesthetic and the fistula tract should be probed by an experienced surgeon. When the fistula opens on the perianal skin of the anterior anus, the tract passes radially, directly to the anal canal. However, when the opening is posterior to a line drawn between the 3 o'clock and 9 o'clock positions (Fig. 21.10), then the tract usually passes circumferentially backwards to the midline and enters the anal canal at the 6 o'clock position. This is known as Goodsall's rule and can help define the extent of the course of a fistula.

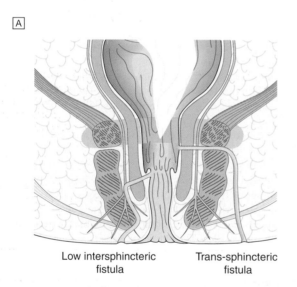

Low intersphincteric fistula   Trans-sphincteric fistula

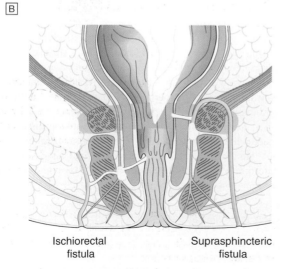

Ischiorectal fistula   Suprasphincteric fistula

Fig. 21.9 Categories of fistula-in-ano.
[A] Low intersphincteric and trans-sphinteric. [B] Ischiorectal and suprasphincteric.

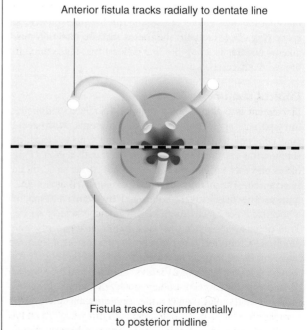

Anterior fistula tracks radially to dentate line

Fistula tracks circumferentially to posterior midline

Fig. 21.10 Goodsall's rule.

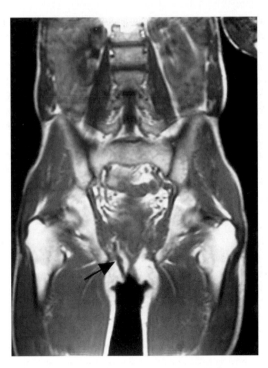

Fig. 21.11 Coronal MRI scan of complex pelvirectal fistula (arrow).

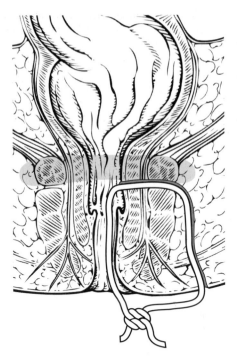

Fig. 21.12 A seton encircling a trans-sphincteric fistula.
A seton is a piece of surgical thread, suture material or specialized tie that is passed through the fistula. It is tied in a loop to allow the fistula to drain (loose seton) and/or to cut slowly through the sphincter muscle, with the muscle healing behind the advancing seton (tight seton).

21

It is essential to avoid inducing further fistulae by ill-advised probing of the region. It is important to determine whether the fistula is low or high (Fig. 21.9), as the prognosis and treatment are different for each. Investigation of most fistulae requires formal examination under anaesthesia (EUA), but complex cases merit detailed investigation to define the extent of the tracts using magnetic resonance imaging (MRI). A complex high fistula involving the pelvirectal space is shown in Figure 21.11. Endo-anal ultrasound also may be useful. A barium follow-through and colonoscopy may be indicated when inflammatory bowel disease is suspected.

Management

Treatment is determined by the course of the fistula tract. Usually, low fistulae can simply be laid open and allowed to heal. However, where a significant proportion of the internal and/or external sphincter is involved, then laying open the tract will result in faecal incontinence. In such complex cases, the fistula tract can be probed and a seton passed along its length (Fig. 21.12) to allow the fistula to drain. Once it is drained, a tighter seton can be applied that will gradually cut out through the sphincters, allowing them to heal behind the seton. This approach keeps the ends of the sphincters together and so minimizes the chances of inducing incontinence. Another approach to high fistulae is to raise a flap of the rectal wall and upper internal sphincter. The flap is advanced downwards to close the internal opening and the external part simply heals, as it has no faecal stream maintaining the sepsis and the tract. This is known as an anorectal advancement flap. In some complex cases, a defunctioning colostomy may be necessary.

> **BOX 21.6   FISTULA-IN-ANO**
>
> - Most are primary idiopathic but inflammatory bowel disease should be considered in recurrent and resistant cases
> - Low fistulae should be laid open; complex high fistulae require repair and/or seton insertion

MISCELLANEOUS BENIGN PERIANAL LUMPS

PERIANAL HAEMATOMA

Perianal haematoma is a painful condition caused by subcutaneous haemorrhage and formation of thrombus in the superficial space between the anoderm and the anal sphincter. A localized lump forms at the anal verge, due to blood tracking subcutaneously from haemorrhoids after the passage of a hard bowel motion. It can also arise in patients with a bleeding diathesis or those on anticoagulants. It is important to recognize the condition because it is readily treated by surgical drainage under local anaesthetic, with almost instantaneous relief. The condition will settle eventually without surgical intervention, but recognizing the haematoma will spare the patient many days of an exquisitely tender anus.

Perianal haematoma is easily recognized by the presence of a well-circumscribed, bluish dome-shaped lump under the perianal skin. The main differential diagnosis is prolapsed, thrombosed haemorrhoids, and so it is essential

331

21

to make an accurate diagnosis, as inappropriate incision of haemorrhoids will result in considerable bleeding. Perianal haematoma should be readily differentiated from perianal abscess by nature of the colour and by the surrounding erythema and induration.

ANAL WARTS

Anal warts cause discomfort, pain, pruritus ani and difficulty with perianal hygiene. Warts are also associated with an increased risk of squamous carcinoma because they are usually associated with human papillomavirus (HPV). The lesions may be very extensive or relatively sparse.

After viral infection and the development of an initial crop of warts, they may be spread extensively by scratching, which is provoked by the associated pruritus ani. Many cases resolve spontaneously, but those requiring treatment can usually be managed effectively by the application of podophyllin. More extensive cases may require surgical excision, and very extensive cases associated with dysplasia may require excision and skin grafting, combined with a temporary colostomy.

FIBROEPITHELIAL ANAL POLYP

Fibroepithelial anal polyp is hypertrophic epithelium arising on a stalk from the anal canal itself; histologically, it is comprised of keratinized squamous epithelium supported by scarred, fibrotic subcutaneous tissue. Hence it is not a neoplasm. The clinical history may suggest haemorrhoids as the main differential diagnosis, but this is easily discounted by examination, which will reveal the polyp on a stalk. The main differential diagnosis on digital examination and proctoscopy is of a prolapsing rectal adenomatous polyp on a long stalk, but this arises above the dentate line. Biopsy will confirm the nature of the polyp, as rectal polyp is comprised of adenomatous glandular tissue, rather than the squamous epithelium of the fibroepithelial type.

Patients with fibroepithelial polyp may present with a prolapsing anal lesion, discomfort on defaecation, or pruritus ani associated with faecal-stained mucus causing irritation to the delicate perianal skin. Anal polyps are usually associated with a previous history of perianal disease, including haemorrhoids or fissure-in-ano. Occasionally, there is no preceding history and in these circumstances it is likely that the patient has had asymptomatic haemorrhoidal disease. Treatment of symptomatic polyps is by simple excision under general anaesthetic.

ANAL SKIN TAGS

Prolapse of haemorrhoids is usually followed by a degree of regression, and may leave irregular skin at the anal verge, known as anal skin tags. Haemorrhoids often present with minor anal skin tags, but it is important to stress that the tags themselves are not haemorrhoids. Although the anus may not look particularly tidy, there is no indication to operate unless the patient is having significant problems with perianal hygiene or the lesions are causing pruritus. Anal tags associated with haemorrhoids that merit surgery can be removed at the same time as haemorrhoidectomy.

ANAL CANCER

Anal cancer is uncommon in comparison with colorectal cancer, with only around 600 incident cases annually in the UK. Over 85% of anal cancers are squamous in origin and arise from the keratinized squamous epithelium of the anal margin, or of the pecten, or from the non-keratinized squamous epithelium of the anal transitional zone immediately above the dentate line. Anal verge tumours often present earlier than canal tumours because the patient becomes aware of a mass or irregular area at the anal margin. Around 5% of tumours are adenocarcinomas and these arise from the glandular epithelium of the upper anal canal. These are distinct from low anorectal adenocarcinoma. Most patients with anal cancer present in the sixth or seventh decade, but younger cases are well recognized, particularly in females. Other rarer tumours include melanoma, lymphoma and sarcoma.

There is a strong association between anal cancer and infection with HPV types 16 and 18. Anogenital warts are also a risk factor for anal cancer, as is anal intercourse. HIV infection is also a predisposing factor, owing to immunosuppression and susceptibility to viral infection. The pre-malignant lesion, anal intraepithelial neoplasia (AIN), is probably the precursor of most anal carcinomas and is analogous to cervical intraepithelial neoplasia (CIN), the precursor lesion of cervical cancer. The level of AIN (1–3) is dependent on the degree of cytological atypia and the depth of that atypia in the epidermis. A high proportion of AIN 3 progresses to carcinoma and is shown in Figure 21.13. It is important to perform a

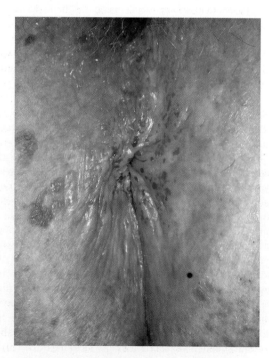

Fig. 21.13 The most severe degree of anal intraepithelial neoplasia (AIN 3), the precursor of most anal squamous cancer.

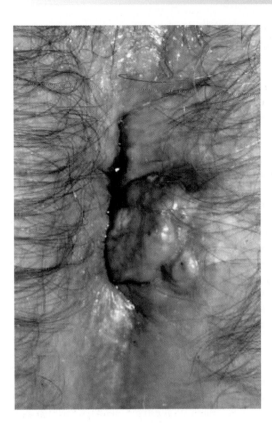

Fig. 21.14 Squamous carcinoma of the anal verge.

Table 21.1 TNM STAGING OF ANAL CANCER

T (Tumour)
- T_X — Primary tumour cannot be assessed
- T_0 — No evidence of primary tumour
- T_1 — < 2 cm
- T_2 — 2–5 cm
- T_3 — > 5 cm
- T_{4a} — Invading vaginal mucosa
- T_{4b} — Invading structures other than skin, or rectal or vaginal mucosa (i.e. local spread to muscle or bone)

N (node)
- N_X — Regional lymph nodes cannot be assessed
- N_0 — No regional lymph node metastasis
- N_1 — Metastasis in perirectal lymph node(s)
- N_2 — Metastasis in unilateral internal iliac and/or inguinal lymph node(s)
- N_3 — Metastasis in perirectal and inguinal lymph nodes and/or bilateral internal iliac and/or inguinal lymph nodes

M (Metastases)
- M_X — Distant metastasis cannot be assessed
- M_0 — No distant metastasis
- M_1 — Distant metastasis

cervical smear in patients with proven anal cancer. There is also an association with vulval intraepithelial neoplasia (VIN), which also has a common HPV aetiology.

Clinical features and assessment

Anal cancer is frequently misdiagnosed in the early stages because of its rarity and because symptoms due to benign anal conditions are highly prevalent. Early cancer may be confused with fissures, piles and warts. Nevertheless, because of accessibility, anal tumours are readily detectable by careful clinical examination; anal pain/discomfort, bleeding or discharge into the underwear, and pruritus ani should be sought. Advanced tumours that have spread to the anal sphincters may present with incontinence. Clinical examination of anal cancer at the margin reveals an ulcerated discoid lesion at the anal verge (Fig. 21.14). Cancer of the anal canal may not be visible, although extensive lesions may protrude to the anal verge by direct spread. Careful examination under anaesthetic is required to allow tumour biopsy and sigmoidoscopy. Biopsy is essential to confirm the diagnosis, but also to determine the tissue of origin, as the treatment for squamous carcinoma varies from that for adenocarcinoma.

Staging

Staging is important for prognosis and also guides treatment approaches. The TNM staging system for anal cancer is shown in Table 21.1. The lymph nodes most commonly involved are the inguinal groups, particularly for anal verge cancers. Canal tumours may spread proximally to the mesorectal nodes or to the internal iliac nodes via the middle rectal lymph nodes. Lymphadenopathy alone is not sufficient to confirm lymph node spread, and accessible nodes should be biopsied because reactive changes due to infection are common. Examination under anaesthetic is an important part of clinical staging, as the tumour is often painful and the anus tender to digital examination. CT and MRI are essential; endo-anal ultrasound may be helpful but usually needs to be performed under anaesthetic.

Management

It is important to detect anal cancer at an early stage, as extensive local invasion and metastatic disease are associated with a poor outcome. Modern treatment of anal cancer is multidisciplinary, with surgeon and radiotherapist working collaboratively in the assessment and treatment on an individual basis. For early, well-circumscribed superficial (T_1N_0) carcinomas, wide surgical excision is the optimal treatment, as it avoids the morbidity of chemo-radiotherapy. However, for T_2, T_3 and T_4 tumours, current standard treatment is radiotherapy to the anal canal and inguinal lymph nodes, combined with 5-fluorouracil (5-FU) and mitomycin C (EBM 21.3). Newer regimens of radiotherapy, combined with 5-FU and cisplatinum, are also being introduced. The usual approach is external beam radiotherapy, but radioactive implants such as selectron wires are also used in selected cases. Surgery has no place as

EBM 21.3 ANAL CANCER

'Chemoradiation is the primary treatment modality for anal canal and T_2, T_3 and T_4 tumours. Abdomino-perineal resection is reserved for salvage procedures in cases of relapse after chemoradiation.'

21

BOX 21.7   ANAL CARCINOMA

- Anal carcinoma is associated with human papillomavirus types 16 and 18
- Anal intraepithelial neoplasia (AIN) is a malignant precursor
- Local surgical excision is the treatment of choice for T_1N_0 lesions
- Chemo-radiotherapy is the treatment of choice for T_2 and above and those with involved lymph nodes
- Abdominoperineal resection is reserved for failures of chemoradiation

---

primary treatment of these lesions but does play an important part in the management of advanced disease. Surgery is reserved for radiotherapy treatment failures, when 'salvage' abdominoperineal excision of the anus and rectum may afford a cure in some cases and alleviate symptoms in others.

Modern multi-modality approaches involving tailored surgery and chemoradiation have radically improved the morbidity of treatment by avoiding abdominoperineal resection and permanent colostomy for many patients; the 5-year survival rate is now around 65%.

RECTAL PROLAPSE

Rectal prolapse is a distressing condition that can affect young and older adults, as well as children. The term rectal prolapse encompasses three types of abnormal protrusion of all, or part of, the rectal wall:

- A *full-thickness* rectal prolapse includes the mucosa and the muscular layers.
- *Mucosal* prolapse, as the name suggests, involves only the mucosal lining of the rectum.
- *Occult* rectal prolapse refers to intussusception of the rectal wall but without the prolapse protruding through the anal canal. This term also refers to the much rarer condition of *solitary rectal ulcer syndrome*, which is a prolapse of the full thickness of only the anterior rectal wall, although the terms occult rectal prolapse and solitary rectal ulcer syndrome are not synonymous.

The pathological process that results in rectal prolapse is incompletely understood. However, certain factors are clearly implicated in predisposing to the condition. Mucosal prolapse should not be confused with full-thickness prolapse. It is often associated with a degree of haemorrhoids, but whether these are causal or simply the result of a common aetiology is not understood. The majority of cases of full-thickness rectal prolapse occur in elderly women, with no obvious aetiological basis. Weight loss in the elderly with loss of fat supporting the rectum, combined with degeneration of collagen fibres and weakness of the musculature of the pelvic floor, results in loss of the anorectal angle and laxity of the rectal wall (Fig. 21.2). In many cases, there is a deep rectovaginal pouch with a long loop of sigmoid colon that pushes down into the rectovaginal pouch and contributes to the prolapse. Occasionally,

there is a clear history of childbirth injury but many patients are nulliparous.

Chronic constipation and straining at stool are the most common aetiological factors in young adults, although spinal injury, psychiatric illness, multiple sclerosis, spinal injuries and spinal tumour are predisposing factors. In children, the lack of a sacral hollow, combined with constipation and excessive straining at stool, is responsible for evagination of the rectum and protrusion of the prolapse through the anus. In children with cystic fibrosis, excessive coughing contributes to elevated intra-abdominal pressure.

Clinical features and assessment

Patients present with an uncomfortable sensation of 'something coming down' the back passage. Initially, this is only on defaecation, but eventually the rectum remains constantly prolapsed and will not reduce spontaneously. The patient may be able to reduce the prolapse digitally. Constipation is usually an accompanying feature. There is often a degree of faecal incontinence and there may be mucous discharge into the underwear. Blood-stained mucus is also common when the rectum remains prolapsed. The prolapse may become ulcerated and may become strangulated. In extreme cases, there may be associated uterine prolapse, alluding to the fact that the underlying aetiology relates to weakness of the entire pelvic floor.

Examination will confirm the diagnosis in most cases and this may involve asking the patient to attempt to produce the prolapse by straining on a commode. A typical example of a full-thickness rectal prolapse is shown in Figure 21.15. Digital examination reveals a patulous anus, poor sphincter tone and evidence of a weak pelvic floor on straining. Rigid sigmoidoscopy will reveal cases of occult prolapse.

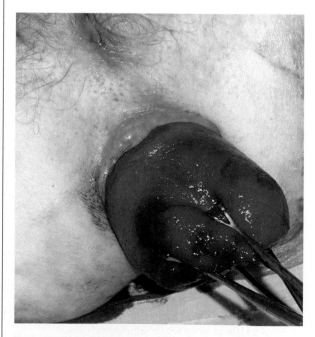

Fig. 21.15   Full-thickness rectal prolapse at operation prior to repair.

Usually, there is no need for further investigation, but if the history is of short duration, consideration should be given to the presence of a spinal tumour, a spinal stenosis or a prolapsed intervertebral disc. In occult rectal prolapse, radiological assessment using a defaecating proctogram may help secure the diagnosis. Conditions that might be mistaken for a rectal prolapse include large fourth-degree haemorrhoids, prolapsing rectal neoplasia, anal warts, anal skin tags and fibroepithelial anal polyp. On the basis of symptoms alone, the differential diagnosis of rectal prolapse includes rectal cancer and inflammatory bowel disease, and these should be excluded by appropriate investigations.

Management

Childhood prolapse

Rectal prolapse in children is effectively treated in almost all cases by attention to maintaining a regular bowel habit with stool softeners, combined with digital reduction of the prolapse by the parents. The condition is self-limiting and surgery is rarely indicated.

Mucosal rectal prolapse

In adults, mucosal rectal prolapse can be treated by sub-mucosal injection of sclerosant, by photocoagulation or by applying Barron's bands to the prolapsed area. In resistant cases, a limited excision of the area, similar to a haemorrhoidectomy, is effective.

Full-thickness rectal prolapse

Surgery is the only effective treatment for established full-thickness rectal prolapse. However, none of the available surgical options is wholly satisfactory. The aim of surgery is to treat the prolapse and improve the associated incontinence. Operations for rectal prolapse can be undertaken employing perineal or abdominal approaches:

- *Perineal approaches* aim to fixate or excise the prolapse surgically from below. 'Delorme's procedure' involves the excision of the mucosa lining the prolapse, with plication of the muscle tube, and 'perineal rectosigmoidectomy' entails excision through the anus of the prolapsed rectum and lower part of the sigmoid. The latter may be combined with a repair of the pelvic floor (Altmeier procedure).
- *Abdominal approaches* aim to fix the rectum to the sacral wall with sutures or foreign material. The abdominal approach may also include resection of the redundant sigmoid colon, particularly when constipation is a predominant feature, because rectal fixation usually aggravates the constipation.

BOX 21.8   RECTAL PROLAPSE

- Rectal prolapse can occur at any age but is most common in the elderly
- Diagnosis is clinical
- Treatment is surgical: either perineal or transabdominal (recurrence rates are highest for perineal procedures)

Solitary rectal ulcer syndrome

This rare condition is difficult to treat effectively because there is usually a psychological overlay. Patients with solitary rectal ulcer syndrome tend to be aged 20–40 years and are often professional men or women. The condition is associated with an introspective and anxious personality. Patients with this condition spend an inordinate amount of time in the toilet trying to move their bowels. The diagnosis is confirmed by visualizing the anterior ulcer in the low rectum, and biopsy shows the typical features of submucosal fibrosis, hypertrophy of the muscularis mucosae and overlying ulceration. Management involves the use of stool softeners and other conservative measures, along with input from a psychologist. Biofeedback may have a place in suitable patients who are compliant, but surgery should be avoided if at all possible.

ANAL INCONTINENCE

Anal continence can be affected adversely by any combination of structural damage to the musculature, disruption of the nerve supply, and marked intestinal hurry with defaecatory urgency (such as in ulcerative colitis). Damage to the internal or external sphincters can occur during childbirth. It can also be a consequence of perianal sepsis or the surgery required to treat it. Peripartum nerve injury or neurodegenerative disease can affect the pudendal nerves, eventually leading to denervation and atrophy of the striated muscle of the external sphincter, the puborectalis sling and the levator ani.

Faecal incontinence is both distressing and socially disabling, and yet patients are often very reluctant and embarrassed to discuss it with their relatives or their GP. The prevalence of incontinence is probably underestimated, although it has been variously documented as 2–5% in population studies and as high as 10% of all adult females. There are a variety of specific aetiological factors but the majority of cases are 'idiopathic', most commonly affecting older parous women. Aetiological factors associated with anal incontinence are listed in Table 21.2.

The substantial majority of patients presenting to colorectal surgeons are women with a past history of obstetric problems and difficult deliveries. The underlying mechanism of subsequent incontinence in such cases is complex. Although full-thickness obstetric tears are rare, significant sphincter defects have been observed to occur in 10–30% of women as a consequence of childbirth. Prolonged labour has been implicated in damage to the nerve supply to the pelvic floor, principally the internal pudendal nerves. Denervation of the pelvic floor results in atrophy of the sphincter complex and the levator ani in later life. Most incontinent women have a combination of sphincter muscle damage and the secondary effects of denervation.

Clinical features and assessment

A full history is essential, with particular reference to obstetric history and any past perianal operations. Incontinence should be graded using established scoring systems, which all take into account the degree and number

21

Table 21.2   AETIOLOGY OF ANAL INCONTINENCE

Trauma
- Sphincter injury during childbirth (including episiotomy)
- Accidental trauma (e.g. road traffic accident, bicycle injury)
- Surgical trauma (injudicious fistula surgery, drainage of perianal abscess or haemorrhoidectomy)
- Perianal sepsis

Congenital
- Anorectal atresia (usually treated surgically in childhood)
- Spinal dysraphism (spina bifida)

Neurological
- Denervation of pelvic floor following childbirth
- Multiple sclerosis
- Low spinal or sacral tumour
- Spinal trauma
- Dementia

Miscellaneous
- Rectal prolapse
- Haemorrhoids
- Rectal cancer invading sphincter
- Perianal Crohn's disease
- Faecal impaction
- Relative incontinence due to intestinal hurry (e.g. inflammatory bowel disease)
- Psychiatric or behavioural problems (including encopresis)

---

of episodes of incontinence to gas, liquid or solid stool. Coexisting disease should be documented and neurological symptoms sought. A defaecation history should be sought, including the degree of defaecatory urgency. A history of coexisting urinary incontinence suggests a generalized problem, most likely neurogenic in origin. Examination to determine sphincter tone, the presence of previous scars and the state of the rectovaginal septum should be undertaken. Poor anal sensation suggests a neurogenic basis for the incontinence. Other anorectal causes of incontinence, as listed in Table 21.2, should be excluded where possible, and by rigid sigmoidoscopy in all cases. It is important to remember that any cause of intestinal hurry (such as colonic cancer) can render incontinent a patient who had previously been coping with a more formed stool, and so colonoscopy or barium enema is indicated in the assessment of older patients. Endo-anal ultrasound scanning of the sphincters allows delineation of the presence and extent of any sphincter defect. Anorectal physiology studies document resting and squeeze anal sphincter pressures, and also define whether there is a predominant neurogenic element. Where there is any concern from the history or clinical examination regarding a spinal lesion, MRI should be performed.

Management
The underlying causes of incontinence (Table 21.2) should be managed appropriately. However, it is women with 'idiopathic' faecal incontinence who constitute the majority of cases dealt with by colorectal surgeons. Where there is clear evidence of a sphincter defect in a young woman, overlapping sphincter repair is often highly successful in selected patients. However, those with an element of

denervation tend to have poorer results. In older women, who almost universally have a combination of sphincter and nerve damage, conservative measures should be instigated in the first instance. Stool-bulking agents should be combined with loperamide to give the patient a degree of constipation. When there is a predominant neurogenic basis, there is often rectal irritability, resulting in faecal urgency. This can be damped using 25 mg of amitriptyline at night. Such conservative measures should be combined with regular emptying of the rectum using stimulant suppositories or enemas. In many cases, these simple measures have a dramatic effect on the patient's quality of life, and although minor degrees of incontinence will continue, this approach is acceptable and effective for many patients.

In a minority of patients with idiopathic faecal incontinence, further surgery is indicated because the results of anterior sphincter repair alone are very disappointing in the long term. Complex total floor repairs have been performed with some success in a limited proportion of patients. Other surgical approaches include transferring the gracilis muscle on a proximal pedicle to wrap it subcutaneously around the anal canal. An electrical stimulator is implanted, which delivers an electrical signal to convert the muscle to a slow twitch type. This allows long-term tonic contraction of the gracilis muscle to maintain continence. The procedure has an acceptable level of success in around 50% of patients, but at a cost of major surgery and potentially major complications. Implantable artificial anal sphincters have been developed and these are placed to encircle the anorectal region. Results from the use of the available devices are encouraging but, as with any foreign material, there is a propensity for infection and many have to be removed. Nevertheless, prosthetic devices may have some place in the future management of anal incontinence.

Another surgical option for the patient with anal incontinence is the creation of a permanent colostomy. Although this might be seen as an admission of failure, a well-sited stoma and professional input from a stoma care specialist can transform a patient's life, from being afraid to leave the house to leading a virtually normal existence.

The management of anal incontinence remains imperfect, but it is clear that patients should be managed by specialist surgeons. This allows a full investigative work-up and tailoring of management for individual patients. In such a setting, the management of anal incontinence can be highly successful. Improvements in obstetric practice are

---

BOX 21.9   FAECAL INCONTINENCE

- Faecal incontinence is most common in females
- Childbirth injury is the most common aetiology
- It may be associated with a neurological disorder, trauma and perianal sepsis or surgery
- Results of surgery for discrete sphincter injuries (the minority) are excellent
- Results of surgery for most cases are poor
- Most patients respond well to conservative management with stool bulking, antidiarrhoeal agents and enemas
- Complex surgery may be indicated in a minority of cases
- Colostomy may be the only option for some debilitated patients

---

needed to avoid sphincter and nerve damage during child-birth. There is a real need for research to determine risk factors for obstetric injury. Unfortunately, progress in this area is hampered by the fact that it is many decades after the initial insult before patients present with anal incontinence.

PRURITUS ANI

The condition can be a minor, short-lived episode but may be an all-consuming obsession for some patients. It is a particular problem at night and some patients may unconsciously scratch the perianal region during sleep, resulting in further trauma and irritation. Pruritus ani is a common complaint and may be a symptom of many anorectal disorders, including haemorrhoids, fistulae, fissures, faecal incontinence, anal carcinoma and rectal pro-lapse. Dermatological conditions can also be associated with pruritus ani, and these include psoriasis, dermatitis, lichen planus and anal warts; skin infections can also be respon-sible. Fungal infections should be considered, including candida and tinea, especially in the diabetic patient.

Management
Underlying conditions, such as anal cancer, perianal fistula and haemorrhoids, should be treated and diabetes mellitus excluded. If there is evidence of fungal infection, this should be treated with antifungal creams. In cases where all other contributing disorders have been excluded and the condition is idiopathic, full explanation and support for the patient are essential. The cycle of trauma to the delicate perianal skin, followed by irritation and subsequent scratching, should be explained in detail. Strong advice on avoiding scratching and a requirement for a great deal of willpower are essential. In some cases, it may be necessary for the patient to wear cotton gloves in bed, to avoid subconscious nocturnal scratching. The use of perfumed soap and strong antiseptics or lotions should be discouraged. The avoidance of nylon undergarments is important to minimize sweating. Particular attention should be paid to the diet, as certain foods (e.g. spicy foods or alcohol) may be responsible. Explanation should be given of the need to avoid over-zealous cleansing of the perianal region after defaecation. Gentle cleaning with toilet paper, followed by washing with mild soap, may be necessary, but it is important to take care to avoid trauma during drying. A simple barrier cream such as is used for nappy rash may be appropriate in some patients, but generally it is best to avoid relying on creams. Overall, it is possible to improve the symptoms of idiopathic pruritus ani in almost all patients, but it requires a commitment to continued support and advice to achieve this. It may take several months before symptoms come under control.

PILONIDAL DISEASE

Pilonidal disease is characterized by chronic inflammation in one or more sinuses in the midline of the natal cleft that contain hair and debris (Fig. 21.16). The superficial part of

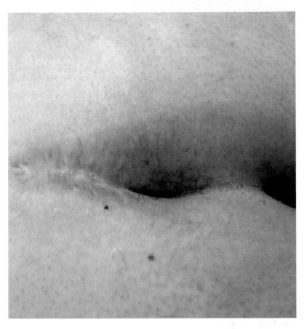

Fig. 21.16 Pilonidal sinus in the natal cleft.

the midline sinus is lined with squamous epithelium, but the tracts themselves are lined with granulation tissue resulting from the associated infection. Pilonidal disease is more common in males than females, and affects around 2% of the population between the ages of 15 and 35. However, it is very rare after the age of 40, suggesting that there is an aetiological relationship with age and skin character. The disease is almost unheard of before puberty, when sex hor-mones act on hair follicles and sebaceous glands. There is enlargement of a hair follicle, which allows the accumu-lation of extraneous hairs that are caught in the natal cleft itself. A foreign-body reaction is set up, with the result that there is a chronic discharging sinus that attracts other debris and hairs. A sedentary occupation, particularly where sweating is common, is a predisposing factor. The condition was described in large numbers of American troops in the Vietnam war, owing to the use of Jeeps in the warm climate.

Clinical features
Many people have asymptomatic pilonidal sinuses and so it is important to treat the condition only if it is causing problems, in view of the high prevalence and the fact that it seldom presents after the fourth decade. When symptomatic, the disease is characterized by midline pits in the natal cleft discharging mucopurulent material, which may smell mildly offensive and may be blood-stained. There is often tenderness on pressure and the patient may avoid long periods of sitting, such as car journeys. When a sinus becomes infected and the pus is loculated, the disease presents as pilonidal abscess, with the abscess typically pointing just off the midline. However, there is invariably a communication with a midline sinus containing hair and granulation tissue. Occasionally, pilonidal sinus may present with extensive and complex branching sinus tracts. In these

cases, it is important to consider perianal Crohn's disease, and careful examination of the anal canal is essential.

Management

The treatment of pilonidal disease includes conservative and surgical management. Conservative management comprises attention to natal cleft hygiene and hair removal by depilatory creams or by careful shaving. Antibiotics have a place in the early stages of abscess formation and may avert the need for incision and drainage of an established abscess. Hair removal from the sinus tract itself on a regular basis allows the sinus to drain and avoid the collection of hair and debris.

Surgical drainage is indicated for established abscess and the incision should avoid the midline to minimize the likelihood of recurrence. Debilitating, chronically discharging sinus tracts also merit surgery and there are a number of surgical options. The tracts can be laid open, the granulations removed with a curette and the resultant defects dressed until they heal from the base. Tracts can also be excised and closed primarily with sutures, although the wound is prone to break down and heal by second intention. Unfortunately, the treatment of pilonidal disease is characterized by frequent recurrence, due partly to inadequate or inappropriate surgery in some cases, but mostly to the fact that the underlying aetiology is still present: namely, the natal cleft and a predisposed skin type. Recurrent disease can be treated using rotation flaps to replace the pitted skin with fresh skin from the buttock. For complex recurrent disease, ablation of the natal cleft using a flap procedure is highly effective but leaves a fairly large unsightly scar. It is important to advise the patient to keep the natal cleft free of hair by depilation after any successful surgical treatment.

BOX 21.10   PILONIDAL DISEASE

- Pilonidal disease is due to hair creating chronic inflammatory sinuses in the natal cleft
- Abscess should be drained
- Symptomatic tracts should be excised
- Recurrence is common and can be dealt with by closure of the natal cleft or other plastic surgical technique

BOX 21.11   SYMPTOMS ASSOCIATED WITH DISORDERS OF THE ANORECTUM

- Bleeding
- Perianal pain
- Discharge
- Pruritus ani
- Anal incontinence
- Prolapse

BOX 21.12   DISORDERS OF THE ANORECTUM

- Haemorrhoids
- Anal fissure
- Anorectal abscess
- Fistula-in-ano
- Perianal haematoma
- Rectal prolapse
- Anal neoplasms
- Functional disorders of sphincters and pelvic floor
- Pilonidal disease

Section 5
SURGICAL SPECIALTIES

J.D. WATSON

Plastic and reconstructive surgery

INTRODUCTION

Plastic and reconstructive surgery is concerned with the restitution of form and function after trauma and ablative surgery. The techniques by which this is achieved are applicable to virtually every surgical subspecialty and are not limited to any single anatomical region or system. The 'reconstructive ladder' is broad, simple and widely applicable at its base, but narrow, technically demanding and complex at its top (Fig. 22.1). It is important to distinguish plastic and reconstructive surgery from cosmetic, or aesthetic, surgery. In the latter, the techniques of the former are applied to improve appearance but not physical function, although there may be considerable psychological benefit.

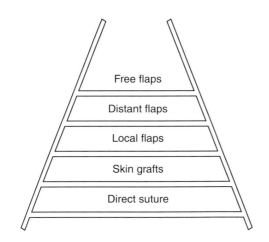

Free flaps

Distant flaps

Local flaps

Skin grafts

Direct suture

Fig. 22.1   Reconstructive ladder.

STRUCTURE AND FUNCTIONS OF SKIN

Skin consists of epidermis and dermis. The epidermis is a layer of keratinized, stratified squamous epithelium (Fig. 22.2) that sends three appendages (hair follicles, sweat glands and sebaceous glands) into the underlying dermis. Because of their deep location, the appendages escape destruction in partial-thickness burns and are a source of new cells for reconstitution of the epidermis. The basal germinal layer of the epidermis generates keratin-producing cells (keratinocytes), which become increasingly keratinized and flattened as they migrate to the surface, where they are shed. The basal layer also contains pigment cells (melanocytes) that produce melanin, which is passed to the keratinocytes and protects the basal layer from ultraviolet light.

The dermis is composed of collagen, elastic fibres and fat. It supports blood vessels, lymphatics, nerves and the epidermal appendages. The junction between the epidermis and the dermis is undulating where dermal papillae push up towards the epidermis.

The three types of epidermal appendage extend into the dermis and, in some places, into the subcutaneous tissues. Hair follicles produce hair, the colour of which is determined by melanocytes within the follicle. The sebaceous glands secrete sebum into the hair follicles, which lubricates the skin and hair. The sweat glands are coiled tubular glands lying within the dermis and are of two types; eccrine sweat glands secrete salt and water on to the entire skin surface, while apocrine glands secrete a musty-smelling fluid in the axilla, eyelids, ears, nipple and areola, genital areas and the perianal region. Hidradenitis suppurativa affects the latter.

The nails are flat, horny structures composed of keratin. They arise from a matrix of germinal cells, which can be seen as a white crescent (lunula) at the nail base. If a nail is avulsed, a new nail grows from this matrix. If the matrix

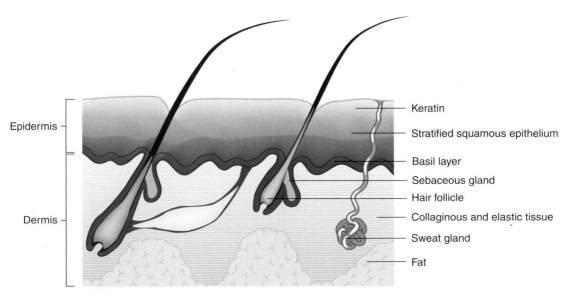

Fig. 22.2   Structure of skin.

22

is destroyed, nail regeneration is impossible, and the layer of epidermal cells covering the nailbed thickens to form a keratinized protective layer.

WOUNDS

A wound may be defined as disruption of the normal continuity of bodily structures due to trauma, which may be penetrating or non-penetrating. In both cases, inspection of the body surface may give little indication of the extent of underlying damage.

TYPES OF WOUND

Wounds can be classified according to the mechanism of injury:

- *Incised wounds.* A sharp instrument causes these; if there is associated tearing of tissues, the wound is said to be lacerated.
- *Abrasions.* These result from friction damage to the body surface and are characterized by superficial bruising and loss of a varying thickness of skin and underlying tissue. Dirt and foreign bodies are frequently embedded in the tissues and can give rise to traumatic tattooing: for example, in coal miners.
- *Crush injuries.* These are due to severe pressure. Even though the skin may not be breached, there can be massive tissue destruction. Oedema can make wound closure impossible. Increasing pressure within fascial compartments can cause ischaemic necrosis of muscle and other structures (compartment syndrome).
- *Degloving injuries.* These result from shearing forces that cause parallel tissue planes to move against each other: for example, when a hand is caught between rollers or in moving machinery. Large areas of apparently intact skin may be deprived of their blood supply by rupture of feeding vessels.
- *Gunshot wounds.* These may be low-velocity (e.g. shotguns) or high-velocity (e.g. military rifles). Bullets fired from high-velocity rifles cause massive tissue destruction after skin penetration.
- *Burns.* These are caused not only by heat but also by electricity, irradiation and chemicals.

Table 22.1   PHASES OF WOUND HEALING
Lag phase (2–3 days)
• Inflammatory response
Incremental or proliferative phase (approximately 3 weeks)
• Fibroblast migration
• Capillary ingrowth (granulation tissue)
• Collagen synthesis with rapid gain in tensile strength
• Wound contraction
Plateau or maturation phase (approximately 6 months)
• Organization of scar
• Slow final gain in tensile strength (80% of original strength)

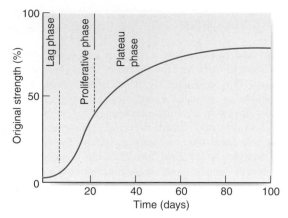

Fig. 22.3   Phases of wound healing.

PRINCIPLES OF WOUND HEALING

The essential features of healing are common to wounds of almost all soft tissues, and result in the formation of a scar. Soft tissue healing can be subdivided into three phases (Table 22.1) according to the development of tensile strength (Fig. 22.3).

Lag phase
The lag phase is the delay of 2–3 days that elapses before fibroblasts begin to manufacture collagen to support the wound. It is characterized by an inflammatory response to injury, during which capillary permeability increases and a protein-rich exudate accumulates. It is from this exudate that collagen is later synthesized. Inflammatory cells migrate into the area, dead tissue is removed by macrophages, and capillaries at the wound edges begin to proliferate.

Incremental phase
During the incremental or proliferative phase, there is progressive collagen synthesis by fibroblasts and a corresponding increase in tensile strength. Increased collagen turnover in areas remote from the wound suggests that there may also be a systemic stimulus for fibroblast activity. Collagen synthesis increases over a period of about 3 weeks, during which the gain in tensile strength accelerates. Old collagen undergoes lysis and new collagen is laid down.

Plateau or maturation phase
After 3 weeks, the gain in tensile strength levels off as the rate of collagen breakdown first approaches and then temporarily surpasses its synthesis. Excess collagen is removed during this final clearing-up process and the number of fibroblasts and inflammatory cells declines. Orientation of collagen fibres in the direction of local mechanical forces increases tensile strength for some 6 months. However, skin and fascia usually recover only 80% of their original tensile strength.

At the time of suture removal, the edges of the newly healed wound should be directly apposed and flat. Thereafter, for up to 3 months, the scar may become progressively raised, red and thickened. It can then remain static for a further 3 months, before slowly improving to become narrow, flat and pale. These changes vary with age, race, the direction of scar and the degree of dermal damage.

In children, scars take longer to resolve, whereas in the elderly they tend to mature and fade very quickly.

Hypertrophic scars

This is an exaggeration of the normal maturation process. Such wounds are very raised, red and firm, but never continue to worsen after 6 months. They are particularly common in children and after deep dermal burns. Unless under tension, they eventually resolve, often after several years. Resolution can be hastened by elastic pressure garments, steroid injections or the application of silicone gel. These scars should not be excised.

Keloids

These are similar to hypertrophic scars, except that they continue to enlarge after 6 months and invade neighbouring uninvolved skin. They are most likely to occur across the upper chest, shoulders and earlobes, and are common in black patients. They are difficult to treat successfully. If the measures described above fail, intralesional excision

followed immediately by low-dose radiotherapy is sometimes considered.

Epidermis

Epithelium heals by regeneration and not by scar formation. Epithelial cells at the edge of the wound lose their adhesion to each other and migrate across the wound until they meet cells from the other side. As they migrate, they are replaced by new cells formed by the division of basal cells near the wound edge. The cells that have migrated undergo mitosis and the new epithelium thickens, eventually forming normal epithelial cover for the scar produced by the dermis.

Primary and secondary intention

Wounds may heal by primary intention if the edges are closely approximated: for example, by accurate suturing. In this situation, epithelial cover is quickly achieved and healing of the apposed dermis produces a fine scar (Fig. 22.4). If the wound edges are not apposed, the defect fills with granulation tissue and the restoration of epidermal continuity takes much longer. The advance of epithelial cells across the denuded area may also be hindered by

22

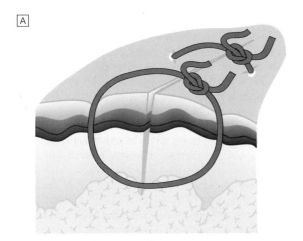

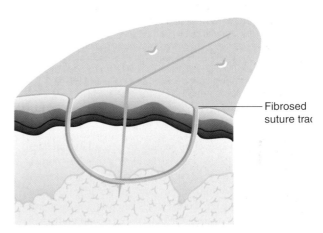

Fibrosed suture trac

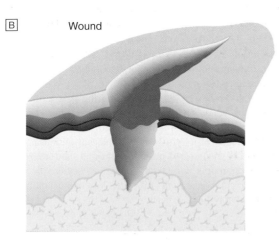

Wound

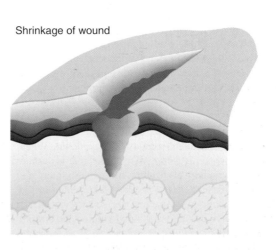

Shrinkage of wound

Fig. 22.4 Wound healing.
A Healing by primary intention. B Healing by secondary intention, showing shrinkage of the wound.

22

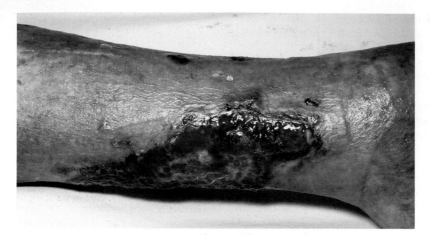

Fig. 22.5   Healing by secondary intention.

BOX 22.1   CLASSIFICATION OF WOUND HEALING

- Healing by first intention is the most efficient method and results when a clean incised surgical wound is meticulously apposed and heals with minimal scarring
- Healing by second intention occurs when wound edges are not apposed and the defect fills with granulation tissue. In the time taken to restore epithelial cover, infection supervenes, fibrosis is excessive and the resulting scar is unsightly
- The term 'healing by third intention' describes the situation where a wound healing by second intention (e.g. a neglected traumatic wound or a burn) is treated by excising its margins and then apposing them or covering the area with a skin graft. The final cosmetic result may be better than if the wound had been left to heal by second intention

---

infection. This is known as healing by secondary intention and usually results in delayed healing, excessive fibrosis and an ugly scar (Fig. 22.5). If a wound has begun to heal by secondary intention, it may still be possible to speed healing by excising the wound edges and bringing them into apposition, or by covering the defect with a skin graft.

FACTORS INFLUENCING WOUND HEALING

Many of the factors influencing healing are interrelated: for example, the site of the wound, its blood supply, and the level of tissue oxygenation. Although some adverse factors, such as advanced age, cannot be influenced, others, such as surgical technique, nutritional status and the presence of intercurrent disease, can be modified or eliminated.

Blood supply

Wounds in ischaemic tissue heal slowly or not at all. They are prone to infection and frequently break down. When this occurs, the ischaemic wound may not be able to sustain the metabolic demands of healing by second intention. Arterial oxygen tension (PaO_2) is a key determinant of the rate of collagen synthesis. Anaemia per se may not affect healing if the patient has a normal blood volume and arterial oxygen tension. Poor surgical technique, such as crushing tissue with forceps, approximating wound edges under tension and tying sutures too tightly, can render well-

vascularized tissue ischaemic and lead to wound breakdown.

Infection

The general risks of wound infection depend upon age, the presence of intercurrent infection, steroid administration, diabetes mellitus, disordered nutrition, and cardiovascular and respiratory disease. Local factors are also important. Bacterial contamination can be minimized by careful skin preparation and meticulous aseptic technique, but some wounds are more likely to be contaminated than others. Despite every precaution, bacteria may enter wounds from the atmosphere, from internal foci of sepsis or from the lumen of transected organs. In some cases, contamination occurs in the post-operative period. Provided contamination is not gross and local blood supply is good, natural defences are usually able to prevent and contain overt infection. Devitalized tissues, haematomas and the presence of foreign material such as sutures and prostheses favour bacterial survival and growth. Common infecting organisms are staphylococci, streptococci, coliforms and anaerobes. Overcrowding of wards and excessive use of operating theatres increase the bacterial population of the atmosphere and hence the risk of wound infection. The failure of medical and nursing staff to wash their hands before and after touching and examining each patient is perhaps the greatest source of cross-contamination.

When wound contamination is anticipated, topical antibacterial chemicals or topical and systemic antibiotics can be used prophylactically. For example, a short course of systemic antibiotics (often a single dose) is normally used to reduce the risk of infection during gastrointestinal surgery and when prosthetic material (hip joint, cardiac valves, arterial bypass) is being inserted. In acute traumatic wounds, tetanus prophylaxis is routine, but antibiotics are not normally necessary provided prompt and thorough surgical treatment is undertaken. However, if there has been a delay in the treatment of such a wound, antibiotic prophylaxis may be necessary.

Age

Wounds in the elderly may heal poorly because of impaired blood supply, poor nutritional status or intercurrent disease.

However, as mentioned above, they tend to form 'good' scars.

Site of wound

Surgical incisions placed in the lines of least tissue tension are subject to minimal distraction and should heal promptly, leaving a fine scar. On the face, these lines run at right angles to the direction of underlying muscles and form the lines of facial expression.

Nutritional status

Malnutrition has to be severe before healing is affected. Protein availability is most important, and wound dehiscence and infection are common when the serum albumin is low. Healing problems should be anticipated if recent weight loss exceeds 20%. Vitamin C is essential for proline hydroxylation and collagen synthesis. The number of fibroblasts is not reduced in scorbutic states. Zinc is a co-factor for important enzymes involved in healing, and its deficiency retards healing. Supplements of ascorbic acid and zinc are effective in patients with known deficiencies, but do not improve healing in normal subjects.

Intercurrent disease

Healing may be affected by the disease itself or by its treatment. Cachectic patients with severe malnutrition (as seen in advanced cancer) have marked impairment of healing. Diabetes mellitus impairs healing by reducing tissue resistance to infection and by causing peripheral vascular insufficiency and neuropathy. Haemorrhagic diatheses increase the risk of haematoma formation and wound infection. Obstructive airway disease lowers arterial PO_2 and so affects healing. Abdominal wound dehiscence is more common in patients with respiratory disease because of the strain put on the wound during coughing. Corticosteroid therapy reduces the inflammatory response, impairs collagen synthesis and decreases resistance to infection. The effect of steroids on wound healing is most marked if they are given within 3 days of injury. Immunosuppressive therapy impairs healing by reducing resistance to infection. Such patients are already compromised by their underlying disorder. As radiotherapy greatly reduces the vascularity of the tissues, the healing of wounds in irradiated areas is often impaired. Chemotherapy also inhibits wound healing.

Surgical technique

Where possible, skin incisions are placed in the line of least tissue tension. Meticulous aseptic technique and gentle handling are mandatory. Accurate apposition of wound edges favours healing by first intention. Dead spaces in the depth of the wound must be avoided, as bleeding and the accumulation of exudate encourage infection. Correct suturing of the deeper layers often allows the skin edges to fall together without tension, so that superficial sutures or adhesive tape can achieve skin apposition. Deep sutures should obliterate any potential dead space. If this is not possible, the space must be drained. Drains should also be used in contaminated wounds and those where exudate is expected. Drains may be connected to a suction apparatus or

---

BOX 22.2   FACTORS AFFECTING WOUND HEALING

- The site of the wound and its orientation relative to tissue tension lines are major determinants of healing
- Wounds with a good blood supply (e.g. head and neck wounds) heal well
- Infection is a major adverse factor and the risk of infection is influenced by:
  General factors such as the patient's age, presence of intercurrent infection, nutritional status and cardiorespiratory disease
  Local factors including bacterial contamination, antibacterial prophylaxis, aseptic technique, degree of trauma, presence of devitalized tissue, haematoma and foreign bodies
- Intercurrent disease may impair healing. Important factors include:
  Malnutrition
  Diabetes mellitus
  Haemorrhagic diatheses
  Hypoxia (e.g. obstructive airways disease)
  Corticosteroid therapy
  Immunosuppression
  Radiotherapy
- Surgical technical factors that have a major influence on wound healing include:
  Gentle tissue handling
  Avoidance of undue trauma
  Accurate tissue apposition
  Meticulous haemostasis
  Appropriate choice of suture material

22

allowed to empty by gravity. The drain site is a potential portal of entry for infection and drains should be removed as soon as possible, especially when prosthetic material has been implanted.

Choice of suture and suture materials

The choice of suture materials is important. Foreign material in the tissues predisposes to infection. The finest sutures that will hold the wound edges together should be used. Wounds are often subjected to stress post-operatively and, whereas 5/0 or 6/0 sutures are appropriate for the face, stronger ones (3/0 or 4/0) are needed for incisions near joints and still stronger ones for the abdominal wall. The suture should be strong enough to support the wound until tensile strength has recovered sufficiently to prevent breakdown. Absorbable materials are preferred for buried layers, but non-absorbable sutures may be needed in some situations: for example, in the aponeurotic layer of an abdominal wound.

WOUND INFECTION

Classification

Surgical procedures can be classified according to the likelihood of contamination and wound infection as 'clean', 'clean-contaminated' and 'contaminated':

- *Clean procedures* are those in which wound contamination is not expected and should not occur. An incision for a clean elective procedure should not become infected, provided no infective focus is encountered and no viscus is entered. In clean

22

operations, the wound infection rate should be less than 1%.

- *Clean-contaminated procedures* are those in which no frank focus of infection is encountered but where a significant risk of infection is nevertheless present, perhaps because of the opening of a viscus, such as the colon. Infection rates in excess of 5% may suggest a breakdown in ward and operating theatre routine.
- *Contaminated or 'dirty' wounds* are those in which gross contamination is inevitable and the risk of wound infection is high; an example is emergency surgery for perforated diverticular disease, or drainage of a subphrenic abscess.

Antibiotic prophylaxis is appropriate for the latter two types of operation.

Clinical features

Wound infection usually becomes evident 3–4 days after surgery. The first signs are usually superficial cellulitis around the margins of the wound, or swelling of the wound with some serous discharge from between the sutures. Fluctuation is occasionally elicited when there is an abscess or liquefying haematoma. Crepitus may be present if gas-forming organisms are involved. In some cases of deep infection, there are no local signs, although the patient may have pyrexia and increased wound tenderness. Systemic upset is variable, usually amounting to only moderate pyrexia and leucocytosis. Toxaemia, bacteraemia and septicaemia can complicate serious wound infection, especially where there is an accumulation of pus. The differential diagnosis includes other causes of post-operative pyrexia, wound haematoma and wound dehiscence. Wound haematoma may result from reactive bleeding during the first 24–48 hours after an operation. It causes swelling and discomfort, but only minimal pyrexia and few systemic signs.

Prevention

The risk of wound infection is reduced by careful patient preparation, the prophylactic use of antibiotics in high-risk patients, and meticulous attention to good operating theatre techniques. Severely contaminated wounds are sometimes best closed by delayed primary suture; most gunshot wounds are treated in this way. Skin sutures may be inserted at this time but are not tied for several days, by which time it should be clear that infection has been avoided. Antibiotic therapy is essential for grossly contaminated wounds. The aim is to achieve high tissue concentrations as soon as possible. The choice of antibiotic is determined by the nature of the infection. Topical agents such as povidone-iodine may also be used to combat infection in contaminated wounds. Radical excision of the wound margins, thorough mechanical cleansing and delayed suture may also be required.

Management

A wound swab or specimen of pus is routinely sent for bacteriological culture and sensitivity determination. In urgent cases, a Gram stain may be useful. The state of

immunity against tetanus is assessed and appropriate action taken. Trivial superficial cellulitis can be managed expectantly. The area of redness is 'mapped out' with an indelible pen so that its extent can be monitored. Spreading cellulitis is an indication for antibiotic therapy. Many infected wounds heal rapidly without further surgery, particularly if the original skin incision is placed in the line of least tissue tension. The problem is often to keep the wound open, rather than to achieve closure. If it appears that spontaneous wound closure will take a long time, secondary suture or skin grafting can be considered to speed healing, but only once it is clear that infection has been eradicated. The presence of clean healthy granulation tissue in the wound is usually a good indication that closure can be undertaken.

INVOLVEMENT OF OTHER STRUCTURES

All wounds must be inspected carefully in good light to assess the extent of devitalization and injury to other structures. However, it is important to appreciate that a small, apparently innocent wound may conceal extensive damage to deeper structures. Body cavities may have been penetrated, or tendons, nerves and blood vessels divided. Damage to muscles, tendons or nerves is assessed by checking relevant motor and sensory function. If the injury involves a limb, the distal circulation must be checked. Where appropriate, X-rays will help to establish whether peritoneal, pericardial or pleural cavities have been entered, and whether there is underlying bony injury.

Provided there is no deep damage, small, relatively uncontaminated wounds can be treated under local anaesthesia in the A&E department on an outpatient basis. The wound margins are cleaned with a mild antiseptic such as cetrimide and the wound is irrigated copiously with sterile saline. Any devitalized tissue is removed, deep tissues are sutured with absorbable material and the skin margins are closed.

More extensive or severely contaminated wounds usually require inpatient treatment, with exploration and debridement under general anaesthesia. The wound and its margins are cleansed, and pieces of grit, soil and other obvious foreign material picked out. All devitalized tissue is trimmed back until bleeding occurs. This process is known as debridement. In areas of poor vascularity such as the leg, or if there is severe contamination, crushing or a fracture, the wound margins are formally excised (Fig. 22.6). Bleeding from the wound margin is not a certain indication of its ultimate survival, as impaired venous drainage can lead to progressive necrosis, particularly after a crushing or degloving injury. If there is any doubt, the wound should not be sutured and a 'second-look' dressing change should be undertaken under anaesthesia after 48 hours.

Primary closure should also be avoided if there is significant delay in treating a grossly contaminated wound: that is, more than 6 hours without antibiotic cover. If primary closure is attempted, wound infection and breakdown are likely and there is a risk of anaerobic infection, which may threaten both life and limb. It is also too late for

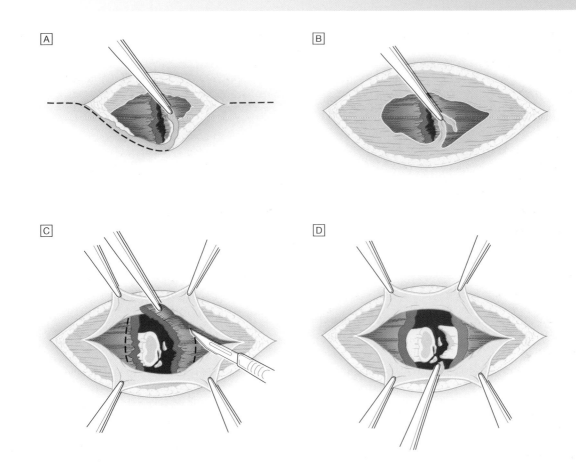

Fig. 22.6 Technique of wound excision in the presence of a compound fracture.

BOX 22.3   PRINCIPLES OF MANAGEMENT OF CONTAMINATED TRAUMATIC WOUNDS

- Contaminated wounds should be debrided under general anaesthesia
- The contaminated wound and its margins must be cleansed thoroughly, and grit, soil and foreign bodies/materials removed
- Devitalized tissue is formally excised until bleeding is encountered
- Primary closure is avoided if there has been gross contamination and when treatment has been delayed for more than 6 hours. Inappropriate attempts to achieve primary closure increase the risk of wound infection and expose the patient to the risks of anaerobic infection (tetanus and gas gangrene)
- Wounds left open may be suitable for delayed primary suture after 2–3 days, or for later excision and secondary suture (with or without skin grafting)
- Appropriate protection against tetanus must be afforded and the use of antibiotics should be considered

---

formal excision, as bacteria will have penetrated the tissues, but foreign bodies and dead tissue should be removed in the usual way. The wound is dressed and antibiotics are started. The dressing is changed daily, and if the wound is clean, in 2 or 3 days delayed primary suture may be carried out. If closure is delayed until granulation tissue has formed, this is usually excised and secondary suture performed. If this is not possible, split-skin grafts (see below) can be applied to the granulations.

Provided that surgical treatment is carried out early, prophylactic antibiotics are only required for deeply penetrating wounds, especially those from dog and human bites or those caused by nails, where adequate debridement may be impossible. However, the early use of antibiotics in situations where a delay in surgical treatment is anticipated may allow primary suture of wounds after 8–12 hours, an interval that is normally considered safe.

DEVITALIZED SKIN FLAPS

A common emergency problem is posed by the patient, usually an elderly woman, who falls and raises a triangular flap over the surface of the tibia (pretibial laceration). In some cases, the flap is blue-black in colour and obviously non-viable, but in most cases viability is uncertain. Similar injuries can occur elsewhere in the body. The wound must be cleansed and all non-viable tissue excised. No attempt should be made to suture the flap back into place; because of the post-traumatic oedema this would only be possible under tension, and would lead to death of the flap. If the defect is small, it can be treated conservatively on an

22

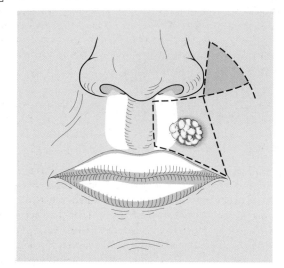 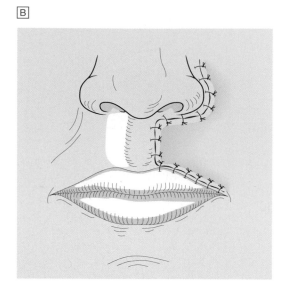

Fig. 22.7 **Local skin flap used to repair a defect after the excision of a skin lesion.**
A Before surgery. B After surgery.

outpatient basis. The wound is dressed, an elastic supporting bandage is applied to the leg (providing the arterial circulation is normal; Ch. 25) and the patient is kept ambulant. The wound will normally take several weeks to heal. Alternatively—and this is essential if the defect is large—a split-skin graft can be applied, either immediately or as a delayed primary procedure.

WOUNDS WITH SKIN LOSS

The aim of wound care is to obtain skin cover and healing as soon as is safely possible, by either primary or delayed primary closure. If skin has been lost as a direct result of trauma, or following the excision of a tumour or necrotic tissue, direct suture may not be possible. If the skin defect is small and at a functionally or aesthetically unimportant site, it may be allowed to heal by secondary intention. However, it is often better to speed healing by importing skin to close the wound. This may be achieved by means of a skin graft, which requires a vascular bed as it has no blood supply of its own, or a flap.

Skin grafts

These may be split-skin or full-thickness. Split-skin grafts are cut with a special guarded freehand knife or an electric dermatome. The donor site heals by re-epithelialization from epithelial appendages in the dermis (the bases of hair follicles and sweat ducts) within 2–3 weeks, depending on the thickness of the graft. To cover very large areas, the graft can be expanded by 'meshing'. The thinner the graft, the more easily it will take on a bed of imperfect vascularity but the poorer the quality of skin will be and the more it will shrink. Split-skin grafts are used to cover wounds after acute trauma, granulating areas and burns, or when the defect is large. A full-thickness graft leaves a donor defect (which needs to be sutured or grafted) as large as the one to be filled and requires a well-vascularized bed to survive. However, such grafts are strong, do not shrink, and look

better than a split-skin graft. They are rarely advisable after acute trauma but are commonly used in reconstructive surgery to close small defects where strength is needed (e.g. on the palm of the hand) or where a good functional and/or cosmetic result is important (e.g. on the lower eyelid). An area where there is skin to spare is chosen for the donor site (e.g. the groin for the former and the area behind the ear or upper eyelid for the latter).

Flaps

Whereas grafts require a vascular bed to survive, flaps bring their own blood supply to the new site. They can therefore be thicker and stronger than grafts and can be applied to avascular areas such as exposed bone, tendon or joints. They are used in acute trauma only if closure is not possible by direct suture or skin grafting, and are more usually reserved for the reconstruction of surgical defects and for secondary reconstruction after trauma. The simplest flaps use local skin and fat (local flaps), and are often a good alternative to grafting for small defects such as those left after the excision of facial tumours (Fig. 22.7). If not enough local tissue is available, a flap may have to be brought from a distance (distant flap) and remain attached temporarily to its original blood supply until it has picked up a new one locally (Fig. 22.8). This usually takes 2–3 weeks, after which the pedicle can be divided. Advances in our knowledge of the blood supply to the skin and underlying muscles have led to the development of many large skin, muscle and composite flaps, which have revolutionized plastic and reconstructive surgery. One example is the use of the transverse rectus abdominis musculocutaneous (TRAM) flap for reconstruction of the breast. The ability to join small blood vessels under the operating microscope now allows the surgeon to close defects in a single stage, even when there is no local tissue available, by free tissue transfer (Fig. 22.9). Other tissues, such as bone, cartilage, nerve and tendon, can also be grafted to restore function and correct deformity after tissue damage or loss.

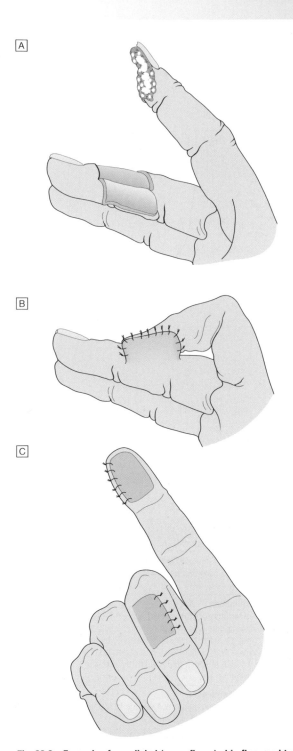

Fig. 22.8 Example of a pedicled (cross finger) skin flap used to cover a defect on the tip of the index finger.
[A] Raised. [B] Inset. [C] Divided.

CRUSHING/DEGLOVING INJURIES AND GUNSHOT WOUNDS

Wounds of this type should never be closed primarily as the tissue destruction is always much greater than at first appears. After thorough irrigation and the removal of any obviously dead tissue and foreign material, such wounds should be lightly packed and dressed. Dressings are removed 48 hours later under anaesthesia and further excision is carried out if necessary. The wound is closed by suture, skin grafting or flap cover, once it is clear that all dead tissue has been removed.

BURNS

MECHANISMS

Burn injuries range from the trivial to severe burns that pose a threat to life, involve a long hospital stay, and carry the risk of permanent disfigurement or impaired function. Most burns follow accidents in the home and could be prevented. They may be caused by flames, hot solids, hot liquids or steam, irradiation, electricity or chemicals. Toddlers are particularly liable to scalding by hot liquids in kitchen accidents, and unguarded fires are a threat to all children. Burns sustained in house fires are often accompanied by smoke inhalation, with injury to the lungs. Alcohol is a common contributing factor in burn injury. In the elderly and infirm, impaired mobility, poor coordination and diminished awareness of pain increase the incidence of burns. Industrial accidents account for most physico-chemical burns, although the accidental or deliberate ingestion of caustic or corrosive chemicals is still an occasional cause of domestic burns.

LOCAL EFFECTS OF BURN INJURY

The local effects result from destruction of the more superficial tissues and the inflammatory response of the deeper tissues (Table 22.2). Fluid is lost from the surface or trapped in blisters, the magnitude of loss depending on the extent of injury. Loss is greatly increased by leakage of fluid from the circulation (see below) where, instead of the normal insensible loss of 15 ml/m^2 body surface/hr, as much as 200 ml/m^2 may be lost during the first few hours. With deeper injuries, the epidermis and dermis are converted into a coagulum of dead tissue known as eschar. In its least severe form, the dermal inflammatory response consists of capillary dilatation, as in the erythema of sunburn. With deeper burns, the damaged capillaries become permeable to protein, and an exudate forms with an electrolytic and protein content only slightly less than that of plasma. Lymphatic drainage fails to keep pace with the rate of exudation and interstitial oedema leads to a reduction in circulating fluid volume. An increase of 2 cm in the diameter of the leg represents the accumulation of over 2 litres of excess interstitial fluid. Exudation is maximal in the first 12 hours, capillary permeability returning to normal within 48 hours.

Destruction of the epidermis removes the barrier to bacterial invasion and opens the door to infection. The burn surface may become contaminated at any time, and wound care must commence when the patient is first seen. Sepsis delays healing, increases energy needs, and may pose a new threat to life, just when the early dangers of hypovolaemia have been overcome.

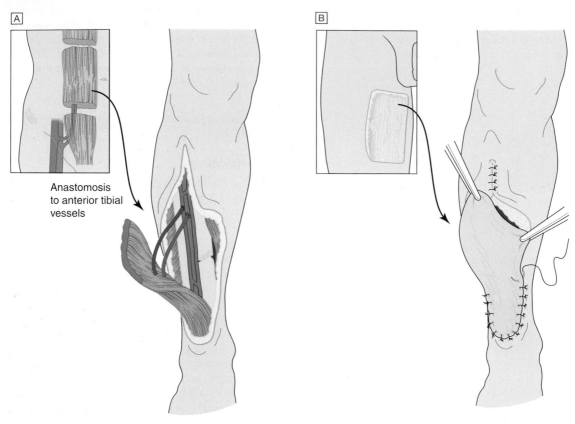

Fig. 22.9 **Example of free tissue transfer based on inferior epigastric vessels.**
Ⓐ Rectus abdominis muscle transferred to shin and its vessels (inferior epigastric vessels) anastomosed to anterior tibial vessels. Ⓑ Muscle covered by split-skin graft.

Table 22.2 EFFECTS OF BURN INJURY
Destruction of tissue
• (Depth depends on heat of causative agent and contact time)
• Loss of barrier to infection
• Fluid loss from surface
• Red cell destruction
Increased capillary permeability
• Oedema
• Loss of circulating fluid volume
• Hypovolaemic shock
Increased metabolic rate

BOX 22.4 CONSEQUENCES OF BURNS
• The morbidity and mortality of burns depend on the site, extent and depth of the burn and on the age and general condition of the patient
Early consequences
• Hypovolaemia (loss of protein, fluid and electrolytes)
• Metabolic derangements (hyponatraemia followed by risk of hypernatraemia, hyperkalaemia followed by hypokalaemia)
• Sepsis, which may be both local and generalized
• Haemolysis with anaemia and need for transfusion
• Hypothermia
Short-term consequences
• Renal failure (acute tubular necrosis due to hypovolaemia, haemoglobinuria and myoglobinuria)
• Respiratory failure (smoke inhalation, airway obstruction, acute respiratory distress syndrome)
• Catabolism and nutritional depletion
• Venous thrombosis
• Curling's ulcer and erosive gastritis
Long-term consequences
• Permanent disfigurement
• Prolonged hospitalization
• Psychological problems
• Impaired function

GENERAL EFFECTS OF BURN INJURY

The general effects of a burn depend upon its size. Large burns lead to water, salt and protein loss, hypovolaemia and increased catabolism. Circulating plasma volume falls as oedema accumulates, and fluid leaks from the burned surface. With large burns, the effect is compounded by a generalized increase in capillary permeability, with widespread oedema. Some red cells are destroyed immediately by a full-thickness burn, but many more are damaged and die later. However, red cell loss is small compared to plasma loss in the early period, and haemoconcentration, reflected by a rising haematocrit, is the norm. The shifts in water and electrolytes are ultimately shared by all body tissues, and if circulatory volume is not restored, hypovolaemic shock ensues. Large burns increase metabolic rate as water losses from the burned surface cause expenditure of calories to provide the heat of evaporation. In severe burns, some 7000 kcal may be expended daily, and a daily weight loss of 0.5 kg is not unusual unless steps are taken to prevent it.

CLASSIFICATION

Burns are classified according to depth as either partial- or full-thickness (Fig. 22.10). In a partial-thickness burn, epithelial cells survive to restore the epidermis. Full-thickness burns destroy all of the epithelial elements.

Superficial partial-thickness burns

Superficial partial-thickness burns involve only the epidermis and the superficial dermis. Pain, swelling and fluid loss can be marked. New epidermal cover is provided by undamaged cells originating from the epidermal appendages. The burn will usually heal in less than 3 weeks, with a perfect final cosmetic result.

Deep partial-thickness burns

In deep partial-thickness (also known as deep-dermal) burns, the epidermis and much of the dermis are destroyed. Restoration of the epidermis then depends on there being intact epithelial cells within the remaining appendages. Pain, swelling and fluid loss are again marked. The burn takes longer than 3 weeks to heal, as fewer epithelial elements survive, and often leaves an ugly hypertrophic scar. Infection often delays healing and can cause further tissue destruction, converting the injury to a full-thickness one.

Full-thickness burns

A full-thickness burn destroys the epidermis and underlying dermis, including the epidermal appendages. The destroyed tissues undergo coagulative necrosis and form an eschar that begins to lift after 2–3 weeks. Unless the raw area is grafted, epidermal cover can only occur through the inward movement and growth of cells from intact skin around the burn, and by contraction of its base. Fibrosis and ugly contracture are thus inevitable in all but small, ungrafted injuries.

Determination of burn depth

There is no foolproof method for the early determination of burn depth; even experienced plastic surgeons may not be able to make an accurate assessment for days or even weeks after injury. However, a number of pointers are valuable.

Mechanisms

Burn depth is proportional to the temperature of the causal agent and to the length of contact time. Scalds from liquids below boiling point usually produce partial-thickness injury, whereas scalds from boiling water and burns due to prolonged contact with hot metal often produce full-thickness damage. Flame burns can be of mixed depth but nearly always include areas of full-thickness loss. Electrical burns are almost always full-thickness, and high-tension electricity can cause devastating necrosis of muscles and other deep tissues.

Appearance

Erythema means that epidermal damage is superficial, and blanching on pressure confirms that dermal capillaries are intact and that the injury is partial-thickness. Blisters are accumulations of fluid superficial to the basal layer of the epidermis and suggest partial-thickness injury. A dead-white appearance frequently indicates full-thickness injury, although at least some of these burns prove to be deep-dermal. A dry, leathery mahogany-coloured eschar with visible thrombosed veins denotes full-thickness destruction.

Sensation

Intact cutaneous sensation implies that the epidermal appendages have survived, as they lie at the same level as cutaneous nerve endings in the dermis. Superficial burns are thus very painful.

PROGNOSIS

Prognosis depends on the following factors.

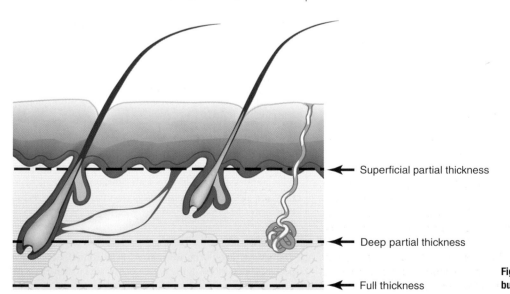

Fig. 22.10 Depth of burn injury.

Superficial partial thickness

Deep partial thickness

Full thickness

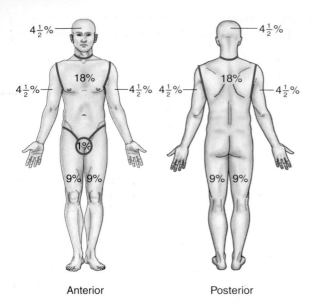

Fig. 22.11 Rule of nines for calculating surface areas of a burn.

Age and general condition

Infants, the elderly, alcoholics and those with other comorbidity fare less well than healthy young adults.

Extent of the burn

The approximate extent of the burn can be quickly calculated in adults by using the 'rule of nines' (Fig. 22.11). Tables are available for more accurate estimations of burn area. The patient's hand and fingers together constitute about 1% of body surface area (BSA). Hypovolaemic shock is anticipated if more than 15% of the surface is burned in adults, or more than 10% in a child. If the sum of an adult patient's age and the percentage area of full-thickness burn comes to more than 80, death is probable. The 'rule of nines' cannot be used in children. This is because of the relatively large head size (about 20% of body surface at birth) and the relatively small limbs (legs are about 13%).

Depth of the burn

Superficial burns of whatever size should heal without scarring within 3 weeks if properly treated. Deep-dermal burns take longer and produce hypertrophic scarring. Full-thickness burns inevitably become infected unless excised early, and in the case of large burns infection may prove life-threatening.

Site of the burn

Burns involving the face, neck, hands, feet or perineum are particularly liable to threaten appearance or function. They require inpatient management.

Associated respiratory injury

This is now extremely common in house fires and usually results from the inhalation of smoke from burning plastic foam upholstery. It is frequently fatal.

Table 22.3 FIRST AID FOR BURNS

• Arrest the burning process
    Extinguish flames
    Remove clothing
    Cool with water
• Ensure adequacy of airway
• Avoid wound contamination
    Clingfilm

Transfer for definitive treatment as soon as possible

MANAGEMENT

First aid

Prompt effective action prevents further damage and may save life or prevent months of suffering. The key principles are to arrest the burning process, ensure an adequate airway and avoid wound contamination (Table 22.3).

Arrest the burning process

Burning clothing is extinguished by smothering the flames in a coat or carpet. The victim is laid flat to avoid flames rising to the head and neck, with inhalation of smoke and fumes. Heat within clothing can continue to burn for many seconds after flames have been extinguished; clothing must therefore be removed or doused with cold water. The same applies to clothing soaked in scalding water, which will continue to cause damage until removed. Cool water is an excellent analgesic and dissipates heat, but common sense must be applied; immersing a child in cold water or covering a patient with cold soaks can cause hypothermia. Cooling counteracts the heat of a burn only if applied immediately after injury. Chemical burns require copious irrigation. If the eyes are involved, prompt and prolonged irrigation may save the patient's sight. Electrical burning is arrested by switching off the current, not by pulling the patient free. If this is not feasible, the patient should be pushed free from the contact using a non-conductor such as a wooden chair.

Ensure an adequate airway

The patient must be moved as quickly as possible into a smoke-free atmosphere. Smoke and fumes can cause asphyxia, often contain poisons and can precipitate respiratory arrest. Mouth-to-mouth ventilation is commenced, if necessary. If cardiac arrest follows electrocution, resuscitation is instituted.

Avoid wound contamination

The burn should be covered with a clean sheet or Clingfilm. Traditional household remedies must be avoided. At best they are messy and interfere with subsequent care; at worst they are destructive, converting a partial injury to a full-thickness one.

Transfer to hospital

The patient should be transferred to hospital as quickly as possible, unless the burn is obviously trivial. Severe burns are best treated in a specialized burns unit from the outset. Hypovolaemia takes time to become manifest and it is easy to misjudge the severity of injury, thereby missing the opportunity for uncomplicated early transfer. Patients embarking on a journey expected to take more than 30 minutes should be accompanied by a trained person. An intravenous infusion should be commenced if the burn is extensive. Transfer of patients with large burns between hospitals should be avoided between 8 and 24 hours after injury. Full-thickness burns are often relatively painless. Partial-thickness injuries can be excruciating and opiates are usually needed. Analgesics must be given intravenously and the dose and route of administration noted.

Adequate ventilation

On arrival at hospital, the maintenance of an adequate airway remains the first priority. Lack of respiratory symptoms on admission is no guarantee that the patient will remain free from airway problems. Every patient who has been exposed to smoke in a closed room should be admitted for observation. Respiratory tract injury is suggested by dyspnoea, cough, hoarseness, cyanosis, coarse crepitations on auscultation, and the presence of soot particles around the nostrils, in the mouth or in the sputum. Endotracheal intubation is advisable if there is anxiety about airway patency, and assisted ventilation may be needed. Tracheostomy is never undertaken lightly in view of the danger of infection of burned tissues around the stoma.

Initial assessment and management

Once airway patency is assured, the time of injury, the type of burn, its previous treatment, and its extent and depth are established. If the burn is over 15% in extent (10% in children), establishing an intravenous infusion takes priority over a detailed history and physical examination. Intravenous therapy may be needed for many days, but there may be few veins available and they must be treated with great respect. It is best to start with the most peripheral vein available in the upper limb, but in shocked patients with vasoconstriction, cannulation of the internal jugular or subclavian vein may be needed. Blood is withdrawn for cross-matching and for determination of haematocrit and urea and electrolyte concentrations. Arterial blood gas analyses are performed and carboxyhaemoglobin levels measured if there is concern about the airway and smoke inhalation. Once an infusion has been established, the pulse rate, blood pressure and core/peripheral temperature difference are monitored. In patients with burns of more than 20%, a catheter is inserted to measure hourly urine output. Severe pain is relieved by intravenous opiates. Tetanus can complicate burns, and tetanus toxoid is given if the patient has not received it recently. In general, patients with burns involving more than 5% of body surface should be admitted to hospital, as should all those with significant full-thickness injury or burns in sites likely to pose particular management problems.

Prevention and treatment of burn shock

The aim of management is to prevent hypovolaemic shock by prompt and adequate fluid replacement (Table 22.4).

Table 22.4   HYPOVOLAEMIC SHOCK AND BURNS
• Anticipate if burn more extensive than 15% (10% in children)
• Prevent by early intravenous resuscitation
• Control pain by adequate intravenous administration of opiates
• Fluid requirements assessed from patient's response
'Formulae' for fluid replacement provide rough guides only

Opinions vary as to the relative amounts of colloid and crystalloid that should be used. Various formulae are available to help calculate replacement needs, but all are merely guides and the amounts of fluid given must be adjusted in the light of the patient's response to resuscitation. In a formula commonly used in the UK, the first 36 hours after injury are divided into six successive periods of 4, 4, 4, 6, 6 and 12 hours. The volume of colloid—for example, purified protein solution (PPS)—to be infused in each period is calculated from the equation:

$$\text{Burn area } (\%) \times \text{body weight (kg)}/2$$

i.e. 0.5 ml/kg for each 1 per cent burn. The need for fluid is greatest in the early hours, but excessive losses may persist for 36–48 hours.

Recently, there has been a tendency to resuscitate major burns using crystalloids rather than colloid. The Parkland formula is now widely used. The fluid volume in millilitres over the first 24 hours is 4 times the weight in kg × %BSA. Half of that volume is given in the first 8 hours, the remainder over the next 16 hours.

Despite renal retention of sodium after injury, there is a tendency to hyponatraemia in the first 2–3 days owing to the secretion of antidiuretic hormone and the sequestration of sodium in oedema. As inflammatory oedema is reabsorbed, the serum sodium concentration returns to normal, and unless water intake is maintained, there is now a danger of hypernatraemia. Tissue destruction releases large amounts of potassium into the extracellular fluid (ECF), but hyperkalaemia is largely prevented by increased renal excretion as part of the metabolic response to injury. Once the first few days have passed, continuing potassium losses can produce hypokalaemia in a patient unable to eat and drink normally.

Water replacement

Daily water losses are replaced using 5% dextrose solution, taking care to avoid water intoxication, especially in young children, in the first few days following injury. Excessive evaporation continues until the burn has re-epithelialized, and a high water intake must be maintained. Although most patients are thirsty, paralytic ileus may occur during the first 48 hours in those with very large burns, so that giving oral fluids too soon can cause gastric distension, vomiting and aspiration. Most patients are able to drink normally after 48 hours and should be encouraged to do so.

Blood transfusion

Blood should not be given in the first 24 hours but may be needed thereafter in patients with large full-thickness burns. Continuing red cell destruction in deep burns with bone

22

marrow suppression can necessitate repeated transfusion. Haemoglobin concentration and haematocrit should be monitored regularly.

Organ failure and burn shock

Organ failure and shock are discussed in detail in Chapter 3, and only those respiratory and renal problems specific to burn shock are considered here.

Respiratory complications

Inhalation of smoke and fumes can cause direct heat damage, carbon monoxide poisoning and damage from other chemicals, all of which predispose to infection. Patients with head and neck burns are best nursed sitting up to encourage the dispersal of oedema. Continued observation is mandatory and physiotherapy is essential to clear bronchial secretions. Chest X-rays and blood gas analyses are repeated regularly in patients with ventilation problems. Arterial hypoxaemia and carbon monoxide poisoning require oxygen therapy, and may necessitate early endotracheal intubation and assisted ventilation. Antibiotics should be prescribed. Tracheostomy is occasionally unavoidable despite the problems associated with its management. Encircling eschar impairing chest or abdominal expansion must be incised (escharotomy) or excised.

Renal failure

Acute tubular necrosis may complicate extensive burns, especially in the elderly, those with pre-existing renal disease and those who develop haemoglobinaemia or myoglobinuria. These pigments appear in the urine after massive red cell destruction or extensive muscle damage (particularly after electrical injury), and can damage the tubules and obstruct urine flow by forming casts. Hourly urine output should be maintained at 30–50 ml in adults. Falling output reflects inadequate resuscitation or impending renal failure (acute tubular necrosis). Measurement of urine osmolality and the response to a test infusion will distinguish between them. Diuretics are used only if oliguria persists despite adequate fluid replacement, when 20% mannitol (1 g/kg) may be infused over 30 minutes.

Nutritional management

Evaporation from open wounds and sepsis is an important cause of increased energy expenditure following a severe burn. Energy expenditure can be reduced by nursing in an environmental temperature of 30–32°C. A high-calorie intake is impractical during the period of hypovolaemic shock, but is encouraged as soon as the patient can drink. The daily caloric intake in adults can be calculated as 20 kcal/kg body weight plus 70 kcal/per cent burn. It is particularly important to provide sufficient protein intake (1 g/kg body weight plus 3 g/per cent burn). In large burns oral intake can usually be supplemented at 48 hours by enteral feeding using a fine-bore nasogastric tube. If the patient's total calculated energy and protein requirements are supplied in this way, weight loss can be limited to less than 10%. Vitamin supplements and iron must also be provided. It is unusual, and often considered undesirable, to use parenteral nutrition in burned patients.

Sepsis

Septicaemia is a constant threat until skin cover has been fully restored, as resistance to infection is low. The wound provides a reservoir of infecting organisms. Catheters, cannulae and tracheostomy wounds are all potential sources of infection. The incidence of septicaemia has been reduced by topical antibacterial agents and early excision and grafting. However, in large burns the risk remains high. Regular monitoring by means of blood cultures is advisable. Systemic antibiotics are not prescribed routinely for fear of producing superinfection with resistant organisms. Their use is reserved for invasive infection and for patients with positive blood cultures.

Curling's ulcer and gastric erosions

Acute duodenal ulceration (Curling's ulcer) and multiple gastric erosions may follow major burns. Early resumption of feeding reduces their incidence, and H_2-receptor antagonists such as ranitidine are prescribed prophylactically.

Local management of burns

Care of the burn wound commences at the time of injury and continues until epithelial cover has been restored. Infection poses the main threat to life once the first 48 hours have passed.

Initial cleansing and debridement

The wound is cleansed meticulously with a mild detergent containing antiseptic and saline as soon as possible after admission. Adherent clothing and loose devitalized tissues are removed. Cleansing must be carried out in an operating theatre or clean dressing room using aseptic technique. Blisters are punctured and serum expressed. Broken blisters are completely deroofed. General anaesthesia may be necessary, but in most cases pain can be relieved by intravenous opiates. In shocked patients, the wound is covered with a sterile drape and further local care is postponed until the circulatory state has stabilized.

Prevention of contamination

Destruction of the epidermis removes the normal barrier to infection. In full-thickness injury, thrombosis of cutaneous vessels impairs the normal response to infection. In large burns, both cellular and humoral immune mechanisms are depressed. Organisms readily colonize the burn wound. If dead tissue is present, they multiply rapidly and invade the surrounding tissues. Staphylococci remain by far the most common infecting organism. *Pseudomonas aeruginosa* remains troublesome in most burn units. Haemolytic streptococci are feared because they can convert superficial into deep burns, and can cause a severe systemic illness.

Once contaminating organisms have been cleared, further contamination can be prevented in a number of ways. The methods described below are not mutually exclusive, and more than one may be used as the patient's needs alter. All dressings are applied using meticulous aseptic technique.

Exposure

After cleansing and debridement, burns to a single surface may be exposed to the air. Evaporation of the protein-rich exudate leaves a dry, adherent crust that is an effective barrier to bacteria as long as it remains intact. Exposure is particularly useful for burns to the face and neck, but can also be used on the trunk and extremities.

Evaporative dressings

These dressings prevent contamination, allow exudate to evaporate and provide comfortable support. After initial cleansing, the wound is covered by a layer of sterile non-adherent dressing, e.g. paraffin gauze or Mepotil, a layer of cotton gauze swabs, a bulky layer of cotton wool or Gamgee, and an outer retaining crepe bandage. The dressing is reviewed daily but left in place for 8–10 days, unless exudate soaks through to the outside.

Semi-occlusive and occlusive dressings

Clingfilm is useful in first aid, but leaks and is too messy for use as a definitive dressing. OpSite is an adhesive film that is effective for small burns; it may also leak initially, and should be covered with a well-padded dressing for 48 hours, after which time it can be patched or replaced as necessary. Many new dressings are now available. Hydrogels and hydrocolloids absorb exudates but offer no particular advantages in acute management. Commercial polythene bags are cheap, sterile when taken from the roll, and useful for treating superficial hand burns. The hands are smeared with liquid paraffin for the first 24–48 hours until a decision as to depth is made. If the decision is made to continue with a conservative regimen, then silver sulfadiazine cream (Flamazine) is applied. The bags are kept in place with a bandage at the wrist. They must be changed at least daily after washing the hand and reapplying the antibacterial cream. Such 'hand bags' allow the patient to continue to use the hand and so prevent stiffness.

Topical antibacterial agents

Silver sulfadiazine cream and povidone-iodine (Betadine) are valuable local antibacterial agents for large burns. To be effective, they must be reapplied daily. They are not necessary or cost-effective for minor burns given proper initial surgical debridement and the use of evaporative dressings.

'Biological' dressings

Freeze-dried xenografts such as porcine skin can be reconstituted for use as temporary occlusive 'biological' dressings, but are very expensive. Amnion or stored homograft skin is now used rarely because of the danger of infection with human immunodeficiency virus (HIV). Sheets of keratinocytes grown in tissue culture are fragile and easily destroyed by infection, limitations which may be overcome in the future by growing the cells on sheets of collagen or synthetic 'dermis'.

Relief of constriction (escharotomy)

The danger of progressive respiratory embarrassment from encircling eschar has already been mentioned. Increasing oedema beneath encircling eschar in the limbs may also imperil the circulation. Relieving incisions (escharotomy), which run from the top to the bottom of circumferential deep burns, may be needed in the first few hours after injury. As these wounds can bleed profusely, it is important to have available methods for controlling haemorrhage, e.g. diathermy and dressings.

Restoration of epidermal cover

Full-thickness and deep-dermal burns of less than 10% are suitable for primary excision of eschar and grafting under general anaesthesia within 48–72 hours of injury. Tangential excision is used for deep-dermal burns. The dead outer layers of skin are shaved away down to the deep-dermal layer and a split-skin graft is applied immediately. More extensive burns can be partially excised and grafted soon after injury, and the remaining areas of skin destruction treated by delayed grafting. After some 2 weeks, eschar begins to separate spontaneously. The process is accelerated by infection and delayed by topical antibacterial agents. As the slough separates, healthy granulation tissue should be revealed, and when all the slough has gone or has been excised, the burn should be ready for grafting. Haemolytic streptococci are a troublesome cause of graft loss, and when such infection is present, grafting must be deferred until the patient has been treated with intravenous penicillin and barrier nursed until three successive wound swabs are negative.

Free skin grafts may be full- or partial-thickness (split-skin), but only split-skin grafts are used to cover acute burns. The grafts may vary in thickness from epidermis only to almost full-thickness; medium-thickness grafts are most commonly used. The donor site forms a new epidermis from residual islands of epithelium, and more skin can be harvested after 14 days. Excess skin can be stored at 4°C for up to 3 weeks.

Full-thickness grafts are used for secondary reconstruction in cosmetically important areas where contraction has to be avoided, or in areas such as the palm of the hands that are subject to repeated trauma.

Functional and cosmetic result

With energetic treatment, it is usually possible to restore skin cover to even the most extensive injury within 3 months, but wound closure is not the end-point. Skin grafts and donor sites must be kept soft and supple by applying moisturizing cream several times a day for many months. Splints may be needed to prevent contractures, and physiotherapy is essential to mobilize joints. Elastic pressure garments help to prevent the build-up of hypertrophic scars. In spite of all this care, reconstructive procedures may be required for many years to correct contractures or rebuild missing or distorted features. Severely burned patients often have difficulty coming to terms with their disfigurement

---

BOX 22.5 KEY QUESTIONS WHEN EXAMINING SKIN SWELLINGS

- Is the swelling located in the skin or in the subcutaneous tissues, i.e. can the overlying skin be pinched up and moved independently of the swelling?
- Is the swelling epidermal or dermal? Epithelial swellings create irregularity of skin surface, whereas dermal swellings do not
- Is the swelling pigmented? Pigmentation most often (although not always) indicates melanocytic activity

and limitations to their way of life. Long-term support, with counselling from surgeon and supporting staff, is invaluable.

SKIN AND SOFT TISSUE LESIONS

DIAGNOSIS OF SKIN SWELLINGS

In addition to describing the site and size of the lesion, it is necessary to determine whether it arises from the skin or is deep to it. If it comes from the skin, then it arises from either the epidermis or the dermis. Surface changes indicate an epidermal origin, whereas the surface is stretched over dermal lesions but remains normal. Ulceration may occur later as a result of pressure necrosis. The colour of a skin lesion is also an important feature in its diagnosis.

CYSTS

Sebaceous cysts

Sebaceous (or epidermoid) cysts are dermal swellings covered by epidermis (Fig. 22.12). They have a thin wall of flattened epidermal cells and contain cheesy white epithelial debris and sebum. They form soft smooth hemispherical swellings over which the skin cannot be moved. A small surface punctum is often visible. If infection supervenes, the cyst becomes hot, red and painful. Infected cysts are incised to allow the infected material to escape. Excision is deferred until the inflammation has settled. In some cases, the inflammation destroys the cyst lining so that excision is not necessary.

Dermoid cysts

Dermoid cysts arise from nests of epidermal cells that have been sequestered in the dermis during development or implanted as a result of trauma. Congenital dermoid cysts are found at sites of embryonic fusion, notably on the face, the base of the nose, the forehead and the occiput. External angular dermoid is the most common congenital dermoid cyst and lies at the junction of the outer and upper margins

Table 22.5 CLASSIFICATION OF SKIN TUMOURS	
Cell/tissue of origin	**Type of tumour**
EPIDERMAL NEOPLASMS (COMMON)	
From basal germinal cells	Papilloma
	Infective wart
	Senile wart
	Pedunculated papilloma
	Keratoacanthoma
	Premalignant keratosis
	Carcinoma in situ
	Epidermoid cancer
	Basal cell cancer (rodent ulcer)
	Squamous cell cancer
From melanocytes	Benign pigmented mole
	Common mole
	Giant hairy mole
	Blue naevus
	Halo naevus
	Malignant melanoma
	Melanotic freckle (lentigo maligna)
	Superficial spreading melanoma
	Nodular melanoma
	Other forms of melanoma
DERMAL NEOPLASMS (RARE)	Fibroma
	Lipoma
	Neurofibroma

of the orbit, in the line of fusion of the maxilla and frontal bones. Implantation dermoid cysts are found at sites of injury, notably the palmar surfaces of the hands and fingers. They are lined by squamous epithelium and contain sebum, degenerate cells and, in some cases, hair. A soft rubbery swelling forms deep to the skin. The cyst may be fixed deeply, particularly when situated on the face. Implantation dermoids can be removed under local anaesthesia. Congenital dermoids usually require formal dissection under general anaesthesia, as they may extend deeply; for example, an external angular dermoid can extend within the cranium.

TUMOURS OF THE SKIN

Skin tumours may arise from the epidermis or the dermis (Table 22.5). Epidermal tumours are common and can arise from basal germinal cells or melanocytes. Dermal tumours arising from connective tissue elements are rare. The remainder of this section will be devoted to the more common epidermal neoplasms.

EPIDERMAL NEOPLASMS ARISING FROM BASAL GERMINAL CELLS

Papillomas

Papillomas (or warts) are common benign skin neoplasms.

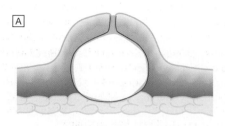

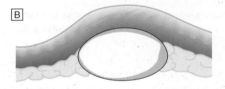

Fig. 22.12 Types of cyst.
[A] Sebaceous (epidermoid). [B] Dermoid.

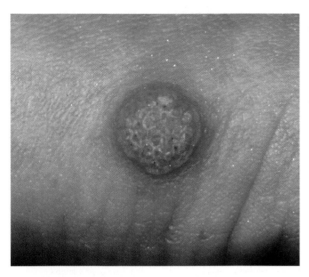

Fig. 22.13 Verruca vulgaris.
Infective warts affecting the hands.

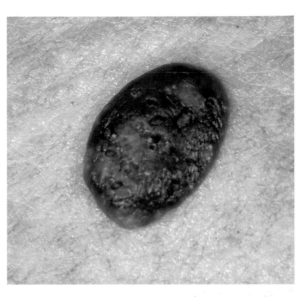

Fig. 22.15 Senile wart or seborrhoeic keratosis.

22

Infective warts

These are common and caused by viral infection. They are found most commonly on the hands and fingers of young children and adults. They spread by direct inoculation and are often multiple. They form greyish-brown, round or oval elevated lesions with a filiform surface and keratinized projections (Fig. 22.13), and may be studded with spots of blood. They often regress spontaneously but can be removed by caustics (acetic acid) or freezing (liquid nitrogen or CO_2 snow). Plantar warts (verruca plantaris) are particularly troublesome infective warts acquired in swimming pools and showers. They are found under the heel and metatarsal heads. They are flush with the surface (Fig. 22.14) and may be intensely painful. If persistent, they are treated by curettage or freezing. Infective warts in the perineum and on the penis may be of venereal origin and are associated with gonorrhoea, syphilis, HIV infection and lymphogranuloma. Infective warts are also common in immunosuppressed patients.

Senile warts

These are basal cell papillomas and are common in the elderly (Fig. 22.15). They form a yellowish-brown or black greasy plaque (synonym: seborrhoeic keratosis) with a cracked surface that falls off in pieces. Senile warts are often multiple, commonly affect the upper back and trunk, and are best treated by curettage.

Pedunculated papillomas

These simple non-infective papillomas form a flesh-coloured spherical warty mass on a stalk of normal epithelium. If small, they can be dealt with by grasping with fine forceps, pulling out from the skin surface and cutting off with scissors; a stitch is rarely required. If they are large, the papilloma and its pedicle are removed formally with an ellipse of normal skin.

Keratoacanthoma (molluscum sebaceum)

This lesion can be confused with squamous cancer because of its clinical appearance. It grows rapidly over 4–6 weeks and then involutes. Histologically, it has a well-defined 'shoulder', but even under the microscope it may resemble a squamous carcinoma. The distinction between the two is the history. Keratoacanthoma occurs most commonly on the face as a hemispherical nodule with a friable red centre crusted with keratin (Fig. 22.16). It is found mainly in those over 50 years of age. It heals after shedding its central core, but can also be eradicated by curettage.

Actinic (solar) keratosis

This is a premalignant keratosis and is characterized by small, single or multiple, firm warty spots on the face, back of the neck and hands (Fig. 22.17). Such keratoses are particularly common in older, fair-skinned people who have been exposed to excessive sunlight. The scaly lesions drop off periodically to leave a shallow premalignant ulcer. The keratoses should be biopsied to exclude frank malignancy, and then treated by freezing.

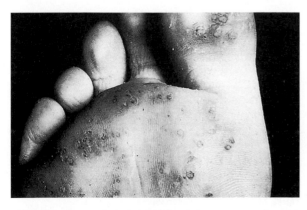

Fig. 22.14   Verruca plantaris (plantar warts).
A plaque of closely grouped warts on the sole of the foot.

22

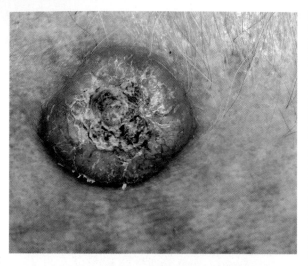

Fig. 22.16 Keratoacanthoma affecting the temple of an elderly man.

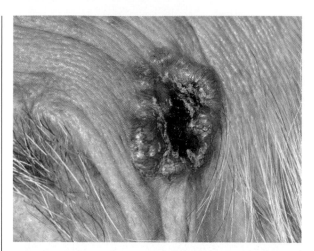

Fig. 22.18 Basal cell carcinoma (rodent ulcer).
Note the raised pearly edge.

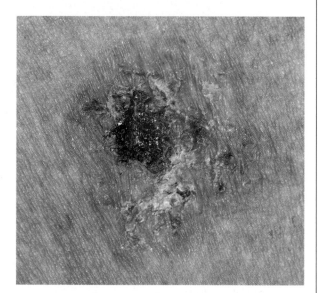

Fig. 22.17 Actinic keratosis.

Intraepidermal cancer (carcinoma in situ)

This non-invasive form of skin cancer forms a discrete, often solitary, raised brown or red fissured plaque which is keratinized. Histologically, the plaques are composed of hyperplastic atypical epithelial cells, but there is no evidence of invasion through the basement membrane. Intraepidermal skin cancer is also known as Bowen's disease and, when it affects the penis or vulva, as erythroplasia of de Queyrat.

Cancer of the epidermis

Epidermal cancer occurs primarily on exposed areas and in those with poor natural protection against sunlight. Albinos and patients with xeroderma pigmentosa (a congenital defect leading to undue sensitivity to sunlight) are at particularly high risk, whereas skin cancer is rare in black-, brown- and yellow-skinned races. Chronic skin irritation by chemicals (e.g. arsenic, tar and soot), chronic ulceration

(e.g. old burns or varicose ulcers) and exposure to other forms of radiation are also established causes. Epidermoid cancer is particularly common in those over 50 years of age. There are two distinct pathological forms: basal cell and squamous cell carcinoma.

Basal cell carcinoma (rodent ulcer)

Rodent ulcers are slow-growing and locally invasive; for all practical purposes, they never metastasize. They almost all arise in the skin of the middle third of the face, typically on the nose, inner canthus of the eye, forehead and eyelids (Fig. 22.18). The earliest lesion is a hard pearly nodule, dimpled in its centre and covered by thin telangiectatic skin. Cystic degeneration may make the lesion raised and translucent. A number of clinical types are recognized, being described as cystic, nodular, sclerosing, morphoeic, centrally healing and 'field fire'. Over a period of years, the rodent ulcer repeatedly scales over and breaks down. Growth is extremely slow. Occasionally, the tumour is highly invasive and can burrow deeply, despite little apparent surface activity. All suspicious lesions must be biopsied. Surgical excision or radiotherapy can be used for definitive

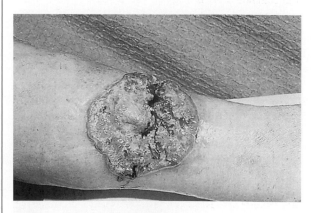

Fig. 22.19 Squamous cell carcinoma.
A warty nodule with induration of the adjacent skin.

treatment, but the latter is contraindicated if the lesion is close to the eye or overlies cartilage. Complex reconstructive surgery may be needed to restore structure and function in patients who present late.

Squamous cell carcinoma

This tumour may affect any area (Fig. 22.19) but is particularly common on exposed parts such as the ear, cheeks, lower lips and backs of the hands. It commonly develops in an area of epithelial hyperplasia or keratosis. In mucosa, such as the lips, the analogous change is leucoplakia. The lesion starts as a hard erythematous nodule, which proliferates to form a cauliflower-like excrescence or ulcerates to form a malignant ulcer with a raised fixed hard edge. The cancer grows more quickly than a rodent ulcer but more slowly than a keratoacanthoma. The regional nodes can be involved early. The choice of treatment (surgery or radiotherapy) depends on the tumour's size, site and aggressiveness. Palpable lymph nodes are an indication for regional lymphadenectomy by block dissection. This may be followed by adjuvant radiotherapy if histology shows extracapsular spread. Chemotherapy is of limited value.

EPIDERMAL NEOPLASMS ARISING FROM MELANOCYTES

Benign pigmented moles

The number of melanocytes is relatively fixed (approximately 2000 million), regardless of the colour of the individual, but the amount of pigment produced obviously varies greatly. As a developmental abnormality, conglomerates of melanocytes may migrate to the dermis or epidermis to form a melanocytic naevus or mole. The naevus cells can cause a variety of pigmented spots and swellings (naevi) according to their site and activity (Fig. 22.20). Moles showing melanocyte activity at the junction of epidermis and dermis (junctional change) are common in childhood; all moles on the soles and palms are of this type. Migration of sheets of naevus cells to the dermis produces a dermal naevus; migration to both dermis and epidermis produces a compound naevus.

Common moles

The common mole is a flat or slightly raised brown-black lesion covered by normal epidermis. It has a period of active growth during childhood as a result of junctional activity, but usually becomes quiescent at puberty and may later atrophy. If naevus cells migrate to the dermis, the lesion becomes firm and raised, and there is often aberrant hair growth. The epidermis remains smooth if it remains uninvolved, but can become soft and roughened in a compound naevus. As only 1 in 100 000 moles becomes malignant, they need not normally be removed. Active growth in childhood need not cause concern, but growth after puberty demands removal. An increase in pigmentation, scaliness, itching and bleeding may also give rise to anxiety about malignancy and indicate the need for excision. Any mole that develops these characteristics should be removed. Further treatment depends on the histological appearances (see below).

Normal

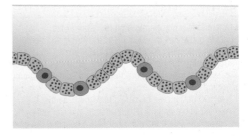

Junctional naevus

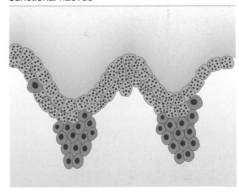

Dermal naevus

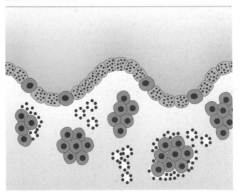

Compound naevus

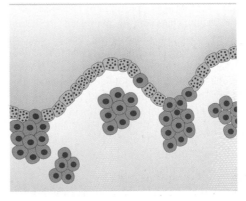

Fig. 22.20   Histopathological types of benign mole.

Giant hairy naevus

Unlike the common mole, this lesion is present at birth. It can cover a large area, which may correspond to a

22

BOX 22.6 EPIDERMAL NEOPLASMS ARISING FROM MELANOCYTES

- A mole is due to a conglomeration of melanocytes
- Melanocyte activity at the junction of epidermis and dermis (i.e. junctional activity) is common in childhood
- Migration of melanocytes into the dermis produces a dermal naevus, while migration to both dermis and epidermis produces a compound naevus
- Only 1 in 100 000 moles becomes malignant, so that the presence of a mole is not in itself an indication for removal. Active growth in childhood need not cause concern, but growth thereafter should
- Excision is indicated if a mole shows an increase in pigmentation, scaliness, itching or bleeding. A 3 mm excision margin is adequate in the first instance

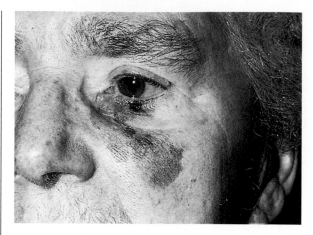

Fig. 22.21 Melanotic freckle on the face of an elderly man.

dermatome. Typical sites are the bathing-trunk area and face. The risk of malignant change is small but such moles should be kept under observation, and in some cases there may be cosmetic indications for excision.

Blue naevus

This intradermal naevus can appear blue because the melanin-containing cells are deep in the dermis. It can develop at any time from birth to middle age.

Halo naevus

This pigmented naevus is surrounded by a white circle of depigmentation associated with lymphocytic infiltration.

Malignant melanoma

Malignant melanomas predominantly affect fair-skinned people. They are rare in blacks but can occasionally affect the depigmented areas such as the palms, soles and mucosa. Exposure to sunlight is the major precipitating factor. In Scotland the incidence is 8 per 100 000 individuals per year, compared to 40 per 100 000 in Queensland, Australia. The incidence has increased world-wide, and in Scotland there has been a 100% increase over the last 10 years. Malignant melanomas are more common in females, with a higher incidence on the legs, presumably because of greater exposure. About half of all malignant melanomas are thought to arise in pre-existing naevi. The average individual has 14 melanocytic naevi and the risk of any one of them becoming malignant is very small. However, the greater the number of moles, the greater the risk, particularly in those with a family history of malignant melanoma. The essential feature of malignant melanoma is invasion of the dermis by proliferating melanocytes with large nuclei, prominent nucleoli and frequent mitoses. Three distinct clinicopathological types of malignant melanoma are described.

Hutchison's melanotic freckle (lentigo maligna)

One in 10 malignant melanomas arises in a melanotic or senile freckle. They occur most commonly on the face of elderly women (Fig. 22.21), beginning as a brown-red patch that grows slowly, advancing and receding over the years. The edge of the lesion appears serrated but its margin with normal skin remains abrupt. Kaleidoscopic pigmentation of the surface is typical. This premalignant phase may last for 10–15 years. The first sign of malignancy is a brownish-red papule that develops eccentrically within the freckle and indicates vertical extension of melanocytes into the dermis in the form of a lentigo maligna melanoma.

Superficial spreading melanoma

This is the most common type of malignant melanoma (Fig. 22.22). It occurs on the trunk and exposed parts, and is most common in middle age. During a pre-invasive phase, which lasts for at most 1 or 2 years, malignant cells spread outwards (horizontal growth phase) in the epidermis in all directions. The surface is slightly raised, the outline is indistinct, pigmentation is patchy and there may be a wide range of colours. Invasion of the dermis (vertical growth phase) occurs while the lesion is still relatively small and produces an indurated nodule, which soon ulcerates or bleeds.

Nodular melanoma

This elevated, deeply pigmented melanoma can occur at any site and at any age. Nodular melanomas are particularly common in females on the leg. They may occur at the site of a pre-existing benign naevus. Nodular melanomas are vertically invasive from the start and there is no initial intra-epidermal spread and therefore no surrounding pigmented macule. The nodule enlarges steadily, both centrifugally and on the surface. Surface spread is detected by the destruction

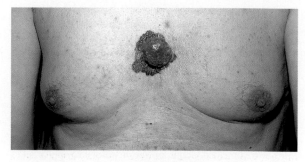

Fig. 22.22 Superficial spreading melanoma.

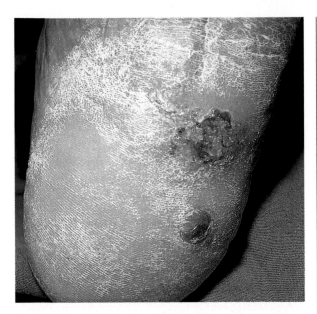

Fig. 22.23 Acral lentiginous melanoma arising on the sole of the foot.

BOX 22.7   MALIGNANT MELANOMA

- Malignant melanoma is predominantly, but not exclusively, a disease of fair-skinned individuals
- Exposure to sunlight is the key aetiological factor
- The lesion is more common in females, reflecting the higher incidence of malignant melanomas of the lower leg
- 50% of all malignant melanomas arise in a pre-existing naevus
- The essential feature of malignancy is invasion of the dermis by proliferating melanocytes (which show large nuclei, prominent nucleoli and frequent mitoses)
- Malignant melanoma spreads rapidly by the lymphatic system and the blood stream. 'In transit' metastases may develop in the lymphatics of the skin and subcutaneous tissues

Table 22.6   PROGNOSIS IN RELATION TO THE STAGE AND DEPTH OF MALIGNANT MELANOMA

Clinical stage	5-year survival rate (%)
I Primary lesion only	70
Breslow depth (mm)	
< 1.5	93
1.5–3.5	60
> 3.5	48
II Primary lesion + regional lymph node or satellite deposit	30
III Metastatic disease	0

of normal skin lines. The lesion darkens progressively and the surface over the area of active growth becomes jet black and glossy. Bleeding may follow trivial injury and is noted as spots of blood on clothes. Crusting, scab formation, itching, irritation and ulceration are typical. Satellite nodules may form around neglected lesions.

Other types of malignant melanoma

Not all melanomas are deeply pigmented. Amelanotic melanomas are rare, pale pink lesions that can grow rapidly. Careful histological examination will demonstrate pigment in virtually every case. Acral lentiginous melanoma is seen on the soles and palms (Fig. 22.23). It resembles superficial spreading melanoma in its behaviour, although the thick skin of the affected regions may mask some of the features and cause late presentation, with nodularity and ulceration. Subungual melanomas typically affect the thumb or great toe of the middle-aged and elderly, causing chronic inflammation beneath the nail. Pigmentation is not usually visible in the early stages and the lesion is often misdiagnosed as a paronychia or ingrowing toenail.

Spread of malignant melanoma

Malignant melanomas spread readily via the lymphatics and blood stream. In transit metastases may develop in the subcutaneous or intracutaneous lymphatics, and form painless discoloured nodules in the line of the lymphatics between the primary and the regional nodes. Lymph node metastases often present as firm enlargement of a node that remains untethered and mobile. The disease then spreads to adjacent regional and central nodes. Blood-borne metastases can occur at any site but are common in the brain, liver, lungs, skin and subcutaneous tissues. Extensive metastatic growth may be associated with the excretion of melanin or its precursor (5-S-cystine L-dopa) in the urine. In about 5% of cases, metastases are present in the absence of a recognizable primary site.

Clinical and pathological staging

Three clinical stages are recognized and staging has major prognostic implications (Table 22.6). For lesions in clinical stage I, the most reliable prognostic indicator is the depth of the lesion (Fig. 22.24); the more superficial the lesion, the better the prognosis. Depth can be measured by reference to the normal layers of skin (Clark) or by a micrometer gauge (Breslow). As the skin layers may be distorted by the tumour, the Breslow system is usually preferred. Mitotic activity also influences prognosis, and tumours can be graded according to the number of mitotic figures in each field. Lymphocytic response and features of regression can also influence prognosis. Melanotic freckles and superficial spreading melanomas tend to remain superficial and so have a better prognosis than nodular melanomas.

Management of malignant melanoma

A biopsy is essential to confirm the diagnosis. Thereafter, the depth and stage of the disease are assessed to define the most appropriate form of treatment. Small pigmented lesions are excised with a margin of 3 mm of normal skin, usually under local anaesthesia. Surgical excision is used to treat stage I lesions. Wide excision with a margin of normal skin of at least 5 cm was once routine but has been shown to be unnecessary, particularly for the more superficial melanomas. Breslow depth is now used as the determinant of clearance margin, using a formula of 1 cm clearance for every millimetre of depth up to 3 cm. A

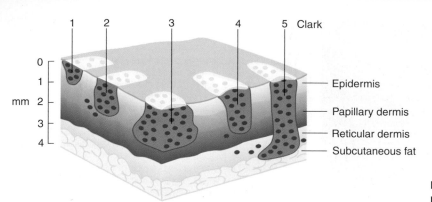

Fig. 22.24 Methods of grading malignant melanoma according to depth of invasion.

smaller margin may be acceptable to avoid mutilation: for example, on the face. The tumour and surrounding skin are excised down to the deep fascia so that the entire depth of subcutaneous fat can be removed. Smaller defects can usually be closed primarily. Large defects have to be covered with a split-skin graft or flap. A block dissection of regional lymph nodes carries significant morbidity and is no longer carried out routinely. However, if the nodes are involved (clinical stage II), or if the primary tumour overlies the nodes, block dissection can be performed at the time of primary surgery. Isolated limb perfusion with cytotoxic drugs can be used in patients with recurrent disease in a single limb. The treatment of metastatic melanoma remains unsatisfactory. The key to the successful management of malignant melanoma is early diagnosis and appropriate surgical excision, with reconstruction as appropriate.

Sentinel lymph node biopsy

This technique is becoming increasingly used in the staging of melanoma. The sentinel lymph node is defined as the first node in the lymphatic basin that drains the lesion and is the node at greatest risk of the development of metastases. Biopsy of this node can assist in staging patients at risk of metastatic disease. Current practice is for patients with a positive sentinel node to proceed to radical node dissection.

BOX 22.8   MANAGEMENT OF MALIGNANT MELANOMA

- The depth of the lesion is a key prognostic factor and can be assessed by micrometer (Breslow) or by reference to normal layers of the skin (Clark). Superficial spreading melanomas and melanotic freckles have a better prognosis than nodular melanomas
- Excision biopsy is essential to confirm malignancy, assess depth and stage, and define the optimal method of treatment
- Once malignancy is confirmed, an excision margin of 1 cm for every 1 mm of Breslow depth is advised. The lesion is excised down to the deep fascia to remove all subcutaneous fat. Skin grafting may be required to close the defect
- Lymph node or satellite deposits reduce 5-year survival rates from 70% to 30%, but patients with distant metastases are not expected to survive for 5 years
- Block dissection of regional lymph nodes is no longer practised routinely but may be indicated if the nodes are obviously involved or located close to the primary lesion

---

As yet, it has not been shown to give any survival advantage but is the subject of ongoing clinical trials.

VASCULAR NEOPLASMS (HAEMANGIOMAS)

The histological classification of haemangiomas is complex and they are best differentiated by their clinical behaviour: that is, whether they regress or persist.

Involuting haemangiomas

These true neoplasms arise from endothelial cells. They appear at or within weeks of birth, and predominantly affect the head and neck. Superficial involuting haemangiomas form a bright-red raised mass with an irregular bosselated surface (strawberry naevus); deeper lesions form a soft, blue-black tumour covered by normal skin. Active growth continues for about 6 months. The tumour then remains static until the child is 2 or 3 years of age, when it shrinks and loses its colour. The lesion usually disappears before the child is 7 years of age and should be left alone unless it involves the periorbital skin.

Non-involuting haemangiomas

These hamartomas are due to abnormal blood vessel formation, and are of two main types.

Port-wine stain

This bright-red patchy lesion often overlies the area of distribution of a peripheral nerve. The lesion neither grows nor involutes, and good cosmetic results can be achieved by laser therapy.

Cavernous haemangioma

This bluish-purple elevated mass appears in early childhood. It empties on pressure and then refills, and histologically consists of mature vein-like structures. It is treated by excision. Cirsoid aneurysm is a variant in which the mass of vein-like structures is fed directly by arterial blood and becomes tortuous, dilated and pulsating. The scalp is a common site and the mass may erode the skull. Penetrating channels may connect the scalp lesion with a similar malformation in the extradural space. Angiography is essential to show the extent of the lesion and outline its arterial supply. Angiographic embolization may be useful prior to ligation of the feeding vessels and excision of the lesion.

TUMOURS OF NERVES

Neurilemmoma

This is an encapsulated solitary benign tumour that origi- nates from the Schwann cells of a nerve sheath and forms a subcutaneous swelling in the course of the nerve. It is laterally mobile but fixed in the direction of the nerve. It may cause radiating pain in the distribution of the involved nerve. Most neurilemmomas occur superficially in the neck or limbs. They grow slowly, have no malignant potential, and are readily treated by excision. Excision can result in loss of nerve function.

Neurofibroma

This is regarded as a hamartoma of nerve tissue. Such lesions may be solitary, but more commonly they are multi- ple in von Recklinghausen's disease (neurofibromatosis). This autosomal disorder is present at birth or becomes apparent in early childhood. Multiple dermal and sub- cutaneous nodules arise from peripheral nerves in asso- ciation with patches of dermal pigmentation ('café au lait' spots). The tumours can cause bony deformities, particularly of the spine. They are potentially malignant, transforming to neurofibrosarcoma. An increase in size of existing swellings, or the appearance of new swellings suggests malignant change.

TUMOURS OF MUSCLE AND CONNECTIVE TISSUES

Lipoma

A lipoma is a slow-growing benign tumour of fatty tissue that forms a lobulated soft mass enclosed by a thin fibrous capsule. Large lipomas rarely undergo sarcomatous change. Although lipomas can occur in the dermis, most arise from the fatty tissue between the skin and deep fascia. Typical features are their soft fluctuant feel, their lobulation, and the free mobility of overlying skin. Lipomas may also arise from fat in the intermuscular septa, where they form a diffuse firm swelling under the deep fascia, which is more prominent when the related muscle is contracted. They may cause discomfort. Unless it is small and asymptomatic, a lipoma should be removed, either by surgical excision or by liposuction.

Liposarcoma

Liposarcoma is the most common sarcoma of middle age. It may occur in any fatty tissue but is most common in the retroperitoneum and legs. Wide surgical excision is recommended but can be difficult for retroperitoneal tumours; post-operative radiotherapy and chemotherapy are advised but are of doubtful worth. Most liposarcomas grow slowly and recurrence may take a long time to develop.

Fibrosarcoma

This tumour arises from fibrous tissue at any site but is most common in the lower limbs or buttocks. It forms a large, deep firm mass. Wide excision is the initial treatment of choice; radiation therapy may be indicated in the palliation of recurrence.

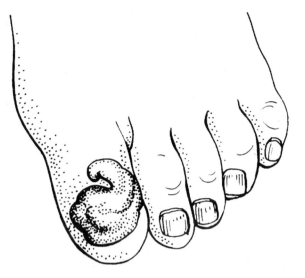

Fig. 22.25   Onychogryphosis.

Rhabdomyosarcoma

This greyish-pink, soft, fleshy lobulated or well- circumscribed tumour arises from striated muscle. It is more common in children, is highly malignant, and requires treatment by radical excision and/or radiotherapy. Amputation of a limb may be unavoidable.

DISORDERS OF THE NAILS

Onychogryphosis (hooked nail)

This overgrowth of the nail resembles an ox or goat horn. The big toenail is most commonly affected (Fig. 22.25). Simple avulsion of the nail does not prevent recurrence, and excision of the nailbed is required. A flap of skin is reflected from the base of the nail and the germinal layer removed. Care must be taken to excise the edges of this layer completely or troublesome spikes of nail continue to grow. An alternative to excision of the nailbed is to cauterize it with phenol.

Ingrowing toenail

This is caused by the sharp edges of the nail impinging on the surrounding skin folds (Fig. 6.8). The skin is split and infection follows. The condition is painful and made worse by misguided attempts to cut the nail back at the corners. The patient usually comes for help once infection has occurred. An attempt is made to 'lift out' the ingrowing portion of the nail with a pledget of gauze soaked in antiseptic. The patient is then instructed to cut the nail square, or shorter in the centre than at the edges, and to avoid wearing narrow shoes. Once infection has spread under the nail or the nail has become deeply embedded, it is best to avulse it under general anaesthesia. Antiseptic footbaths then allow the infection to resolve rapidly. The patient is instructed on the correct way to cut the new nail. If the condition recurs, the nailbed must be ablated surgically or with phenol (Fig. 22.26).

22

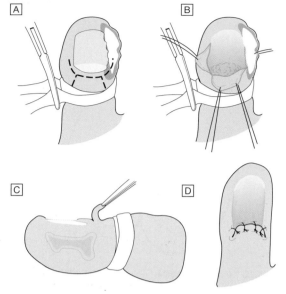

Fig. 22.26   Operation for ablation of the nailbed.
A Skin incision. B Nail avulsed and skin flaps raised. C Excision of nailbed. D Skin flaps sutured.

Nailfold infections (paronychia)

Pain, redness and swelling at the side and base of a nail are the first signs of paronychia. This may extend around the nail to produce a horseshoe swelling of the nailfold. Extension under the nail and into the underlying pulp space may occur (Fig. 22.27). A minor paronychia will usually

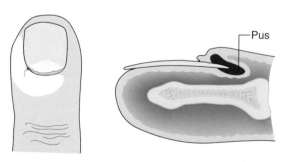

Fig. 22.27   Paronychia.
The longitudinal section shows the relation of pus to the nailbed.

EBM 22.1   BURNS

'Mortality is related to the size (% body surface area, BSA) and age of the patient.

$$\text{Mortality} = \frac{\%\text{BSA} + \text{age}}{100}$$

Large burns > 15% in adults (> 10% in children) require intravenous resuscitation.'

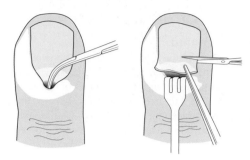

Fig. 22.28   Surgical treatment of paronychia.

resolve spontaneously, but if the infection is spreading, an antibiotic should be prescribed. The development of a tense shiny swelling indicates suppuration and the need for surgical drainage. A single unilateral incision may suffice, but if the infection extends under the nail, a flap of skin should be reflected from the nailbase, which is then excised to allow free drainage (Fig. 22.28). A simple Vaseline gauze dressing is applied. Failure of an acute paronychia to resolve leads to chronic thickening of the nailfold. Fungal infection is a common cause of chronic paronychia, and nail scrapings are essential for diagnosis. The possibility of a subungual melanoma must always be kept in mind.

EBM 22.2   MELANOMA

'Health-care professionals and members of the public should be aware of the risk factors for melanoma.'
'A superficial shave biopsy should not be carried out on suspicious pigmented lesions.'
'Excision margins for primary melanoma:
　< 1 mm ⇓ 1 cm
　1–2 mm ⇓ 1–2 cm
　2–4 mm ⇓ 2 cm
　> 4 mm ⇓ 2 cm'
'Elective lymph node dissection should not be carried out routinely in patients with primary melanoma.'
'Sentinel lymph node biopsy should be considered as a staging technique in appropriate patients, i.e. primary ≥ 1 mm or < 1 mm but Clark level 4.'

23

J.M. DIXON

The breast

ANATOMY AND PHYSIOLOGY

OVERVIEW

The breast is an appendage of skin and is a modified sweat gland. It is composed of glandular tissue, fibrous or supporting tissue, and fat. The functional unit of the breast is the terminal duct lobular unit, and any secretions produced in the terminal duct lobular unit drain towards the nipple into 12–15 major subareolar ducts. Although often described as being segmental like an orange, the glandular and ductal structures of the breast interweave to form a composite mass. In the resting state, the terminal duct lobular unit secretes watery fluid that is reabsorbed as it passes through the ductules and ducts. This rarely reaches the surface of the nipple because the nipple ducts are blocked or plugged by keratin. If the keratin becomes dislodged, then this physiological secretion can be seen on the surface of the nipple. It varies in colour from white to yellow to green to blue/black, and can be produced in up to two-thirds of non-pregnant women by gentle cleaning of the nipple and massage of the breast.

ANATOMY

The breast lies between the skin and the pectoral fascia, to which it is loosely attached. It extends from the clavicle superiorly down on to the abdominal wall, where it extends over the rectus abdominis, external oblique and serratus anterior muscles. The axillary tail of the breast runs between the pectoral muscles and latissimus dorsi to blend with the axillary fat. The breast is supplied by the lateral thoracic artery or the lateral thoracic branch of the axillary artery superolaterally, and by perforating branches of the internal mammary artery superomedially. The functioning unit of the breast, the terminal duct lobular unit, is lined, as are the draining ducts, by a single layer of columnar epithelial cells surrounded by myoepithelial cells. The major subareolar ducts in their terminal portion are lined by stratified squamous epithelium.

The main route of lymphatic spread of breast cancer is to the axillary nodes, which are situated below the axillary vein. On average, there are 20 nodes in the axilla below the axillary vein (Fig. 23.1). These are separated into three levels by their relation to the pectoralis minor muscle. Nodes lateral to the pectoralis minor are considered level I, those beneath are classified as level II, and the nodes medial to pectoralis minor are level III. Level I nodes, which are nearest the breast, are usually affected first by breast cancer. In less than 5% of patients, levels II or III nodes are involved without level I nodes being affected. Lymph also drains to the internal mammary nodes. Occasionally, the main route of lymph drainage of a cancer is to the interpectoral nodes situated between the pectoralis major and minor muscles.

CONGENITAL ABNORMALITIES

These are most commonly the result of persistent extramammary portions of the breast ridge. In the sixth week of embryonal development, a bilateral ridge called the 'milk line' develops and extends from the axilla to the groin. Segments coalesce into nests of cells and, in humans, all

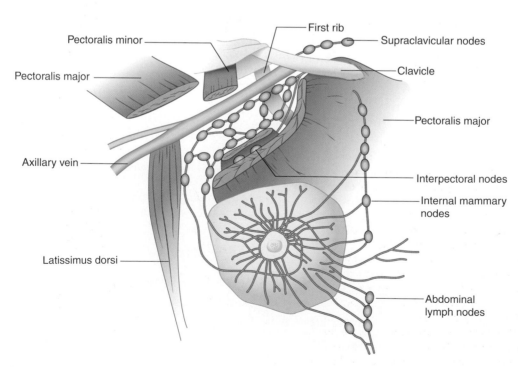

Fig. 23.1   Lymph node drainage of the breast.

but one of these nests opposite the fifth intercostal space disappear. In 1–5% of people, one or more of the other nests persists as supernumerary or accessory nipples or, less frequently, as breasts. The most common site for an accessory nipple is in the milk line between the normal breast and the umbilicus; the most common site for an accessory breast is the lower axilla. Supernumerary nipples or breasts rarely require treatment unless they are unsightly. Accessory breast tissue is subject to the same diseases found in normally placed breasts.

Some degree of breast asymmetry is normal, the left usually being the larger of the two. One breast can be absent or hypoplastic, and this is often associated with pectoral muscle defects. Some patients have abnormalities of the pectoralis muscle and absence or hypoplasia of the breast, associated with a characteristic deformity of the upper limb; this cluster of anomalies is called Poland's syndrome. Abnormalities of the chest wall, such as pectus excavatum and scoliosis of the thoracic spine, can make normal breasts look asymmetric. True asymmetry can be treated by augmentation of the smaller breast, reduction or elevation of the larger breast, or a combination of the two.

HORMONAL CONTROL OF BREAST DEVELOPMENT AND FUNCTION

Enlargement of the breast bud in the first week or two of life occurs in approximately 60% of newborn babies; the gland may reach several centimetres in size before regressing. This is because circulating maternal oestrogens cause one or both breasts to enlarge and secrete a colostrum-like fluid (witch's milk) from the nipple. The swelling usually subsides within a few weeks and the breasts then normally remain dormant until puberty, when the onset of cyclical hormonal activity stimulates growth.

The life cycle of the breast consists of three main periods: development (and early reproductive life), mature reproductive life and involution. Development occurs at puberty and involves proliferation of ducts and ductules associated with very rudimentary lobule formation. The breast then undergoes regular changes in relation to the menstrual cycle. During pregnancy, the breast approximately doubles in weight, and lobules and ducts proliferate in preparation for milk production. Lobular development only becomes marked during pregnancy. Milk production during pregnancy is inhibited by ovarian and placental steroids. Delivery reduces the amount of circulating oestrogen and increases the sensitivity of the breast epithelium to prolactin. Suckling stimulates the release of prolactin and oxytocin, with oxytocin stimulating the myoepithelial cells to eject milk into the terminal ducts. By the age of 30, ageing or involution is evident and continues to the menopause and beyond. During involution, glandular tissue and fibrous tissue atrophy and the shape of the breasts changes as they become more ptotic or droopy. Microscopic changes in the glandular tissue that occur during involution include fibrosis, the formation of small cysts (microcysts) and a focal increase in the number of glandular elements (adenosis). These changes were previously considered abnormal and were called fibrocystic disease or fibroadenosis. However, they occur as part of normal breast ageing or involution and should not be considered as disease.

EVALUATION OF THE PATIENT WITH BREAST DISEASE

CLINICAL FEATURES

Approximately 25% of all surgical referrals relate to breast problems. In the UK, 1 in 4 women will attend a breast clinic, and 1 in 10 will develop breast cancer at some point in their lives. The most common symptoms are a breast lump, which may or may not be painful; an area of lumpiness; pain alone; nipple discharge; nipple retraction; a strong family history of breast cancer; breast distortion; swelling or inflammation; or a scaling nipple or eczema. The most important pointer to the diagnosis is the age of the patient. Although malignant disease can occur in young women, benign conditions are much more common. The duration of any symptom is important; breast cancers usually grow slowly, but cysts may appear overnight. Details of risk factors, including family history and current medication, can be obtained using a simple questionnaire that the patient can complete while waiting to be seen in the outpatient clinic.

CLINICAL EXAMINATION

The patient is asked to undress to the waist and sit facing the examiner. Inspection should take place in good light with the patient's arms by her side, above her head, and then pressing on her hips (Fig. 23.2). Skin dimpling or a change

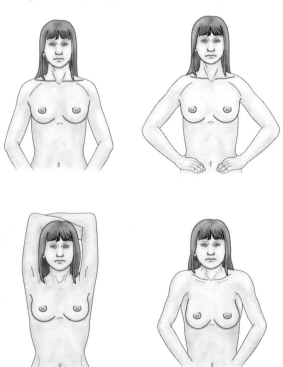

Fig. 23.2　Clinical inspection of the breast.

23

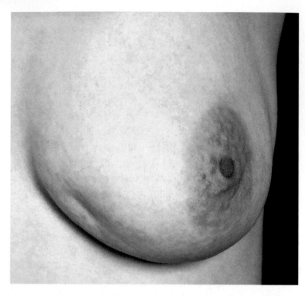

Fig. 23.3 Skin dimpling in the lower inner quadrant of the left breast associated with breast cancer.

and outline of the mass. Deep fixation is assessed by asking the patient to tense the pectoralis major muscle; this is accomplished by asking her to press her hands on her hips. All palpable lesions should be measured with callipers and the size and site (using the clock) recorded in the hospital notes.

If the patient complains of a nipple discharge, an attempt should be made to reproduce the discharge and to determine whether it arises from a single or multiple ducts. Any discharge should be tested for haemoglobin. Only marked or moderate amounts of haemoglobin in a nipple discharge are significant.

ASSESSMENT OF REGIONAL NODES

Once the breast has been palpated, the nodal areas are checked (Fig. 23.5). Clinical assessment of axillary nodes is not always accurate. Palpable nodes can be identified in up to 30% of patients with no clinically significant breast disease, while up to 25% of patients with breast cancer who have no palpable nodes on examination will be found histologically to have metastatic disease in the axillary nodes. The supraclavicular nodes are best examined from behind.

of contour is present in a high percentage of patients with breast cancer (Fig. 23.3). Breast palpation is performed with the patient lying flat with her arms above or under her head. All the breast tissue is examined, using the fingertips to detect any abnormality (Fig. 23.4). Any abnormal area is then examined in more detail, to determine the texture

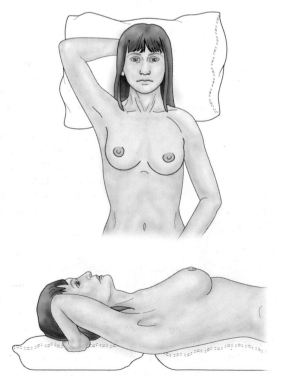

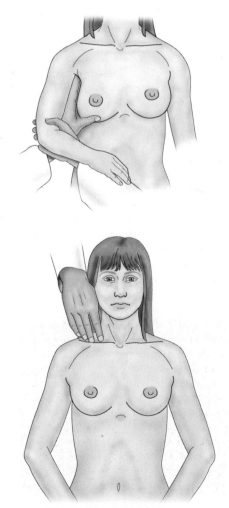

Fig. 23.4   Clinical examination of the breast.

Fig. 23.5   Examination of the regional nodes.

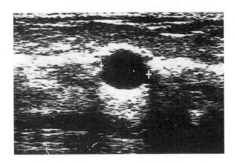

Fig. 23.6   Ultrasound of a cyst.

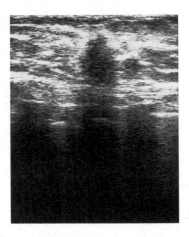

Fig. 23.8   Ultrasound of a cancer.

23

IMAGING

Mammography

This requires compression of the breast between two plates and is uncomfortable. By using high-resolution films and X-rays of low penetrating power, the radiation dose is kept as low as possible (0.5–1.5 mGy per film). Two views, an oblique and a craniocaudal, are usually obtained. Mammography allows the detection of mass lesions, areas of parenchymal distortion and microcalcification. Because the breasts are relatively radiodense in women under 35 years of age, mammography is rarely of value in this group.

Ultrasonography

High-frequency waves are beamed through the breast and reflections are detected and turned into images. Cysts show up as transparent objects (Fig. 23.6) and other benign lesions tend to have well-demarcated edges (Fig. 23.7), whereas cancers usually have an indistinct outline and absorb sound, resulting in a posterior acoustic shadow (Fig. 23.8).

Magnetic resonance imaging (MRI)

This is an accurate way of imaging the breast. It has a high sensitivity for breast cancer and may be of value in demonstrating the extent of both invasive and non-invasive disease. It is particularly useful in the conserved breast to determine whether a mammographic lesion at the site of previous surgery is due to scar or to recurrence. It is

---

EBM 23.1   SCREENING FOR BREAST CANCER BY MRI
'MRI is more effective than mammography at screening women < 50 years who are at very high risk of breast cancer either because they carry a BRCA1 or BRCA2 mutation or because of their family history.' *MARIBS Study Group. Lancet 2005; 365:1769–1778*

currently being evaluated as a screening tool for high-risk women between the ages of 35 and 50 (EBM 23.1). MRI is the optimum method of imaging breast implants and detecting implant leakage or rupture.

CYTOLOGY AND BIOPSY

Fine-needle aspiration cytology

Needle aspiration can differentiate between solid and cystic lesions. If the lesion is cystic, the fluid is aspirated and, providing it is not blood-stained, discarded. Aspiration of solid lesions requires skill to obtain sufficient cells for cytological analysis and expertise is needed to interpret the smears. Aspiration is usually performed with a 21- or 23-gauge needle attached to a syringe. The needle is introduced into the lesion and suction applied by withdrawing the plunger; multiple passes are then made through the lesion. The plunger is then released and the material spread on to microscope slides. These are then either air-dried or fixed in alcohol and later stained. In some units, a report is available within 30 minutes.

Core biopsy

Several cores are removed from a mass or an area of microcalcification by means of a cutting needle technique (Fig. 23.9). A 14-gauge needle combined with a mechanical gun produces satisfactory samples and allows the procedure to be performed single-handed. Core biopsy can be performed using palpation to guide biopsy but is most successful when image guidance is employed (ultrasound for mass lesions, stereotactic biopsy for calcifications which are usually impalpable). Vacuum-assisted core biopsy devices

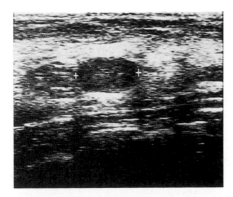

Fig. 23.7   Ultrasound of a fibroadenoma.

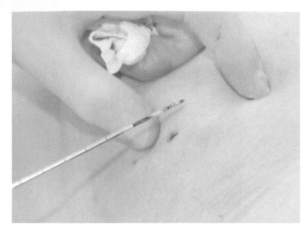

Fig. 23.9   Core biopsy being performed.

allow several large cores to be removed without withdrawing the needle from the breast, and have some advantages when biopsying areas of indeterminate microcalcifications detected on screening.

Open biopsy

An open biopsy should only be performed in patients who have been appropriately investigated by imaging, fine-needle aspiration cytology and/or core biopsy. Breast biopsy is a morbid procedure and one-fifth of patients who have a biopsy performed develop a further lump under the scar, or pain specifically related to the operation site. Biopsy can be performed under local or general anaesthesia. The removal of impalpable lesions requires localization by a hooked wire. Following excision, the specimen is X-rayed to confirm that the appropriate area has been removed.

Frozen section

The routine use of frozen sections to diagnose breast cancer is no longer practised. Frozen sections can be used to assess lymph nodes, but in this situation the sensitivity (the ability to detect cancer in the lymph nodes) is only 80%.

ONE-STOP CLINICS

The combination of clinical examination, imaging (mammography with or without ultrasonography for women over 35 years, and ultrasonography for women under 35 years) and fine-needle aspiration cytology and/or core biopsy is known as triple assessment. Patients presenting with breast symptoms can now have triple assessment performed and reported during a single clinic visit. This allows patients with benign disease to be reassured, and in many cases discharged.

ACCURACY OF INVESTIGATIONS

False-positive results occur with all diagnostic techniques. The sensitivity of clinical examination and mammography varies with age, and only two-thirds of cancers in women under 50 years of age are considered suspicious or definitely malignant on clinical examination or mammography (Table 23.1). Image-guided core biopsy is the most accurate and efficient of the various techniques used to diagnose breast masses.

DISORDERS OF DEVELOPMENT

Most benign breast conditions occur during development, cyclical activity or involution, and are so common that they are best considered as aberrations rather than true disease (Table 23.2).

JUVENILE HYPERTROPHY

Uncontrolled overgrowth of breast tissue occurs occasionally in adolescent girls, whose breast development initially begins normally at puberty and is followed by rapid breast growth. These changes are usually bilateral, but may be limited to one breast or part of one breast. This process is often referred to as virginal or juvenile hypertrophy (Fig. 23.10). However, it is not hypertrophy, as there is an increase in the amount of stromal tissue rather than in the number of lobules or ducts. This excessive growth is an aberration rather than a true disease, and presenting symptoms are large breasts and pain in the shoulders, neck and back or under the bra straps. Treatment is by reduction mammoplasty.

Table 23.1   ACCURACY OF INVESTIGATIONS IN THE DIAGNOSIS OF SYMPTOMATIC BREAST DISEASE IN SPECIALIST CLINICS

	Clinical examination	Mammography	Ultrasonography	Fine-needle aspiration cytology	Core biopsy
Sensitivity for cancers[1]	86%	86%	90%	95%	90–98%[4]
Specificity for benign disease[2]	90%	90%	92%	95%	95%
Positive predictive value for cancers[3]	95%	95%	95%	99.8%	100%

[1] % of cancers detected by test as malignant or probably malignant (that is, complete sensitivity).
[2] % of benign disease detected by test as benign.
[3] % of lesions diagnosed as malignant by test that are cancers (that is, absolute positive predictive value).
[4] Sensitivity increases if core biopsy is image-guided.

Table 23.2 ABERRATIONS OF NORMAL BREAST DEVELOPMENT AND INVOLUTION

Age (years)	Normal process	Aberration
< 25	Breast development	
	Stromal	Juvenile hypertrophy
	Lobular	Fibroadenoma
25–40	Cyclical activity	Cyclical mastalgia
		Cyclical nodularity (diffuse or focal)
35–55	Involution	
	Lobular	Palpable cysts
	Stromal	Sclerosing lesions
	Ductal	Duct ectasia

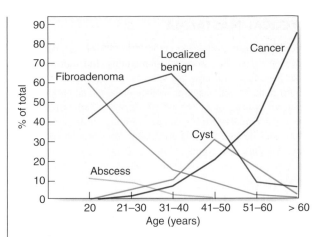

Fig. 23.11 Percentage of patients in 10-year age groups with a discrete breast lump who have common benign conditions and breast cancer.

23

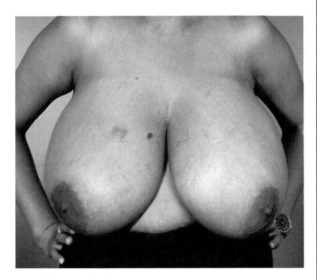

Fig. 23.10 Juvenile hypertrophy.

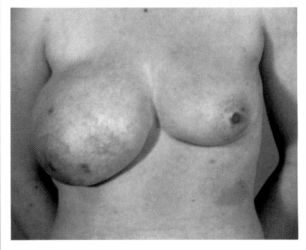

Fig. 23.12 Juvenile fibroadenoma.

FIBROADENOMA

Fibroadenomas are classified in most texts as benign tumours, but are best considered as aberrations of development rather than true neoplasms. The reasons are that fibroadenomas develop from a single lobule rather than from a single cell, and show hormonal dependence similar to that of normal breast tissue, lactating during pregnancy and involuting in the perimenopausal period. Fibroadenomas are most commonly seen immediately following the period of breast development and growth in the 15–25-year age group (Fig. 23.11). They are usually well-circumscribed, firm, smooth, mobile lumps, and may be multiple or bilateral. Although a small number of fibroadenomas increase in size, most do not and over one-third become smaller or disappear within 2 years. Fibroadenomas have a characteristic appearance with easily visualized margins on ultrasound (Fig. 23.7). Large or giant fibroadenomas (> 5 cm) are infrequent but are more commonly seen in women from certain African countries. Occasionally, a fibroadenoma in an adolescent girl undergoes rapid growth, a condition called juvenile fibroadenoma (Fig. 23.12). Once a diagnosis of fibroadenoma has been established on core

biopsy, and provided the lesion measures less than 4 cm, options for management include observation or excision; fibroadenomas over 4 cm in diameter should be excised to ensure that phyllodes tumours are not missed (see below). A carcinoma arising in a fibroadenoma is rare, and patients with simple fibroadenomas are not at significantly increased risk of developing breast cancer.

DISORDERS OF CYCLICAL CHANGE

Premenstrual nodularity and breast discomfort are so common that they are considered part of the normal cyclical changes. When premenstrual pain is severe, interferes with daily activities and influences quality of life, then this is classified as moderate or severe cyclical mastalgia. There is no association between cyclical breast pain and any underlying histological abnormality. The cause of cyclical mastalgia is unknown. Another common and significant problem is non-cyclical mastalgia.

23

CYCLICAL MASTALGIA

Evening primrose oil was previously used for breast pain but the original studies were of poor quality and more recent ones have failed to show any benefit. It is no longer used for breast pain. Effective agents include danazol and tamoxifen. Danazol is used in a dose of 100 mg/day. Tamoxifen in a dose of 10 mg/day for breast pain, although it does not have a product licence for this condition, improves the pain in 80% of patients. Agnus castis, a fruit extract, has also been shown in randomized studies to be effective in cyclical breast pain.

NODULARITY

Lumpiness and nodularity in the breast can be diffuse or focal. Diffuse nodularity is normal, particularly premenstrually. It is now appreciated that the normal breast is lumpy. In the past, women with lumpy breasts were regarded as having fibroadenosis or fibrocystic disease, but this diffuse nodularity is not associated with any underlying pathological abnormality and so these terms are inappropriate. Focal nodularity is a common cause of a breast lump and is seen in women of all ages (Fig. 23.11). Patients with focal nodularity often report that the lump fluctuates in size in relation to the menstrual cycle. Breast cancer should be excluded in patients with localized asymmetric areas of nodularity, using triple assessment.

NON-CYCLICAL BREAST PAIN

Localized pain in the chest wall, referred pain and diffuse true breast pain must be differentiated. Examining a patient on her side to move the breast away from the chest wall is the best way of demonstrating that the ribs or chest wall muscle are the site of origin of the pain. Oral non-steroidal anti-inflammatory agents (NSAIDs) are usually effective in improving chest-wall pain. Up to 60% of patients with a persistent localized painful area in the chest wall can be effectively treated by infiltration of local anaesthetic and steroid (2 ml 0.5% bupivacaine and 1 ml containing 40 mg of methylprednisolone).

DISORDERS OF INVOLUTION

Aberrations of the normal ageing process include cyst formation, areas of scarring (sclerosis), duct ectasia and epithelial hyperplasia.

PALPABLE BREAST CYSTS

Approximately 7% of women in developed countries develop a palpable breast cyst at some time in their life. Cysts constitute approximately 15% of all discrete breast masses. They are distended, involuted lobules and are most frequently seen in the perimenopausal period (Fig. 23.11). Clinically, they are smooth discrete lumps that can be painful and are sometimes visible. Mammographically, they have characteristic haloes and are easily diagnosed by

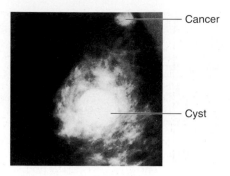

Fig. 23.13   Mammogram of a cyst and a cancer.

ultrasonography (Fig. 23.6). Symptomatic palpable cysts are treated by aspiration and, provided the fluid is not blood-stained, it is discarded. If aspiration results in the disappearance of the mass, then the patient can be reassured. Cysts that contain blood-stained fluid require excision to exclude an associated intracystic cancer. These cancers are rare and are usually evident on ultrasound. Most cysts are asymptomatic and, provided they are appropriately investigated by ultrasound, do not need aspiration. All patients with cysts should have mammography, preferably before cyst aspiration, as between 1 and 3% will have a cancer, usually remote from the cyst, visible on mammography (Fig. 23.13). Patients with cysts have a slightly increased risk of developing breast cancer, but the magnitude of this risk is not considered of clinical significance.

SCLEROSIS

Areas of excessive fibrosis or sclerosis can occur as part of stromal involution. These lesions are of clinical importance only because they produce stellate lesions that mimic breast cancer mammographically, and so can cause diagnostic problems during screening. Sclerosing lesions include radial scars, complex sclerosing lesions and sclerosing adenosis.

DUCT ECTASIA

The major subareolar ducts dilate and shorten with age; when symptomatic, this is known as duct ectasia. By the age of 70, 40% of women are affected, some of whom present with nipple discharge or retraction. The discharge is usually cheesy and the retraction is classically slit-like (Fig. 23.14), which contrasts with breast cancer, in which the whole nipple is pulled in (Fig. 23.15). Surgery is indicated if the discharge is troublesome or if the patient wishes the nipple to be everted.

EPITHELIAL HYPERPLASIA

An increase in the number of cells lining the terminal duct lobular unit is known as epithelial hyperplasia, the degree of which is graded as mild, moderate or florid. If the hyperplastic cells show cellular atypia, the condition

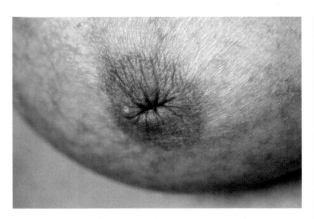

Fig. 23.14 Duct ectasia showing slit-like nipple retraction.

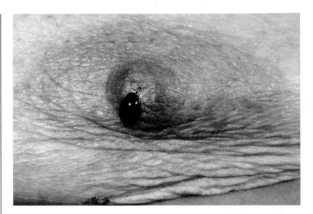

Fig. 23.16 Blood-stained nipple discharge.

23

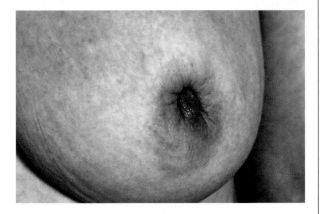

Fig. 23.15 Asymmetric nipple inversion in a patient with breast cancer.

is called atypical hyperplasia. Women with atypical hyperplasia have a significant increase in their risk of breast cancer. The absolute risk for a woman with atypical hyperplasia without a first-degree relative with breast cancer is 8% at 10 years; for women with a first-degree relative with breast cancer it is 20–25% at 15 years.

BENIGN NEOPLASMS

DUCT PAPILLOMAS

These can be single or multiple. They are very common, and should be considered as aberrations rather than true neoplasms as they show minimal malignant potential. They can cause persistent and troublesome nipple discharge, which can be either frankly blood-stained (Fig. 23.16), or serous and containing moderate or large amounts of blood on testing. Treatment comprises removal of the discharging duct (microdochectomy), which removes the papilloma (if this is the cause) and allows exclusion of an underlying neoplasm, seen in approximately 5% of women who present with a blood-stained nipple discharge.

LIPOMAS

These are soft, lobulated, radiolucent lesions and are common. Interest lies in their confusion with pseudolipoma (a soft mass that can be felt around a cancer, caused by indrawing of surrounding fat).

PHYLLODES TUMOURS

These rare fibro-epithelial neoplasms may be malignant in their behaviour, although most are benign. They present as localized discrete masses that clinically feel like fibro-adenomas, although they tend to be larger (> 4 cm). Up to 20% of benign phyllodes tumours recur locally following simple excision. In more malignant lesions it is the sarcomatous element that recurs; approximately one-quarter of lesions reported as malignant metastasize. Treatment of phyllodes tumours, whether malignant or benign, is wide excision. If the lesion is large, mastectomy may be needed to ensure complete removal.

Other benign tumours that occur in the breast include granular cell tumours, neurofibroma and leiomyoma.

BREAST INFECTION

Breast infection is less common than it used to be. It is seen occasionally in neonates but most commonly affects women between the ages of 18 and 50. In this age group, infection can be divided into lactational and non-lactational. Infection can also affect the skin overlying the breast, when it can be a primary event or secondary to a lesion in the skin (such as a sebaceous cyst or an underlying condition such as hidradenitis suppurativa).

The principles of treating breast infection are:

- Give appropriate antibiotics early to reduce the incidence of abscess formation (Table 23.3).
- If an abscess is suspected, confirm pus is present by ultrasound or aspiration before embarking on surgical drainage.

BOX 23.1 BENIGN BREAST DISEASE

- Is more common than breast cancer
- Can be difficult to differentiate from breast cancer
- Inappropriate treatment of benign conditions is associated with significant morbidity
- Occurs against the background of breast development (age < 25), cyclical activity (up to menopause) and involution (following the menopause)
- The only benign condition associated with a significant increased risk of subsequent breast cancer is atypical hyperplasia

---

- Exclude breast cancer using imaging and core biopsy in an inflammatory lesion that is solid and that does not settle despite adequate antibiotic treatment.

Most breast abscesses can be managed by repeated aspiration (preferably guided by ultrasound), combined with oral antibiotics or incision and drainage under local anaesthetic. Few abscesses, except those in children, require drainage under general anaesthesia. Placement of a drain or packing the abscess cavity after incision and drainage is unnecessary.

LACTATING INFECTION

Improvements in maternal and infant hygiene have considerably reduced the incidence of infection associated with breastfeeding. When infection does occur, it usually develops within the first 6 weeks of breastfeeding or, occasionally, during weaning. Presenting features are pain, swelling, tenderness and a cracked nipple or skin abrasion. *Staphylococcus aureus* is the most common organism, although *Staph. epidermidis* and streptococci are occasionally implicated. Drainage of milk from the affected segment is often reduced, with the resultant stagnant milk becoming infected. Early infection is treated with flucloxacillin or co-amoxiclav. An established abscess should be treated by recurrent aspiration, or by incision and drainage (Fig. 23.17). Women should be encouraged to breastfeed, as this promotes milk drainage from the affected segment. Rarely, milk flow needs to be stopped using cabergoline, a prolactin antagonist.

NON-LACTATING INFECTION

This can be separated into infections that occur centrally in the peri-areolar region and those affecting the periphery of the breast.

Central (peri-areolar) infection

This is most commonly seen in young women (mean age 32 years). The underlying cause is periductal mastitis. It used to be thought that recurrent infection was related to duct ectasia and that the contents of ectatic ducts leaked into the surrounding tissue to cause periductal inflammation. This is now known to be incorrect. Current evidence suggests that smoking is important in the aetiology of non-lactational infection, 90% of women who present with periductal mastitis or its complications being smokers. Substances in cigarette smoke either directly or indirectly damage the subareolar breast ducts, and the damaged tissue then becomes infected by either aerobic or anaerobic organisms. Initial presentation is with peri-areolar inflammation, with or without an associated mass, or with an established abscess. Clinical features include breast pain, erythema, peri-areolar swelling and tenderness, and/or nipple retraction; these occur in relation to the affected duct.

Treatment is with appropriate antibiotics (Table 23.3). Abscesses are managed by aspiration or incision and drainage. Infection associated with periductal mastitis is commonly recurrent because treatment does not remove the damaged subareolar duct(s). Following drainage of a non-lactating abscess, up to one-third of patients develop a mammary duct fistula. Recurrent episodes of peri-areolar infection require excision of the diseased duct(s) (total duct excision).

Mammary duct fistula

This is a communication between the skin—usually at the areolar margin—and a major sub-areolar duct (Fig. 23.18). Treatment is by excision of the fistula and diseased duct(s) under antibiotic cover.

Peripheral non-lactating abscesses

These are less common than peri-areolar abscesses and are sometimes associated with an underlying condition, such as diabetes, rheumatoid arthritis, steroid treatment, granulomatous lobular mastitis or trauma. Infection associated with granulomatous lobular mastitis can be a particular problem, as there is a strong tendency for this condition to persist and recur despite surgery. This condition usually affects young parous women, who develop large areas of inflammation with multiple simultaneous peripheral abscesses. Peripheral abscesses should be treated by recurrent aspiration with antibiotics (Table 23.3), or incision and drainage under local anaesthesia.

Table 23.3 ANTIBIOTICS MOST APPROPRIATE FOR TREATING BREAST INFECTIONS*

Type of infection	No allergy to penicillin	Allergy to penicillin
Lactating and skin-associated Non-lactating	Flucloxacillin (500 mg 6-hourly) Co-amoxiclav (375 mg 8-hourly)	Clarithromycin (500 mg 12-hourly) Combination of clarithromycin (500 mg 12-hourly) with metronidazole (200 mg 8-hourly)

* Doses are for adults.

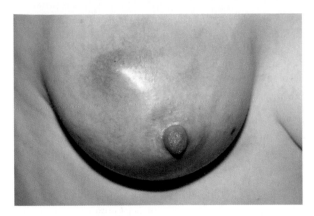

Fig. 23.17 Lactating breast abscess.

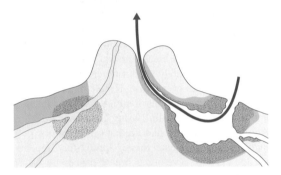

Fig. 23.18 Mammary duct fistula and periductal mastitis.

Table 23.4 ESTABLISHED AND PROBABLE RISK FACTORS FOR BREAST CANCER

Factor	Relative risk	High-risk group
Age	> 10	Elderly
Geographical location	5	Developed country
Age at first full pregnancy	3	First child in early 40s
Previous benign disease	4–5	Atypical hyperplasia
Cancer in other breast	> 4	Women treated for breast cancer
Socioeconomic group	2	Social classes I and II
Diet	1.5	High intake of saturated fat
Exposure to ionizing radiation	3	Abnormal exposure in young females after age 10
Taking exogenous hormones		
Oral contraceptives	1.24	Current use
Combined hormone replacement therapy	2.3	Use for ≥ 10 years
Family history	≥2	Breast cancer in first-degree relative

BOX 23.2 BREAST INFECTION

- Antibiotics should be given early to reduce abscess formation
- Hospital referral is indicated if infection does not settle rapidly on antibiotics
- If an abscess is suspected, this should be confirmed by ultrasound or aspiration
- If the lesion is solid on ultrasound or aspiration a core biopsy should be performed to exclude an underlying inflammatory carcinoma

SKIN-ASSOCIATED INFECTION

Primary infection of the skin most commonly affects the lower half of the breast and can be recurrent in women who either are overweight or have large breasts. It is more common after previous surgery or radiotherapy. Treatment is with antibiotics (Table 23.3) and drainage or aspiration of abscesses. Women with recurrent infection should be advised about weight reduction and keeping the area as clean and dry as possible.

Sebaceous cysts are common in the skin of the breast and may become infected. Some recurrent infections in the skin of the lower part of the breast are due to hidradenitis suppurativa, which is more common in smokers. This condition, which affects the apocrine glands of the breast, is difficult to treat. Excision of the affected skin is effective at stopping further infection in about half of patients.

BREAST CANCER

EPIDEMIOLOGY

Over 1 million new cases of breast cancer are diagnosed each year world-wide. It is the most common malignancy in women and comprises 18% of all female cancers. In the UK, approximately 1 in 10 women will develop breast cancer. The known risk factors for breast cancer are shown in Table 23.4.

The incidence of breast cancer increases with age, doubling every 10 years until the menopause, when the rate of increase slows dramatically (Fig. 23.19). Compared with lung cancer, the incidence of breast cancer is higher at young ages. There is a variation in incidence by up to a factor of 5 between different countries. Studies of migrants from Japan, a low-risk area, to Hawaii show that the rates of breast cancer in migrants become the same as the rate in the host country within one or two generations. This suggests that environmental rather than genetic factors are important in the aetiology. Women who start menstruating early in life, or who have a late menopause, have a slightly increased risk of developing breast cancer. Young age at first delivery protects against breast cancer. The risk of breast cancer in women who have their first child after the age of 30 is twice that of women who have their first child before the age of 20. Breast cancer is also increased in nulliparous women, who have a risk approximately 2.4 times that of women having their first child before the age of 20. The highest risk is in women who have a first pregnancy over the age of 40 years. Breastfeeding has a small protective effect and women who have breastfed have a slightly reduced incidence of breast cancer.

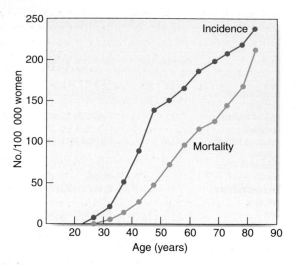

Fig. 23.19 Percentage of all deaths in women attributable to breast cancer.

Women with severe atypical hyperplasia have a four- to five-fold higher risk of developing breast cancer than women who have no proliferative changes. A doubling of breast cancer was observed among teenage girls exposed to radiation during the Second World War. Women treated by radiation therapy for lymphoma during adolescence and teenage years are also at significant risk of developing early-onset breast cancer. Although there is a close correlation between the incidence of breast cancer and dietary fat intake in populations, the true relationship does not appear to be particularly strong or consistent. A high alcohol intake may also increase breast cancer risk. Patients who take the oral contraceptive pill have an increased relative risk of breast cancer while they are on the pill 1.24 times that of the general population. This rapidly falls to normal after stopping the pill. Hormone replacement therapy (HRT) increases breast cancer risk. Combined oestrogen and progestogen HRT is associated with a greater risk than preparations containing oestrogen alone (Table 23.5).

Up to 10% of breast cancers in developed countries are due to genetic predisposition. The genetic contribution is mainly through single genes inherited as autosomal dominants but with limited penetrance. Not all gene carriers develop breast cancer. Human breast cancer genes that have been identified and that affect different families include *BRCA1* on chromosome 17, *BRCA2* on chromosome 13, *p53* on chromosome 17 and *PTEN* on chromosome 10. Throughout the USA and most of Europe, germline mutations in *BRCA1* and *BRCA2* are believed to occur in just over 1 in 1000 of the population.

In some populations, e.g. Ashkenazi Jews and Icelanders, particular mutations in *BRCA1* and *BRCA2* may be relatively common. In 'breast cancer families', there is also an increased risk of other tumours, notably ovarian cancer. Most *BRCA1* and *BRCA2* mutations confer a 50–60% lifetime risk of breast cancer. Environmental factors probably modify inherited breast cancer risk, and other genes probably interact with *BRCA1* and *BRCA2* to modify risk. Pointers to an inherited disposition are a first-degree relative who developed breast cancer, particularly bilateral cancer, under the age of 40 years, numerous female relatives with breast cancer, or a close female relative who has had ovarian cancer. Options for high-risk women include regular screening, prevention using hormonal agents such as tamoxifen, raloxifene and aromatase inhibitors, or prophylactic bilateral mastectomy. Tamoxifen appears to reduce the risk of developing breast cancer by 40–50%, whereas surgery reduces the risk by over 90%.

TYPES OF BREAST CANCER

Breast cancers are derived from the epithelial cells that line the terminal duct lobular unit. Cancer cells that remain within the basement membrane of the lobule and the draining ducts are classified as in situ or non-invasive. An invasive cancer is one in which cells have moved outside the basement membrane of the ducts and lobules into the surrounding adjacent normal tissue. Both in situ and invasive cancers have characteristic patterns by which they are classified.

Non-invasive

Two main types of non-invasive cancer can be recognized on the basis of cell type. Ductal carcinoma in situ (DCIS) is the most common form (Fig. 23.20), making up to 3–4% of symptomatic and 17–25% of screen-detected cancers. Screen-detected DCIS is most commonly associated with microcalcifications on mammograms (Fig. 23.21), which can be either localized or widespread. Lobular carcinoma in situ (LCIS) (Fig. 23.22) is usually an incidental finding and is generally treated by regular follow-up, as these women are at significant risk of developing invasive cancer in either breast.

Invasive

The most commonly used classification of invasive cancers divides them into ductal and lobular types and was based on the belief that ductal carcinomas arise in ducts and lobular carcinomas in lobules. This is now known to be incorrect,

Table 23.5 RELATIONSHIP OF HRT TO BREAST CANCER DEVELOPMENT: RELATIVE RISK OF BREAST CANCER RELATED TO TYPE AND RECENCY OF HRT USE*	
Patient group	**Relative risk (95% confidence intervals)**
Never used HRT	1.0 (0.96–1.04)
All previous users	1.01 (0.95–1.08)
Current users of:	
Oestrogen only	1.3 (1.22–1.38)
Oestrogen/progestogen combinations	2.0 (1.91–2.09)

* Lancet 2003; 362:419–427.

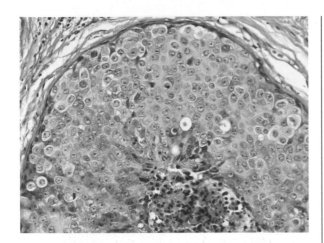

Fig. 23.20 Ductal carcinoma in situ.
This is characterized by cells with irregularly shaped and often angular nuclei with variable amounts of chromatin. The cells themselves are variable in size and the necrosis seen in the lumen is a frequent finding.

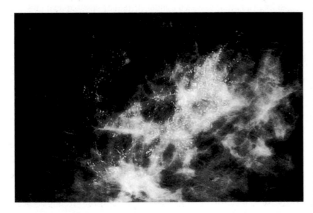

Fig. 23.21 Diffuse microcalcification in the breast affected by ductal carcinoma in situ.

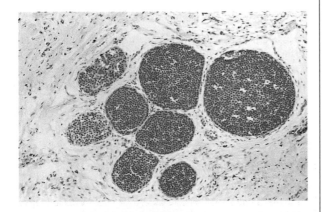

Fig. 23.22 Lobular carcinoma in situ.
This is characterized by regular cells with regular round or oval nuclei. (Compare this with DCIS.)

as almost all cancers arise in the terminal duct lobular unit. The two types behave differently, however, so the classification remains in use. Certain invasive ductal carcinomas show distinct patterns of growth and are classified separately as tumours of 'special type'; this includes tubular, cribriform, mucinous and medullary cancers. Tubular and mucinous cancers are well differentiated and have a better than average prognosis. Mucinous cancers are rare circumscribed tumours characterized by tumour cells that produce mucin; these also have a good prognosis. Medullary cancers are circumscribed and soft, and consist of aggregates of high-grade pleomorphic cells surrounded by lymphoid cells. Invasive lobular cancer accounts for up to 10% of invasive cancers and is characterized by a diffuse pattern of spread that causes problems with clinical and mammographic detection. These tumours are often large at diagnosis and have an increased rate of bilaterality.

Tumours of 'no special type' are graded on the presence or absence of glands, the extent of nuclear pleomorphism and the mitotic rate of the tumour. Grade I are the most differentiated and have the best prognosis, grade II have an intermediate prognosis, and grade III or high-grade cancers have a poor prognosis. The presence of tumour cells in lymphatics or blood vessels is a marker of aggressive disease and is associated with an increased rate of both local and systemic recurrence.

SCREENING FOR BREAST CANCER

Randomized controlled trials have shown that screening by mammography can significantly reduce mortality from breast cancer (EBM 23.2). Mortality is reduced by up to 40% in women who attend for screening, with the greatest benefit being seen in women aged over 50. Published data from combined Swedish trials have shown an overall reduction in breast cancer mortality of 29% in the first 12 years after screening of women over 50, with a smaller, 13% reduction in younger women. To be effective, attendance at screening programmes has to be greater than 70%. Ideally, screening should incorporate the 50–70-year age group.

The most appropriate interval between mammographic screens is yet to be determined. In the UK, screening takes place every 3 years in women aged 50–70 but the rate of cancers diagnosed between the second and third years after the initial screen climbs rapidly, suggesting that this interval may be too long, at least for women aged 50–60. Patients are currently screened by two-view mammography.

EBM 23.2 BREAST SCREENING BY MAMMOGRAPHY

'Mammography is at present the best screening tool available. Randomized controlled trials have shown screening by mammography reduces mortality from breast cancer by 40% in those who attend. Benefit is greatest in women aged 50–70 years. Two-view mammography should be performed at each screening visit.'

Nystrom L, et al. Lancet 1993; 341(8851):973–978

23

23

About two-thirds of screen-detected abnormalities are shown to be unimportant on further mammographic or ultrasound imaging. Among women aged 50–70, approximately 60 cancers are detected for every 10 000 attending for their initial screen. At subsequent screens, 35 cancers should be identified for every 10 000 attenders. Up to 70% of important abnormalities are impalpable, and for these, image-guided (ultrasound or stereotactic radiography) core biopsy or fine-needle aspiration cytology is necessary to establish a diagnosis. Compared with symptomatic cancers, screen-detected cancers are smaller and more likely to be non-invasive. The ability of screening to influence mortality from breast cancer (EBM 23.3) indicates that early diagnosis identifies the cancer at an earlier stage of evolution, when metastasis is less likely to have occurred.

MAMMOGRAPHIC FEATURES OF BREAST CANCER

Mammographically, a cancer most commonly appears as a dense opacity with an irregular outline from which spicules pass into the surrounding tissue (Fig. 23.23). Associated features include microcalcifications, which can occur within or outside the lesion, skin tethering or thickening, distortion of the shape of the breast or overlying skin, and tenting or direct involvement of underlying muscle. Involved lymph nodes can also sometimes be seen (Fig. 23.24). Microcalcification alone is a feature of DCIS.

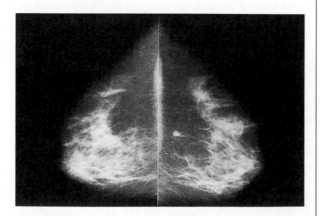

Fig. 23.23   Mammogram of a cancer detected at breast screening.
A small lesion at the back of the left breast.

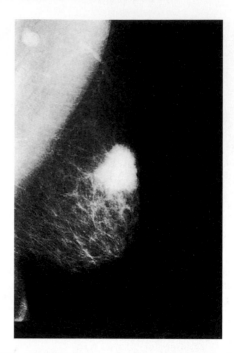

Fig. 23.24   Mammogram of a cancer (irregular dense mass) and involved axillary nodes (see localized density in the axillary tail).

STAGING

When invasive cancer is diagnosed, the extent of the disease should be assessed. The currently used TNM (tumour, nodes and metastases) system depends on clinical measurements and clinical assessment of lymph node status, both of which are inaccurate (Table 23.6). To improve the TNM system, a separate pathological classification has been added. Patients with small breast cancers (< 4 cm) have a low incidence of detectable metastatic disease and, unless they have specific symptoms, should not undergo investigations to search for metastases. Patients with larger or more locally advanced breast cancers are more likely to have metastases and should be considered for bone scans and liver ultrasounds. A simpler classification of breast cancer separates patients into three groups: operable, locally advanced and metastatic.

THE CURABILITY OF BREAST CANCER

Almost half the women with operable breast cancer treated by surgery, with or without radiotherapy, die from metastatic disease. This suggests that in most cases the cancer has already spread at the time of presentation. Invasive breast cancers spread via lymphatics and the blood stream. The first lymph node that drains the tumour, called the sentinel node, is most commonly a level I axillary node. However, in 5% of women the sentinel node is in the internal mammary chain. In most patients with internal mammary node metastases, axillary nodes are also involved. Rarely (usually in medial tumours), the internal mammary nodes are the only regional nodes involved. It was believed that haematogenous spread took place after lymph node involvement, but it is now appreciated that lymph nodes do not act as a filter and that the presence of nodal

Table 23.6   TNM STAGING FOR BREAST CANCER

T (Primary tumour)
- T_X Primary tumour cannot be assessed
- T_0 No evidence of primary tumour
- T_{1s} Carcinoma in situ: intraductal carcinoma, lobular carcinoma in situ, or Paget's disease of the nipple with no associated tumour mass[1]
- T_1 Tumour 2.0 cm or less in greatest dimension[2]
- T_{1a} 0.5 cm or less in greatest dimension
- T_{1b} More than 0.5 cm but not more than 1.0 cm in greatest dimension
- T_{1c} More than 1.0 cm but not more than 2.0 cm in greatest dimension
- T_2 Tumour more than 2.0 cm but not more than 5.0 cm in greatest dimension[2]
- T_3 Tumour more than 5.0 cm in greatest dimension[2]
- T_4 Tumour of any size with direct extension to chest wall or skin
- T_{4a} Extension to chest wall
- T_{4b} Oedema (including peau d'orange), ulceration of the skin of the breast or satellite nodules confined to the same breast
- T_{4c} Both of the above (T_{4a} and T_{4b})
- T_{4d} Inflammatory carcinoma

N (Regional lymph nodes)
- N_X Cannot be assessed (e.g. previously removed)
- N_0 No regional lymph node metastasis
- N_1 Movable ipsilateral axillary lymph node(s)
- N_2 Ipsilateral lymph node(s) fixed to one another or to other structures
- N_3 Ipsilateral internal mammary lymph node(s)

M (Distant metastases)
- M_X Cannot be assessed
- M_0 No distant metastasis
- M_1 Distant metastasis present (includes metastasis to ipsilateral supraclavicular lymph nodes)

Note: Chest wall includes ribs, intercostal muscles and serratus anterior muscle, but not pectoral muscle.

[1] Paget's disease associated with tumour mass is classified according to the size of the tumour.
[2] Dimpling of the skin, nipple retraction or other skin changes may occur in T_1, T_2 or T_3 without changing the classification.

metastases usually means the cancer has spread systemically. Metastasis can occur at any site, but the most commonly affected organs are the bony skeleton, lungs, liver, brain, ovaries and peritoneal cavity.

Prognostic factors

Factors related to prognosis include:

- the stage of the tumour at diagnosis: principally, its size and the involvement of the axillary lymph nodes or the presence of clinically evident metastases

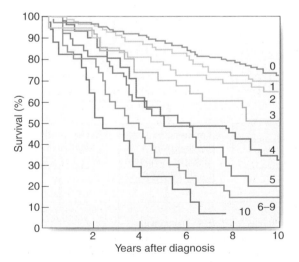

Fig. 23.25   Relation between number of involved axillary lymph nodes and survival after breast cancer.

- biological factors that relate to tumour aggressiveness. These include histological grade, histological type, the presence of lymphatic or vascular invasion, markers or proliferation, and hormone receptor content.

The single most important prognostic factor is the number of axillary lymph nodes involved (Fig. 23.25). It is possible to combine independent prognostic factors to form an index that allows the identification of groups with different prognoses. The Nottingham Prognostic Index (Table 23.7) is the most widely used and incorporates three factors: tumour size, node status and histological grade.

- Tumour size is the pathological size of the tumour in centimetres.
- Node status is scored 1 if no nodes are involved, 2 if 1–3 nodes are involved, and 3 if four or more nodes are involved.
- Grade I tumours are scored as 1, grade II tumours are scored as 2 and grade III tumours are scored as 3.

PRESENTATION OF BREAST CANCER

The most common presentation is with a breast lump or lumpiness, which is usually painless. Any discrete lump, no matter how small or mobile, can be a cancer. The investigation of a breast lump is shown in Figure 23.26. Malignant lesions are usually firm and irregular and often produce visible signs of breast asymmetry, such as flattening, dimpling or puckering of the overlying skin, or retraction or alteration in nipple contour. Approximately 50% of breast

23

Table 23.7 NOTTINGHAM PROGNOSTIC INDEX (NPI) AND SURVIVAL

NPI = (0.2 × size in cm)
+ lymph node stage (score 1 for no nodes, 2 for 1–3 nodes, 3 for ≥ 4 nodes)
+ grade (score 1 for grade I, 2 for grade II, 3 for grade III)
Originally, the NPI was used to divide women into good, intermediate or poor prognostic groups; several confirmatory studies have led to a refined NPI with five categories

Group	Index value	10-year survival (%)
Excellent (EPG)	≤ 2.4	98
Good (GPG)	≤ 3.4	90
Moderate I (MPGI)	≤ 4.4	83
Moderate II (MPGII)	< 5.4	75
Poor (PPG)	> 5.4	47

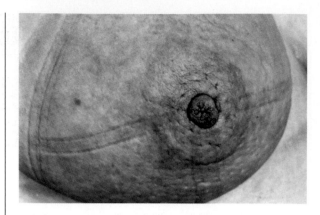

Fig. 23.27 Peau d'orange of the skin around the nipple in a patient with inflammatory carcinoma.

cancers are located in the upper outer quadrant of the breast. Diagnosis of breast lumps is a particular problem in young women, in whom the breasts are dense and lumpier and cancer is rare. Some patients present with skin ulceration, with direct infiltration of the skin by tumour or with oedema (Fig. 23.27) of the overlying skin. These are features of locally advanced breast cancer.

Breast pain alone is a rare presenting feature of breast cancer; 2.7% of patients with breast pain have cancer, whereas 4.6% of patients presenting with breast cancer have pain as their only symptom. Nipple discharge, which is either blood-stained or contains moderate or large amounts of blood on testing, can be a presenting feature of breast cancer. However, only 5–10% of patients who have a blood-stained or blood-containing discharge will have an underlying malignancy. The investigation of patients who present with nipple discharge is shown in Figure 23.28. Patients with breast cancer occasionally present with a

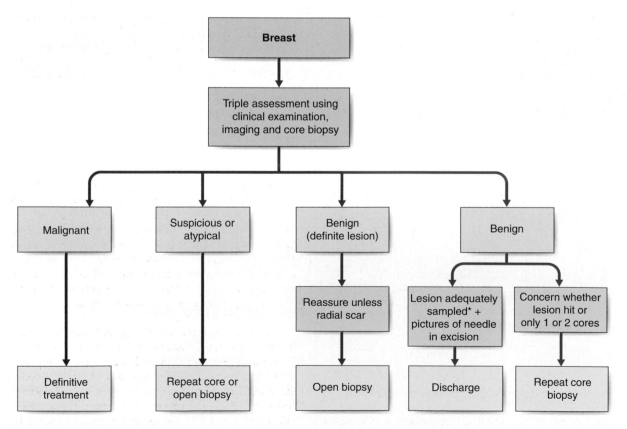

Fig. 23.26 Investigation of a breast mass.

* A minimum of three cores is required, preferably image-guided, to be certain the lesion is adequately sampled.

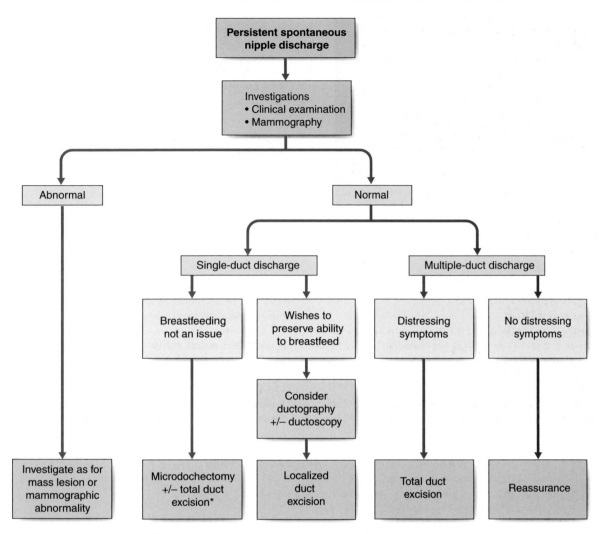

Fig. 23.28 Investigation of nipple discharge.
* Some surgeons prefer total duct excision in women > 45 to reduce the incidence of further discharge from ducts.

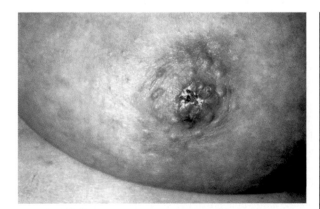

Fig. 23.29 Paget's disease.

dry scaling or red weeping appearance of the nipple known as Paget's disease; this signifies an underlying invasive or non-invasive cancer (Fig. 23.29) and should be

differentiated from eczema (Fig. 23.30). Paget's disease always affects the nipple and only involves the areola as a secondary event, whereas eczema primarily involves the areola and only secondarily affects the nipple. Approximately 1–2% of patients with breast cancer present with Paget's disease. In half of these, it is associated with an underlying mass lesion, and 90% of such patients will have an invasive cancer. Of the patients without a mass lesion, 30% have an invasive cancer and the rest have in situ disease alone.

Patients can also present initially with palpable axillary nodes or signs and symptoms of distant metastatic disease: for example, palpable supraclavicular nodes, bone pain, a cough or breathlessness, lethargy and tiredness, jaundice and headaches, or a sudden onset of grand mal seizures. Fewer than 1 in 300 patients with breast cancer present with nodal metastases and an occult primary cancer. Up to 70% of women shown histologically to have metastatic adenocarcinoma in the axillary nodes will have an occult

23

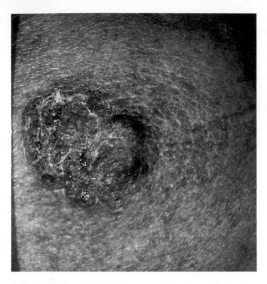

Fig. 23.30 Eczema of the nipple.

breast cancer. Most of these cancers will be visible on mammography or, if not, can be visualized by MRI of the breast.

MANAGEMENT OF OPERABLE BREAST CANCER

In situ breast cancer
Localized DCIS (less than 4 cm in maximum dimension) should be treated by complete wide excision, ensuring that surrounding normal tissue is present at all lateral margins. Following wide excision alone, approximately 2% per year will recur; half of these will be further in situ disease, the other half being invasive. For this reason, following wide excision, patients should be considered for post-operative radiotherapy. Patients with small areas of DCIS or who have low or intermediate grade DCIS that have been completely excised do not require radiotherapy. Tamoxifen appears to reduce both the risk of recurrence and the rate of development of contralateral cancer in those women with oestrogen receptor-positive disease. It is not without side-effects and its use for DCIS is not widespread. Current studies are evaluating the role of aromatase inhibitors in reducing recurrence. DCIS that is incompletely excised

---

BOX 23.3 DUCTAL CARCINOMA IN SITU (DCIS)

- Localized disease is treated by wide local excision to clear margins
- All patients other than those at low risk of recurrence should be considered for adjuvant radiotherapy to the breast following wide local excision
- Tamoxifen reduces all breast cancer events following wide excision, but its exact role in reducing local recurrence following conservative treatment is not clear
- The value of aromatase inhibitors is being investigated
- Widespread (> 4 cm) areas of DCIS are treated by mastectomy ± reconstruction

---

EBM 23.4   BREAST CONSERVATION IN OPERABLE CANCERS

'Breast-conserving surgery followed by radiotherapy is as effective as mastectomy for small operable breast cancer.'
Fisher B, et al. N Engl J Med 2002; 347(16):1270–1271.

EBM 23.5   RADIOTHERAPY AFTER SURGERY FOR BREAST CANCER

'Radiotherapy reduces local recurrence after surgery and reduces deaths from breast cancer.'
Morrow M, Harris JR. In: Harris JR, et al., eds. Diseases of the breast. 3rd edn. Philadelphia: Lippincott, Williams & Wilkins; 2004:719–744.

requires re-excision or mastectomy. Widespread (≥ 4 cm) or multifocal DCIS should be treated by mastectomy, with or without immediate breast reconstruction.

Operable breast tumours
Operable breast tumours are those restricted to the breast or associated with mobile axillary lymph nodes on the same side: T_1, T_2, T_3, N_0, N_1, M_0. As only a minority of patients are cured by loco-regional treatments alone, all should be considered for systemic therapy after local therapy (EBMs 23.4 and 23.5).

Local therapy
There are currently two accepted methods of local therapy for operable breast cancer.

Breast-conserving treatment (wide local excision and radiotherapy)
This involves excising the tumour with a 1 cm margin of macroscopically normal tissue. Breast conservation is usually only suitable for single cancers measuring less than 4 cm in diameter. Complete excision of all invasive and non-invasive cancer is necessary. Wide excision should be combined with an axillary node staging procedure. This involves either removing the first node or nodes draining the tumour (sentinel node biopsy), sampling (removing four nodes from the lower axilla) or axillary clearance (removing all nodes at levels I, II and III). To identify the sentinel node(s), blue dye and/or radioisotope is injected either around the cancer or under the nipple. The sentinel node can be seen on scintigraphy, can be identified with a hand-held probe, or is stained blue. When blue dye and radioactively labelled sulphur colloid or albumin techniques are combined, one or more sentinel nodes will be identified in approximately 97% of patients, and this sentinel node is accurate in determining the presence of any involved nodes in the axilla in approximately 98% of patients.

The cosmetic outcome following breast conservation relates to psychological wellbeing. Patients who have a good cosmetic result have low levels of anxiety and depression and improved body image and self-esteem. The larger the volume of tissue excised, the poorer the cosmetic result.

BOX 23.4 BREAST CONSERVATION

- Suitable for localized, unifocal operable breast cancers in which there is no evidence of metastatic disease beyond regional nodes; excision must leave a reasonable cosmetic result to produce benefits compared with mastectomy
- Includes wide local excision of the cancer to clear histological margins, axillary surgery (sentinel node biopsy, sampling or clearance of the axillary nodes) and whole-breast radiotherapy consisting of a 45–50 Gy dose of radiotherapy applied to the whole breast, with an optional 10–15 Gy boost to the tumour bed

---

BOX 23.5 MASTECTOMY

- Is appropriate for large or multifocal operable breast cancers or in patients with extensive non-invasive disease, an incomplete excision after attempted breast-conserving surgery or some women with central tumour
- Consists of total removal of the breast together with sentinel node biopsy, axillary node sampling or axillary clearance
- Should be followed by chest-wall radiotherapy in those women identified to be at significantly increased risk of local recurrence

---

The aim of breast-conserving surgery is to remove the cancer completely in as small a volume of tissue as possible.

Wide excision should be followed by radical radiotherapy using megavoltage equipment to deliver 45–50 Gy to the whole breast. An additional boost of 10–15 Gy by electrons of appropriate energy, or an iridium-192 (^{192}Ir) implant, is given to the tumour bed in women under 50 years of age or those with close margins. For patients with involved nodes identified by a sentinel node biopsy or an axillary node sampling procedure, the remaining axillary nodes should be removed or treated by radiotherapy to the axilla and/or the medial supraclavicular fossa.

Mastectomy

This is an alternative method of local treatment. It is indicated in patients:

- where radiotherapy is not available or when there is a wish to avoid radiotherapy
- who elect to have a mastectomy
- who have more than one focus of cancer in their breast
- who have a localized invasive cancer but a large area of surrounding non-invasive disease
- when breast conservation would produce an unacceptable cosmetic result. (This includes some central lesions directly underneath the nipple, and most cancers measuring more than 4 cm in diameter.) Breast-conserving surgery is possible in these women if they have shrinkage following initial systemic therapy, or if the breast defect is filled with a latissimus dorsi flap (Fig. 23.31).

Mastectomy removes all breast tissue with some overlying skin (usually including the nipple), but leaves the chest wall muscles intact. If reconstruction is being performed, minimal skin around the tumour is excised. Mastectomy should be combined with some form of axillary surgery. Radiotherapy is given after mastectomy to patients who are at high risk of local recurrence. Risk factors for local recurrence after mastectomy include axillary lymph node involvement, lymphatic or vascular invasion by tumour, a grade III cancer, a cancer more than 4 cm in diameter (pathological measurement), or a tumour that involves the pectoral fascia or pectoral muscle.

Systemic therapy

Systemic treatment may be given as adjuvant therapy after surgery and/or radiotherapy, or as primary or neoadjuvant treatment before surgery and/or radiotherapy. The effectiveness of adjuvant treatment has been shown in clinical trials (EBM 23.6). Randomized studies comparing primary systemic treatment with adjuvant treatment have shown similar survivals, with a higher rate of breast conserving surgery in patients having initial medical treatment. Adjuvant treatments consist of chemotherapy or hormonal therapy. For chemotherapy, a combination of drugs is more effective than a single one and the optimal benefit seems to come from at least four cycles of post-operative chemotherapy. The benefits of chemotherapy are greatest in women under the age of 50 (Table 23.8); a smaller but still significant benefit is seen in older women. Commonly used regimens include AC (adriamycin, cyclophosphamide) or FEC (5-fluorouracil, epirubicin and cyclophosphamide) alone, or four courses of epirubicin alone, or FEC followed by four courses of CMF (cyclophosphamide, methotrexate and 5-fluorouracil). The taxanes (taxol and taxotere) are also effective in the adjuvant setting in regimens combined with

---

EBM 23.6 ADJUVANT SYSTEMIC TREATMENT FOR BREAST CANCER

'Adjuvant systemic treatment reduces the risk of relapse by 30–40%. In hormone receptor-positive breast cancer, reducing oestrogen levels or using an oestrogen antagonist is effective at reducing recurrence and improving survival in all ages. Chemotherapy reduces risk of recurrence and reduces deaths from breast cancer, the greatest benefit being in younger women and those with hormone receptor-negative cancer.'

Early Breast Cancer Trialists' Collaborative Group (EBCTCG). Lancet 2005; 365:1687–1717.

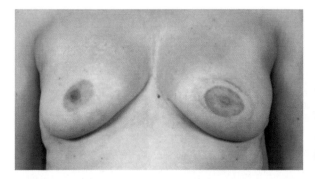

Fig. 23.31 A patient who had a left mastectomy and breast reconstruction with a latissimus dorsi reconstruction.
The patient also had a nipple reconstruction with tattooing.

Table 23.8 REDUCTION IN RECURRENCE AND MORTALITY IN POLYCHEMOTHERAPY TRIALS

Age	Reduction in annual odds of recurrence (% ± SD)	Reduction in annual odds of death (% ± SD)
< 40	37 ± 7	27 ± 8
40–49	34 ± 5	27 ± 5
50–59	22 ± 4	14 ± 4
60–69	18 ± 4	8 ± 4
All ages	23 ± 8	15 ± 2

23

an anthracycline such as AT (adriamycin, taxotere/taxol) or ET (epirubicin and taxotere/taxol).

Adjuvant hormonal treatments consist of oophorectomy, tamoxifen and the aromatase inhibitors letrozole, anastrozole and exemestane. Oophorectomy is only of benefit in women under 50 years of age and produces survival benefits of similar magnitude to those obtained by polychemotherapy in younger women. It can be achieved surgically, by radiation or by the administration of gonadotrophin-releasing hormone (GnRh) analogues such as goserelin. Tamoxifen is a partial oestrogen agonist that is given in a dose of 20 mg once daily. At least 5 years of tamoxifen should be given. It reduces the risk of contralateral breast cancer by between 40 and 50%. The benefits of tamoxifen and oophorectomy are greatest in patients with tumours that are rich in oestrogen receptors. Tamoxifen is effective in both pre- and post-menopausal women. The aromatase inhibitors, which block the conversion of androgens to oestrogen in post-menopausal women, appear more effective than tamoxifen. They can be given immediately after surgery, after 2 years of tamoxifen or after 5 years of tamoxifen to reduce recurrence rate and improve survival. The current view is that aromatase inhibitors should be included as part of the adjuvant therapy programme of most post-menopausal women with hormone receptor-positive breast cancer. Overall, 10–15% of cancers over-express the oncogene *HER2* and these cancers have a worse prognosis than those that are *HER2*-negative. A humanized monoclonal antibody (trastuzumab) has been shown to reduce the risk of cancer recurrence by up to 50% in women whose cancers over-express *HER2* (EBM 23.7). Adjuvant systemic therapy is effective in patients at both low and high risk of recurrence, but the absolute gains in survival are greatest in the latter. Risk can be calculated using the Nottingham Prognostic Index (Table 23.7) or can be based on individual factors (Table 23.9). An outline of the use of adjuvant treatment in different groups is presented in Table 23.10.

BOX 23.6 ADJUVANT THERAPY

Following surgery and/or radiotherapy for operable breast cancer, patients should receive adjuvant systemic therapy, which can be either hormonal therapy or chemotherapy.

Examples of hormonal therapy

- Pre-menopausal women: tamoxifen, goserelin, or both together
- Post-menopausal women: tamoxifen or aromatase inhibitors, or tamoxifen followed by an aromatase inhibitor

Chemotherapy

- Commonly used regimens are AC, FEC, Epi CMF, AT, ET*

Positive factors influencing the use of chemotherapy

- Young age (especially < 50 years)
- Axillary node positivity
- Large tumour size
- Histological features
  Grade III
  Lymphatic/vascular invasion
- Negative oestrogen receptor

---

* Defined in text.

EBM 23.7 EFFECT OF TRASTUZUMAB ON BREAST CANCER

'Trastuzumab given to patients whose cancer over-expresses the oncogene HER2 reduces recurrence by up to 50%'

Piccart-Gebhart MJ, et al. N Engl J Med 2005; 353:1659–1672.
Romond EH, et al. N Engl J Med 2005; 353:1673–1684.

Table 23.9 DEFINITIONS OF RISK GROUPS AND ASSOCIATED RISK OF RELAPSE

Risk group	Age and tumour characteristic	Survival without relapse at 5 years (%)
NODE-NEGATIVE PATIENTS		
Low	> 35 yrs, tumour ≤ 1 cm in diameter	> 90
Intermediate	≤ 35 yrs, tumour ≤ 1cm in diameter	75–80
	> 35 yrs, tumour > 1 cm grade I or II	
High	≤ 35 yrs, tumour > 1 cm grade I or II	50–60
	Any age, tumour > 1 cm grade III	
NODE-POSITIVE PATIENTS		
Low + intermediate	> 35 yrs, 1–3 positive nodes	40–50
High	≤ 35 yrs, 1–3 positive nodes	20–30
	> 35 yrs, 4–9 positive	
Very high	≤ 35 yrs, 4+ nodes involved	10–15
	> 35 yrs, 10+ nodes involved	

Table 23.10 SUGGESTED ADJUVANT TREATMENT FOR PATIENTS WITH BREAST CANCER[1]		
Risk group	**Pre-menopausal**	**Post-menopausal**
Very low-risk	Nil or tamoxifen	Nil or tamoxifen
Low-risk ER+	Tamoxifen ± OS[2]	Tamoxifen
Low-risk ER-	Chemotherapy	Chemotherapy
Moderate-risk ER+	Chemotherapy + tamoxifen ± OS	Chemotherapy + Al/tam[3]
Moderate-risk ER-	Chemotherapy	Chemotherapy
High-risk	Chemotherapy + tamoxifen + OS (if ER+)	Chemotherapy + Al/tam[3]

[1]Patients whose tumours over-express *HER2* should also be considered for adjuvant trastuzumab.
[2]Ovarian suppression (OS): either luteinizing hormone releasing hormone (LHRH) analogue or surgical oophorectomy.
[3]With the data showing superiority of aromatase inhibitors (Als) over tamoxifen, the former are being increasingly used either as first-line treatments in high-risk women or in sequence with tamoxifen.

(ER = oestrogen receptor)

Primary systemic therapy

The use of primary medical (neoadjuvant) or pre-operative treatment for operable breast cancer can allow large tumours that would otherwise require a mastectomy to become suitable for breast-conserving surgery. Both the primary tumour and lymph node metastases can be shown to respond. With conventional chemotherapy regimens, approximately 70% of patients will demonstrate tumour shrinkage of over 50%. Although chemotherapy is most commonly used as pre-operative treatment, particularly in pre-menopausal women, primary hormonal therapy is being increasingly used in post-menopausal women with strongly oestrogen receptor-positive breast cancers. Response rates of over 75% are reported. Randomized studies have suggested that the aromatase inhibitor, letrozole, produces significantly better responses in the neoadjuvant setting than tamoxifen, and this is currently the first-line agent of choice in this setting.

COMPLICATIONS OF TREATMENT

Haematoma and infection are uncommon (less than 5%) after breast surgery. Removal of all the axillary nodes often damages the intercostobrachial nerve, which results in numbness and paraesthesia down the upper inner aspect of the arm. Other nerves that can potentially be damaged during axillary surgery are the long thoracic nerve, damage to which causes winging of the scapula, and the thoracodorsal nerve, which can lead to atrophy of the latissimus dorsi muscle and prominence of the scapula. Axillary surgery is associated with some short-term reduction in shoulder movement and about 5% of women develop a frozen shoulder. Approximately 5% of patients treated by a full axillary dissection develop lymphoedema. The treatment of lymphoedema is unsatisfactory and is best managed by bandaging and a supportive elastic arm stocking.

Radiotherapy

Following radiotherapy, the skin develops an erythematous reaction, which often lasts for 3–4 weeks. Patients should avoid exposing the area to direct sunlight for several months. Subsequent exposure is possible with an appropriate sunscreen. Following radiotherapy to the axilla, some patients develop fibrosis around the shoulder, which can lead to some restriction in their range of movement.

Chemotherapy

Although hair loss is the most common concern of patients before starting chemotherapy, 80% report fatigue and lethargy as the most troublesome side-effects. The occurrence of alopecia with some chemotherapy regimens may be reduced by scalp cooling. Nausea and vomiting are unpleasant side-effects but in most patients can be controlled with appropriate antiemetic drugs. Trastuzumab, when combined with anthracycline-containing chemotherapy, can result in cardiac failure in a small but significant number of patients.

Hormonal treatments

The side-effects of hormonal treatments are greatest in pre-menopausal patients. Only 3% of patients stop taking tamoxifen because of side-effects, but vaginal dryness or vaginal discharge, loss of libido and hot flushes all have a considerable impact on quality of life. Aromatase inhibitors in post-menopausal women cause fewer hot flushes than tamoxifen and fewer vaginal problems, but more muscular aches and pains and fractures.

PSYCHOLOGICAL ASPECTS

Most women who present with breast lumps are emotionally distressed. When the doctor is breaking bad news to the patient, the first step should be to check the patient's idea of what is wrong. Almost two-thirds of patients with breast cancer already suspect that their lump is malignant. In patients with proven malignancy, the doctor's role is to confirm to the patient that their diagnosis is correct, pause to let this sink in, acknowledge their distress and establish what concerns are contributing to this distress. When a patient is unaware that she has cancer, the doctor should break the news more slowly. Only once a patient's distress and concerns are addressed, should reassurance, information and advice be offered. Counselling is essential and most specialist units employ nurse counsellors who ensure that the patient is fully informed about the nature of the disease and its treatment, who provide advice on prostheses after surgery, and who recognize and support patients with significant psychiatric problems.

Up to 30% of women with breast cancer develop an anxiety state or depressive illness within a year of diagnosis, which is 3–4 times the expected rate. After mastectomy, 20–30% of patients develop persisting problems with body image and sexual difficulties. Breast-conserving surgery reduces problems with body image. Psychiatric morbidity is increased when radiotherapy or chemotherapy is used. Few patients mention psychological problems to

Table 23.11 CLINICAL FEATURES OF LOCALLY ADVANCED BREAST CANCER
Skin • Ulceration • Satellite nodules • Dermal infiltration • Peau d'orange • Erythema over tumour
Chest wall • Tumour fixation to Ribs Intercostal muscles Serratus anterior
Axillary nodes • Nodes fixed to one another or to other structures

BOX 23.7 LOCALLY ADVANCED BREAST CANCER
• For the majority, consider systemic chemotherapy or, in the elderly or those who have indolent hormone-sensitive cancers, prescribe hormonal therapy • Radiotherapy can be used following primary chemotherapy, or can be given concurrently with hormonal therapy • Consider surgery if the disease becomes operable following primary systemic therapy, or in patients with locally advanced breast cancers that have occurred because of either a delay in diagnosis or their position in the breast, e.g. superficial or at the breast margin. Surgery is also possible in those with inoperable disease after radiotherapy

their doctor because they think it is unacceptable to do so. Doctors can promote the disclosure of such problems by being empathetic, making educated guesses about how patients are feeling, and summarizing what they have disclosed.

There is evidence that patients benefit psychologically from immediate breast reconstruction. One option for reconstruction is to insert an implant behind the chest wall muscles at the time of mastectomy. The problem with this approach is that the size of implant that can be inserted is limited and symmetry is difficult to obtain. Another option is to place a tissue expander behind the pectoral muscles. Small amounts of fluid are injected regularly into the expander over a period of months before replacing it, at a second operation, with a permanent prosthesis. Alternative options include using myocutaneous flaps; the most commonly used are the latissimus dorsi myocutaneous flap with or without an implant (Fig. 23.31), and the rectus abdominis myocutaneous flap alone.

FOLLOW-UP

Patients treated by wide local excision and radiotherapy have an approximate 1% per year rate of local recurrence in the treated breast. Those with cancer in one breast are also at risk of cancer in the other breast (0.4–0.6% per year). The majority of local recurrences after mastectomy occur within

the first few years. The aim of follow-up is to detect local recurrence at a stage when it is treatable, to support the patient psychologically and to discuss problems associated with adjuvant therapy. Patients should have an annual clinical examination and mammography of one or both breasts every 1–2 years. No investigations should be performed to detect asymptomatic metastases, as there is no evidence that this influences survival.

MANAGEMENT OF LOCALLY ADVANCED BREAST CANCER

Locally advanced breast cancer (LABC) is characterized by features suggesting infiltration of the skin or chest wall by tumour or matted involved axillary nodes (Table 23.11). It has a variable natural history, with reported 5-year survivals of between 1 and 30%. The median survival was previously about 2–2.5 years but this has improved with better systemic therapy. LABC can arise because of its position in the breast (for example, peripheral), neglect (some patients do not present to hospital for months or years after they notice a mass) or biological aggressiveness. The latter includes inflammatory cancers that present with erythema and/or widespread peau d'orange affecting the breast skin. The peau d'orange is because of lymphatic obstruction by cancer cells in lymphatics or in lymph nodes (Fig. 23.27). Inflammatory carcinomas are uncommon and are characterized by brawny, oedematous, indurated and erythematous skin changes (Fig. 23.32). They have the worst prognosis of all LABCs.

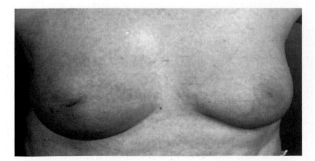
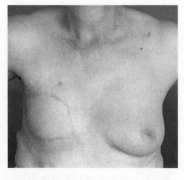

Fig. 23.32 Inflammatory breast cancer.
A Inflammatory breast cancer at diagnosis. B Following chemotherapy and radiotherapy, then surgery to excise residual disease using myocutaneous flap for skin closure.

Local and regional relapse is a major problem in LABC and affects more than half of patients. By treating patients initially with systemic therapy, followed by surgery and radiotherapy or radiotherapy alone, improvements in local control have been achieved. Systemic treatment consists of either chemotherapy (inflammatory cancers, oestrogen receptor-negative tumours and rapidly progressive disease) or hormonal treatment (slow or indolent disease, oestrogen receptor-positive cancers, or women who are elderly or unfit). Following systemic therapy, the disease may become operable, at which point surgery, usually mastectomy, is followed by radiotherapy. In women whose disease remains inoperable following systemic treatment, radiotherapy is given. This is followed by surgery in some women in whom viable resectable cancer remains following radiotherapy (Fig. 23.32). Systemic therapy, either chemotherapy (for 3–4 months) or hormone treatment (usually for 5 years), is often given after surgery.

BREAST CANCER IN PREGNANCY

Overall, 1–2% of breast cancer occurs during pregnancy. It affects 1–3 of every 10 000 pregnancies. Although there is no evidence that breast cancer occurring during pregnancy is more aggressive, up to 65% have involved axillary nodes because the diagnosis is often delayed. Treatment during the first two trimesters is with mastectomy. Radiotherapy should not be delivered during pregnancy. Chemotherapy can be given but is associated with a small risk of fetal damage. Breast cancer during the third trimester can be managed either by immediate surgery or by monitoring the tumour and delivering the baby early at 32 weeks, and then instituting treatment after delivery.

Pregnancy after treatment for breast cancer
There is only limited information on the effect of pregnancy on the outcome of patients with breast cancer, but the available data show no detrimental effect.

MANAGEMENT OF METASTATIC OR ADVANCED BREAST CANCER

The average period of survival after a diagnosis of metastatic disease is 20–30 months, but this varies widely between patients. The survival of patients with bone-only disease is over 2 years, with a median survival of patients with lung, liver and brain metastases of 10, 8 and 3 months, respectively. A patient may present with metastatic breast carcinoma or can develop metastases following treatment of an apparently localized breast cancer. The aim of treatment is to produce effective symptom control with minimal side-effects. This ideal is only achieved in the 40–50% of patients whose cancers respond to hormonal therapy or chemotherapy. There is no evidence that treating asymptomatic metastases improves overall survival, and chemotherapy is normally given only to symptomatic patients.

Chemotherapy
With chemotherapy, a balance must be achieved between a high response rate and limiting side-effects. The best palliation is obtained with regimens that produce the highest response rates. The most commonly used drugs are the anthracyclines, adriamycin and epirubicin. Taxanes (taxol and taxotere) are also commonly used. Overall rates of response to chemotherapy are approximately 40–60%, with a median time to relapse of 6–10 months. Subsequent courses have response rates of less than 25%.

Hormonal treatment
A variety of hormonal interventions are available for use in metastatic breast cancer (Table 23.12). In pre-menopausal women these include oophorectomy (surgical, radiation- or drug-induced by GnRh analogues) combined with tamoxifen. Options in post-menopausal women include the new aromatase inhibitors (anastrozole, letrozole and exemestane) and the progestogens (such as medroxyprogesterone acetate or megestrol acetate). First-line treatment is with letrozole or anastrozole. Objective responses to hormonal treatments are seen in 30% of all patients and in 50–60% of those

23

BOX 23.8   METASTATIC BREAST CANCER

- The primary aim is to improve symptoms and both the quantity and quality of life
- Consider hormone therapy if there is a long disease-free interval and the tumour is hormone receptor-positive
- Consider chemotherapy if there is a short disease-free interval, vital organs are affected and the tumour is oestrogen receptor-negative

---

Table 23.12   HORMONAL TREATMENT OF METASTATIC BREAST CANCER

Pre-menopausal
- Ovarian suppression
- Gonadotrophin-releasing hormone analogues
- Oophorectomy
- Radiation menopause
- Tamoxifen
- Ovarian suppression + tamoxifen[1]
- Ovarian suppression + an aromatase inhibitor

Post-menopausal
- Aromatase inhibitor[2], progestins, e.g. megestrol or medroxyprogesterone acetate
- Exemestane[3]
- Fulvestrant[4]

Note These agents can be used in any order.

[1]There is evidence that combined ovarian suppression plus an anti-oestrogen is superior to single-agent treatment in pre-menopausal women.
[2]Letrozole or anastrozole are first-line agents in post-menopausal women. Data for letrozole is more impressive than for anastrozole.
[3]A steroidal aromatase inhibitor (e.g. exemestane) can have efficacy even if a tumour is resistant to the non-steroidal aromatase inhibitors letrozole and anastrozole.
[4]Licensed in England, Wales and Northern Ireland, but not Scotland; continues to be evaluated in trials.

with oestrogen receptor-positive tumours. Response rates of 25% are seen when using second-line hormonal agents, although fewer than 15% of patients who show no response to first-line treatment will have a response to second-line agents. Approximately 10–15% of patients respond to third-line endocrine agents.

Immunotherapy

The humanized monoclonal antibody trastuzumab, raised against *HER2*, increases both the rate and duration of response of patients with metastatic disease when combined with chemotherapy in patients with tumours over-expressing *HER2*.

Specific problems

Bone disease

Three-quarters of patients who develop secondary breast cancer have disease involving the bony skeleton. Widespread bony disease responds well to hormonal treatment, but in young patients cytotoxic agents may be required. Treatment of localized pain includes external beam radiotherapy and analgesics, including NSAIDs and opiates. Pathological fractures due to bone disease should be avoided and can be predicted by a sharp increase in pain over a few days or weeks. When X-rays show that fracture is likely, a combination of internal fixation and radiotherapy should be used. Options for widespread bony pain include the use of bisphosphonates (which reduce osteoclast activity) and sequential upper and lower body hemiradiotherapy or radioactive strontium.

Hypercalcaemia

This is seen in up to 40% of patients with bony metastases. Symptoms include nausea, constipation, thirst, polyuria, personality change, muscle weakness and bone pain. Treatment consists of hydration with saline (about 3 litres given over 24 hours) and the administration of intravenous bisphosphonates, followed by a change in systemic anticancer therapy.

Marrow infiltration

A leuco-erythroblastic blood picture (immature cells in the peripheral blood) suggests extensive marrow infiltration. Chemotherapy is generally required, although hormones can be effective in oestrogen receptor-rich disease. Chemotherapy should be given initially in reduced doses with careful monitoring and adequate supportive care.

Spinal cord compression

This is most often seen in patients with thoracic spinal metastases. It must be recognized early and treated promptly. Patients with isolated metastases causing cord compression, and who are fit, should be treated by surgery followed by post-operative radiotherapy and appropriate systemic therapy. In the remaining patients, treatment consists of steroids and fractionated radiotherapy.

Pleural effusion

Up to half of patients with metastatic breast cancer will develop a malignant pleural effusion. Cytological exami-

---

> **BOX 23.9 METASTATIC DISEASE: SPECIFIC PROBLEMS**
>
> - Bone metastases may require local radiotherapy, bisphosphonates or orthopaedic intervention, combined with systemic hormonal therapy or chemotherapy
> - Hypercalcaemia causes nausea, constipation, thirst, polyuria, weakness, pain and personality change, and is treated by rehydration followed by bisphosphonates
> - Spinal cord compression should be treated by surgical decompression if appropriate, or by steroids and radiotherapy
> - Pleural effusions should be treated by tube drainage, followed by instillation of bleomycin, tetracycline or talc
> - Discrete lung metastases may not cause acute symptoms but lymphangitis carcinomatosa can cause severe bronchospasm and dyspnoea, which may be relieved by steroids, bronchodilators and chemotherapy
> - Liver metastases present most commonly with general debility, nausea and lack of appetite; they are usually treated by chemotherapy but hormone therapy with aromatase inhibitors is now an option
> - Brain metastases are treated initially with steroids, followed by radiation. Surgery can be used for isolated single metastases

nation of aspirated fluid reveals malignant cells in only 85% of patients. Aspiration of pleural effusions is ineffective treatment, as between 97 and 100% of patients will re-accumulate fluid. In contrast, tube drainage alone is effective in controlling effusions in over one-third of patients. The instillation of bleomycin, tetracycline or talc to cause pleurodesis reduces recurrence.

Liver metastases

Right upper quadrant pain, general debility, tiredness, a feeling of nausea and lack of appetite, and the onset of jaundice are all symptoms suggestive of liver infiltration. Chemotherapy is usually indicated, except in postmenopausal patients with oestrogen receptor-rich tumours in whom the new aromatase inhibitors can be effective. Where jaundice is due to nodal disease at the porta hepatis, a stent inserted in the common bile duct using endoscopic retrograde pancreatography (ERCP) should be considered.

Brain metastases

These should be suspected in any patient with breast cancer who presents with focal neurological symptoms. CT or MRI can detect even small volumes of disease. Initial treatment consists of high-dose corticosteroids (16 mg daily of dexamethasone), followed by radiotherapy. The greatest benefits of radiotherapy are seen in patients whose neurological symptoms improve following steroid treatment, but the long-term results of treatment are disappointing. A small group of patients with solitary brain metastases, and without evidence of involvement at other sites, are suitable for local excision followed by post-operative radiotherapy and appropriate systemic treatment. A few of these patients remain well without other evidence of disease for many years.

23

MISCELLANEOUS TUMOURS OF THE BREAST

Lymphoma

This is rare in the breast. Staging investigations are necessary because patients will usually have disease elsewhere. Characteristically, lymphoma presents as a discrete smooth rubbery mass. Small localized breast lymphomas can be treated by wide excision, axillary node sampling, radiotherapy and chemotherapy. Larger lesions should be treated by radiotherapy and chemotherapy after biopsy.

Sarcomas

Sarcomas can develop in breast tissue and can affect the skin overlying the breast. Rarely, they are induced by radiotherapy to the chest wall. Sarcomas are treated by excision. As many of these tumours are large at diagnosis, mastectomy is generally necessary. Radiotherapy should be given to the chest wall after excisional surgery, but there is no evidence that adjuvant chemotherapy is of benefit.

Malignant phyllodes tumours

Previously called cystosarcoma phyllodes, these present as large lobulated lesions that can involve the overlying skin. Initial treatment is by wide excision or mastectomy. The roles of radiotherapy and chemotherapy in these lesions are unclear.

Secondary tumours

Metastases from tumours elsewhere, e.g. bronchus, thyroid, melanoma or the opposite breast, produce a well-defined mass both clinically and mammographically.

MALE BREAST

GYNAECOMASTIA

Gynaecomastia (the growth of breast tissue in males to any extent in all ages) is entirely benign and usually reversible. It commonly occurs at puberty and in old age and is seen in 30–60% of boys aged 10–16. In this age group it usually requires no treatment, as 80% resolve spontaneously within 2 years (Fig. 23.33). Embarrassment or persistent enlargement is an indication for surgery. Senescent gynaecomastia usually affects men between 50 and 80, and in most cases does not appear to be associated with any endocrine abnormality. Causes include excess alcohol intake and drugs including cannabis, cirrhosis, hypogonadism and,

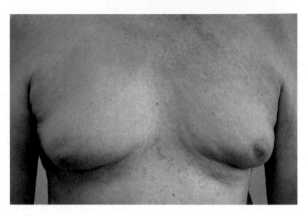

Fig. 23.33   Gynaecomastia.

rarely, testicular tumours. Rapidly progressive gynaecomastia is an indication for an assessment of hormonal profile. A history of recent progressive breast enlargement without pain and tenderness, or an easily identifiable cause, should raise the suspicion of breast cancer. If there is a localized mass, then further investigations should be performed. Surgery consists of excision of glandular tissue combined with liposuction or liposuction alone and is reserved for patients with significant social embarrassment.

MALE BREAST CANCER

Fewer than 0.5% of all breast cancers occur in men, and breast cancer comprises 0.7% of all male cancers. The peak incidence in males is 5–10 years later than in women. Klinefelter's syndrome and a strong family history are the only known risk factors. Male breast cancers can be associated with *BRCA2* gene mutations. Cancer usually presents with an eccentric breast mass or retraction of the overlying skin. Direct involvement of the skin occurs more often in male breast cancer because of the smaller breast volume compared to the female breast, and so the disease is more likely to be advanced at diagnosis. Mammography and core biopsy or fine-needle aspiration cytology confirms the diagnosis. Treatment for localized breast cancer is by total mastectomy and the removal of axillary nodes, usually followed by post-operative radiotherapy to the chest wall. Wide local excision, axillary surgery and post-operative radiotherapy can be used to treat some small breast cancers. Adjuvant tamoxifen is effective at reducing recurrence. Adjuvant chemotherapy should be considered for fit patients with tumours that have nodal involvement or are oestrogen receptor-negative.

T.W.J. LENNARD

Endocrine surgery

INTRODUCTION

In surgical endocrine disease, thyroid disorders are common, adrenal disease is uncommon and parathyroid disease is rare.

THYROID GLAND

SURGICAL ANATOMY AND DEVELOPMENT

The thyroid gland develops from the thyroglossal duct, which grows downwards from the pharynx through the developing hyoid bone. On the front of the trachea, the duct bifurcates and fuses with elements from the fourth branchial arch, from which the parafollicular (C) cells are derived.

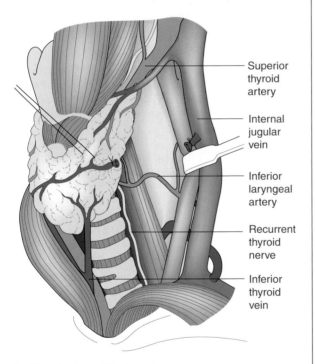

Fig. 24.1 Anatomy of the thyroid gland.
The middle thyroid vein has been divided to allow forward rotation of the left lobe of the gland.

The duct is normally obliterated in early fetal life but can persist in part to produce a thyroglossal cyst. The upper end of the duct is identified in adults as the foramen caecum at the junction of the anterior two-thirds and the posterior third of the tongue. Arrest of descent of the duct may result in an ectopic thyroid (e.g. lingual thyroid).

There are two pairs of parathyroid glands. The upper glands arise from the fourth branchial arch and are usually found at the back of the thyroid above the inferior thyroid artery. The lower glands arise from the third arch (in association with the thymus) and are less constant in position. They are usually found posterior to the lower pole of the thyroid lobes but can lie within the gland, some distance below it, in the upper mediastinum or within the thymus.

The right and left lobes of the thyroid lie on the front and sides of the trachea and larynx at the level of the 5–7th cervical vertebrae (Fig. 24.1). The two lobes are connected by a narrow isthmus, which overlies the second and third tracheal rings. The thyroid normally weighs 15–30 g and is invested by the pre-tracheal fascia, which binds it to the larynx, cricoid cartilage and trachea (Fig. 24.2). The strap muscles (sternohyoid and sternothyroid) lie in front of the pre-tracheal fascia and must be separated to gain access to the gland. It is difficult to feel the normal thyroid gland except at puberty and during pregnancy, when physiological enlargement occurs.

The superior thyroid artery runs down to the upper pole of the gland as a branch of the external carotid artery, whereas the inferior thyroid artery runs across to the lower pole from the thyrocervical trunk (a branch of the subclavian artery). As it nears the gland, the inferior thyroid artery usually passes in front of the recurrent laryngeal nerve, but may branch around it. Blood from the thyroid drains through superior, middle and inferior thyroid veins into the internal jugular and innominate veins. Lymphatics drain laterally to the deep cervical chain and downwards to pre-tracheal and mediastinal nodes. The recurrent laryngeal nerve is a branch of the vagus, which passes upwards in the groove between the oesophagus and trachea to enter the larynx and supply all of its intrinsic muscles except the cricothyroid. The superior laryngeal nerve (also a branch of the vagus) runs with the superior thyroid vessels and supplies the cricothyroid muscles (external branch), which tense the vocal cords. The recurrent nerve also supplies sensation to the larynx below the vocal cords. The internal branch

24

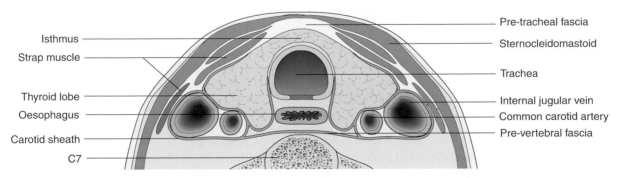

Fig. 24.2 Transverse section of the neck at the level of the 7th cervical vertebra to show the arrangement of the deep cervical fascia.

24

of the superior laryngeal nerve provides sensation above the cords. Normal sensory and motor function within the larynx is necessary for speech and coughing. Both nerves are at risk of damage during thyroid surgery and the consequences, if permanent, can be disabling.

THYROID FUNCTION

Histologically, the gland is made up of follicles containing colloid, which on haematoxylin and eosin staining appears pink. The follicles are spheroids lined by cuboidal epithelium (thyrocytes). The parafollicular or C cells may be seen between follicles. The gland has an exceedingly rich blood supply. The thyrocytes secrete triiodothyronine (T_3) and thyroxine (T_4). T_3 is the active hormone, and T_4 is converted to T_3 in the periphery.

Secretion of T_3 and T_4 is controlled by thyroid-stimulating hormone (TSH), which is secreted by the anterior pituitary. TSH release is in turn controlled by thyrotropin-releasing hormone (TRH) from the hypothalamus. Circulating levels of T_3 and T_4 exert a negative feedback effect on the hypothalamus and anterior pituitary. The parafollicular cells produce calcitonin. This can be measured in the blood and is normally secreted in small amounts. Secretion is increased after food. Calcitonin lowers the serum calcium but it is not an essential hormone and does not require replacement after total thyroidectomy.

ASSESSMENT OF THYROID DISEASE

Measurement of T_3, T_4 and TSH gives a biochemical estimation of thyroid function. TSH is totally suppressed in thyrotoxicosis and elevated in hypothyroidism. Pregnancy or oestrogen administration increases the level of thyroid-binding globulin, so that estimation of the ratio of free to bound hormone may be needed. TRH and TSH stimulation tests may be required to determine the site of failure of production of thyroid hormones.

The thyroid can be imaged best by ultrasonography or radioisotope scanning (^{99m}Tc-sodium pertechnetate behaves like iodine and is 'trapped' by the gland). The main value of scanning is to differentiate between 'hot' (actively functioning), 'cool' (normally functioning) and 'cold' (non-functioning) thyroid nodules. Total isotope uptake also reflects thyroid activity.

Magnetic resonance imaging (MRI) and computed tomography (CT) provide excellent means of determining the extent of goitre. Fine-needle aspiration cytology is used to determine the nature of thyroid nodules. Thyroid antibodies detected in significant titre may indicate autoimmune thyroid disease.

ENLARGEMENT OF THE THYROID GLAND (GOITRE)

Clinical features

Goitre is a visible or palpable enlargement of the thyroid (Fig. 24.3). The swelling appears in the lower part of the neck and retains the shape of the normal gland (*thyreos*—Greek for shield). The swelling characteristically moves

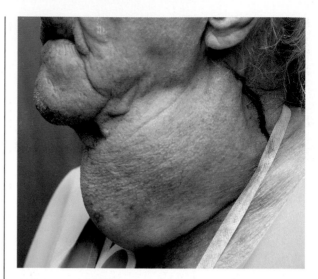

Fig. 24.3　Massive goitre.

upwards on swallowing because of the gland's attachment to the trachea. Careful observation usually allows this physical sign to be detected during a spontaneous swallow. Patients in consultation are often nervous and have a dry mouth, and to ask them to swallow repeatedly is unnecessary unless water can be provided.

'Physiological' enlargement

Transient enlargement may occur during puberty or pregnancy.

NON-TOXIC NODULAR GOITRE

Aetiology

This common disease occurs endemically in areas of iodine deficiency, but can be sporadic or a reaction to drugs. It occurs much more commonly in females. In the past, lack of iodine in the diet was a common cause of thyroid enlargement, but 'endemic goitres' in areas such as Wales and Derbyshire are now rare because table salt is iodized. In areas of the world where iodine intake cannot be guaranteed, iodized oil emulsion can be injected.

Pathology

In iodine deficiency, the gland initially enlarges diffusely as the follicles fill with colloid. Later, multiple nodules develop, some of which contain abundant colloid; others show degenerative changes, with the formation of cysts, areas of old and new haemorrhage, and even calcification. The goitre varies greatly in size, from little more than normal to weighing several hundred grams. The whole gland may be involved, or the changes may be confined to one lobe.

Clinical features

Most multinodular goitres are asymptomatic. Others cause tracheal compression and dyspnoea, particularly when they extend behind the sternum (retrosternal goitre). Oesophageal compression can cause dysphagia. Very rarely,

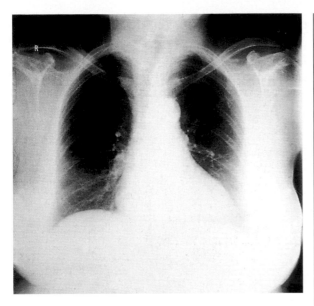

Fig. 24.4 X-ray of the thoracic inlet showing a retrosternal goitre with marked deviation of the trachea to the right.

bleeding into a nodule may cause pain and rapid enlargement and, in the case of retrosternal goitre, respiratory distress. The thyroid is visibly enlarged and multiple nodules are usually palpable. Sometimes only one nodule is palpable, giving the erroneous impression of a solitary nodule.

Investigations
In the case of retrosternal goitre, plain films of the thoracic inlet may reveal tracheal deviation (Fig. 24.4). Only a CT scan will show tracheal compression. The presence of stridor should alert the physician to the presence of compromise of the tracheal lumen (Fig. 24.5). T_3, T_4 and TSH are usually normal. Isotope scans are most often unhelpful.

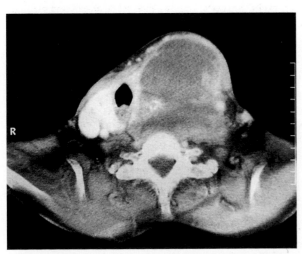

Fig. 24.5 CT scan of the neck of an 80-year-old woman with massive enlargement of the left thyroid lobe, causing marked tracheal deviation and narrowing.

Management
The administration of thyroxine occasionally prevents further enlargement by suppressing TSH secretion, but regression of the goitre is unusual. Large goitres and those causing symptoms of compression require total or subtotal thyroidectomy. Some patients request surgery for cosmetic reasons. Thyroxine may be used post-operatively to suppress TSH secretion and prevent the enlargement of any residual gland. Patients may be willing to accept total thyroidectomy and lifelong replacement therapy as preferable to the chance of recurrence and the need for reoperation.

THYROTOXIC GOITRE

Diffuse thyroid enlargement can result from stimulation by TSH or TSH-like proteins, resulting in increased production of T_3 and T_4 and thyrotoxicosis. However, most goitres occur in individuals who have normal function. The combination of goitre and hyperfunction is an indication for surgical treatment.

THYROIDITIS

Subacute thyroiditis (de Quervain's disease)
This rare condition is associated with an influenza-like illness, during which there is painful diffuse swelling of the gland. Thyroid antibodies may appear in the serum. The disease may be due to a viral infection and usually resolves, although occasionally it runs an intermittent course.

Autoimmune thyroiditis (Hashimoto's disease)

Aetiology
This condition is believed to be due to the destruction of thyroid follicles by immunocompetent lymphocytes. Antibodies are detected in the serum against thyroglobulin, thyroid cell cytosol and microsomes. Histologically, there is marked lymphocytic infiltration around destroyed follicles.

Clinical features
The patient is usually euthyroid, but thyrotoxicosis can occur. In the long term, the patient becomes hypothyroid. Post-menopausal women are most commonly affected (female:male ratio 10:1). The thyroid is diffusely enlarged and firm. A nodular form may be confused with multinodular goitre. Lymphoma may occur in a thyroid that has been affected by long-standing Hashimoto's disease.

Investigations
The diagnosis depends on demonstrating high titres of circulating antithyroid antibodies, particularly to microsomal components of the follicle cells. Biopsy for cytology helps to confirm the diagnosis.

Management
Thyroxine causes regression of small goitres, but thyroidectomy is needed when a large goitre is causing compression symptoms. Surgery can be difficult because of the firm nature of the gland and inflammation of the surrounding structures. There is a higher than normal risk of damage to the recurrent laryngeal nerves or parathyroid glands.

24

Riedel's thyroiditis

In this very rare condition the thyroid is replaced by dense fibrous tissue, resulting in a firm painless swelling and tracheal compression. The cause is unknown. Surgical decompression of the trachea may be required.

SOLITARY THYROID NODULES

Slow-growing and painless clinically 'solitary' nodules are common, although 50% of them are really part of a multinodular goitre. Of the true solitary nodules, half are benign adenomas and the rest are cysts or differentiated

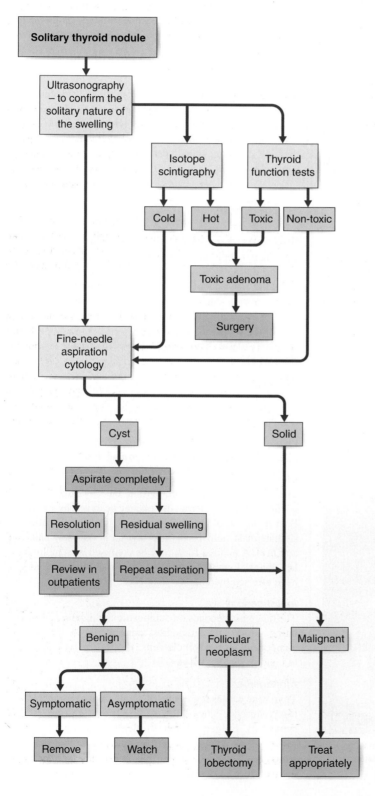

Fig. 24.6 Algorithm for the management of a patient with a suspected solitary thyroid nodule.

BOX 24.1   GOITRES

- Physiological enlargement of the thyroid gland may occur during puberty or pregnancy
- Non-toxic nodular goitre can be associated with iodine deficiency and drug reactions; it is usually asymptomatic but can cause compression symptoms
- Thyrotoxic goitre results from stimulation of the gland by TSH or TSH-like proteins, resulting in excessive production of T_3 and T_4. About 25% of cases of thyrotoxicosis are due to a toxic multinodular goitre (in which a long-standing non-toxic goitre develops one or more hyperactive nodules that function independently of TSH levels)
- Thyroiditis can produce diffuse painful swelling that may be subacute (de Quervain's disease) or autoimmune (Hashimoto's disease). Riedel's thyroiditis is a very rare cause of painless thyroid swelling and tracheal compression, in which the gland is replaced by fibrous tissue
- A solitary thyroid nodule often proves to be a conspicuous palpable nodule in a gland affected by multinodular goitre. True solitary nodules may be adenomas, cysts or cancers, conditions that are distinguished by fine-needle aspiration cytology, ultrasonography, isotope scans and function tests
- Thyroid cancers can produce a goitre, particularly in the case of medullary carcinoma of the thyroid and lymphoma

---

cancers. The pivotal diagnostic test is fine-needle aspiration cytology, complemented by ultrasonography, isotope scans and thyroid function tests (Fig. 24.6). Cysts can be aspirated and, provided that they do not refill and that the cytology is negative for neoplastic cells, they need not be removed. Very rarely, a cyst contains a carcinoma (often papillary) within its wall, and blood-stained aspirate or a residual swelling after aspiration should raise this possibility. A cytopathologist cannot distinguish between a follicular adenoma and follicular carcinoma; this can only be achieved on definitive histopathology by looking for capsular or vascular invasion. Surgery is needed if aspiration reveals a follicular neoplasm. Intra-operative frozen section does not always provide a definitive diagnosis, but the demonstration of carcinoma means that more extensive surgery is needed. In some patients, carcinoma is only revealed on definitive histopathological examination, and reoperation may then be indicated, to remove any remaining thyroid tissue.

OTHER FORMS OF NEOPLASIA

All forms of thyroid cancer can produce a goitre. Lymphoma and anaplastic tumours may cause diffuse thyroid swellings. Medullary and follicular tumours are often solitary swellings.

HYPERTHYROIDISM

Thyrotoxicosis results from the overproduction of T_3 and T_4 and, because of the feedback mechanism, serum TSH levels are reduced or undetectable. The three conditions that may produce thyrotoxicosis are primary thyrotoxicosis (Graves' disease), toxic multinodular goitre and toxic adenoma.

PRIMARY THYROTOXICOSIS (GRAVES' DISEASE)

Pathophysiology

This condition accounts for 75% of cases. It is an autoimmune disease in which TSH receptors in the thyroid are stimulated by circulating thyroid-stimulating immunoglobulins (TSI). The gland is uniformly hyperactive, very vascular and usually symmetrically enlarged, although not to a great degree. Histologically, there is marked epithelial proliferation, with papillary projections into follicles devoid of colloid. TSI can cross the placental barrier, so that neonatal thyrotoxicosis can occur.

Clinical features

The patient is usually a young female (male:female ratio 1:8) and the condition can be familial. The thyroid is usually moderately and diffusely enlarged and soft, and because of its vascularity a bruit may be audible. High circulating levels of T_3 and T_4 increase the basal metabolic rate and potentiate the actions of the sympathetic nervous system.

Metabolic effects

The patient feels hot at rest and is intolerant of warmth. The skin is moist and warm because of peripheral vasodilatation and excess sweating. Weight loss is the rule, despite an increased appetite. Cardiac output is increased to meet the metabolic demands.

Sympathetic effects

Tachycardia is present, even during sleep. Palpitations can be troublesome, and cardiac irregularities and arrhythmias (especially atrial fibrillation) are common in older patients. The hands exhibit a fine tremor. The upper eyelids are retracted (the levator palpebrae superioris has some non-striated muscle which is innervated by the sympathetic nervous system) and there is lid lag. Gastrointestinal motility is increased. There is general hyperkinesia; anxiety and psychiatric disturbance may occur.

Other features

Exophthalmos is usual but not invariable (Fig. 24.7). Ophthalmoplegia, pretibial myxoedema, proximal muscle

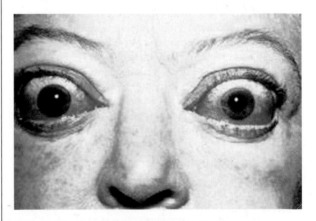

Fig. 24.7   Thyroid-associated ophthalmopathy.
(Courtesy of Prof Michael Sheppard, University of Birmingham Medical School.)

myopathy and finger clubbing are sometimes present. Menstrual irregularity and infertility can occur.

Diagnosis

The diagnosis is usually obvious clinically, although in patients with anxiety, distinction from neurosis can be difficult. Raised T_3 and T_4 levels, coupled with low TSH levels, are confirmatory. The TSH response to intravenous injection of TRH is absent owing to atrophy of the TSH-producing cells of the pituitary.

Management

Antithyroid drugs

These drugs block the incorporation of iodine into tyrosine and so prevent the synthesis of T_3 and T_4. Carbimazole, given in full blocking doses (30–60 mg daily in four divided doses), can render the patient euthyroid within 4–6 weeks. However, up to 60% of patients will relapse within 2 years of stopping treatment.

Radioactive iodine

Many consider this to be the treatment of choice. As long as it is not used in pregnancy, the risks of genetic damage are minimal in both patients and their offspring. If ablative doses of iodine are used, patients require thyroxine replacement, but can lead an otherwise normal life with little risk of recurrence.

Surgery

Thyroidectomy is a highly successful form of treatment for many patients, especially younger ones. In experienced hands, operative mortality and morbidity are low. Patients may be cured by surgery, and recurrence is usually due to the removal of insufficient glandular tissue. Hypothyroidism occurs in 50% or more of patients, and low T_3 and T_4 levels with high TSH levels persisting for more than 6 months signal the need for lifelong thyroid hormone replacement.

Before surgery, patients must be rendered euthyroid with antithyroid drugs. Iodine can be given before surgery to reduce vascularity. Beta-adrenergic blocking drugs can be used as an alternative means of countering the effects of thyrotoxicosis before operation. They block sympathetic over-activity and make the gland less vascular. Cardiac failure, obstructive airways disease and diabetes (where they may mask hypoglycaemic symptoms) are contraindications to the use of β-blockers. Propranolol is given in a dose of 40–80 mg 6-hourly, the aim being to reduce the pulse rate to below 80 beats per minute (bpm). Long-acting preparations may be preferred. The drug is continued on the morning of operation and for 7 days thereafter to avoid 'thyroid storm' or 'thyrotoxic crisis'. Excessive sweating or tachycardia after operation is an indication to increase the dose. Increasingly, total thyroidectomy is performed in preference to subtotal.

TOXIC MULTINODULAR GOITRE AND TOXIC ADENOMA

Pathophysiology

A toxic multinodular goitre is responsible for thyrotoxicosis in about 25% of patients. There is usually a long-standing non-toxic goitre in which one or more nodules become hyperactive and begin to function independently of TSH levels. A single functioning adenoma is a rare cause of thyrotoxicosis (1–2% of patients). The adenoma secretes thyroid hormones autonomously, TSH secretion is completely suppressed, and the remainder of the gland is non-functional.

Clinical features

Toxic multinodular goitre is more common in older women, and cardiac complications such as arrhythmias are particularly frequent. Exophthalmos is rare. Patients with a toxic adenoma hardly ever have exophthalmos, ophthalmoplegia or myopathy.

Diagnosis

In a toxic multinodular goitre, the isotope scan demonstrates one or more areas of increased uptake. In toxic adenoma, the nodule is 'hot' and the remainder of the gland is 'cold'.

Management

Treatment consists of removal of the hyperfunctioning glandular tissue by subtotal thyroidectomy (multinodular goitre) or lobectomy (toxic adenoma), or radioiodine.

MALIGNANT TUMOURS OF THE THYROID

Thyroid cancer accounts for less than 1% of all forms of malignancy. As with all thyroid disease, females are more often affected (male:female ratio 1:3). The two main types of thyroid carcinoma are papillary (50%) and follicular (30%), with the remainder comprising medullary carcinoma, anaplastic carcinoma and lymphoma. The incidence of thyroid cancer is increased by exposure to ionizing radiation: for example, following the Chernobyl disaster.

PAPILLARY CARCINOMA

Clinical features

This tumour is rare after the age of 40 years and presents as a slow-growing solitary thyroid swelling that is not particularly hard. Enlarged lymph nodes are palpable in one-third of patients and may be the only finding in some patients with a microscopic primary (a situation once misinterpreted as a 'lateral aberrant thyroid'). Distant metastases are rare. Occasionally, papillary carcinoma is discovered as an incidental finding in a gland that has been removed for other reasons. Histologically, complex papillary folds lined by several layers of cuboidal cells project into what appear to be cystic spaces.

Management

The disease is commonly multifocal, so that total or near-total thyroidectomy is indicated. Involved lymph nodes are removed but radical neck dissection is unnecessary. Hormone replacement therapy (T_3, 20 µg 6–8-hourly, or thyroxine 150 µg/day) is given and its adequacy monitored by measuring TSH. Widespread metastases are rare but

24

may be amenable to radioactive iodine therapy. The disease has an excellent prognosis, with 10-year survival rates approaching 90%.

FOLLICULAR CARCINOMA

Clinical features

This disease typically presents as a solitary thyroid nodule in patients aged 30–50 years. Lymph node metastases are much less common than haematogenous spread, and 20% of patients have deposits in the lungs, bone or liver. Histologically, malignant cells are arranged in solid masses with rudimentary acini. Vascular and capsular invasion characterize this neoplasm and distinguish it from a benign follicular adenoma.

Management

Treatment consists of total thyroidectomy with preservation of the parathyroids. If a post-operative radioisotope scan (tracer dose) reveals increased uptake in the skeleton or neck, therapeutic doses of radioiodine are given. T_4 is administered routinely to suppress TSH secretion. Plasma thyroglobulin levels should be undetectable after surgery and radioiodine therapy. Subsequent detection of thyroglobulin indicates recurrent disease. The disease is more aggressive than papillary carcinoma and the 10-year survival rate is 50%.

ANAPLASTIC CARCINOMA

Clinical features

These rapidly growing, highly malignant tumours tend to occur in older patients. Local invasion may involve the recurrent laryngeal nerve(s) and cause hoarseness, or compress the trachea and cause dyspnoea and stridor, and/or compress the oesophagus and cause dysphagia. Invasion of the cervical sympathetic nerves may cause Horner's syndrome (contraction of the pupil, enophthalmos, narrowing of the palpebral fissure and loss of sweating on the face and neck). Pulmonary metastases are common. Death usually occurs within 6 months of diagnosis.

Management

Resection is rarely possible but surgery can relieve tracheal compression. Radiotherapy and chemotherapy are of marginal value.

MEDULLARY CARCINOMA

Clinical features

This tumour arises from the parafollicular C cells. There is hard enlargement of one or both thyroid lobes, and in 50% of patients the cervical lymph nodes are involved. The tumour may occur sporadically or as part of an inherited multiple endocrine neoplasia (MEN) syndrome type II (Sipple's syndrome). Calcitonin levels are elevated, and can be used to monitor progress and screen relatives. The

gene causing the inherited form of this tumour is the *Ret* proto-oncogene, and the finding of this mutation allows the diagnosis to be made at any age. Prophylactic thyroidectomy for affected children is recommended from the age of 5 years in MEN IIa, but at 1 year for MEN IIb.

Management

Treatment consists of total thyroidectomy and dissection of the lymph nodes in the central compartment of the neck. Medullary carcinoma in MEN IIb syndrome is particularly aggressive, and those affected rarely live beyond 30–40 years of age. Other forms—for example, pure inherited medullary thyroid cancer occurring without other endocrine tumours—can be very indolent.

LYMPHOMA

Primary lymphoma of the thyroid is a rare complication of autoimmune thyroiditis. It can also occur as a primary tumour that originates in an otherwise normal gland. It is amenable to treatment by radiotherapy and chemotherapy, but patients often require core biopsy of the gland to characterize the type of lymphoma. CT is used to stage the disease fully.

BOX 24.2 THYROID CANCER

- Thyroid cancers may arise from the epithelium (papillary 50% or follicular 30%). Anaplastic parafollicular C cells (medullary carcinoma) or lymphoreticular tissue (lymphoma) make up the other tumours of the gland
- Papillary cancers are rare after the age of 40 years, are often multifocal and spread to lymph nodes, but rarely disseminate widely. Total or near-total thyroidectomy with the removal of involved nodes is followed by T_4 replacement therapy. Ten-year survival rates approach 90%
- Follicular carcinoma occurs in the 30–50-year age group, spreads preferentially via the blood stream, and is treated by total thyroidectomy. Residual neck or skeletal radioisotope uptake signals the need for radio-iodine therapy. T_4 is used routinely to suppress TSH production. The 10-year survival rate is 50%
- Anaplastic carcinoma occurs in older patients, spreads locally and frequently gives rise to pulmonary metastases. Curative resection is rarely possible, radiotherapy/chemotherapy is of little value, and most patients die within 1 year
- Medullary carcinomas secrete calcitonin, may involve both lobes, and involve neck nodes. They may be sporadic or part of MEN II. Treatment consists of total thyroidectomy and node dissection, and prognosis can be poor

The most relevant websites and publications for the management of thyroid cancer are:

- www.aace.com/pub/guidelines/index.php American Association of Endocrine Surgeons, *thyroid_carcinoma guidelines.*
- www.baes.info/Thyroid.htm British Association of Endocrine Surgeons.
- www.british-thyroid-association.org National thyroid cancer guidelines group of the British Thyroid Association.
- Northern Cancer Network. Guidelines for management of thyroid cancer. Clinical Oncology 2000; 12:373–391.

24

THYROIDECTOMY

Technique

The gland is exposed through a transverse skin-crease incision placed 2–3 cm above the sternal notch. The deep cervical fascia is divided longitudinally in the midline and the strap muscles are separated. Each lobe is mobilized by dividing first the vessels supplying the superior pole, then the middle and inferior thyroid veins, and finally the inferior thyroid artery. The recurrent laryngeal nerves should be identified, so that they can be protected from injury. The amount of thyroid tissue removed depends on the indication for operation. Care is taken to preserve the parathyroid glands. Haemostasis must be meticulous and drains are unnecessary. The layers of the neck are reconstituted with interrupted absorbable sutures and the skin is approximated with skin clips, a subcuticular suture or steristrips. Skin clips and steristrips can be removed on the second post-operative day. Minimally invasive techniques are being explored as a means of performing thyroidectomy.

Complications

Haemorrhage

Early secondary haemorrhage should not occur if meticulous haemostasis is achieved before closure. If bleeding does occur, it can compress structures in the thoracic inlet, leading to venous engorgement, tracheal compression and asphyxia. The wound must be reopened urgently and the patient intubated and taken back to theatre for exploration of the wound, removal of haematoma and control of bleeding.

Nerve damage

The external branch of the superior laryngeal nerve may be damaged during ligation of the vascular pedicle at the upper pole of the thyroid. Inability to tense the vocal cord results in a weak, hoarse deep voice. Anaesthesia of the mucous membrane of the upper larynx allows foreign bodies to enter the larynx more readily. Damage to the recurrent laryngeal nerve is more serious. Traction or bruising of this nerve causes temporary paralysis of a vocal cord in 5% of patients undergoing thyroidectomy, but recovery within 3 months is the rule. Division of the nerve paralyses the cord in the 'cadaveric' position (i.e. midway between the closed and open positions). The normal cord on the other side compensates by crossing the midline in phonation, but the voice is altered in timbre and weak. Some degree of stridor, especially on exertion, may be noted.

Bilateral nerve injury results in stridor and ineffective coughing when the endotracheal tube is withdrawn at the end of the operation. The tube is reinserted immediately and, if there is no early improvement, tracheostomy may be required. The paralysis is originally flaccid, but fibrosis draws the cords together and, even if tracheostomy has been avoided, increasing dyspnoea on exertion may be troublesome. Laryngoplasty may be needed to reconstitute the cords, but if this fails, permanent tracheostomy may be unavoidable.

Hypothyroidism

Thyroid function is monitored after surgery in case replacement therapy is needed. The risk of hypothyroidism depends on the type of disease and extent of surgery. After total thyroidectomy, replacement therapy may commence the following day. A standard dose for adults is 150 μg thyroxine daily, adjusted according to clinical findings and thyroid function tests.

Hypoparathyroidism

Bruising or accidental removal of the parathyroid glands leads to hypoparathyroidism, manifest by hypocalcaemia and symptoms of increased neuromuscular excitability. Early symptoms are tingling or numbness around the mouth and in the fingers. Hypercontractility can be demonstrated in the muscles of facial expression by tapping the facial (VII) nerve over the parotid gland (Chvostek's sign). In extreme cases, tetany may develop. Serum calcium must be checked 24 hours after thyroid surgery. Hypocalcaemic symptoms, or a serum calcium less than 2.0 mmol/l, require calcium supplements. Severe hypoparathyroidism may require vitamin D therapy as well. Serum calcium checks are required, with gradual withdrawal of supplements as the parathyroids recover. If supplementation is still necessary at 12 months, then the patient is likely to require lifelong treatment.

Scar complications

The scar can become hypertrophic or keloid, particularly when the incision has been placed low in the neck. Recurrent keloid formation is common after excision of the scar (with or without steroid infiltration), and reoperation is not advised lightly.

Patient information

A forewarned patient is much less aggrieved than one who learns about previously unmentioned complications on the first post-operative day. Full informed consent should describe the potential complications and should be obtained by the surgeon who will carry out the procedure. Surgeons should be able to provide patients with their own complication rates, and information on how these compare with national averages. It is important to couch the advice in readily understood terms. Remember that the patient is unlikely to have heard of the parathyroid glands, let alone know what they do. The starting point must certainly be at the beginning, and explanations should be given in simple language. The advice must be full and honest, but should not frighten the patient. Written advice may be provided for reading and digestion at home. The patient may be well informed, having 'surfed' the Internet, or may have obtained totally inaccurate and inappropriate information from this source.

PARATHYROID GLANDS

SURGICAL ANATOMY

The development of the parathyroid glands was considered earlier in the chapter. These glands receive a rich blood supply from the inferior thyroid artery, the branches of

Table 24.1   CAUSES OF HYPERCALCAEMIA

Hyperparathyroidism
- Primary
- Secondary
- Tertiary

Increased calcium absorption
- Vitamin D excess
- Sarcoidosis
- Drugs (e.g. diuretics, lithium)

Excessive bone breakdown
- Metastatic disease (particularly breast cancer)
- Myeloma
- Immobilization following multiple fractures

Ectopic secretion of parathyroid-like hormone
- Cancer of bronchus
- Cancer of breast

Table 24.2   CAUSES OF HYPOCALCAEMIA

Hypoparathyroidism
- Thyroid surgery
- Parathyroid surgery

Hypoproteinaemia
- Nephrosis (excessive protein loss)
- Malnutrition (inadequate intake)
- Cirrhosis (deficient synthesis)
- Severe inflammation (e.g. burns, acute pancreatitis)

Vitamin D deficiency
- Pseudohypoparathyroidism

which are a valuable guide to their position. Histologically, the glands contain chief cells (classified as dark, light and water-clear) that secrete parathormone (PTH). After the age of 5–7 years, eosinophilic cells appear; their function is unknown.

CALCIUM METABOLISM

Plasma calcium levels are kept constant in the range 2.25–2.6 mmol/l by regulating the amounts absorbed from the intestine, deposited in or withdrawn from bone, and excreted in the urine. PTH and vitamin D are the main regulators, with minimal modulation by calcitonin.

Hypercalcaemia and hypocalcaemia
Hypercalcaemia is a common biochemical abnormality and may be due to many causes other than excess PTH secretion (Table 24.1). Similarly, hypocalcaemia may be due to causes other than parathyroid removal or damage (Table 24.2).

PRIMARY HYPERPARATHYROIDISM

Pathology
In 90% of patients, primary hyperparathyroidism is due to an adenoma, in 10% it results from hyperplasia (usually affecting all four glands), and in less than 1% it results from parathyroid carcinoma. Adenomas are normally small spherical brown nodules but can be 10 times larger than the normal gland. Most are single, but 20% of patients have multiple adenomas. Histologically, there is a mixed pattern of cells in which chief cells predominate. Hyperplasia is due to an increase in the number of chief cells and, by definition, the gland must be at least twice the upper limit of normal: that is, weigh more than 70 mg.

Clinical features
Women are affected twice as often as men. The disease usually presents in middle age and is increasingly being diagnosed in asymptomatic patients who happen to be found to have hypercalcaemia on routine biochemical estimations. If clinical manifestations occur, renal and bone effects predominate. Renal effects include nephrocalcinosis (speckled calcification) and the formation of urinary calculi owing to increased excretion of calcium and phosphate. Polyuria is an early sign of hyperparathyroidism. Serum calcium levels must be checked repeatedly in all patients with urinary calculi, especially when these are recurrent, if hyperparathyroidism is to be diagnosed in time to avoid renal damage.

Bone damage used to be common but is now rarely seen as the disease is diagnosed earlier. Gross demineralization, subperiosteal bone resorption (seen typically in the middle and distal phalanges of the fingers), cysts in the long bones and jaw, and the moth-eaten appearance of the skull gave rise to the descriptive term 'osteitis fibrosa cystica'. Multiple pathological fractures were also once common.

Other manifestations of hyperparathyroidism include peptic ulceration, acute and chronic pancreatitis, lethargy, muscle weakness and psychotic symptoms. The clinical picture of florid hyperparathyroidism is often summarized as one of 'bones, stones and groans'. Rarely, patients present with a hypercalcaemic crisis characterized by marked hypercalcaemia (> 3.5 mmol/l), mental confusion, nausea and vomiting. The vomiting increases pre-existing dehydration, leading to higher levels of serum calcium, more confusion and prostration, more dehydration, and so on. Urgent expert attention is required to reverse this vicious downward spiral. The most pressing need is to correct the dehydration. The calcium may be further reduced by the use of diphosphonates.

Diagnosis
If hyperparathyroidism is suspected, serum calcium and PTH levels must be measured on more than one occasion. PTH levels may be normal, but the detection of PTH in a patient with hypercalcaemia supports the diagnosis of primary hyperparathyroidism. Other supportive findings include a low serum phosphate, hyperchloraemia (and an abnormal Cl/PO_4 ratio), and a raised 24-hour urinary calcium excretion. A low urinary calcium excretion should alert the clinician to the possibility of familial hypercalcaemic hypocalciuria, a disease of the renal tubules in which the parathyroids are normal. Alkaline phosphatase (skeletal) levels may be raised, even if there is no radiological evidence of bone disease.

24

24

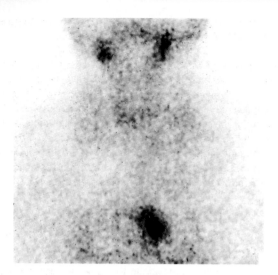

Fig. 24.8 Thallium–technetium subtraction scan showing excess thallium uptake in a mediastinal parathyroid adenoma.

Management

The aim of treatment is to identify and remove overactive parathyroid tissue. The surgical approach is similar to that used for thyroidectomy. Each lobe of the thyroid is mobilized, and all four glands are identified and inspected. Normal parathyroids are smooth and brownish-tan in colour. They are small, especially if suppressed by over-production of PTH from an adenoma. Enlarged glands are nodular. Immediate frozen section examination is used to establish the diagnosis and make certain that parathyroid, rather than thyroid, thymus or fat, has been identified and removed.

Various methods have been used to localize abnormal glands in an attempt to make surgical exploration more focused. These include ultrasonography, CT, MRI, isotope scintigraphy, arteriography and selective venous sampling for PTH assays. However, none is capable of bettering the results of bilateral neck exploration by an experienced parathyroid surgeon. As in thyroid surgery, some have used minimally invasive techniques to explore the neck, using intra-operative PTH assays to confirm removal of the localized adenoma.

In the majority of patients, only one gland is enlarged and this is removed. If two or more glands are enlarged, they should be removed. If all four glands are thought to be hyperplastic, then all but a portion of one gland should be removed. The integrity of the recurrent laryngeal nerves must be assured. If exploration fails to identify an adenoma or hyperplasia, the incision is closed. Reoperation is considered after (re)confirming the diagnosis and attempting to localize the gland by thallium–technetium scan (Fig. 24.8), sestamibi scintigraphy, MRI scans or selective venous catheterization with PTH measurement. Recurrent hyperparathyroidism is approached in the same way.

SECONDARY AND TERTIARY HYPERPARATHYROIDISM

In secondary hyperparathyroidism, there is over-secretion of PTH in response to low plasma levels of ionized calcium, usually because of renal disease or malabsorption. This is an increasing problem in patients on long-term dialysis for chronic renal failure. It is managed initially by giving 1-α-hydroxyvitamin D_3 (alfacalcidol) to increase calcium absorption and provide negative feedback on the parathyroids.

Excessive PTH secretion in secondary hyperparathyroidism may become autonomous; it is then termed tertiary hyperparathyroidism. This may occur after renal transplantation. Total parathyroidectomy may be needed, with autotransplantation of parathyroid tissue (equivalent in size to one normal gland) into an arm muscle (where it can be readily located if problems persist). Postoperatively, alfacalcidol and calcium are continued to heal bone disease and reduce the risk of recurrent hyperparathyroidism.

HYPOPARATHYROIDISM

Hypoparathyroidism may occur temporarily after parathyroidectomy until the suppressed residual glands assume normal function. A fall in ionized calcium levels gives rise to paraesthesiae ('pins and needles') in the hands and feet, and muscle cramps and spasms (tetany) that cause bunching and flexion of the fingers and toes. Respiratory obstruction with stridor due to spasm of the laryngeal muscles can prove fatal. Clinical signs include Chvostek's sign (twitching of the facial muscles on tapping of the facial nerve), Trousseau's sign (spasm of hand and forearm muscles after applying a tourniquet to occlude the pulse) and Erb's sign (hyperexcitability of muscles on electrical stimulation). The patient is lethargic and depressed. Blood levels of ionized calcium and PTH are low, and the electrocardiogram (ECG) shows a lengthened Q–T interval. Acute hypoparathyroidism is treated with intravenous calcium gluconate (20 ml of a 10% solution given 4-hourly until calcium levels rise). Oral calcium (effervescent calcium gluconate) and vitamin D (cholecalciferol 20 000

U daily) are prescribed for maintenance. Calcium levels must be monitored regularly.

PARATHYROIDECTOMY

Patient information

In order to provide informed consent, it is important that patients understand several aspects of the glands and the disease, specifically:

- the variable position of the glands
- the function of the glands
- the results of hyperfunction: renal effects, bone disease and systemic effects
- that only one gland is likely to be diseased and overactive, and that this is not cancerous
- that surgery will attempt to remove the abnormal gland but may fail to locate it because it is in an ectopic position
- that there may be a need for calcium and vitamin D supplements after surgery.

PITUITARY GLAND

SURGICAL ANATOMY

The pituitary gland is small and weighs about 500 mg. It is enclosed within a bony shell, the sella turcica, which is sealed superiorly by a fold of dura mater, the diaphragma sellae. The pituitary stalk connects the pituitary to the hypothalamus. The pituitary has two parts: the anterior pituitary (adenohypophysis) and the posterior pituitary (neurohypophysis) (Fig. 24.9).

ANTERIOR PITUITARY

The anterior pituitary develops from an epithelial outgrowth from the pharynx (Rathke's pouch). Some cells are thought to be of neural crest origin and belong to the APUD (amine and precursor uptake and decarboxylation) system. The anterior pituitary contains solid cords of secreting cells that used to be classified as acidophil, basophil or chromophobe on staining with haematoxylin and eosin. On the basis of immunofluorescence and other specific stains, these are now subdivided into cell types that secrete (Fig. 24.10):

- the polypeptides: growth hormone (GH), prolactin (PRL) and adrenocorticotrophic hormone (ACTH)
- the glycoproteins: luteinizing hormone (LH), follicle-stimulating hormone (FSH) and TSH.

The hypophysial stalk contains a portal venous system that connects capillaries in the median eminence of the hypothalamus with capillaries and sinusoids of the anterior pituitary. This system carries neurosecretory hormones that stimulate or inhibit specific endocrine cells in the pituitary. The most important messengers are GH-releasing and inhibiting factors, corticotrophin-releasing factor (CRF), gonadotrophin-releasing hormone (GnRH), TRH and prolactin-inhibiting factor (PIF). If the portal tract is divided, the secretion of all anterior pituitary hormones is suppressed, with the exception of prolactin, the secretion of which is increased. A number of feedback loops ensure that the secretion of pituitary hormones is adjusted to need.

TUMOURS OF THE ANTERIOR PITUITARY

Pathophysiology

Functioning pituitary adenomas may result from over-stimulation by hypothalamic factors. Initially small and confined within the gland (microadenomas), they grow

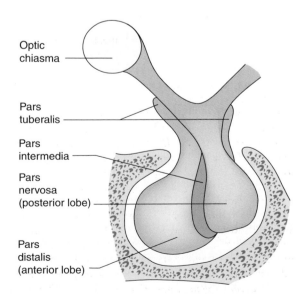

Optic chiasma

Pars tuberalis

Pars intermedia

Pars nervosa (posterior lobe)

Pars distalis (anterior lobe)

Fig. 24.9   Sagittal section through the pituitary gland.

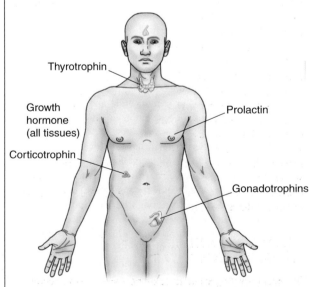

Thyrotrophin

Growth hormone (all tissues)

Corticotrophin

Prolactin

Gonadotrophins

Fig. 24.10   The anterior pituitary hormones and their target organs.

24

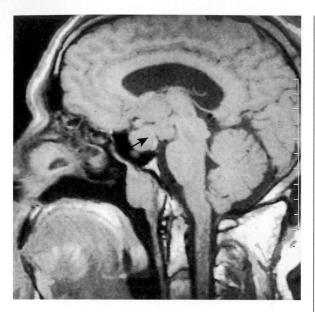

Fig. 24.11   MRI scan showing a pituitary tumour.

slowly and can ultimately expand the sella turcica. Eccentric enlargement is common and asymmetry of the pituitary fossa can often be detected by lateral tomograms. Upward extension of the adenoma may stretch the diaphragm or herniate through it, to compress the optic chiasma and cause visual defects. It is therefore important that pituitary adenomas are detected before they enlarge the fossa or extend above it. CT with contrast enhancement or MRI (Fig. 24.11) can be used to reveal the tumour and delineate its extent. Three endocrine syndromes caused by anterior pituitary disorders have surgical relevance.

Acromegaly

Excess secretion of GH occurs most often in early adult life and results in overgrowth of the soft tissues of the hands, feet and face. This gives the patient 'large extremities' and a characteristically coarse face, with bulging supra-orbital ridges and a protruding jaw. Endochondral ossification and periosteal new bone formation account for some of these changes. All viscera are enlarged and there is muscle hypertrophy, although muscle weakness and cardiac failure develop later. The skin is coarse and greasy and acne is common. Headaches, sweating and the carpal tunnel syndrome often develop. Glucose tolerance is impaired and galactorrhoea can occur in females. GH and somatomedin levels are increased, and glucose or a meal does not suppress their secretion.

Treatment is directed at restoring GH levels to normal. External radiation achieves this in 70% of patients, but only after 10 years. Radioactive implants act more quickly (see below). For small adenomas, trans-sphenoidal removal is the treatment of choice. Although bromocriptine inhibits GH release, it achieves normal levels in only 20% of patients with acromegaly. Somatostatin analogues offer a more effective way of normalizing GH levels and can be used to reduce the size of macroadenomas or to treat recurrent or residual tumour.

Hyperprolactinaemia

Prolactin is the most common hormone secreted by pituitary tumours. Hypersecretion results in galactorrhoea and amenorrhoea (owing to the suppression of gonadotrophin secretion) in young women, whereas in men gynaecomastia and impotence may occur. Basal levels of prolactin are high, the nocturnal increase is absent, and the response to TRH and metoclopramide is diminished. It is important to exclude other causes of hyperprolactinaemia, notably the administration of drugs such as metoclopramide.

To preserve pituitary function in younger patients, small adenomas are enucleated and larger tumours are treated by bromocriptine, with monitoring to ensure that tumour expansion does not threaten visual integrity.

Cushing's disease

This may be due to a functioning adenoma of ACTH-secreting cells. Only 15% of patients show expansion of the pituitary fossa. Removal of the microadenoma or its irradiation will relieve symptoms. Unsuccessful surgery may require bilateral adrenalectomy (removal of end organs) to terminate the syndrome of hypercortisolism, with its widespread destructive systemic effects.

SURGICAL HYPOPHYSECTOMY

The trans-sphenoidal approach is preferred for the removal of a normal-sized gland or enucleation of a small adenoma. An operating microscope is used to approach the gland through the sphenoidal or ethmoidal sinuses (Fig. 24.12). The pituitary stalk is divided low, so that diabetes insipidus is rare. By placing a free flap of muscle in the fossa, cerebrospinal fluid (CSF) rhinorrhoea is prevented. The transcranial approach is a major neurosurgical procedure that results in loss of the sense of smell and the development of diabetes insipidus. It is now reserved for the removal of large tumours with suprasellar extension, often in combination with a trans-sphenoidal approach.

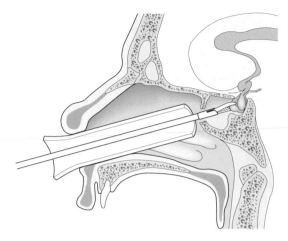

Fig. 24.12   Trans-sphenoidal removal of a pituitary adenoma.

RADIATION THERAPY

External radiation

The pituitary is comparatively radioresistant and at least 100 Gy are needed to affect the function of a normal gland. Smaller doses (40–50 Gy) are used to treat acromegaly and Cushing's disease. A rotational technique avoids excessive irradiation of surrounding neural tissue. Larger doses can be delivered by the narrow focused beam of heavy particles that are generated by a cyclotron.

Internal irradiation

Radioactive sources can be implanted, under radiological control, via the trans-sphenoidal or transethmoidal routes (Fig. 24.13), although trans-sphenoidal surgery is now preferred. ^{90}Yttrium is a β-particle emitter of high energy and short half-life (64 hours), and was once commonly used. Diabetes insipidus followed only if the hypothalamic nuclei were irradiated; CSF rhinorrhoea was an occasional complication.

MAINTENANCE THERAPY

After total hypophysectomy, replacement therapy is required for life: that is, hydrocortisone 20 mg each morning and 10 mg each evening. All episodes of stress or trauma, including hypophysectomy itself, require additional cortisol or cortisone to cover the metabolic response. Patients are advised to wear a band or bracelet advising medical attendants that they are receiving steroid replacement therapy. Aldosterone secretion is unaffected and there is no need for mineralocorticoid replacement. TSH secretion is suppressed and hypothyroidism is avoided by giving thyroxine. Diabetes insipidus is a common but often transient complication of pituitary surgery or the insertion of radioactive implants. Intramuscular injection or intranasal delivery of the vasopressin analogue, desmopressin (DDAVP), relieves polyuria.

THE POSTERIOR PITUITARY

Pathophysiology

The neurohypophysis is part of a secretory and storage unit that includes the nerve cells of the supraoptic and paraventricular hypothalamic nuclei (Fig. 24.14). Fibres pass from these nuclei via the hypothalamo–hypophysial tract to the median eminence of the hypothalamus and posterior pituitary. The nerve cells secrete arginine vasopressin (antidiuretic hormone, ADH) and oxytocin, both of which pass down the nerve fibres to be stored in vesicles in the pituitary. The close anatomical relationship of the anterior and posterior pituitary has functional significance in that oxytocin release during lactation is paralleled by increased TSH and prolactin production, and the posterior pituitary may influence prolactin secretion by dopamine release.

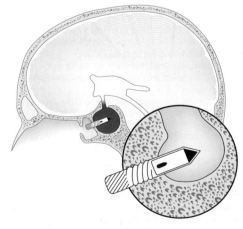

Fig. 24.13   Implantation of radioactive ^{90}yttrium into the pituitary fossa.

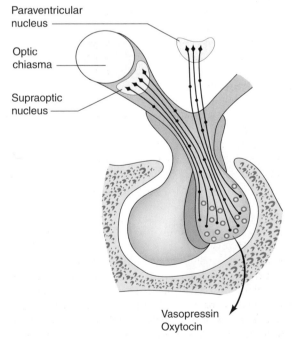

Paraventricular nucleus

Optic chiasma

Supraoptic nucleus

Vasopressin
Oxytocin

Fig. 24.14   The neurohypophysial system.

24

24

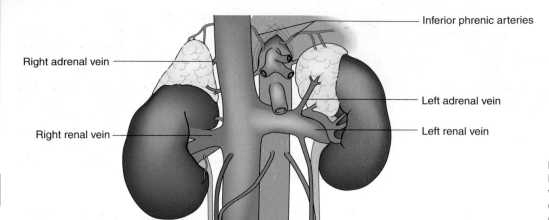

Inferior phrenic arteries

Right adrenal vein

Right renal vein

Left adrenal vein

Left renal vein

**Fig. 24.15
Blood supply and
venous drainage
of the adrenal
glands.**

ADRENAL GLAND

SURGICAL ANATOMY AND DEVELOPMENT

Each adrenal gland weighs approximately 4 g and lies immediately above and medial to the kidneys. The glands are not easily accessible to the surgeon. The right adrenal lies in close contact with the inferior vena cava, into which it drains by a short wide vein that can be difficult to ligate at operation. The left adrenal vein drains into the left renal vein (Fig. 24.15). The glands are supplied by small vessels that arise from the aorta and the renal and inferior phrenic arteries.

Each gland has an outer cortex and inner medulla. The cortex, like the gonads, is derived from mesoderm, whereas the medulla is derived from the chromaffin ectodermal cells of the neural crest. The cortex secretes corticosteroids. The medulla is part of the sympathetic nervous system. Its APUD cells secrete the catecholamines, adrenaline (epinephrine), noradrenaline (norepinephrine) and dopamine, and are supplied by pre-ganglionic sympathetic nerves.

ADRENAL CORTEX

Cortical function

Microscopically, the adrenal cortex has three zones (Fig. 24.16). The outer zona glomerulosa secretes the

mineralocorticoid, aldosterone. The zona fasciculata and zona reticularis act as a functional unit and secrete gluco-corticoids (cortisol and corticosterone) (Fig. 24.17), andro-genic steroids (androstenedione, 11-hydroxy-androstenedione

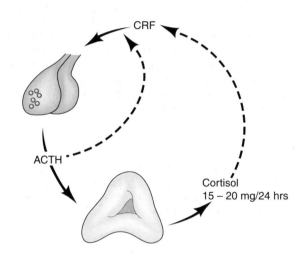

CRF

ACTH

Cortisol
15 – 20 mg/24 hrs

Fig. 24.17   Feedback loop in the control of cortisol secretion.
(ACTH = adrenocorticotrophic hormone; CRF = corticotrophin-releasing factor)

BOX 24.5   ADRENOCORTICAL HORMONES

- Cortisol secretion is controlled by pituitary adrenocorticotrophic hormone (ACTH). Cortisol protects against stress, maintains blood pressure and aids recovery from injury/shock. Its metabolic activities include protein breakdown, increased gluconeogenesis, reduced glucose utilization and mobilization/redistribution of fat and water
- In excess, cortisol has mineralocorticoid activity, can cause psychosis, and has anti-inflammatory effects (used in transplantation immunosuppression)
- Aldosterone secretion is controlled mainly by angiotensin levels (and thus by renin release from the juxtaglomerular apparatus during decreased perfusion)
- Aldosterone conserves sodium (by facilitating its exchange for potassium and hydrogen ions in the kidney) and is a major determinant of extracellular fluid conservation
- Androgenic steroids and dehydroepiandrosterone sulphate (DHA-S) are also secreted by the adrenal cortex. DHA-S is converted to testosterone and oestrogen by fat and liver, and this peripheral aromatization is the main source of oestrogen in post-menopausal women

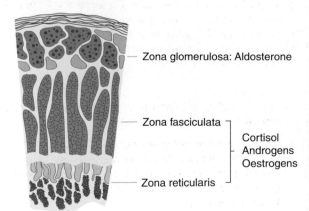

Zona glomerulosa: Aldosterone

Zona fasciculata

Cortisol
Androgens
Oestrogens

Zona reticularis

Fig. 24.16   Functional zones of the adrenal cortex.

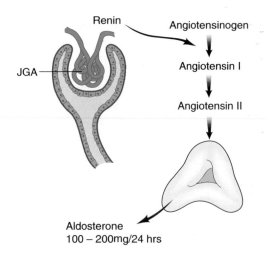

Fig. 24.18 Control of aldosterone secretion by the adrenal cortex. (JGA = juxtaglomerular apparatus)

and testosterone) and the inactive androgen and oestrogen precursor, dehydroepiandrosterone sulphate (DHA-S). Precursors of aldosterone (Fig. 24.18) are also synthesized by the fasciculata–reticularis zone, as are small amounts of progesterone and oestrogen. Only a fraction of the amount of hormone needed daily is stored in the cortex. The hormones are, therefore, secreted 'to order' and circulate either free (5%) or bound to α-globulin.

CUSHING'S SYNDROME

This syndrome was first described by the American neuro-surgeon, Harvey Cushing. It results from any prolonged and inappropriate exposure to cortisol and has the causes described below (Fig. 24.19).

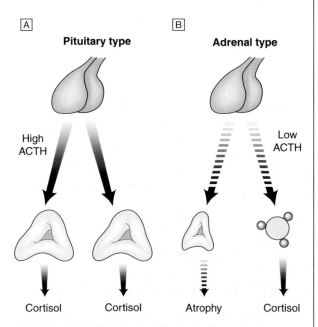

Fig. 24.19 Types of Cushing's syndrome.
[A] Over-stimulation of the normal adrenal glands by excess ACTH.
[B] Over-secretion of cortisol by a functioning tumour of the left adrenal gland, leading to suppression of function in the opposite gland.

Tumours of the adrenal cortex (20%)

Benign adenoma is the most common adrenal cause of Cushing's syndrome. It is almost invariably unilateral and is more common in females. Histologically, the tumour contains clear cells like those of the zona fasciculata, or compact cells like those of the zona reticularis. Autonomous cortisol secretion inhibits ACTH production, so that the contralateral gland becomes atrophic and ceases to function.

Adrenal carcinoma is a rare cause of Cushing's syndrome that occurs more frequently in young adults and children. The tumour grows to a large size and has frequently metastasized by the time of presentation.

Pituitary disease (80%)

Pituitary tumours causing Cushing's syndrome are usually basophil or sometimes chromophobe adenomas of ACTH-secreting cells. They range from tiny 'microadenomas' to large and even invasive tumours. Because of the continued ACTH secretion, both adrenals become hyperplastic. When Cushing's syndrome is caused by a pituitary tumour, it is referred to as Cushing's disease.

Ectopic ACTH production

Inappropriate secretion of ACTH-like peptide by tumours of non-pituitary origin (e.g. pancreas, bronchus, thymus) is a rare cause.

Iatrogenic

Cushing's syndrome can be a major side-effect of thera-peutic steroid use. Adrenal atrophy occurs if the steroid dosage is considerable and prolonged in duration.

Clinical features

Cushing's syndrome occurs most frequently in young women. The most striking feature is truncal obesity, a 'buffalo hump' (due to redistribution of water and fat) and 'mooning' of the face (Fig. 24.20). Cushing's original description was a 'tomato head, potato body and four matches as limbs'. As a result of protein loss, the skin becomes thin, with purple striae, dusky cyanosis and visible dermal vessels. Proximal muscle weakness is prominent. Other features include increased capillary fragility, purpura, osteoporosis, acne, loss of libido, hirsutism, diabetes, hyper-tension and amenorrhoea. The clinical signs develop insidiously over years and sometimes are only fully appreciated when the patients and their family review old photographs. In some cases, the disease runs a fulminant course, particularly when due to an adrenal carcinoma or ectopic ACTH secretion. Electrolyte disturbances, cachexia, pigmentation, severe diabetes and psychosis are common in these patients.

Investigations

Before proceeding to adrenalectomy, the surgeon must be convinced that:

- Cortisol secretion is beyond normal control. In Cushing's syndrome plasma cortisol levels are high, diurnal variation is lost and secretion is not suppressed by low-dose dexamethasone or increased by insulin-induced hypoglycaemia.
- The primary problem is in the adrenal. In patients with a functioning adrenal tumour, ACTH cannot be detected

24

24

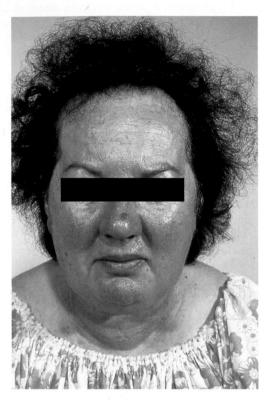

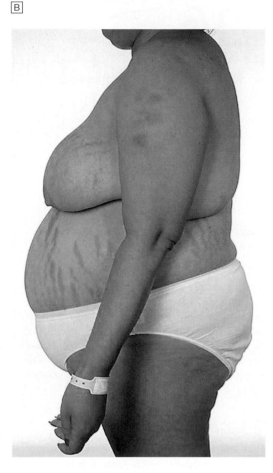

Fig. 24.20
Features of Cushing's syndrome.
A Moon face and puffy eyes. B Papery skin with striae and a propensity to bruising, muscle wasting of limbs and centripetal obesity. (Courtesy of Prof Michael Sheppard, University of Birmingham Medical School.)

in the plasma, and urinary excretion of cortisol is not suppressed by high-dose dexamethasone (Fig. 24.21).

- Pituitary and ectopic sources of excessive ACTH production have been excluded. In Cushing's disease due to a pituitary adenoma, plasma ACTH levels are inappropriately high and urinary cortisol excretion is suppressed by dexamethasone. In ectopic ACTH syndrome, the ACTH levels are often exceedingly high and there is an associated electrolyte disturbance. These patients may also have cancer cachexia.
- Attempts have been made to localize the lesion by techniques such as CT (Fig. 24.22) or isotope scintigraphy using radiolabelled iodocholesterol (Fig. 24.23).

Management

Adrenal adenoma
Adrenal adenomas are rarely bilateral and unilateral adrenalectomy is indicated. As the other adrenal is suppressed and atrophic, cortisone replacement is needed until the pituitary–adrenal axis recovers. This may take up to 2 years, and steroids must not be reduced or discontinued until a low-dose dexamethasone test shows normal function in the remaining gland.

Adrenal carcinoma
Adrenal carcinomas should be completely removed whenever possible; debulking may be helpful if chemotherapy is to be used. Patients often present late, with large tumours and lung metastases. Chemotherapy with mitotane or p-p-DDD may be tried, but this is a toxic drug and is often poorly tolerated. The therapeutic gain may be small.

Pituitary disease
The symptoms of bilateral adrenal hyperplasia due to pituitary hyperfunction can be relieved by bilateral adrenalectomy, but at the price of lifelong steroid therapy. Furthermore, adrenalectomy removes all feedback control, so that over-production of ACTH and melanocyte-stimulating hormone (MSH) produces characteristic skin pigmentation, and continued growth of the adenoma

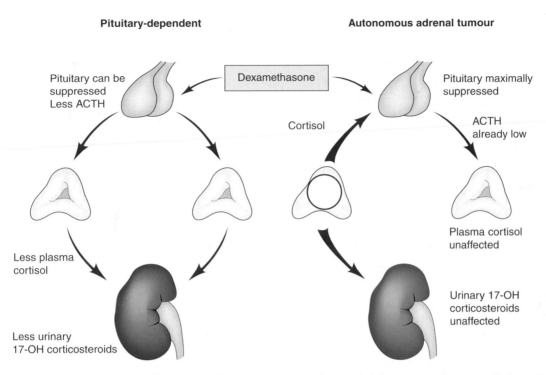

Pituitary-dependent

Autonomous adrenal tumour

Dexamethasone

Pituitary can be suppressed Less ACTH

Pituitary maximally suppressed

Cortisol

ACTH already low

Less plasma cortisol

Plasma cortisol unaffected

Less urinary 17-OH corticosteroids

Urinary 17-OH corticosteroids unaffected

Fig. 24.21   The principle of the dexamethasone test in differentiating between adrenal and pituitary causes of excess cortisol secretion.

BOX 24.6   CUSHING'S SYNDROME

- Cushing's syndrome results from inappropriate secretion of cortisol
- The syndrome may be caused by tumours of the adrenal cortex (20%), tumours of the anterior pituitary (80%) or ectopic ACTH production (rare), or may be a side-effect consequent upon the use of steroids for therapy
- The main clinical features are truncal obesity, buffalo hump, mooning of the face ('tomato head, potato body, four matchsticks as limbs'), thinning of the skin, livid striae and proximal muscle weakness
- An adrenal tumour is usually treated by unilateral adrenalectomy, but cortisone replacement is needed until the suppressed contralateral adrenal recovers
- Before proceeding to adrenalectomy, the surgeon should confirm that cortisol secretion is beyond normal control, that the primary problem is not pituitary or ectopic ACTH production, and that attempts have been made to localize the adrenal lesion (CT scan and radioisotope scan with iodocholesterol)
- Pituitary disease is best treated by pituitary surgery (or irradiation) rather than by bilateral adrenalectomy. This avoids continued growth of the pituitary tumour, problems due to ACTH and MSH production (pigmentation, Nelson's syndrome), and the side-effects of adrenalectomy

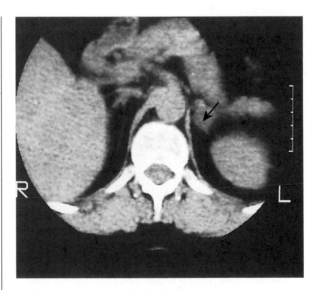

Fig. 24.22   CT scan of an adrenal tumour.

---

may compress the optic chiasma (Nelson's syndrome). Pituitary irradiation or surgery avoids the side-effects of adrenalectomy, and microsurgical removal of the adenoma is now the treatment of choice after pre-operative preparation with adrenal antagonists.

HYPERALDOSTERONISM

Primary hyperaldosteronism (Conn's syndrome)

This is usually due to a benign adenoma and is most common in young or middle-aged women. The adenoma is

24

24

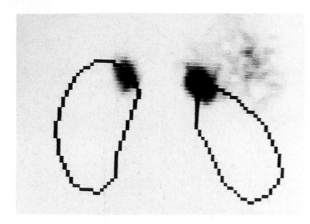

Fig. 24.23 Bilateral uptake of radio-labelled iodocholesterol in a patient with Cushing's disease.

small, single, canary yellow on bisection and composed of cells of the glomerulosa type. Only rarely is the syndrome due to bilateral adrenal hyperplasia or multiple microadenomas. The high circulating levels of aldosterone suppress renin secretion—a helpful biochemical diagnostic observation.

Clinical features

Retention of sodium increases plasma volume and produces hypertension, often in association with headaches and visual disturbance (although serious retinopathy is uncommon). Potassium loss leads to worsening hypokalaemia, episodes of muscle weakness and nocturnal polyuria. Unrecognized, the syndrome progresses to severe hypokalaemic alkalosis, with periodic muscle paralysis, paraesthesia and tetany.

Diagnosis

Low serum potassium in a hypertensive patient should signal the possibility of hyperaldosteronism. Diagnosis then rests on the following:

- *Confirm hypokalaemia.* This may require repeated blood sampling without an occluding cuff; 24-hour urine collections usually show increased potassium excretion.
- *Demonstrate hypersecretion of aldosterone.* Plasma and/or urinary aldosterone levels are measured at 4-hourly intervals to allow for diurnal variations. Giving the aldosterone antagonist, spironolactone, should reduce blood pressure and reverse hypokalaemia.
- *Exclude secondary hyperaldosteronism.* Measurement of plasma renin is the critical investigation; renin levels are increased in secondary hyperaldosteronism but undetectable in the primary disease. Spironolactone causes further increases in renin levels in secondary hyperaldosteronism.
- *Localize the adenoma.* If primary hyperaldosteronism is confirmed biochemically, attempts should then be made to localize the adenoma by CT or scanning with radiolabelled iodocholesterol. Failure to 'see' an adenoma may mean that there is no discrete tumour

and that the patient has bilateral cortical hyperplasia. Plasma cortisol levels should always be measured to exclude Cushing's syndrome. Selective adrenal vein sampling to determine aldosterone levels may be required to help localize small adenomas to one or other gland.

Management

Primary hyperaldosteronism due to an adenoma is treated by removal of the affected gland *after* correcting the hypokalaemia with oral potassium and spironolactone. Hyperaldosteronism due to adrenal hyperplasia can be cured by bilateral adrenalectomy, but at such a high price that long-term drug treatment is preferable.

Secondary hyperaldosteronism

Hyperaldosteronism is most commonly secondary to excessive renin secretion (and stimulation of the zona glomerulosa by angiotensin) in chronic liver, renal or cardiac disease.

ADRENOGENITAL SYNDROME (ADRENAL VIRILISM)

Pathophysiology

This syndrome is due to one of a number of genetically determined enzyme defects that impair cortisol synthesis. The resultant increase in pituitary ACTH production causes adrenal hyperplasia and inappropriate adrenal androgen secretion.

Clinical features

The effects depend on the patient's sex and age. Female infants show enlargement of the clitoris and varying fusion of the labial folds. Later, other signs of virilism appear, leading to precocious heterosexual puberty. Young boys have precocious isosexual puberty. In both sexes, growth is at first rapid, but the epiphyses fuse early so that the final height is stunted. Excess muscle growth produces an 'infant Hercules' appearance. Milder forms of the disease may affect older girls and cause hirsutism and acne.

Management

The patient is given cortisol for replacement purposes and to suppress ACTH production. Surgical correction of the genital abnormality may be needed. Rarely, virilism is due to an adrenal tumour, which is usually large and malignant.

ADRENAL FEMINIZATION

Exceptionally, a tumour of the adrenal cortex may secrete oestrogens. Such tumours are usually large and malignant. In the female, there is sexual precocity; in the male, there is feminization, with gynaecomastia, decreased libido and testicular atrophy. Treatment consists of removing the tumour, although recurrence and metastatic spread are common.

ADRENAL MEDULLA

Pathophysiology

The adrenal medulla is not essential for life. There are other collections of chromaffin cells in paraganglia in the retroperitoneum, mediastinum and neck that release noradrenaline (norepinephrine). The normal adrenal medulla secretes catecholamines in the ratio 80% adrenaline to 20% noradrenaline. It also secretes the noradrenaline precursor, dopamine. Small amounts of catecholamines are excreted in the urine in free and conjugated form. Larger amounts are excreted as metnoradrenaline and 3-methoxy-4-hydroxymandelic acid (VMA).

PHAEOCHROMOCYTOMA

Pathology

Phaeochromocytomas are tumours either of the adrenal medulla (90%) that secrete large amounts of adrenaline (epinephrine) and noradrenaline (norepinephrine), or of the extra-adrenal paraganglionic tissue (10%) that secrete only noradrenaline. Virtually all (99%) arise within the abdomen, 10% are multiple and 10% are malignant. Benign tumours are usually chocolate-brown and highly vascular. Associated conditions are neurofibromatosis, medullary carcinoma of the thyroid (as part of MEN type II), duodenal ulcer and renal artery stenosis. If it presents in pregnancy, phaeochromocytoma can be mistaken for hypertension of pregnancy and may cause maternal and fetal mortality.

Clinical features

Phaeochromocytomas usually present before the age of 50 years. Excess noradrenaline secretion causes hypertension; adrenaline excess has metabolic effects (e.g. diabetes and thyrotoxicosis), and may even give rise to hypotension. Paroxysmal hypertension is a very characteristic symptom; it is due to the sudden release of catecholamines and may be precipitated by abdominal pressure, exercise or postural change. During an attack the blood pressure may rise to 200/100 mmHg and there is headache, palpitation, sweating, extreme anxiety, and chest and abdominal pain. Pallor, dilated pupils and tachycardia are prominent features. In some patients, persistent and severe hypertension develops at the age of 30–40 years, often in association with severe retinopathy, which can cause optic atrophy and blindness. Glycosuria is common. The skin may be mottled, with tingling of the extremities. Extra-adrenal phaeochromocytomas are always associated with persistent hypertension. On rare occasions, the tumour is in the bladder, and micturition may precipitate a syncopal attack. A few patients present with predominantly metabolic effects, such as those found in thyrotoxicosis. Occasionally, a phaeochromocytoma may cause sudden and unexplained death after trauma or during surgery, owing to severe hypertension causing a cerebrovascular accident or by precipitating a fatal arrhythmia.

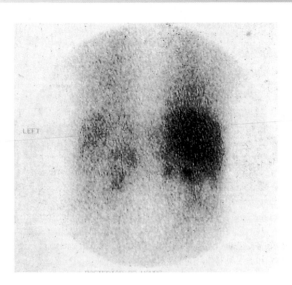

Fig. 24.24 Markedly excessive uptake of meta-iodobenzylguanidine (MIBG) in a huge right-sided phaeochromocytoma.

Investigations

All young hypertensive patients should be screened for a catecholamine-secreting tumour. Twenty-four hour collections of urine should be analysed for free catecholamine, metadrenaline and VMA output. A CT scan may show the tumour. It may also be demonstrated by scintigraphy after giving radio-iodine-labelled metaiodobenzylguanidine (MIBG), a substance which is taken up by catecholamine precursors (Fig. 24.24). Abdominal ultrasonography, intravenous urography with tomography, arteriography and selective venous sampling are no longer used for localization. Preliminary blockade (see below) is essential if invasive angiography is used.

Management

Surgical removal of the tumour is the treatment of choice. The use of α- and β-blocking drugs has greatly reduced

---

BOX 24.7 PHAEOCHROMOCYTOMA

- Phaeochromocytomas are usually benign tumours of the adrenal medulla (90% of patients) but 10% arise in extra-adrenal paraganglionic tissue, 10% are multiple and 10% are malignant (the '10% tumour')
- Phaeochromocytomas may be associated with neurofibromatosis, medullary carcinoma of the thyroid (MEN II), duodenal ulcer and renal artery stenosis
- The tumour presents clinically with hypertension, which is often paroxysmal, and with metabolic effects such as diabetes mellitus
- All young hypertensive patients should be screened for phaeochromocytoma; urinary 3-methoxy-4-hydroxymandelic acid (VMA), and catecholamine determination is the most reliable method of diagnosis
- The location of a phaeochromocytoma is best defined by CT and radiolabelled metaiodobenzylguanidine (MIBG) scanning
- Treatment consists of adrenalectomy after careful preparation to control blood pressure and heart rate and to re-expand blood volume (by α-adrenergic blockade with β-blockade)

24

the risk of hypertensive attacks, tachycardia and arrhythmias during induction of anaesthesia or tumour handling. The patient should come to operation with blood pressure and pulse rate controlled. Adrenergic blockade also allows restoration of blood volume, so that sudden hypotension after removal of the tumour is unusual. To achieve blockade, an α-adrenergic receptor blocker such as doxazosin should be used. A typical starting dose would be 1 mg 12-hourly, building up to 6 or 8 mg a day until hypertension is controlled and postural symptoms occur. The benefit of this drug over longer-acting agents such as phenoxybenzamine is that once the tumour has been removed there is less residual hypotension.

Once and only once α-blockade has been established, unopposed β effects, such as tachycardia, may become evident and are treated with a β-blocker such as propranolol. Beta-blockade should not be instituted first, as this may allow unopposed α-agonist effects, which may make hypertension worse and precipitate heart failure.

Atropine and thiopental are best avoided, and enflurane is the preferred anaesthetic. Pulse and blood pressure are monitored throughout surgery, and blood volume must be maintained. Short-acting α- and β-blocking agents and sodium nitroprusside (which acts directly on vessels independent of adrenergic receptors and gives additional control of hypertension) should be available.

NON-ENDOCRINE ADRENAL MEDULLARY TUMOURS

Ganglioneuromas
These are benign, firm, well-encapsulated tumours of ganglion cells. They grow slowly, may become large and can cause diarrhoea. Surgical excision gives excellent results.

Neuroblastomas
These are highly malignant tumours arising from sympathetic nervous tissue. They are one of the most common malignant tumours of infancy and childhood, and metastasize widely. About 75% secrete catecholamines. Treatment by radical excision, radiotherapy and chemotherapy offers the only hope of cure, although spontaneous regression has been reported.

ADRENAL 'INCIDENTALOMA'

The increasing use of imaging modalities such as CT or MRI has led to adrenal tumours being discovered incidentally in patients being investigated for other reasons. In such cases, it is important to determine whether there is cortical or medullary hyperfunction, by the use of appropriate biochemical tests as detailed above. If there is no hyperfunction and the swelling is less than 3.5 cm in diameter, further investigation and exploration are unwarranted. The lesion is likely to be a benign non-functioning cortical adenoma. Endocrine hyperfunction, a swelling larger than 3.5 cm or the suspicion of malignancy is an indication for further assessment and exploration.

ADRENALECTOMY

Indications
Normal adrenal glands were once removed as palliative treatment in post-menopausal women with breast cancer (to remove the source of DHA-S and prevent its peripheral conversion to oestrogen). Aromatase inhibitors (e.g. aminoglutethimide) have made this approach obsolete.

Indications for adrenalectomy now include adrenal adenomas producing Cushing's syndrome, Conn's syndrome or excess catecholamines (phaeochromocytoma). Bilateral adrenalectomy may be needed for bilateral tumours, nodular hyperplasia producing Conn's or Cushing's syndrome, and if pituitary surgery fails to cure Cushing's disease.

Technique
Whether approached from in front, from the side or from behind, the adrenals are inaccessible. The anterior transperitoneal route requires a large incision, inevitably causes ileus, has a high incidence of wound and respiratory complications (especially in patients with Cushing's syndrome), and is now seldom used.

Large tumours may be malignant and are best approached through a flank incision, after removing a rib to allow access; if possible, the diaphragm, pleura and peritoneum are left intact.

The posterior approach through the bed of the 11th or 12th rib is technically more difficult, but has lower morbidity and patients have a quicker return to normal activity. If the pleura is breached in the course of adrenalectomy, it can be repaired on closing the wound, ensuring that the lung is fully inflated. There is no need for pleural or wound drains.

Adrenalectomy can best be carried out using minimally invasive techniques. The usual route is anteriorly, beneath the costal margins, transperitoneally with reflection of liver on the right and spleen, pancreas and colon on the left. The adrenal vein can often be divided early in laparoscopic surgery which, especially with phaeochromocytomas, means that dangerous levels of catecholamines are prevented from gaining access to the circulation, thereby reducing the perturbations in blood pressure that characterize open procedures with direct manipulation of the tumour. It is occasionally necessary to convert to an open procedure if bleeding is encountered or there are other technical or access problems.

Replacement therapy
Corticosteroid replacement is needed for life after bilateral total adrenalectomy, but may not be needed permanently after unilateral adrenalectomy. Replacement is best achieved by a combination of oral hydrocortisone (30 mg daily in divided doses) and the mineralocorticoid fludrocortisone acetate (0.1 mg daily). If both adrenals are removed or the remaining adrenal is non-functional, the operation must be covered by commencing steroid replacement at the time of surgery. Adequacy of replacement is assessed by monitoring blood pressure in the erect and supine position, by

serum electrolyte determinations and by patient well-being.

Hydrocortisone sodium succinate is water-soluble and can be given by intravenous infusion during the first 24 hours. Further doses are given intravenously until the patient can take oral steroid. It cannot be overemphasized that blood pressure is the best guide to therapy. If hypotension occurs, 100 mg hydrocortisone sodium succinate is given immediately by intravenous injection, followed by 100 mg every 6–8 hours in a saline infusion. All adrenalectomized patients must be warned to increase the dose of steroid if stress or infection occurs. Failure to anticipate the need for added steroid may precipitate an 'adrenal crisis', with acute hypotension and collapse. Such patients should carry a 'steroid card' giving details of dosage and possible complications, and should be able to recognize the symptoms of adrenal insufficiency (i.e. loss of appetite, nausea, cramps, muscle pains and malaise). If such symptoms occur, the patient should take an extra two tablets of hydrocortisone and seek urgent medical help.

Patient information

Although adrenal cortical function is vital for life, patients are unlikely to have heard of the adrenal glands. Patient awareness is to some extent governed by disease frequency, and so, for example, most will understand the rudiments of diabetes or cancer of the breast because these are very frequently encountered disorders. By contrast, adrenal tumours occur at a rate of about 1 per million population per annum. Patients may have an awareness of cortisone or adrenaline from contexts of other disease and fright/flight reactions, respectively.

In advising patients about adrenal or pituitary surgery, then, the starting point must indeed be at the very beginning. Explain why they may not have heard of the adrenal glands, draw diagrams to show where the glands lie, and explain basic function in terms of the hormones produced and what effects they have.

It is necessary to discuss the technicalities of surgery and the approach to be used, and to forewarn patients that a laparoscopic procedure may have to be converted to an open one.

Complications should be minimal, but it is nevertheless worth mentioning blood loss and drains.

One of the most important features to describe will be any requirement for steroid replacement therapy (necessary after bilateral adrenalectomy, unilateral adrenalectomy for an adenoma producing Cushing's syndrome, and after pituitary surgery) and the need for dosage increase at times of stress (e.g. other surgery) or intercurrent illness (e.g. pneumonia).

OTHER SURGICAL ENDOCRINE SYNDROMES

APUDOMAS AND MULTIPLE ENDOCRINE NEOPLASIA

The APUD cell series

Distributed throughout the body (anterior pituitary, adrenal medulla, thyroid gland and intestine) are *a*mine *precursor uptake* and *decarboxylation* (APUD) cells that have in common the capacity to synthesize and store amines (e.g. ACTH, catecholamines, calcitonin, secretin, gastrin, cholecystokinin, enteroglucagon, somatostatin, vasoactive intestinal peptide). Hyperplasia and tumour of any APUD cell can produce specific endocrine syndromes.

Multiple endocrine neoplasia (MEN) syndromes

In MEN syndromes, which are inherited as autosomal dominant traits of variable penetrance and expression, patients develop benign or malignant tumours in more than one endocrine gland.

MEN type I

This is characterized by hyperplasia and/or tumours of the parathyroid, pancreatic islets and anterior pituitary. There may also be non-functioning tumours of the thyroid, pituitary, adrenal cortex and soft tissues (lipomas), and functioning carcinoid tumours of the gut or lungs. The earliest biochemical sign in affected individuals is hypercalcaemia from hyperparathyroidism or hyperprolactinaemia from an asymptomatic pituitary tumour. Families are often uncovered when an index patient presents dramatically with small bowel perforation or bleeding due to the Zollinger–Ellison syndrome (see below), or with hypoglycaemia due to an insulinoma of the pancreas. Family members should be screened by measurement of fasting serum calcium and other hormonal markers such as prolactin. Some of the mutational events on chromosome 21 can be detected. A bracelet may be worn to alert medical attendants to the condition. Treatment is directed at the dominant clinical or biochemical feature. For example, pancreatic endocrine tumours are localized by ultrasonography or CT and removed as necessary. Hypercalcaemia is treated by parathyroid surgery. Diseased glands are excised, and four-gland hyperplasia may be treated by excising all four glands and by prescribing calcium replacement therapy.

MEN type II

This is characterized by medullary carcinoma of the thyroid, phaeochromocytoma and parathyroid hyperplasia. Genetic diagnosis, based on a mutation in *Ret* proto-oncogene chromosome 10, obviates the need for biochemical testing in family members. Unlike in MEN I, there is advantage in prophylactic surgery with affected individuals undergoing thyroidectomy at the age of 5 or earlier. Continued screening for phaeochromocytoma (see below) is also required. Kindred members not showing the mutation can be dismissed from follow-up and can be reassured that they will not pass on the genetic abnormality to their offspring. Phaeochromocytomas are diagnosed by urinary VMA and catecholamine excretion, and localized by CT and MIBG scanning. Surgical treatment of the adrenal medullary abnormality must take precedence over the treatment of thyroid and parathyroid disease, as anaesthesia and surgery in patients with undiagnosed or untreated phaeochromocytoma can be life-threatening.

24

CARCINOID TUMOURS AND THE CARCINOID SYNDROME

Carcinoid tumours are most frequently found incidentally in the appendix of a patient undergoing appendicectomy for acute appendicitis, and account for 85% of all appendiceal tumours. They are usually less than 1 cm in diameter and are dealt with by appendicectomy, as metastases are exceptional in this situation. Carcinoid tumours larger than 2 cm in diameter are rare, but may have spread to lymph nodes and are best treated by right hemicolectomy. Liver metastases are extremely rare in patients with appendiceal carcinoids. Carcinoids occurring in the small intestine frequently spread to lymph nodes, and in 10% of cases there are liver metastases by the time the patient presents with obstructive symptoms or bleeding. Carcinoids in any site produce 5-hydroxytryptamine (5-HT) and other biologically active amines and peptides. In the case of gut carcinoids, these products are normally inactivated by the liver, but liver secondaries secrete these substances directly into the systemic circulation, giving rise to a carcinoid syndrome: periodic flushing, diarrhoea, bronchoconstriction, wheezing and distinctive red-purple discoloration of the face. Right-sided heart disease, notably pulmonary stenosis, may result and can prove fatal.

The diagnosis of carcinoid syndrome is confirmed by detecting 5-hydroxyindoleacetic acid (a breakdown product of 5-HT) in the urine. If the primary tumour is causing symptoms, it should be removed surgically if possible (e.g. right hemicolectomy, small bowel resection, lung resection). Hepatic metastases can be dealt with by excising the involved liver lobe or enucleating the deposits in an attempt to gain symptomatic relief. Alternatively, hepatic metastases may be de-arterialized by hepatic artery ligation or angiographic embolization.

Attempts have been made to relieve symptoms by blocking 5-HT synthesis (e.g. α-methyldopa) or action (e.g. methysergide), but the prevention of 5-HT release by somatostatin analogues or α-adrenergic antagonists may be more useful. Long-acting somatostatin analogues are now available and, instead of a need for once- or twice-daily injections of octreotide subcutaneously, 1 month's effective therapy can be achieved by an intramuscular injection of a depot preparation. Octreotide preparations are expensive but may bring dramatic symptomatic relief. Chemotherapy (e.g. 5-fluorouracil) is sometimes effective. Interferon is also sometimes used, but the side-effects can be troublesome.

24

R.T.A. CHALMERS
T.J. CLEVELAND
A.W. BRADBURY

Vascular and endovascular surgery

INTRODUCTION

The management of patients with vascular disease requires a multidisciplinary approach involving vascular surgeons, vascular interventional radiologists, anaesthetists, physicians (angiologists), nursing and rehabilitation specialists, physiotherapists, occupational therapists and orthotists. Standard surgical procedures have been complemented, and in some cases replaced, by less invasive percutaneous endoluminal interventions. As the population ages and the risk factors for vascular disease show no sign of diminishing, the health and socioeconomic burden of arterial and venous disease will continue to increase.

PATHOPHYSIOLOGY OF ARTERIAL DISEASE

PATHOLOGY

Most patients presenting to vascular surgeons have atherosclerosis. This condition involves the following: endothelial cell injury; subendothelial deposition of lipids and inflammatory cells; smooth muscle cell migration and proliferation; and plaque haemorrhage, rupture and thrombosis (Fig. 25.1).

Endothelial injury

Chemical injury
The main risk factor for the development of atherosclerosis is smoking. Hypercholesterolaemia and hypertriglyceridaemia are also important risk factors. Arterial disease is also far more common in diabetics, who have disordered glucose and lipid metabolism.

Physical injury
Atheroma often appears first where blood flow exerts high levels of shear stress on the arterial wall: for example, at bifurcations. Hypertension, which increases this stress, is an important predisposing factor for arterial disease.

Lipid deposition
Injury increases the permeability of the endothelium to lipids and inflammatory cells, which become deposited in the subendothelial layer. At this point, the atheroma forms a discoloured but flat yellow patch (fatty streak). In

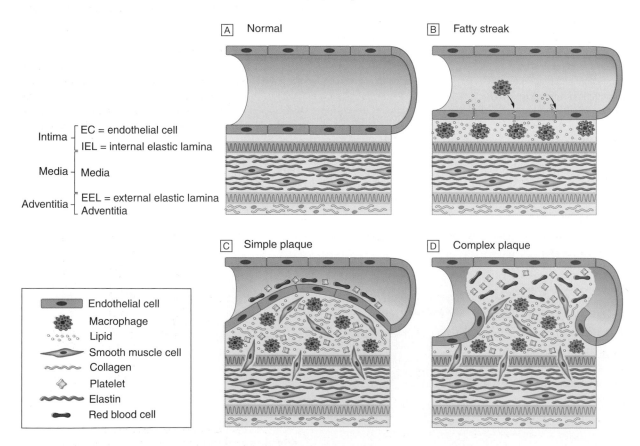

Fig. 25.1 Pathophysiology of atherosclerosis.
A Normal arterial wall. The intima, comprising a single layer of endothelial cells, rests upon a basement membrane and the internal elastic lamina. The media comprises smooth muscle cells and elastin, and the adventitia consists of collagenous tissue and vasa vasorum. B Fatty streak. Injured endothelial cells permit the sequestration of lipids and macrophages in the subendothelial space. C Simple plaque. Through the internal elastic lamina, smooth muscle cells enter the media, where they proliferate, take on the characteristics of fibroblasts and produce collagen. D Complex plaque. The endothelial cap has ruptured, leading to acute thrombosis and distal embolization.

developed countries, many young adults will have such lesions, which may progress to atherosclerosis.

Inflammatory cell infiltrate

Leucocytes adhere to the overlying damaged endothelium, migrate into the subendothelial space, digest lipid and become 'foam' cells, and liberate free radicals and proteases that destroy the arterial wall. They also liberate cytokines, which attract further leucocytes and smooth muscle cells from the media. The overlying endothelium becomes increasingly 'sticky', leading to platelet deposition and thrombosis.

Smooth muscle cells

Smooth muscle cells migrate from the media into the subendothelial space and begin to proliferate. They take on the properties of fibroblasts and lay down collagen. At this stage, the atheroma is raised and encroaches upon the lumen of the artery.

Plaque rupture

At this point, the plaque often comprises a thin 'cap' of endothelium stretched over a mass of lipid and inflammatory and smooth muscle cells. Intraplaque haemorrhage, from immature new blood vessels that infiltrate the lesion (angiogenesis), weakens the plaque. Further chemical and/or physical injury can lead to rupture and the exposure of highly thrombotic plaque contents to the flowing blood. This results in acute thrombotic occlusion of the vessel and/or distal embolization. It is very important to appreciate that it is this sudden decompensation that leads to the most serious and dramatic clinical presentations of arterial disease, and that rupture can occur in a plaque that has hitherto been completely asymptomatic.

CLINICAL FEATURES

The clinical manifestations of arterial disease depend upon:

- the site of the disease
- whether the artery is an end-artery or well collateralized
- the speed with which the disease develops
- whether the underlying process is haemodynamic, thrombotic, atheroembolic or thromboembolic, or due to aneurysmal dilatation or dissection
- the presence of other comorbidity and the general condition of the patient.

Anatomical site

The patient's symptoms and signs will obviously depend upon the territory supplied by the affected artery:

- *coronary arteries*: angina, myocardial infarction (MI)
- *cerebral circulation*: stroke, transient ischaemic attack (TIA), amaurosis fugax, vertebrobasilar insufficiency (VBI)
- *renal arteries*: hypertension, renal failure
- *mesenteric arteries*: mesenteric angina, acute intestinal ischaemia
- *limbs*: intermittent claudication (IC), chronic critical limb ischaemia (CLI), acute limb ischaemia.

Collateral supply

The clinical picture also depends upon whether the affected artery is essentially the only supply to the distal tissue (e.g. coronary artery and myocardium), or whether it is one of several arteries supplying the part (e.g. carotid artery and brain). This may vary between patients. For example, in a patient with a complete circle of Willis, the occlusion of one carotid artery may be asymptomatic. In a patient where there is no such cross-circulation, occlusion is likely to cause a stroke.

Speed of onset

Where atheroma develops slowly over months or years, a collateral supply to the distal part is likely to develop, such that when the main artery finally occludes, there may be little change in the patient's clinical status. The most common example is where the profunda (deep) femoral artery collateralizes around a diseased superficial femoral artery in patients with IC (see below). By contrast, the sudden occlusion of a previously normal artery is likely to cause severe distal ischaemia.

Mechanism of injury

The mechanism of injury has a major influence on the clinical presentation, prognosis and treatment of arterial disease (Fig. 25.2).

Haemodynamic mechanism

An atheromatous plaque must reduce the cross-sectional diameter of an artery by about 70% to cause an appreciable drop in flow and pressure at rest, a so-called 'critical stenosis'. However, on exertion—for example, walking—a much lesser stenosis may become 'critical'. The reason for

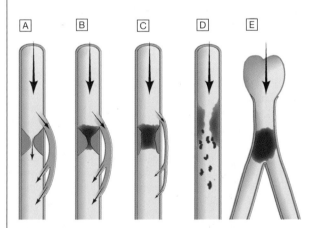

Fig. 25.2 Mechanisms of injury in atherosclerotic disease.
A Critical stenosis of main artery compensated for by collateral vessels; only symptomatic on exercise. B Acute thrombosis of a critical stenosis; little change in clinical status because of well-developed collaterals. C Acute thrombosis of a non-critical stenosis; severe symptoms because collateral supply is poorly developed. D Atheroembolism from ruptured, ulcerated plaque. E Thromboembolism from the heart; severe ischaemia because of lack of collateral supply.

this is that the pressure drop across a stenosis is proportional to the square of the velocity of the blood entering that stenosis; on exercise, blood velocity increases markedly. The clinical consequence of this is that the lesion only becomes flow-limiting, and therefore symptomatic, on exertion. This type of mechanism tends to have a relatively benign course. IC is a common example.

Thrombosis

By the time a 'critical' stenosis occludes, the collateral supply may be so well developed that the event is clinically silent. However, if a plaque that has been causing little or no haemodynamic impairment suddenly ruptures, then acute thrombosis of the vessel can have severe consequences. Such an event can cause MI (coronary arteries) or stroke (internal carotid artery) in a previously asymptomatic patient.

Atheroembolism

The effect that embolizing plaque contents (predominantly cholesterol) or adherent thrombus (predominantly platelets) have upon the distal circulation depends upon the factors outlined above, as well as the embolic load. Perhaps the best-known example is atheroembolism from a carotid plaque, which can cause small, discrete areas of cerebral and retinal ischaemia that manifest clinically as TIA and amaurosis fugax. If the embolic load is high, however, these emboli may cause irreversible occlusion of major distal vessels, leading to stroke and retinal infarction (monocular blindness).

Thromboembolism

The most common source of thromboembolism is the left atrium, in association with atrial fibrillation (AF). The clinical consequences are usually dramatic, as the thrombus load is often large and tends suddenly and completely to occlude a large or medium-sized vessel that has previously been healthy, and for which there is therefore no collateral supply. This is an important cause of stroke and acute limb ischaemia.

CHRONIC LOWER LIMB ARTERIAL DISEASE

ANATOMY

The lower limb arterial tree comprises the aorto-iliac segment above the inguinal ligament ('inflow'), the femoro-popliteal segment and the infra-popliteal segment ('outflow') (Fig. 25.3).

CLINICAL FEATURES

Symptoms

Chronic lower limb ischaemia presents as two distinct clinical entities: intermittent claudication and critical limb ischaemia. They have different epidemiologies, natural histories, treatments and prognoses (see below).

Examination findings

On examination, the chronically ischaemic limb is usually characterized by:

- skin that is thin and dry
- pallor, particularly on elevation. Upon dependency, the foot becomes bright red; this is known as dependent rubor or 'sunset foot', and is due to reactive hyperaemia (Buerger's test)
- superficial veins that fill sluggishly in the horizontal position and empty upon minimal elevation (venous guttering)
- nails that are brittle and crumbly
- muscle wasting
- reduced temperature
- pulses that are weak or absent and sometimes associated with thrills on palpation and bruits on auscultation.

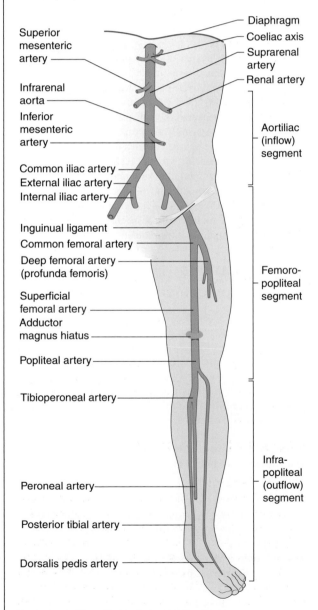

Fig. 25.3 Aortic and lower limb arterial anatomy.

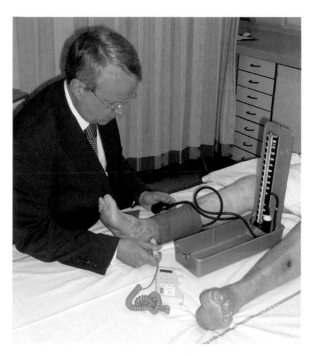

Fig. 25.4   Measurement of ankle:brachial pressure index (ABPI) using Doppler ultrasound.
(Courtesy of Professor Andrew Bradbury.)

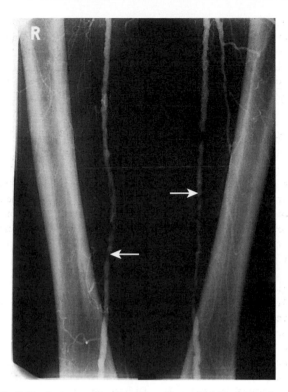

Fig. 25.5   Angiogram showing diffuse disease in both right and left superficial femoral arteries (arrows).

Pulse status

All patients admitted to hospital must have their pulse status recorded. In IC and CLI, the popliteal and pedal pulses are usually absent. If there is aorto-iliac disease, then one or both femoral pulses will be weak or absent. The presence of a thrill and/or bruit denotes turbulent flow.

Ankle:brachial pressure index

The severity of ischaemia can be estimated by determining the ratio between the ankle and brachial blood pressures. The latter is recorded in the normal way, the former using a cuff and a hand-held Doppler device (Fig. 25.4). In health, the ankle:brachial pressure index (ABPI) should be at least 1; that is, the pressure at the ankle should be at least as high as that in the arm. Patients with IC usually have an ABPI of 0.5–0.9, and those with CLI usually have an ABPI of less than 0.5.

INTERMITTENT CLAUDICATION

Clinical features

IC usually leads to pain in the muscles of the calf because the disease most often affects the superficial femoral artery (Fig. 25.5). If the iliac arteries are affected as well, then the pain may also be felt in the thigh and even the buttock. The pain comes on after a reasonably constant 'claudication distance', and subsides rapidly and completely on cessation of walking. Resumption of walking causes the pain to return. These and other features distinguish it from neurogenic and venous claudication (Table 25.1).

Typically, the earliest lesion is usually a stenosis in the superficial femoral artery (SFA) in the region of the adductor canal (Fig. 25.6A), which leads to IC after walking several hundred metres. Ankle pulses are palpable but diminished, and a bruit may be heard at or below the adductor canal. Ankle systolic pressures are often normal at rest but reduced following exercise.

Over the next few months or years, the collateral vessels of the profunda system enlarge to carry a higher proportion of the blood flow to the leg. In the majority of patients, symptoms gradually improve or even disappear. Thrombotic occlusion of the SFA (Fig. 25.6B) leads to a sudden deterioration in walking distance. Ankle and popliteal pulses are now absent.

Further development of the collateral circulation leads to an improvement in symptoms. This phase of moderate claudication may remain apparently stable for several years. However, unless there is a change in the patient's lifestyle, the atherosclerosis may progress to involve other segments (Fig. 25.6C). Claudication is now severe, forcing the patient to stop every 50 metres or so, and the scope for spontaneous improvement is steadily diminishing. As the disease progresses further in terms of severity and extent, symptoms are likely to worsen to a point where CLI develops as a result of multilevel disease (Fig. 25.6D). Such patients will often go on to develop night/rest pain and are at risk of tissue loss (see below).

An understanding of this cyclical pattern of exacerbation and resolution is important, as spontaneous improvement may mislead the patient into thinking all is well and that

25

Table 25.1   DIFFERENTIAL DIAGNOSIS OF CLAUDICATION

	Arterial	Neurogenic	Venous
Pathology	Stenosis or occlusion of major lower limb arteries	Lumbar nerve roots or cauda equina compression (spinal stenosis)	Obstruction to the venous outflow of the leg due to ilio-femoral venous occlusion secondary to deep venous thrombosis
Site of pain	Muscles: usually the calf but may affect thigh and buttock	Ill-defined; whole leg. Shooting in nature; may be associated with tingling and numbness	Whole leg. Bursting in nature
Laterality	Usually unilateral if femoro-popliteal, bilateral if aorto-iliac disease	Often bilateral	Nearly always unilateral
Onset	Gradual onset after walking the 'claudication distance'	Often immediate upon walking or even on standing up	Gradual onset but may be present from the moment walking commences
Relieving features	On cessation of walking, the pain disappears completely in 1–2 minutes	On cessation of walking, the pain may gradually subside over 5–10 minutes. Often the patient has to sit down or lean against something to obtain relief	The subject usually needs to elevate the leg to obtain relief
Colour	Normal or pale	Normal	Cyanosed. Often visible varicose veins and venous skin changes
Temperature	Normal or cool	Normal	Normal or increased
Swelling	Absent	Absent	Always present
Pulses	Reduced or absent	Normal	Present, but may be difficult to feel because of swelling
Straight leg raising	Normal	Limited	Normal

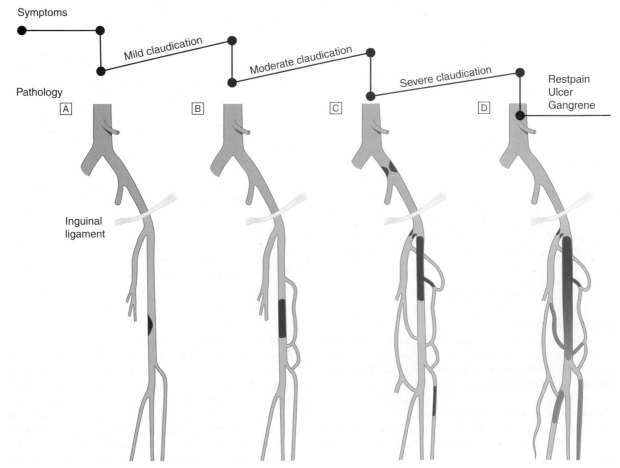

Fig. 25.6   Symptoms and pathology in intermittent claudication.

BOX 25.1   INTERMITTENT CLAUDICATION

- Intermittent claudication is the most common manifestation of peripheral arterial disease, affecting 1 in 20 adults aged over 55 years
- Limb loss is uncommon (1–2% per year), but myocardial infarction and stroke are three times more common than in a non-claudicant population (5–10% per year)
- The mainstays of treatment are risk factor modification, statin, aspirin and exercise. This leads to an improvement in walking distance in the majority of patients; it also increases longevity
- Patients should not normally be considered for surgical or endovascular intervention until they have been compliant with best medical therapy for at least 6 months
- Intervention includes angioplasty, stenting and bypass surgery. Long-term results are much better in the aorto-iliac segment than below the inguinal ligament

there is no longer a need to comply with medical advice (see below).

Epidemiology

IC affects 5% of men aged 55–75 years. Provided patients comply with 'best medical therapy' (BMT, see below), only 1–2% per year will deteriorate to a point where amputation and/or revascularization is required. However, the annual mortality rate is over 5% per year, which is 2–3 times higher than an age- and sex-matched non-claudicant population. This is because IC is a marker of widespread atherosclerosis, and most of these patients succumb to MI, stroke and limb loss. The emphasis is therefore on the preservation of life; in most patients, measures to reduce cardiovascular mortality will also improve the functional status of the limb and thus the patient.

CRITICAL LIMB ISCHAEMIA

Whereas IC is usually due to single-level disease, CLI is caused by multiple lesions affecting different arterial segments (Fig. 25.6D). These patients have tissue loss (ulceration or gangrene), with or without rest pain, and, by definition, have an ankle blood pressure of less than 50 mmHg. Without revascularization, such patients will usually lose their limb—and often their life—in a matter of weeks or months.

Subcritical limb ischaemia (SCLI)

The term SCLI is often used to describe patients who have night and/or rest pain, but not tissue loss. They are in an intermediate group between IC and CLI, and share features of both. A proportion of these patients may respond to BMT, thereby obviating the need for arterial reconstruction to save the limb.

Severe limb ischaemia (SLI)

This term is sometimes used to describe all patients with chronic limb ischaemia that is more severe than IC: that is, CLI and SCLI.

Night and rest pain

Pain develops, typically in the forefoot, about an hour after going to bed. 'Night pain' is due to the accumulation of metabolites, and occurs because the perfusion of the foot falls as a result of the loss of the beneficial effects of gravity, and because the patient's blood pressure and cardiac output also fall during sleep. It is severe and wakes the patient from sleep, but may at first be relieved by hanging the limb out of bed. As the disease progresses, the patient has to get up and walk about to obtain relief. The patient may volunteer a history of gaining relief from the pain by pressing the affected foot into a cold surface such as the kitchen floor.

This happens increasingly frequently through the night, with resulting loss of sleep. The patient then takes to sleeping in a chair, which leads to dependent oedema. This increases interstitial tissue pressure and so further reduces arterial perfusion. The patient is then in a vicious cycle of increasing pain and sleep loss. At this point, even a trivial injury will fail to heal, and the entry of bacteria leads to infection and an increase in the metabolic demands of the foot. The result is the rapid formation of ulcers, gangrene and, without treatment, limb loss and death.

Diabetic vascular disease

Approximately 40% of patients with SLI have diabetes and such patients pose a number of unique problems for vascular specialists:

- Their arteries are often calcified, which may make surgery and angioplasty technically difficult.
- Measured ankle pressures and thus the ABPI may be spuriously high.
- Diabetics have a reduced ability to fight infection.
- Diabetics often have severe multisystem arterial disease (coronary, cerebral and peripheral), which increases the risks of intervention.
- In the lower limbs, diabetic vascular disease has a predilection for the crural (calf) vessels. Although vessels in the foot are often spared, the technical challenge of performing a satisfactory bypass or angioplasty to these small vessels is considerable.
- Diabetics often have coexisting neuropathy, which may lead to foot ulceration in its own right but may also complicate peripheral ischaemia (see below).

The diabetic foot

This refers to the combination of ischaemia, neuropathy and immunocompromise that renders the feet of diabetic patients particularly susceptible to sepsis, ulceration and gangrene. Diabetic neuropathy affects the motor, sensory and autonomic nerves.

Sensory neuropathy

This renders the patient incapable of feeling pain. Minor trauma—for example, from a stone in the shoe—remains unnoticed. Even severe ischaemia and/or tissue loss that would lead a sensate patient to seek urgent medical advice may be completely painless. For this reason, diabetic patients often present late, with extensive destruction of the foot. Sensory neuropathy also affects proprioception such that, upon walking, pressure is taken at unusual sites.

25

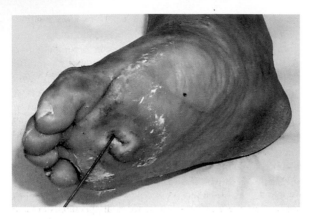

Fig. 25.7 Neuropathic ulceration of the first metatarsal head with sinus entering joint space.

This is thought to underlie the process of joint destruction (Charcot's joints) seen in severe cases and also leads to ulceration.

Motor neuropathy

The normal structure and function of the foot depend not only upon ligaments, but also upon the long and short flexors and extensors of the calf and sole. The latter are affected more than the former by motor neuropathy, leading to weakness and atrophy. The result is that the long extensors of the toes are unopposed and the toes become increasingly dorsiflexed. This exposes the metatarsal heads to abnormal pressure, and they are a frequent site of callus formation and ulceration (Fig. 25.7).

Autonomic neuropathy

This leads to a dry foot deficient in the sweat that normally lubricates the skin and contains antibacterial substances. The result is scaling and fissuring of the skin, and the creation of a portal of entry for bacteria. Abnormal blood flow in the bones of the ankle and foot due to loss of autonomic control may also contribute to osteopenia and bony collapse.

Management

If the blood supply is adequate, then dead tissue can be excised in the expectation that healing will occur, provided infection is controlled and the foot is protected from pressure (so-called off-loading). If there is ischaemia as well, then the priority is to revascularize the foot, if possible. Sadly, many diabetic patients present late, with extensive tissue loss and 'unreconstructable' disease, which accounts for the very high amputation rate.

MANAGEMENT OF LOWER LIMB ISCHAEMIA

Medical management

Patients should be urged to comply with BMT, which comprises:

- Immediate, absolute and permanent cessation from smoking
- Control of hypertension
- Control of hypercholesterolaemia. It is increasingly apparent that, whatever a patient's baseline cholesterol, if there is any manifestation of atherosclerosis, then that level of cholesterol is too high for the individual patient and should be lowered. Thus, almost regardless of baseline cholesterol, patients with clinically apparent atherosclerosis and asymptomatic individuals at risk of developing symptomatic atherosclerosis (e.g. smokers, diabetics) require cholesterol-lowering therapy (EBM 25.1). While dietary advice is important, virtually all patients will require drug therapy, usually with statins, to obtain the necessary fall (around 30% from baseline) in total cholesterol. There is increasing evidence that statins, as well as having cholesterol-lowering properties, also stabilize atheromatous plaques and prevent the development and progression of aneurysmal disease through as yet incompletely understood anti-inflammatory mechanisms.
- Prescription of an antiplatelet agent. This is normally aspirin (75 mg daily), but in the significant proportion of patients who state they are unable to tolerate this, clopidogrel (75 mg daily) is an equally effective alternative. There is no evidence that warfarin is of any benefit for most patients, although those who are in atrial fibrillation may benefit from anticoagulation.
- Regular exercise (if possible).
- Control of obesity. This will help to bring down blood pressure, cholesterol and the 'strain' of walking.
- The identification and active treatment of patients with diabetes. This includes foot care (see below).

Compliance with BMT increases not only walking distance, but also, as it affords very significant protection against cardiovascular events, improves the patient's quality of life and life expectancy. Unfortunately, many patients fail to comply and, in particular, continue to smoke. These patients have a guarded prognosis in terms of both limb loss and premature death. Active intervention, by either endovascular or open surgery, should not normally be considered until the patient has been compliant with BMT for at least 6 months. Obviously, revascularization is in addition to, not instead of, BMT, a point that often has to be emphasized to patients anxious to return to their previous lifestyle.

By the time a patient develops CLI, it is often but by no means always the case that, without revascularization, the limb will be lost. However, this does not in any way

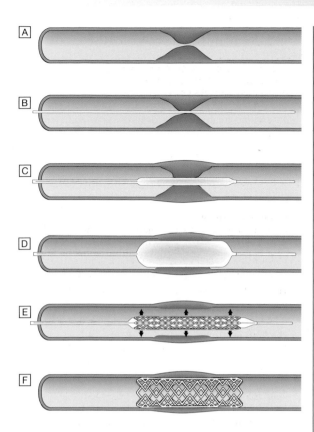

Fig. 25.8 Percutaneous transluminal angioplasty (PTA) and stenting.
[A] Critical arterial stenosis. [B] A guidewire is used to cross the lesion. [C] The guidewire is used to direct a balloon angioplasty catheter across the lesion. [D] The balloon is inflated. [E] A metal stent may be mounted on a catheter. The stent may be self-expanding or require expansion with a balloon. In many cases, the first manoeuvre is to cross the lesion with a stent and in this circumstance steps C and D may be omitted. [F] Metal stent holding open the stenosis.

undermine the value of instituting BMT in such patients. On occasion, BMT may improve the condition of the leg such that intervention is not required or a lesser procedure becomes an option. In those undergoing intervention, BMT undoubtedly reduces the overall risks and increases the success of the procedure.

Endovascular management

Percutaneous transluminal (balloon) angioplasty (PTA) has been used successfully in the iliac, femoral, popliteal and crural arteries. PTA is performed under local anaesthesia. The lesion is identified on duplex ultrasound or arteriography and crossed with a wire. A balloon catheter is introduced over the wire and the balloon inflated (Fig. 25.8). This ruptures the atheromatous plaque, thereby enlarging the lumen. In supra-inguinal (aorto-iliac) occlusions and complex disease, metal stents may be deployed across the lesion to improve patency and reduce distal embolic complications. Endoluminal repair of the aorto-iliac segment is routine practice in most vascular units because of its high patency rates and low morbidity, compared to

open surgery. Infra-inguinal PTA is also widely used in the management of IC and CLI.

Intermittent claudication

Endoluminal treatment (PTA, stent) should be used selectively in patients with IC because it is relatively expensive, it may be associated with a 1–2% morbidity rate and rarely mortality, and many patients have a pattern of disease that is unsuitable. There is particular controversy with regard to its role in the femoro-popliteal segment because of a perceived lack of durability of benefit. Several randomized controlled trials comparing infra-inguinal PTA with other treatments, in particular supervised exercise programmes, are on-going. By contrast, most vascular specialists believe that endoluminal therapy should be considered in most patients with IC due to aorto-iliac disease (absent or reduced femoral pulses) because:

- Such patients tend to be younger, so that their symptoms have a greater impact on their quality of life and livelihood.
- They often may have short-segment disease that is amenable to PTA with or without a stent.
- They often have (relatively) normal infra-inguinal arteries, so that restoring flow in the aorto-iliac segment effects a dramatic improvement in the perfusion to their leg(s).
- They tend to be more symptomatic, with shorter walking distances and bilateral symptoms.
- They may not achieve a satisfactory increase in walking distance with BMT alone, because the ability of the body to collateralize around aorto-iliac disease is not as good as it is around femoro-popliteal disease.
- The long-term patency of PTA and stenting is optimal in high-flow, large-calibre vessels, leading to durable benefit in most patients.

Critical limb ischaemia

Whereas the number of endoluminal procedures performed for IC is falling, the number performed for CLI is increasing. Endoluminal therapy has a number of major theoretical advantages in this group of patients. Specifically, it may be safer, cheaper and quicker than surgery; it may require less hospitalization; it can be repeated; and, even if it is unsuccessful, it may not prejudice the chances of subsequently performing a successful arterial bypass. However, because patients with CLI tend to have complex multilevel disease, many are unsuitable for conventional PTA. Randomized controlled trials comparing the clinical effectiveness and cost-effectiveness of surgery and PTA in this large and extremely challenging patient group are currently under way.

Indications for arterial reconstruction

Intermittent claudication

Most surgeons are reluctant to perform infra-inguinal bypass surgery for IC because:

- The risk of limb loss is very low with BMT.
- Those patients who fail to comply with BMT are those

most likely to press for surgery because of on-going symptoms. However, they are also those at greatest operative risk and those least likely to gain durable benefit from their bypass.

- Surgery is associated with a significant risk of mortality and major morbidity, the size of that risk depending on the procedure but probably exceeding 5% for infra-inguinal bypass and 10% for aorto-bifemoral bypass.
- As most patients have bilateral disease, even if they have unilateral symptoms, successful surgery on one side often reveals limiting symptoms on the other, requiring a second operation. (This is also a problem with unilateral PTA/stenting.)
- Grafts have a finite patency, especially in those who fail to comply with BMT and, in particular, continue to smoke.
- As soon as a bypass graft is inserted, collaterals circumventing the original lesion involute. For this reason, when the graft occludes, usually suddenly, the patient is normally returned to a worse level of ischaemia than before the operation. A patient who was previously a claudicant may now have acute limb-threatening ischaemia, which then forces the surgeon or radiologist to intervene again. Secondary interventions, such as thrombolysis or re-operation, are technically more difficult, are associated with higher risk and enjoy a lower patency rate.

As with PTA and stenting, the balance of risks and benefits is different in patients with aorto-iliac disease. Although the risk of surgery is higher, the long-term patency rates of such grafts are excellent, and one operation deals with both legs. It perhaps goes without saying that, whatever the treatment being considered, patients must be fully appraised of the risks and benefits so that they can give fully informed consent.

Principles of arterial reconstruction

Endarterectomy
This involves the direct removal of atherosclerotic plaque and thrombus (thrombo-endarterectomy). With the advent of prosthetic large-calibre grafts and the successful endovascular treatment of focal disease, endarterectomy is a relatively uncommon operation in modern surgical practice, except at the carotid bifurcation (see below). In the lower limb, common femoral endarterectomy, with or without a profundaplasty, is probably the most common example (Fig. 25.9).

Bypass grafting
For a surgical bypass operation (Fig. 25.10) to be successful in the long term, three conditions must be fulfilled:

- There must be high-flow, high-pressure blood entering the graft (inflow).
- The conduit must be suitable.
- The blood must have somewhere to go when it leaves the graft (outflow).

Two main types of conduit are available:

- autogenous material, most commonly the ipsilateral long saphenous vein
- prosthetic material, most commonly expanded polytetrafluoroethylene (ePTFE) or Dacron.

The main advantage of vein (Table 25.2) is that it is lined by endothelium that is actively antithrombotic and profibrinolytic, and therefore much less liable to induce coagulation than even the most inert of man-made materials. This translates into much better long-term graft patency. Vein is also much more resistant to infection (see below).

Reversed vs. in situ vein bypass
It is generally agreed that, wherever possible, vein should be used for infra-inguinal reconstruction. However, unless the long saphenous vein is reversed before being used as an arterial conduit, its valves will prevent the flow of blood

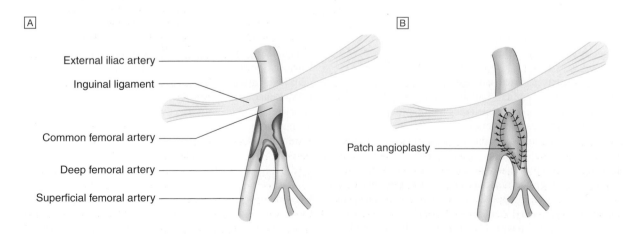

| A |
External iliac artery
Inguinal ligament
Common femoral artery
Deep femoral artery
Superficial femoral artery

| B |
Patch angioplasty

Fig. 25.9 Profundaplasty.
[A] Focal atherosclerotic disease of the left common femoral artery is causing severe ischaemia because it is obstructing flow down the superficial and deep femoral (profunda femoris) arteries. [B] Local endarterectomy and closure of the profunda femoris using a patch (profundaplasty) restores normal flow to both vessels.

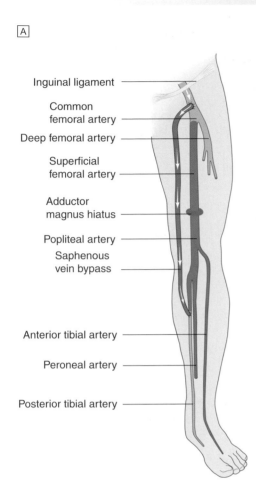

A

Inguinal ligament

Common femoral artery

Deep femoral artery

Superficial femoral artery

Adductor magnus hiatus

Popliteal artery

Saphenous vein bypass

Anterior tibial artery

Peroneal artery

Posterior tibial artery

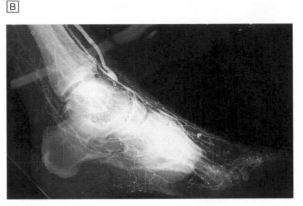

B

Fig. 25.10 Femorodistal bypass graft.
A Diagram showing femoral to posterior tibial bypass graft. B On-table angiogram showing distal end of vein graft anastomosed to the dorsalis pedis artery in the foot.

Table 25.2 AUTOGENOUS AND PROSTHETIC GRAFTS

	Autogenous graft (vein)	Prosthetic graft (ePTFE, Dacron)
Advantages	No cost Superior long-term patency Resistant to infection	Easy to use Available 'off the shelf' in a variety of calibres and lengths
Disadvantages	Only available in small calibre Often diseased (varicose veins) or absent (previous bypass surgery, CABG, varicose vein surgery)	Expensive (£500–1000) per graft No resistance to infection Poor long-term patency below the knee

(ePTFE = expanded polytetrafluoroethylene; CABG = coronary artery bypass graft)

down the leg. Alternatively, the vein can be left as it is but the valves divided; this latter type of graft is called 'in situ' or 'non-reversed'. There are pros and cons to each technique, and no difference in long-term patency between them has ever been demonstrated. The choice depends upon individual patient anatomy and surgeon preference.

Extra-anatomic bypass

In most bypass operations, the new conduit more or less follows the course of the original artery—so-called anatomic bypass (Fig. 25.11). Where this is not possible and/or desirable, a so-called extra-anatomic bypass can be inserted (Fig. 25.12). For example, if only one iliac artery is blocked, and the patient is unfit for abdominal surgery and unsuitable for endoluminal treatment, a femoro-femoral crossover graft can be performed. If both iliac arteries are occluded, then an axillo-bifemoral graft can be inserted. In general, these extra-anatomic grafts do not have as good long-term patency as anatomic aorto-iliac reconstruction. However, they are much lesser procedures and often the

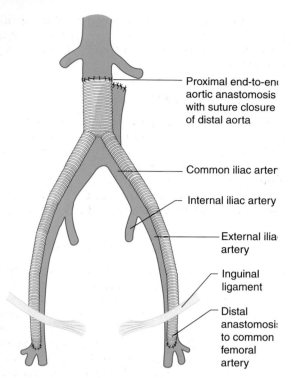

Fig. 25.11   Anatomic aortic bypass.
Reconstruction of an occluded aorto-iliac segment by a bifurcation bypass graft.

Proximal end-to-end aortic anastomosis with suture closure of distal aorta

Common iliac artery

Internal iliac artery

External iliac artery

Inguinal ligament

Distal anastomosis to common femoral artery

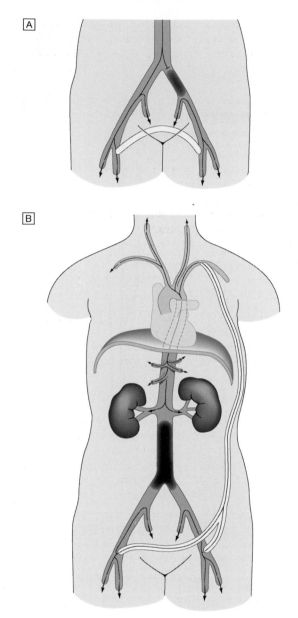

Fig. 25.12   Extra-anatomic bypass.
A Unilateral iliac disease may be treated by femoro-femoral crossover graft. B Bilateral aorto-iliac-disease may be treated with axillo-bifemoral bypass graft.

preferred option in high-risk patients or those that have a limited life expectancy.

Complications of arterial reconstruction

In the early post-operative period (30 days), vascular patients are susceptible to all the general complications of major surgery and anaesthesia. As such patients are usually elderly and unfit with widespread vascular disease, and the operations are lengthy and blood loss is often high, the morbidity of vascular surgery is considerably higher than for most other types of major surgery: for example, gastrointestinal. Meticulous perioperative care is essential for optimal results, and close liaison between the surgeon, the anaesthetist and the intensivist is mandatory.

In the longer term, the major complications are graft occlusion and infection. There are many reasons why a graft may occlude, and the correct management of this situation is a complex issue beyond the scope of this chapter. Suffice to say that the sooner a failed graft is identified and treated, the better, in general, the outcome. Many surgeons perform ultrasound scans of their grafts at regular intervals in the post-operative period, typically at 1, 3, 6, 12, 18 and 24 months. This so-called 'graft surveillance' is designed to pick up technical problems with the graft that are likely to increase the risk of failure. It is generally better to correct a 'failing' graft before it has blocked than to try to resurrect one that has already failed.

Infection of prosthetic grafts is a serious and growing problem, largely due to the increasing prevalence of antibiotic-resistant organisms, including meticillin-resistant

Staphylococcus aureus (MRSA). Once a prosthetic graft is infected, it must be removed to rid the patient of sepsis and/or to prevent the anastomoses coming apart and causing life-threatening haemorrhage. Obviously, this renders the distal part ischaemic and, where possible, a new graft is inserted through fresh uninfected tissue. This can be extremely challenging, and on occasion is impossible. Measures to avoid graft infection include:

- using autogenous material wherever possible
- perioperative antibiotic prophylaxis
- strict aseptic technique in the operating theatre and ward
- washing hands between examining patients

- prescribing antibiotics to patients with grafts in place whenever a bacteraemia might develop: for example, dental extraction, cystoscopy or any gastrointestinal intervention.

AMPUTATION

INDICATIONS

Amputation should only be considered where arterial reconstruction is considered by a vascular surgeon to be inappropriate or impossible.

In some cases, patients are admitted profoundly unwell and septic from spreading gangrene, and immediate amputation may be the only means of saving the patient's life.

LEVEL OF AMPUTATION

This is determined by local blood supply, the status of the joints, the patient's general health and his or her age. The broad principle is to amputate at the lowest level consistent with healing (Fig. 25.13). It is important to conserve the knee joint if at all possible, as the energy required for walking with a below-knee prosthesis is only a fraction of that required with one above the knee. However, if the patient has other comorbidity or disability that would make walking with a prosthesis impossible, there is no point in attempting to conserve the knee joint at the expense of healing. A common situation is where a patient presents with a fixed flexion contracture of the knee. To attempt a below-knee amputation in such a patient is

usually a mistake because the contracture will prevent the patient from ever walking and will also result in the stump wound resting on the bed or chair, leading to poor healing and breakdown.

SURGICAL PRINCIPLES

A number of important principles must be observed if primary healing and satisfactory rehabilitation are to be achieved. The in-hospital mortality for major limb amputation is around 10–20% and can exceed 30% in the elderly undergoing above-knee amputation. The decision to amputate, the level of amputation and the procedure itself require direct input from an experienced vascular surgeon.

REHABILITATION AND LIMB FITTING

At about 1 week, the patient should begin to bear weight on the other limb between parallel bars, and at 10 days to walk with a pneumatic walking aid. If healing is progressing well, a temporary prosthesis can be fitted at about 3 weeks. Final fitting of the artificial limb must await shaping and firming of the stump. Approximately 70% of below-knee amputees and 30% of above-knee amputees eventually walk. It is important to appreciate that, because of the prolonged hospital admission, rehabilitation, home modifications and, in some cases, long-term care, amputation is also a much more expensive option than revascularization leading to limb salvage.

Patients need strong support and their care is a matter of teamwork, with the surgeon, nursing staff, physiotherapist, occupational therapist, prosthetist and social worker all playing vital roles. Amputation for vascular disease has high

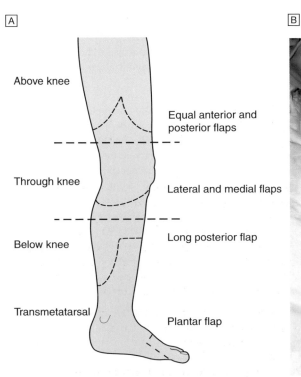

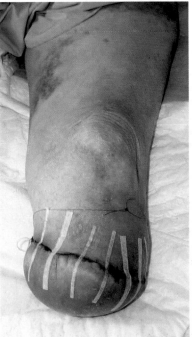

Fig. 25.13 Amputation.
A Levels of amputation and types of flap used to close the residual defect.
B Below-knee amputation.

25

morbidity and mortality and only a few patients remain alive for 5 years.

PHANTOM PAIN

Phantom limb pain can be a troublesome and persistent problem, especially if pain has not been well controlled before and after the operation. With analgesia, reassurance and time, it usually settles. There is some evidence that if the patient goes to theatre pain-free, the risk of phantom pain is much reduced. For this reason, many centres now commence epidural anaesthesia the night before surgery. Input from a pain specialist can be invaluable.

ARTERIAL DISEASE OF THE UPPER LIMB

OVERVIEW

Occlusive arterial disease is 10 times more common in the leg than in the arm. Nevertheless, when the arm is affected, treatment can be difficult, and the loss of an arm (especially the dominant one) is even more devastating for the patient than loss of a leg.

The subclavian artery just proximal to the origin of the vertebral artery is the most common site of disease, especially on the left. This may lead to:

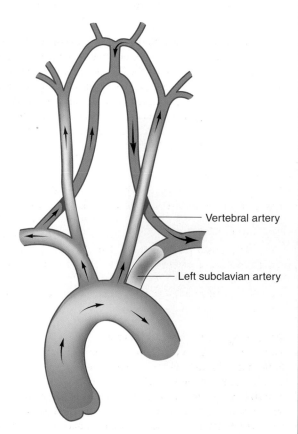

Fig. 25.14 Occlusion of the left subclavian artery, causing 'subclavian steal'.

Vertebral artery

Left subclavian artery

- *Arm claudication.* This is relatively unusual, even when the subclavian artery is completely occluded, because of the very well developed collaterals from the vertebral artery and around the scapula.
- *Atheroembolism to the hand.* Small emboli lodge in the vessels of the fingers and the hand and lead to symptoms that are often mistaken for Raynaud's phenomenon, except that in this case the symptoms are unilateral (see below). Failure to make the diagnosis may eventually lead to amputation.
- *Subclavian steal.* In this circumstance, when the arm is used, blood is 'stolen' from the brain, with retrograde flow via the vertebral artery. This leads to vertebrobasilar ischaemia, characterized by dizziness, cortical blindness and/or collapse when the arm is used (Fig. 25.14).

MANAGEMENT

Most subclavian artery disease can be treated by means of PTA and stenting, as the results are good and surgical access to the area is difficult. If surgery is required, then the usual operation is bypass from the common carotid artery to the subclavian or axillary artery distal to the lesion (carotid–subclavian bypass).

CEREBROVASCULAR DISEASE

DEFINITIONS

Stroke

Stroke may be defined as an episode of focal neurological dysfunction lasting more than 24 hours, of presumed vascular aetiology.

Transient ischaemic attack

When such symptoms last for less than 24 hours, the episode is described as a transient ischaemic attack (TIA).

Amaurosis fugax

This describes transient, usually incomplete, loss of vision in one eye owing to occlusion of a branch of the retinal artery by cholesterol emboli. The patient typically describes it as a veil or curtain coming across the eye, which remains for a few minutes and then disappears. Amaurosis fugax is never synchronously bilateral, as it is almost infinitely improbable that an embolus would enter both retinal arteries at exactly the same time. Bilateral visual loss is usually due to occipital ischaemia secondary to vertebrobasilar insufficiency (see below). Non-synchronous amaurosis fugax is, of course, possible in patients with bilateral carotid disease.

CAROTID ARTERY DISEASE

Pathophysiology

Approximately 80% of strokes are ischaemic and about half of these are thought to be due to atheroembolism from the carotid bifurcation. The origin of the internal carotid artery is particularly prone to atheroma, which is often focal and therefore amenable to local treatment. In general, the tighter the degree of stenosis, the more likely the plaque is to rupture and embolize. Atheroemboli entering the ophthalmic artery lead to amaurosis fugax or permanent monocular blindness on the same side (ipsilateral). If they enter the middle cerebral artery, they may cause hemiparesis and hemisensory loss on the opposite side (contralateral). If the dominant hemisphere is affected, there may also be dysphasia.

Assessment

The presence of a 'carotid' bruit bears no relationship to the severity of underlying internal carotid artery disease and thus the risk of stroke. Such a bruit may arise from the external carotid artery or be transmitted from the heart. Furthermore, in the presence of a very tight internal carotid artery stenosis, flow may be so slow that no audible turbulence is present. It is important to exclude other causes of cerebral ischaemia and haemorrhage.

Colour Doppler (duplex) ultrasound (CDU) is the initial investigation of choice for imaging the carotid arteries. However, CDU is limited by vessel calcification and is very operator-dependent. Magnetic resonance angiography (MRA) provides excellent images and is increasingly used to plan treatment. Computed tomographic angiography also provides good images but involves ionizing radiation and

iodinated contrast. Intra-arterial digital subtraction angiography (IA-DSA) is associated with a small risk of TIA/stroke even in the best of hands, and should normally be reserved for patients with unsuccessful or inconsistent non-invasive imaging (Fig. 25.15), rare nowadays, or those who are undergoing carotid stenting as an alternative to surgery.

Management

Medical therapy

All patients should receive BMT.

Carotid endarterectomy (CEA)

Patients with completed major stroke and no or little recovery are not candidates for carotid intervention; nor are those with an occluded internal carotid artery. However, several large randomized controlled trials have clearly indicated that CEA, in addition to BMT, is associated with a significant reduction in stroke, compared with BMT alone in patients with amaurosis, TIA and stroke with good recovery, provided that:

- there is a high degree of internal carotid artery stenosis (usually taken as a greater than 60–70% diameter reduction)
- the patient is expected to survive at least 2 years
- the intervention can be undertaken with a stroke and/or death rate of less than 5%
- the intervention can be performed soon after the index event, preferably within a month, but certainly within 6 months.

Patients who do not fulfil these criteria should, in most cases, be treated medically. The operation can be performed under general or local anaesthetic. The carotid bifurcation is dissected out, heparin is given and the arteries are clamped. If this leads to cerebral ischaemia, then a shunt is inserted. The plaque is shelled out (the endarterectomy) and the artery repaired with direct suture or a patch graft (patch angioplasty) (Fig. 25.16).

Carotid stenting

Primary carotid stenting, usually using a distal protection device to prevent distal embolization, is currently being evaluated in terms of safety and efficacy (stroke prevention) as an alternative to surgery in several randomized controlled trials. The potential advantages are that the procedure can be performed under local anaesthesia via the femoral artery, possibly with a reduced length of stay, and without a cut in the neck and thus any risk of cranial nerve injury (Fig. 25.17).

Asymptomatic carotid disease

Two randomized controlled trials have now indicated that in patients with asymptomatic high-grade (> 60%) internal carotid artery stenosis, CEA in addition to BMT is probably associated with a significant reduction in TIA and ischaemic stroke (up to 50%), compared with BMT alone (EBM 25.2). As a result of these data, in many parts of the world where health care is largely provided in the private sector for profit and where surgeons are reimbursed

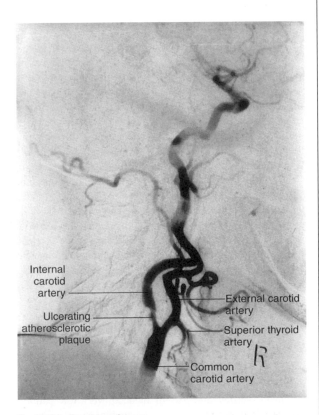

Fig. 25.15 Carotid angiogram.
Intra-arterial digital subtraction angiogram (IA-DSA) showing severe stenosis at the origin of the internal carotid artery.

Labels on figure:
Internal carotid artery
Ulcerating atherosclerotic plaque
External carotid artery
Superior thyroid artery
Common carotid artery

25

25

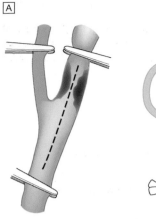
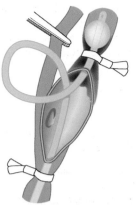
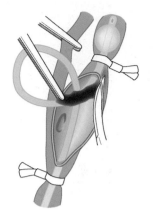
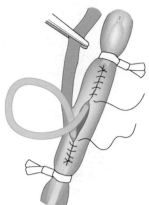

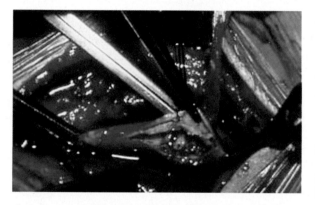

Fig. 25.16   Carotid endarterectomy.
A Diagram showing endarterectomy using a shunt to maintain cerebral blood flow while the occluding plaque is removed. B Operative photograph of plaque being removed at carotid endarterectomy.

BOX 25.2   CAROTID ARTERY DISEASE

- Up to 50% of all ischaemic strokes may be caused by atheroembolism from the carotid bifurcation
- Patients with carotid territory transient ischaemic attacks and amaurosis fugax should be assessed with a view to carotid endarterectomy
- Carotid endarterectomy, in addition to best medical therapy, has been proved to reduce the risk of further ipsilateral ischaemic stroke significantly, compared to best medical therapy alone, in patients with symptomatic internal carotid artery stenosis exceeding 70%
- Carotid endarterectomy for high-grade asymptomatic internal carotid artery stenosis is controversial; such patients should be discussed with a vascular surgeon
- Angioplasty and stenting may be used to treat an increasing proportion of carotid artery disease in the future

---

developing TIA/stroke in the future are actually quite low, perhaps 10% at 5 years. Thus, even if one could halve that risk with CEA, so obtaining an impressive *relative* risk reduction of 50%, the *absolute* risk reduction would be only 5%, or 1% per year. Hence, the number of operations needed to prevent one TIA or stroke is potentially quite large (perhaps 20–30 or more). By contrast, the number of CEAs for symptomatic disease required to prevent one TIA/stroke is probably less than 10. This suggests that undertaking large numbers of asymptomatic CEAs is probably not the best use of public money set aside to improve the health of the nation. There are, as yet, no compelling data to suggest that carotid stenting is of benefit in patients with asymptomatic disease, but even if there were, the same sorts of consideration would apply, as the costs of surgery and stenting are probably similar.

VERTEBROBASILAR DISEASE

The vertebrobasilar system feeds the occipital cortex, cerebellum and brain stem. Patients with vertebrobasilar insufficiency (VBI) may complain of (bilateral) cortical blindness, vertigo and loss of balance. Very few patients have focal, discrete disease amenable to vascular or endovascular intervention, and the mainstay of treatment is medical for the overwhelming majority.

on a 'per case' basis, the numbers of CEAs being performed for asymptomatic disease is increasingly rapidly as the disease is common and can be readily detected on CDU. In the UK and other countries where health care is funded from the public purse and surgeons are salaried, there has been much more reluctance to follow suit. The main reason is that, with or without treatment, the risks of such people

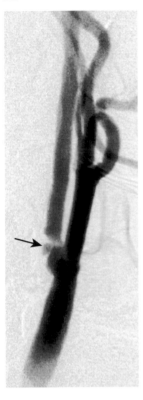
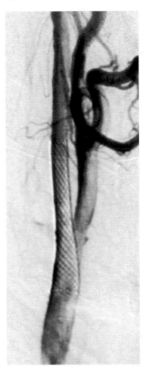

Fig. 25.17 Carotid stenting.
[A] Intra-arterial digital subtraction angiogram showing high-grade internal carotid artery stenosis. [B] The same artery after deployment of a carotid stent.

EBM 25.2 CAROTID ENDARTERECTOMY (CEA) FOR ASYMPTOMATIC CAROTID STENOSIS

'In asymptomatic patients younger than 75 years of age with a carotid diameter reduction of about 70% or more, immediate CEA halved the 5-year stroke risk.'

MRC Asymptomatic Carotid Surgery Trial (ACST) Collaborative Group. Lancet 2004; 363:1491–1502.

RENAL ARTERY DISEASE

ATHEROSCLEROSIS

Critical stenoses impair the perfusion of the juxtaglomerular apparatus, which in turn leads to an increase in renin and angiotensin and in hypertension. The disease may also lead to ischaemic necrosis of the renal parenchyma and progressive renal failure.

It is often difficult to determine whether renal artery disease is merely an incidental finding or is causally linked. Sometimes, the only way of clarifying the situation is to revascularize the kidney and observe what happens. However, this means that a significant proportion of patients may be receiving unnecessary, potentially harmful, treatment.

FIBROMUSCULAR HYPERPLASIA

This is a relatively uncommon and poorly understood stenosing condition that most commonly affects the renal arteries of young and middle-aged women. It may cause hypertension, but rarely renal failure.

MANAGEMENT

Indications for intervention
There are two indications for active intervention in cases of renal artery stenosis:

- control of hypertension that is refractory to medical therapy
- preservation of renal function.

Endovascular therapy
Primary stenting is the treatment of choice for atherosclerotic renal artery disease. PTA is also very effective for fibromuscular dysplasia (FMD). Major complications (1–2%) include acute arterial occlusion, embolization and rupture.

Surgery
Renal artery reconstruction is a major undertaking, with significant associated morbidity and mortality. It is largely reserved for patients who are not treatable by percutaneous means.

MESENTERIC ARTERY DISEASE

The coeliac axis and the superior and inferior mesenteric arteries supply the gastrointestinal tract. Owing to the rich collaterals, it is usually necessary for two of the three vessels to be occluded or critically stenosed before patients develop symptoms and signs of mesenteric vascular insufficiency, often termed 'mesenteric angina'. Typically, the patient develops severe central abdominal pain 15–30 minutes after eating, which may be associated with diarrhoea. Food avoidance leads to significant weight loss, which is universal. The condition can mimic many much more common intra-abdominal pathologies. Surgery is associated with significant morbidity and mortality (5–10%). but the long-term symptom relief is usually excellent. PTA and stenting are being increasingly used, particularly in patients with high operative risk and in those who have limited life expectancy.

Acute mesenteric ischaemia is usually caused by acute occlusion of the superior mesenteric artery (SMA) due to embolus (usually from the heart of a patient in atrial fibrillation) or acute thrombosis on top of pre-existing atherosclerosis. The patient usually presents with sudden onset of excruciating abdominal pain, collapse, bloody diarrhoea and peritonitis. Treatment comprises emergency SMA embolectomy (embolus) or SMA bypass (thrombosis) and resection of non-viable bowel. Unfortunately, extensive bowel necrosis is often present at surgery and mortality exceeds 50%. Endovascular techniques have little to offer, as the exclusion of bowel infarction requires a laparotomy.

25

25

Table 25.3	EMBOLUS VS. THROMBOSIS IN SITU	
Clinical features	Embolus	Thrombosis
Severity	Complete ischaemia (no collaterals)	Incomplete ischaemia (collaterals)
Onset	Seconds or minutes	Hours or days
Limb	Leg 3:1 arm	Leg 10:1 arm
Multiple sites	Up to 15%	Rare
Embolic source	Present (usually AF)	Absent
Previous claudication	Absent	Present
Palpation of artery	Soft; tender	Hard/calcified
Bruits	Absent	Present
Contralateral leg pulses	Present	Absent
Diagnosis	Clinical	Angiography
Management	Embolectomy, warfarin	Medical, bypass, thrombolysis
Prognosis	Loss of life > loss of limb	Loss of limb > loss of life

ACUTE LIMB ISCHAEMIA

AETIOLOGY

Acute limb ischaemia is the most common vascular emergency. It is most frequently caused by acute thrombotic occlusion of a pre-existing stenotic arterial segment (60%), thromboembolism (30%) and trauma, which may be iatrogenic. Distinguishing between thrombosis and embolism is important because investigation, treatment and prognosis are different (Table 25.3). More than 70% of peripheral emboli are due to AF. Thrombosis in situ may arise from acute plaque rupture, hypovolaemia or 'pump failure' (see below).

CLASSIFICATION

Limb ischaemia is classified on the basis of onset and severity (Table 25.4). Incomplete acute ischaemia (e.g. thrombosis in situ) can usually be treated medically, at

Table 25.4	CLASSIFICATION OF LIMB ISCHAEMIA
Terminology	Definition/comment
Onset	
Acute	Ischaemia < 14 days
Acute-on-chronic	Worsening symptoms and signs (< 14 days)
Chronic	Ischaemia stable for > 14 days
Severity (acute, acute-on-chronic)	
Incomplete	Limb not threatened
Complete	Limb threatened
Irreversible	Limb non-viable
Severity (chronic)	
Non-critical	Intermittent claudication
Subcritical	Night/rest pain
Critical	Tissue loss (ulceration +/– gangrene)

Table 25.5	SYMPTOMS AND SIGNS OF ACUTE LIMB ISCHAEMIA	
Symptoms/signs	Comment
Pain	May be absent in complete acute ischaemia; severe pain is also a feature of chronic ischaemia
Pallor	Also a feature of chronic ischaemia
Pulseless	Also a feature of chronic ischaemia
Perishing cold	Unreliable, as the ischaemic limb takes on the ambient temperature
Paraesthesia and paralysis	Loss of function is the most important feature of acute limb ischaemia and denotes a threatened limb that is likely to be lost unless it is revascularized within a few hours

least in the first instance. Complete ischaemia (e.g. embolus) will normally result in extensive tissue necrosis within 6 hours unless the limb is revascularized. Irreversible ischaemia mandates early amputation or, if the patient is unfit, end-of-life care.

CLINICAL FEATURES

Apart from those that indicate 'loss of function', namely *p*aralysis (inability to wiggle toes/fingers) and *p*araesthesia (loss of light touch over the dorsum of the foot/hand), the so-called Ps of acute ischaemia (Table 25.5) are non-specific and/or inconsistently related to its severity and should not be overly relied upon. Acute loss of limb function, of which vascular insufficiency is only one cause, must always be taken very seriously. In the presence of ischaemia, pain on squeezing the calf indicates muscle infarction and impending irreversible ischaemia.

At first, acute complete ischaemia is associated with intense distal arterial spasm and the limb is 'marble' white. As the spasm relaxes over the next few hours and the skin fills with deoxygenated blood, mottling appears. This is light blue or purple, has a fine reticular pattern and blanches on pressure: so-called 'non-fixed mottling'. At this stage, the limb is still salvageable. As ischaemia progresses, blood coagulates in the skin, leading to mottling that is darker in colour, coarser in pattern and does not blanch. Finally, large patches of fixed staining progress to blistering and liquefaction (Fig. 25.18). Attempts at revascularization at this late stage are futile and will lead to life-threatening reperfusion injury (see below).

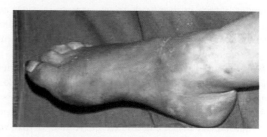

Fig. 25.18 Mottled right foot due to advanced acute limb ischaemia.

MANAGEMENT

All suspected acutely ischaemic limbs must be discussed *immediately* with a vascular surgeon; a few hours can make the difference between death/amputation and complete recovery of limb function. If there are no contraindications, administer an intravenous bolus of heparin to limit propagation of thrombus and protect the collateral circulation. If ischaemia is complete, proceed directly to the operating theatre because angiography will introduce delay, thrombolysis is not an option, lack of collateral flow will prevent visualization of the distal vasculature and the required operation is likely to be embolectomy (preferably under local anaesthesia). If ischaemia is incomplete, obtain pre-operative imaging wherever possible, as simple embolectomy or thrombectomy is unlikely to be successful, thrombolysis may be an option, a 'road-map' for distal bypass is helpful, and it is often possible, at least initially, to manage the patient medically based on the results of imaging.

Acute embolus

Embolic occlusion of the brachial artery is not usually limb-threatening and, in an elderly patient, non-operative treatment is reasonable. Younger patients should undergo embolectomy to prevent subsequent claudication, especially where the dominant arm is affected.

A leg affected by embolus is nearly always threatened and requires immediate surgical revascularization. Femoral embolus is associated with profound ischaemia to the level of the upper thigh because the deep femoral artery is also affected. Acute embolic occlusion of the aortic bifurcation (saddle embolus) leads to absent femoral pulses and a patient who is 'marble' white or mottled to the waist. Patients may also present with paraplegia due to ischaemia of the cauda equina, which may be irreversible. Embolectomy can be performed under local/regional or general anaesthetic (Fig. 25.19). Post-operatively, the patient should continue on heparin. Warfarin reduces the risk of recurrent embolism. The in-hospital mortality from cardiac death and/or recurrent embolism, particularly stroke, is 10–20%.

Thrombosis in situ

There is usually a reason why the limb affected by stable chronic ischaemia suddenly deteriorates due to thrombosis in situ on top of atherosclerosis. Reasons include 'silent' or overt MI (drop in blood pressure); underlying, hitherto asymptomatic, malignancy (increase in thrombogenicity of the blood); septicaemia, particularly pneumococcal and meningococcal; and dehydration from any cause, which may be associated with widespread thrombosis.

Popliteal aneurysm

Popliteal aneurysm can undergo thrombosis or act as a source of emboli. Catheter-directed intra-arterial thrombolysis of the crural vessels is often the treatment of choice, as simple thrombectomy usually leads to early re-thrombosis and the distal run-off is often obliterated, precluding surgical bypass. Once the crural circulation is restored,

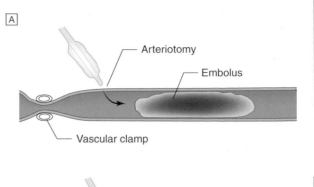
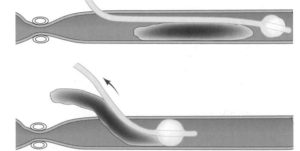

A

Arteriotomy
Embolus
Vascular clamp

25

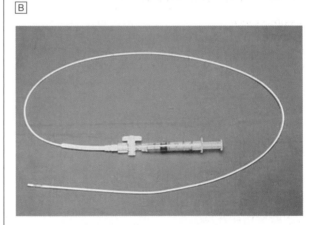

B

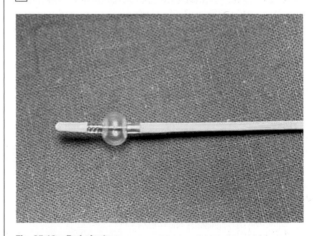

C

Fig. 25.19 Embolectomy.
A Diagram showing removal of an embolus with a balloon catheter. The balloon is inflated once it is beyond the thrombus and then withdrawn. **B** Embolectomy catheter. **C** Tip of embolectomy catheter with balloon inflated.

25

a bypass should be performed to exclude the aneurysm (see below).

Trauma

In the UK, acute traumatic limb ischaemia is frequently iatrogenic. The most common causes of non-iatrogenic injury are limb fractures and dislocations, blunt injuries occurring in the course of road traffic accidents, and stab wounds. The presence of distal pulses does *not* exclude significant arterial injury. Where there is suspicion of major vascular injury, angiography should be performed.

Intra-arterial drug administration

This leads to intense spasm and microvascular thrombosis. The leg is mottled and digital gangrene is not uncommon, but pedal pulses are usually palpable. The mainstay of treatment is supportive care, hydration to minimize renal failure secondary to rhabdomyolysis, and full heparinization. Vascular reconstruction is almost never indicated, but fasciotomy may be required to prevent compartment syndrome (see below).

Thoracic outlet syndrome

Pressure on the subclavian artery from a cervical rib or abnormal soft tissue band may lead to a post-stenotic dilatation lined with thrombosis, predisposing to occlusion or embolization. The distal circulation may be chronically obliterated and digital ischaemia advanced before the diagnosis is made. The diagnosis is made on duplex scan and/or angiography. Treatment options include thrombolysis, thrombectomy/embolectomy, excision of the cervical rib and repair of the aneurysmal segment.

Thrombolysis

This is performed percutaneously under local anaesthetic by interventional radiologists. A catheter is embedded into the distal extent of thrombus and recombinant tissue plasminogen activator (rTPA) is infused. TPA converts plasminogen to plasmin, which dissolves fibrin clot. The technique may be used in embolic occlusion, but if the ischaemia is severe, lysis may be contraindicated because thrombus dissolution often takes several hours. Mechanical thrombectomy or thrombus aspiration may help to accelerate the process. Thrombolysis may dissolve the clot to reveal an underlying lesion amenable to endovascular therapy or surgery. Thrombolysis is associated with a significant major (5%) and minor (15%) complication rate, including stroke (2%), which may be due to intracerebral haemorrhage or ischaemia secondary to atherothromboembolism from the heart or carotid bifurcations.

POST-ISCHAEMIC SYNDROMES

Reperfusion injury

Activated neutrophils, free radicals, enzymes, hydrogen ions, carbon dioxide, potassium and myoglobin released from reperfused tissue can lead to acute respiratory distress syndrome (ARDS), myocardial stunning, endotoxaemia and acute tubular necrosis, and in turn, to multiple organ failure.

Compartment syndrome

Endothelial cell injury during ischaemia leads to increased capillary permeability and oedema on reperfusion. In the calf, where muscles are confined within tight fascial boundaries, the increase in interstitial tissue pressure can lead to continuing muscle necrosis despite apparently adequate arterial inflow: the so-called compartment syndrome. There is swelling and pain on squeezing the calf muscle or moving the ankle or toes. It is very important to remember that palpable pedal pulses do not exclude the syndrome. The key to management is prevention through expeditious revascularization and a low threshold for fasciotomy (Fig. 25.20).

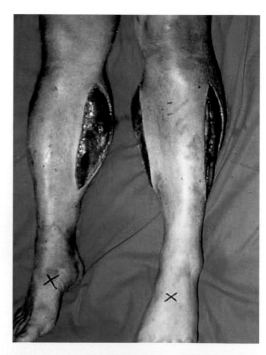

Fig. 25.20 Medial and lateral fasciotomy to decompress compartment syndrome in a patient who presented with bilateral acute limb ischaemia due to saddle embolus.

BOX 25.3   ACUTE LIMB ISCHAEMIA

- Acute limb ischaemia is the most common vascular emergency
- The most common causes are embolus from the left atrium in association with atrial fibrillation and acute thrombosis at a site of long-standing atherosclerotic narrowing
- It is often possible to distinguish these two conditions on clinical grounds alone
- The treatment of embolism is urgent embolectomy, usually without prior angiography
- Patients with thrombosis in situ should undergo angiography, and treatment comprises a combination of medical therapy, thrombolysis, angioplasty and bypass
- Paralysis, paraesthesia and muscle tenderness are the cardinal signs of complete acute ischaemia; when they are present, the limb must be revascularized immediately, if it is to be saved. Always consider a fasciotomy upon successful reperfusion in such cases to avoid compartment syndrome

ANEURYSMAL DISEASE

CLASSIFICATION

An aneurysm may be defined as an abnormal focal dilatation of an endothelial-lined vascular structure (artery, vein, heart chamber). Arterial aneurysms are by far the most common. Aneurysms may be classified according to their site, underlying aetiology and morphology.

Site

Any artery can be affected. The most common site for aneurysmal disease presenting to the vascular surgeon is the infra-renal aorta; others include the popliteal, femoral and subclavian arteries.

Aetiology

Atherosclerotic

Most aneurysms are 'non-specific' in aetiology; in the past they were termed 'atherosclerotic'. However, it is now widely believed that aneurysmal disease is a distinct pathological process from occlusive arterial disease, although they share some of the same risk factors (smoking and hypertension) and may coexist in the same patient.

Mycotic

The term mycotic, meaning fungal, is a misnomer because fungi do not cause aneurysms. The term is used nowadays to include all aneurysms that are believed to be infected. The infection can be primary or secondary to other pathology. Arteries are generally resistant to infection, but

two organisms, *Treponema pallidum* (syphilis) and salmonella, have a particular ability to produce primary mycotic aneurysms. Septic emboli from heart valves affected by subacute bacterial endocarditis may also lodge in the distal vasculature and produce secondary mycotic aneurysms. 'Non-specific' aneurysms and the layers of laminated thrombus within them may become infected in the course of a bacteraemia from another site. Lastly, infection of prosthetic grafts can lead to infected anastomotic aneurysms.

True aneurysms

All three layers of the arterial wall enclose a true aneurysm (Fig. 25.21).

False aneurysms

If the wall of an artery is pierced, the resulting haematoma sometimes remains in continuity with the lumen via the puncture site. A pulsatile swelling then forms, the wall of which consists of compacted thrombus and surrounding connective tissue. Small aneurysms (2–3 cm in diameter) often thrombose spontaneously. Larger aneurysms tend to expand, especially if the patient is on aspirin, heparin or warfarin, and compress surrounding tissues. The most common site is the groin after common femoral artery instrumentation, and this may cause femoral vein compression and deep venous thrombosis (DVT). Surgery is the traditional method of treatment, but ultrasound-guided compression repair and thrombin injection are increasingly used and successful. Where such aneurysms develop in less accessible sites, such as the aorto-iliac segment, then the hole can be sealed using a metal stent covered in graft material (covered stent) introduced percutaneously, usually via the femoral artery.

ABDOMINAL AORTIC ANEURYSM (AAA)

Epidemiology

AAA is present in 5% of men aged over 60 years. In about 70% of cases, only the infra-renal segment is involved. In the remainder, the rest of the abdominal aorta, the thoracic aorta or a combination of both is involved. The incidence of AAA is increasing. It is three times more common in men than in women, and the median age at presentation is 65 years for elective and 75 years for emergency cases.

Clinical features

An AAA may present in the following ways:

- *Asymptomatic (30%)*. The AAA may be detected incidentally on routine physical examination, plain X-ray or, most commonly, abdominal ultrasound scan conducted for another reason. Even a large AAA can be difficult to feel, which explains why so many remain undetected until they rupture. Studies have shown that screening men over the age of 60 for AAA by means of ultrasound results in a reduction in the number of deaths from rupture (EBM 25.3). All patients in whom an incidental finding of an AAA is made should be discussed with a vascular surgeon.

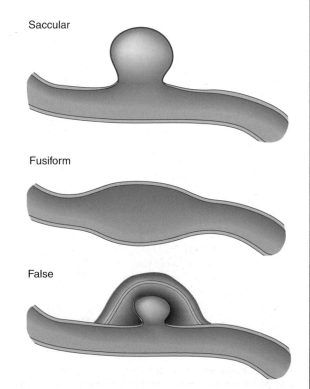

Saccular

Fusiform

False

Fig. 25.21   True and false aneurysms.

25

EBM 25.3   ABDOMINAL AORTIC ANEURYSM (AAA) SCREENING

'For men aged 65–75 years, an invitation to attend for AAA screening reduces AAA-related mortality by about 50%.'

Fleming C, et al. Ann Intern Med 2005; 142(3):203–211. Multi-centre Aneurysm Screening Study (MASS) Group. Lancet 2002; 360:1531–1539.

- *Symptomatic (20%).* AAA may cause pain in the central abdomen, back, loin, iliac fossa or groin. Thrombus within the aneurysm sac may be a source of emboli to the lower limbs. Less commonly, the aneurysm may undergo thrombotic occlusion. AAA may also become inflamed and then compress surrounding structures such as the duodenum, ureter and the inferior vena cava.
- *Rupture (50%).* AAA may rupture, usually into the retroperitoneum, but sometimes into the peritoneal cavity or rarely into surrounding structures, most commonly the inferior vena cava, leading to an aorto-caval fistula.

Investigations

About two-thirds of AAAs are sufficiently calcified to show up on a plain abdominal X-ray (Fig. 25.22). Ultrasound (Fig. 25.23) is the best way of establishing the diagnosis, of obtaining an approximate size, and of following up patients with asymptomatic AAAs that are not yet large enough to warrant surgical repair. CT and angiography (CTA) (Fig. 25.24) will provide much more accurate information about the size and extent of the aneurysm, involvement of visceral arteries and the surrounding structures, and whether there is any other intra-abdominal pathology. It is the standard pre-operative investigation but is not suitable for surveillance because of the ionizing radiation.

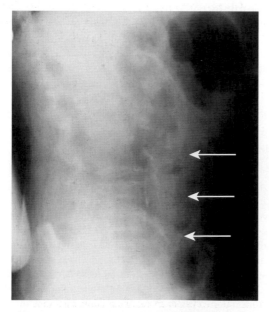

Fig. 25.22   Plain lateral abdominal X-ray showing calcification of the wall of an abdominal aortic aneurysm (arrows).

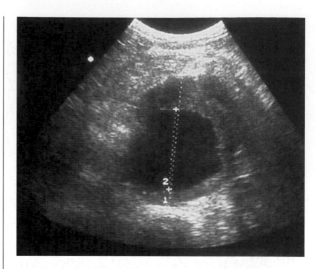

Fig. 25.23   Abdominal ultrasound showing a transverse section through a large abdominal aortic aneurysm.

Asymptomatic AAA

The UK Small Aneurysm Trial and the similar US-based ADAM trials have shown that the risks of open surgery generally outweigh the risks of rupture until an asymptomatic AAA has reached 5.5 cm in antero-posterior maximum diameter. It is, therefore, very unusual in the UK for an AAA smaller than this to be operated upon in the absence of symptoms. Once a small AAA has been detected, the best way of following up the affected patient is by repeated ultrasound scans at 3–6-monthly intervals (depending on the size) within an 'aneurysm surveillance' clinic. In the clinic, patients are started on and encouraged to comply with BMT, which affords the same benefits as it does in patients with occlusive disease (which often coexists). Ultrasound is only accurate to about 0.5 cm and tends to underestimate AAA size. Thus, most surgeons will arrange for a CT scan to be performed when the AAA reaches 5.0 cm, along with other tests designed to assess fitness for surgery. Once the AAA reaches 5.5 cm and assuming the clinical assessment and investigations indicate that the patient is fit for surgery, the surgeon will normally begin discussions with the patient with a view to operative or endovascular repair.

Symptomatic AAA

All symptomatic AAAs should be considered for repair, not only to rid the patient of their symptoms, but also because pain often predates rupture. Distal embolization is a definite indication for repair, even if the AAA is small, as limb loss is common if the AAA is left untreated.

Ruptured AAA

This is the most common emergency presentation of AAA to vascular surgeons in the UK. Patients survive rupture for the following reasons:

- The rupture is usually into the retroperitoneum, which tamponades the leak.

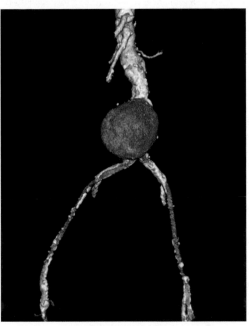

Fig. 25.24
Computed tomography (CT) in abdominal aortic aneurysm.
[A] Transverse section. [B] CT angiography (CTA): 3-D reconstruction.

25

- There is intense vasoconstriction of non-essential circulatory beds.
- The patient develops an intensely prothrombotic state.
- The patient's blood pressure drops, which helps to seal the hole.

Any medical intervention that upsets this delicate balance will convert a relatively stable, salvageable patient into someone unlikely to reach the operating theatre or to survive surgery. Specifically, large volumes of intravenous fluid (saline or plasma expander) increase the patient's blood pressure, impair haemostasis and abolish vasoconstriction, and must therefore not be given. The only way of saving the patient is to clamp the aorta (Fig. 25.25), and there must be no delay in getting the patient to the operating theatre so that this can be done.

Open AAA repair

This entails replacing the aneurysmal segment with a prosthetic graft (Fig. 25.26). The 30-day major morbidity and mortality for this procedure is approximately 10% for elective asymptomatic AAA, 20% for emergency symptomatic AAA and over 50% for ruptured AAA.

Endovascular aneurysm repair (EVAR)

The last 5 years have seen extraordinary progress in the development of EVAR, especially of infra-renal AAA. EVAR involves placing a covered stent inside the aneurysm via a femoral arteriotomy, or percutaneously, under radiological guidance (Figs 25.27 and 25.28). The procedure can be performed under regional (epidural) or even

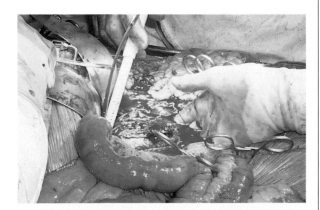

Fig. 25.25   Intra-operative photograph of repair of a ruptured abdominal aortic aneurysm.

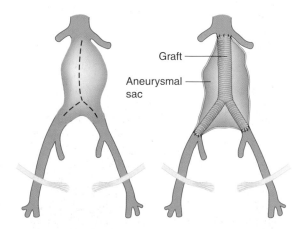

Graft

Aneurysmal sac

Fig. 25.26   Open repair of an abdominal aortic aneurysm.
Diagram showing insertion of a 'trouser' bifurcation graft within the opened aneurysmal sac.

25

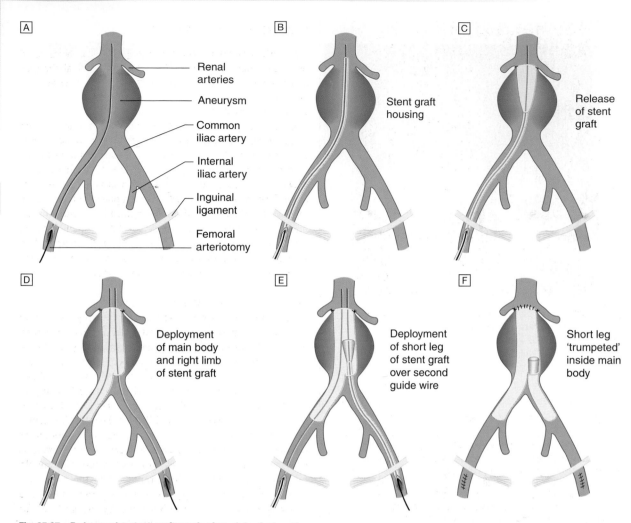

Fig. 25.27 Endovascular stent-graft repair of an abdominal aortic aneurysm.
A A guidewire is passed through the aneurysm via an incision in the right common femoral artery. B A catheter containing the main body of the stent graft is passed over the guidewire and into position within the aneurysm. C The outer cover of the catheter is removed, allowing the upper part of the stent graft to spring open and become attached by hooks to the wall of the aorta just below the renal arteries. D The rest of the catheter is removed, allowing deployment of the main body of the graft and the right (long) limb within the common iliac artery. Note the short (left) limb of the graft. E Via an incision in the left common femoral artery a second guidewire is passed up through the short limb of the stent graft. A second catheter containing the rest of the stent graft is passed over the guidewire and into the main body of the stent graft. As before, retraction of the outer cover allows the top of the second limb of the stent graft to open within the short limb of the main body. F Deployment is complete and the aneurysm sac completely excluded from the circulation. The femoral arteries are closed.

local anaesthesia, and laparotomy and cross-clamping of the aorta are avoided. The patient is often fit to go home within 48 hours, as opposed to the 10 days that are typical following open repair. Patients also make a rapid return to their pre-operative functional status, whereas those who have undergone open repair often take 4–6 months to feel as well as they did before their operation. Perhaps not surprisingly, therefore, the recent EVAR 1 trial has shown that, in patients with asymptomatic AAAs who are suitable and fit for open repair or EVAR, the latter is associated with a marked reduction in hospital mortality and morbidity, reduced hospital stay and improved post-operative quality of life (EBM 25.4). As always, though, there are downsides; specifically, the devices are very expensive (£6000), less than 50% of AAAs are suitable for the procedure with present technology, and there are still questions over durability in that the secondary intervention rate following EVAR is much higher than it is following open repair. The EVAR 2 trial showed that in patients unfit for open surgery, the addition of EVAR to BMT was of no benefit when compared to BMT alone. Over the next 5 years, the technology is likely to continue to improve, such that the morbidity and mortality associated with EVAR will fall even further, the secondary intervention rates will also fall, and most patients can be treated by EVAR, which is likely to become the standard treatment. The technique also has applicability in patients with thoracic and thoraco-abdominal aneurysms and dissection (Fig. 25.29), and several groups have published encouraging results of EVAR for ruptured aortic aneurysms.

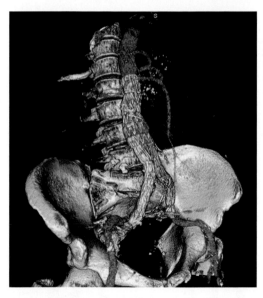

Figure 25.28 3-D CT reconstruction of a stent graft deployed inside an abdominal aortic aneurysm.
(Courtesy of Mr Donald Adam.)

EBM 25.4   ENDOVASCULAR ANEURYSM REPAIR (EVAR)

'Compared with open AAA repair, EVAR is associated with a significant reduction in short-term post-operative morbidity and mortality, which translates into a 3% improvement in AAA-related mortality after 4 years. However, after 4 years, EVAR offers no advantage with respect to all-cause mortality or health-related quality of life (HRQL), is more expensive, and is associated with a greater number of (mostly minor) complications and re-interventions.'

EVAR trial participants. Lancet 2005; 365:2179–2186

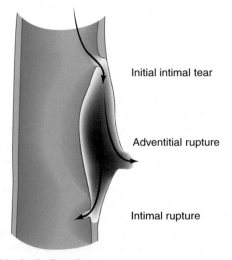

Initial intimal tear

Adventitial rupture

Intimal rupture

Fig. 25.29   Aortic dissection.
(1) Initial intimal tear. (2) Adventitial rupture. (3) Intimal rupture.

PERIPHERAL ANEURYSMS

Any peripheral artery, and very rarely vein, can be affected by aneurysmal dilatation. The aetiology, clinical features and treatment vary depending upon the site of disease.

Iliac aneurysms

Approximately 20% of AAAs extend into one or both common iliac arteries and about a third of these extend into the internal iliac artery; for reasons unknown, the external iliac artery is rarely affected. Isolated iliac aneurysms can also occur. The bifurcation of the aorta is at the level of the umbilicus, so that a pulsatile mass below that level is likely to be iliac in origin. Iliac aneurysms are most often treated in the course of AAA repair. Isolated iliac aneurysms should be considered for endoluminal or surgical repair if they are causing symptoms or have reached twice the normal diameter of the native artery.

Femoral aneurysms

Three types of femoral aneurysm commonly present to the vascular surgeon: iatrogenic false aneurysm (see above), non-specific aneurysm and anastomotic aneurysm. 'Non-specific' aneurysms of the common femoral artery are found in 10% of patients with AAA and as an isolated occurrence. Patients presenting with a femoral aneurysm should have an AAA excluded, if necessary, by ultrasound scan. In 50% of cases they are bilateral. They are frequently asymptomatic but may cause pain and compression of surrounding structures (femoral vein and nerve); rupture is uncommon. If large (> 3 cm) or symptomatic, they should be considered for surgical repair. Anastomotic false aneurysms are increasingly being seen in patients who have previously undergone aorto-bifemoral bypass grafting for occlusive or aneurysmal disease. They may not present until many years after the original surgery, but once present, they usually grow inexorably and require repair. They are usually due to mechanical disruption of the anastomosis as a result of late suture failure or progressive disease of the femoral artery; less commonly, they are due to infection.

Popliteal aneurysms

These are present in 20% of patients with AAA and their presence must be sought, if necessary with ultrasound, in all such patients. Around 50% are bilateral. If a patient presents with a popliteal aneurysm, there is a 50% chance that he or she also has an AAA, which again must be sought. The main complications of popliteal aneurysm are distal embolization and acute thrombosis; the latter is associated with limb loss in up to 50% of cases because the calf vessels are often chronically occluded, which makes surgical bypass difficult. As discussed above, the best treatment is usually thrombolysis, followed by surgical bypass using the long saphenous vein (Fig. 25.30). Sometimes, in severely ischaemic limbs, it is necessary to instil the lytic agent at the same time as operative exclusion and bypass. Rupture of popliteal aneurysms is extremely rare. Occasionally, they can compress the popliteal vein and present as a DVT.

25

25

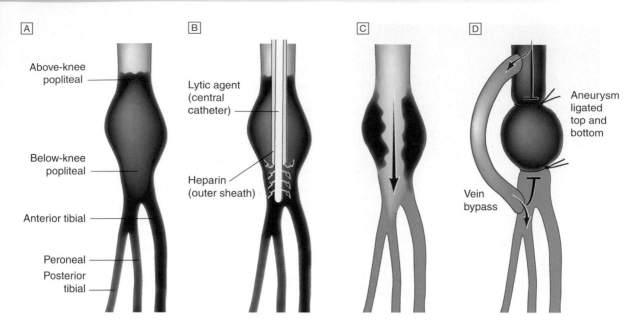

Fig. 25.30 Thrombolytic treatment of a thrombosed popliteal aneurysm.
A Thrombosed popliteal aneurysm associated with complete thrombotic occlusion of the calf vessels. B The interventional radiologist has placed a catheter in the thrombosed aneurysm. The catheter has been introduced via the contralateral femoral artery, percutaneously under local anaesthesia. The outer part of the catheter is used to deliver heparin, and the inner part to deliver lytic agent into the thrombus. C Lysis is complete and flow has been restored to the foot. The catheter has been removed. D The popliteal aneurysm has been bypassed and excluded from the circulation to prevent re-thrombosis.

Subclavian aneurysms

These are usually associated with mechanical compression at the thoracic outlet from a cervical rib. Arterial stenosis causes a jet of high-velocity blood flow just distal to the narrowed area and, for reasons that are not entirely clear, this leads to post-stenotic dilatation (Fig. 25.31). This dilatation can become frankly aneurysmal and lined with thrombus which, as described above with regard to popliteal aneurysm, can lead to thrombotic occlusion and/or distal embolization. This presents as chronic or acute-on-chronic arm ischaemia; a pulsatile supraclavicular mass is often present.

BUERGER'S DISEASE (THROMBOANGIITIS OBLITERANS)

This is an inflammatory obliterative arterial disease that is quite distinct from atherosclerosis. It is rare in Caucasians in the UK but more common in people from the Mediterranean, Asia and North Africa. It usually presents in young (20–30 years) male smokers and characteristically affects the peripheral arteries, giving rise to claudication in the feet or rest pain in the fingers or toes (Fig. 25.32). (Such pain in the feet on walking is often misdiagnosed as musculoskeletal in nature, whereas pain in the fingers or toes is often misdiagnosed as primary Raynaud's phenomenon—see below.) The condition also affects the veins, and superficial thrombophlebitis is common. Wrist and ankle pulses are usually absent, but brachial and popliteal pulses are palpable. Arteriography shows narrowing or occlusion of arteries below the diseased segment, but relatively healthy vessels above that level.

The condition often remits if the patient stops smoking; sympathectomy and prostaglandin infusions may be helpful. If amputation is required, it can often be limited to the digits at first. However, if the patient continues to smoke, then bilateral below-knee amputation is a frequent outcome. Although the disease is rare, it is very important to consider and exclude it in patients presenting with

---

BOX 25.4 ANEURYSMAL DISEASE

- AAAs are present in 5% of men aged over 60 and more than half are asymptomatic and undetected until they rupture
- Ruptured AAA is the 10th most common cause of death in men. Only a third of patients with ruptured AAA reach hospital alive and, of these, only about half survive surgery. The overall mortality for the condition is therefore in excess of 80%. Population screening of men over the age of 60 years with ultrasound reduces the number of ruptured AAAs by up to 50%
- Patients with asymptomatic AAA should be considered for repair if the maximum diameter reaches 5.5 cm and the surgeon believes the operation will be associated with a mortality of less than 5–7%
- An increasingly large number of AAAs *can* be repaired endoluminally using stent grafts
- Thrombosed popliteal aneurysm is a relatively common, but frequently overlooked, cause of acute and acute-on-chronic lower limb ischaemia
- Distal embolization from a subclavian aneurysm may be misdiagnosed as Raynaud's phenomenon, but Raynaud's is always bilateral

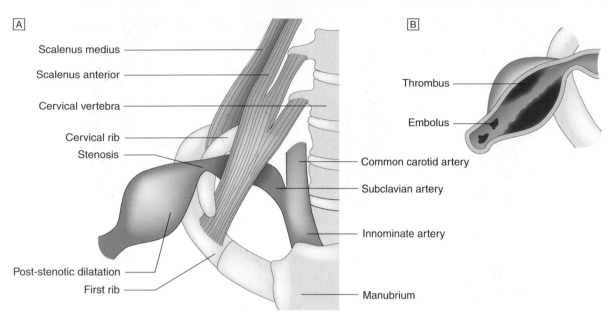

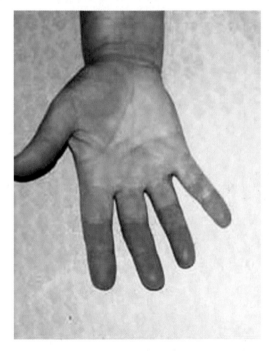

Fig. 25.31   Subclavian aneurysm.
[A] Compression of the subclavian artery by a cervical rib has led to post-stenotic dilatation and aneurysm formation. [B] Thrombus within a subclavian aneurysm acting as a source of distal emboli. [C] Ischaemic right hand due to distal embolization from subclavian aneurysm.

vascular symptoms in their legs and arms, especially if the symptoms are atypical and the patient is young (under 50 years of age). Failure to make the diagnosis often leads to avoidable limb loss and is a source of medicolegal activity.

RAYNAUD'S PHENOMENON

Raynaud's phenomenon describes digital pallor due to vasospasm of the digital arteries, followed by cyanosis owing to the presence of deoxygenated blood, then rubor due to reactive hyperaemia upon restoration of flow, in response to cold and emotional stimuli.

PRIMARY RAYNAUD'S PHENOMENON

This is also called Raynaud's disease. It affects 5–10% of young women in temperate climates, and usually appears between the ages of 15 and 30 years; a family history is common. It does not progress to ulceration or infarction. No investigation is necessary and the patient is given

25

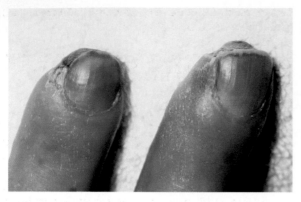

Fig. 25.32 **Fingertip ulceration in a patient affected by Buerger's disease.**

reassurance, advised to avoid exposure to cold, and treated in the first instance with nifedipine (a calcium channel blocker). The underlying cause is unclear.

SECONDARY RAYNAUD'S PHENOMENON

This is also known as Raynaud's syndrome and tends to occur in older people in association with:

- connective tissue disease, most commonly systemic sclerosis
- vibration-induced injury, from the use of power tools (vibration white finger or VWF, hand–arm vibration syndrome or HAVS)

- atherosclerosis, most commonly thoracic outlet obstruction from the cervical rib (see above).

Unlike primary disease that is due to reversible spasm, secondary disease is usually associated with fixed obstruction of the digital arteries. Fingertip ulceration and necrosis are often present. The fingers must be protected from cold and trauma, infection is treated with antibiotics, and surgery is avoided if possible. Vasoactive drugs have no clear benefit. Sympathectomy helps for a year or two. Prostacyclin infusions are sometimes beneficial. In the UK, VWF/HAVS is increasingly recognized as a common industrial occupational disease for which very large sums of money are being paid out in compensation.

PATHOPHYSIOLOGY OF VENOUS DISEASE

ANATOMY

The long (LSV) and short (SSV) saphenous veins and their tributaries (Fig. 25.33) lie outside the deep fascia and carry only 10% of the venous return from the limb. The LSV begins at the medial end of the dorsal venous arch, crosses in front of the medial malleolus and ascends the medial side of the leg. It penetrates the deep (cribriform) fascia 2.5 cm below and lateral to the pubic tubercle, to

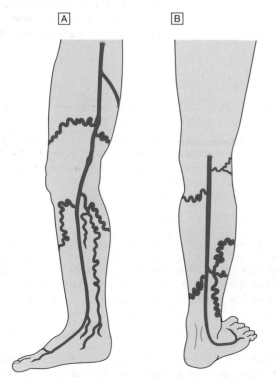

Fig. 25.33 **Diagrammatic representation of varicose veins in the lower limb.**
A Long saphenous system. B Short saphenous system.

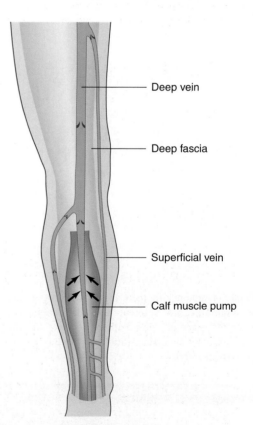

Fig. 25.34 **Diagrammatic representation of the venous drainage of the lower limb.**

enter the common femoral vein at the saphenofemoral junction (SFJ). The SSV starts at the lateral end of the dorsal venous arch, passes posterior to the lateral malleolus, then ascends the median line of the calf to join the popliteal vein at the saphenopopliteal junction (SPJ), usually just above the knee. Anatomical variations are common.

The deep venous system comprises intramuscular veins and axial veins that accompany the main arteries; they are usually paired in the calf. Communicating veins perforate the deep fascia to connect the superficial and deep systems (Fig. 25.34).

PHYSIOLOGY

Weight-bearing compresses the veins in the sole of the foot, which propels blood into the calf ('foot pump'). Pushing off is associated with calf muscle contraction and the compression of venous blood in the muscular sinuses and axial veins; this propels blood further up the leg ('calf pump'). When the leg is lifted off the floor and the muscles relax, blood is prevented from refluxing back down the leg by the closure of valves. During this relaxation phase, blood passes from the superficial to the deep veins via perforators, ready to be expelled during the next step. In motionless standing, the venous pressure at the ankle is approximately 100 mmHg: that is, the hydrostatic pressure exerted by the column of venous blood stretching from the ankle to the right atrium. However, upon walking, the mechanisms described above reduce the ankle pressure to less than 25 mmHg (ambulatory venous pressure, AVP). The symptoms and signs of lower limb venous disease are largely due to failure of these protective mechanisms and the presence of a high AVP.

VARICOSE VEINS

CLASSIFICATION

Trunk varices
These involve the main stem and/or major tributaries of the LSV and SSV, are usually > 4 mm in diameter (and may be much larger) (Fig. 25.35), lie subcutaneously, are palpable, do not usually discolour the overlying skin, and are present in about a third of the adult population. Although 2–3 times more women than men present for treatment, the prevalence is roughly equal between the sexes. There appears to be a familial tendency, and obesity, pregnancy, constipation and prolonged standing may be aggravating factors.

Reticular varices
These lie deep in the dermis, are < 4 mm in diameter, are impalpable, and render the overlying skin dark blue. They are present in about 80% of the adult population, and may or may not be associated with trunk varices.

Telangiectasia
These are also called spider and hyphen web veins. They lie superficially in the dermis, are usually 1 mm or less in diameter, are impalpable, and render the overlying skin purple or bright red. Again, they may be associated with trunk and reticular varices, and are present in 90% of adults. Like reticular veins, they appear to be more common in women, probably because of poorly understood hormonal reasons.

EPIDEMIOLOGY

Varicose veins (VV) are so prevalent that they could almost be considered a variant of normal for a creature that spends its life on two as opposed to four legs. Their prevalence increases markedly with age and they are an almost universal finding in individuals over the age of 60.

CLINICAL FEATURES

The great majority of individuals with VV are asymptomatic, or at least they do not seek treatment. Those that do attend the surgical clinic do so because they are unhappy about the appearance of their leg(s), and/or they associate lower limb symptoms with their VV, and/or they are concerned about developing complications.

Cosmetic issues
Many patients, especially young women, seek treatment because they consider their veins to be unsightly. Possibly because they are embarrassed to admit that cosmesis is the main issue, they frequently complain of various lower limb symptoms as well.

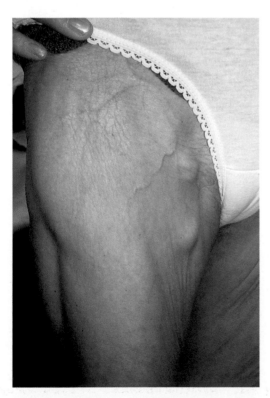

Fig. 25.35 Long saphenous varicose veins and saphena varix.

25

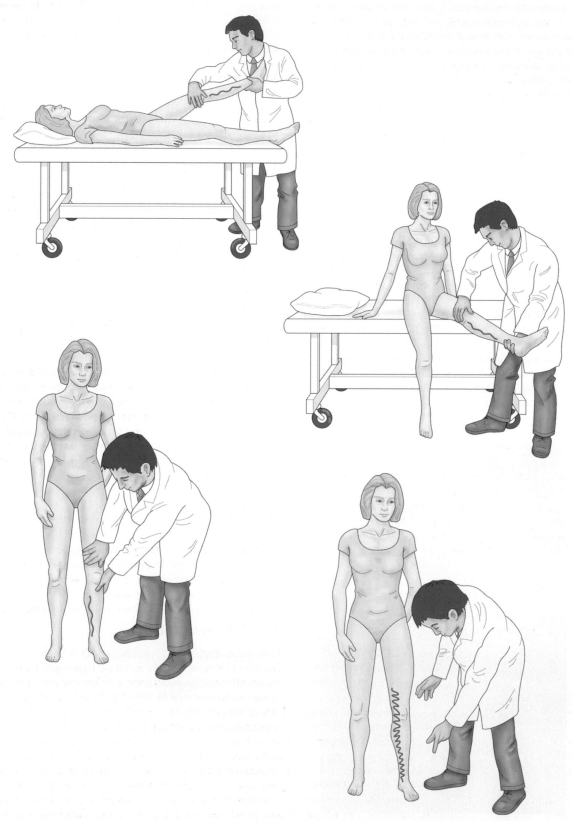

Fig. 25.36 Trendelenburg test to demonstrate saphenofemoral incompetence.

Symptoms

A wide variety of lower limb symptoms have been attributed to VV. Lower limb symptoms are present in about half of the adult population, and there is a weak relationship between these symptoms and venous disease. Experience in the clinic confirms a poor relationship between the size and extent of VV on clinical examination and the presence and severity of symptoms claimed (see above).

Complications

Only a small proportion of patients with VV go on to develop the complications of chronic venous insufficiency (CVI): for example, leg ulcers, haemorrhage and thrombophlebitis. There is on-going controversy as to whether VV are a risk factor for DVT. In young, otherwise healthy individuals, they are probably not. However, in the elderly, in whom VV are more likely to be associated with skin changes of chronic venous insufficiency and in whom they may be a marker for coexistent deep venous disease, they probably are. At present, it is difficult to predict which patients will develop these complications and to know whether early VV surgery would prevent them, because the necessary longitudinal studies have never been done.

Indications for treatment

In correctly selected patients, it is clear that VV surgery is associated with a marked improvement in quality of life and symptom relief. In patients with uncomplicated VV, surgeons must use their own judgement and experience to determine whether the patient truly does have symptoms, whether those symptoms are of venous aetiology, and, if so, whether they are likely to be relieved by surgery.

AETIOLOGY

The aetiology of VV is unclear. The favoured hypothesis is that there is a structural defect in the vein wall, which may, at least in part, be inherited and which causes progressive dilatation in response to increased venous pressure consequent upon our bipedal posture and other factors. This leads to secondary incompetence of the valves, which in turn leads to more stress on the wall and more dilatation. Unlike the deep system, incompetence of superficial valves is only rarely due to post-thrombotic damage.

EXAMINATION

The patient should be examined standing in a warm room. The distribution of varices will usually, but not always, indicate whether they are long or short saphenous or both. Percussion over a varix while palpating with the other hand at a higher or lower level will help trace the pattern. The level at which deep-to-superficial reflux is occurring can be checked by the Trendelenburg test (Fig. 25.36). The leg is elevated and a rubber tourniquet applied just below the saphenofemoral junction. The patient is then asked to stand. Veins fill slowly from arterial inflow but quickly from venous reflux. If venous distension below the tourniquet is controlled, the site of reflux must be above it. By moving the tourniquet to different levels in the limb, the pattern of incompetence can be mapped out. A more effective way to demonstrate reflux is to insonate over the site of incompetence and reflux with a portable continuous-wave Doppler ultrasound probe. This is particularly valuable in obese patients or those with recurrent VV, where the anatomy may be obscure. As ultrasound machines become smaller, more portable, easier to use and cheaper, there is a move towards performing colour duplex examinations in the clinic and dispensing with the hand-held Doppler, as the information gleaned is so much greater and it is possible actually to show the patient what the problem is on the screen in real time.

INVESTIGATIONS

There is considerable debate as to which patients with VV should undergo further investigation. To all intents and purposes, further investigation entails duplex ultrasound, as contrast venography is rarely performed nowadays. Imaging is particularly helpful in the following situations:

- recurrent VV
- short saphenous VV
- where there is a suspicion of deep venous pathology: for example, previous DVT or skin changes of CVI
- atypical distribution.

Severe varicose veins, especially if in children, of atypical distribution or associated with cutaneous haemangioma, soft-tissue hypertrophy or limb overgrowth, should raise the suspicion of congenital arteriovenous malformations. In modern practice, it is increasingly unusual for any patient to undergo interventional treatment for VV without first having had a duplex ultrasound scan, often performed by the surgeon.

MANAGEMENT

Conservative treatment

Elderly patients or those with mild disease can be treated conservatively. Elastic support hose, weight reduction, regular exercise and the avoidance of constricting garments and prolonged standing all help to relieve tiredness and reduce swelling.

Sclerotherapy

Standard injection treatment using liquid sclerosants is commonly used for small varices below the knee that are due to incompetence of local perforators, for small recurrent varices after surgery, and for reticular and spider veins. Such sclerotherapy is not satisfactory for trunk varices associated with saphenofemoral or saphenopopliteal incompetence, as recurrence is inevitable. However, ultrasound-guided foam sclerotherapy (UGFS) appears to be an equally effective alternative to surgery in a proportion of patients. In this procedure, the sclerosant is prepared and used as a foam, and introduced into the LSV or SSV under direct vision using duplex ultrasound control. UGFS can be performed as

25

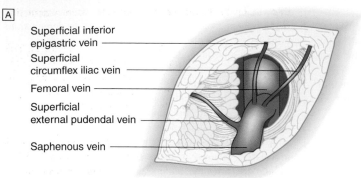

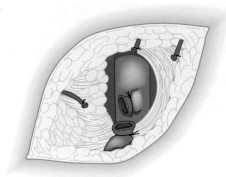

- Superficial inferior epigastric vein
- Superficial circumflex iliac vein
- Femoral vein
- Superficial external pudendal vein
- Saphenous vein

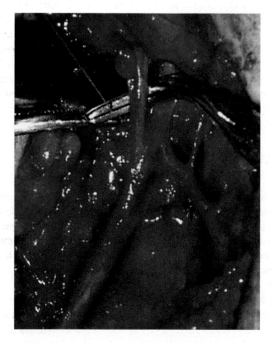

Fig. 25.37 Saphenofemoral disconnection.
A Diagram showing ligation of the tributaries of the long saphenous vein.
B Operative photograph showing proximal long saphenous vein and major tributaries.

an outpatient procedure with no requirement for general anaesthesia, skin incisions or time off work.

Surgery

Varicose vein surgery aims to remove varices and intercept incompetent connections between deep and superficial veins so that further varices do not form. In patients with LSV disease, the SFJ is ligated flush with the femoral vein (Fig. 25.37). Recurrence is very much less likely if the long saphenous vein is stripped out from knee to groin. Care must be taken not to damage the saphenous nerve, which joins and runs with the LSV below the knee. In patients with SSV disease, the SPJ is dealt with in a similar fashion. However, the SSV is not normally stripped for fear of injuring the sural nerve with which it runs. Remaining varices are then avulsed through multiple tiny incisions.

Other new treatments

As well as UGFS, several other novel treatments for VV have been introduced as an alternative to surgery. These involve using radiofrequency or laser light energy to obliterate the LSV or SSV. Their potential advantage is that

they can be performed as an outpatient or day-case procedure without general anaesthetic. However, the technology is expensive, not all patients are suitable, and currently these treatments are not used widely in the UK outside the private sector.

SUPERFICIAL THROMBOPHLEBITIS

Inflammation and thrombosis of a previously normal superficial vein may result from trauma, from irritation from an intravenous infusion or from the injection of noxious agents. Except when it arises in septic puncture sites, superficial thrombophlebitis is usually non-bacterial. When it arises spontaneously, it almost invariably occurs in a VV. Redness and tenderness follow the line of the vein. Thrombosis may spread through communicating channels into the deep veins and give rise to DVT and pulmonary embolism (PE).

Treatment comprises analgesia, anti-inflammatory drugs, support stockings and active exercise. Once the inflammation has settled down, it is usually wise to remove the underlying VV, as recurrence is common. Propagation

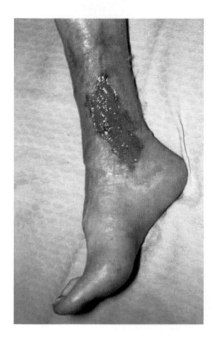

Fig. 25.38 Chronic venous ulcer.

towards the deep veins usually requires heparin therapy, and occasionally emergency thrombectomy or vein ligation. Recurrent migrating superficial phlebitis is occasionally seen in malignant disease.

CHRONIC VENOUS INSUFFICIENCY

PATHOPHYSIOLOGY

Chronic venous insufficiency (CVI) may be defined as the presence of irreversible skin damage in the lower leg as a result of sustained ambulatory venous hypertension. This hypertension is due to failure of the mechanisms (see above) that normally lower venous pressure upon ambulation, namely:

- *Venous reflux due to valvular incompetence (90%).* This may affect the superficial veins, the deep veins or both, and may be due to primary valvular insufficiency (as in VV) or to post-thrombotic damage (see below).
- *Venous obstruction (10%).* This is usually post-thrombotic in nature.

CVI affects 5–10% of the adult population. Chronic venous ulceration, the end result of CVI, affects 2–3% of people over the age of 65, and its treatment accounts for 1–2% of health-care spending in developed countries. In 1992, in the UK, this was estimated to be £400–600 million per annum. The female:male ratio is 3:1. Approximately 70% of all leg ulcers are venous in aetiology. Another 20% are due to mixed arterial and venous disease. In many cases, the situation is aggravated by old age, poor social circumstances, obesity, trauma, immobility, osteoarthritis, rheumatoid arthritis, diabetes and neurological problems: for example, stroke. It is usually possible to differentiate venous (Fig. 25.38) from arterial ulceration on clinical examination alone (Table 25.6).

ASSESSMENT

History

This should include the history of the present and previous episodes of ulceration; previous thrombotic episodes; previous venous and non-venous surgery to the leg, pelvis and abdomen; arterial symptoms; diabetes; autoimmune disease; other medical conditions; locomotor problems; current medications; and allergies.

Examination

This should include a description of the ulcer, concentrating on the features outlined in Table 25.6. Pulse status and ABPI should be recorded. The pattern of venous disease should be

Table 25.6	DIFFERENTIAL DIAGNOSIS OF LEG ULCERATION	
Clinical features	**Arterial ulcer**	**Venous ulcer**
Gender	Men > women	Women > men
Age	Usually presents > 60 years	Typically develops at 40–60 years but patient may not present for medical attention until much older; multiple recurrences are the norm
Risk factors	Smoking, diabetes, hyperlipidaemia and hypertension	Previous DVT, thrombophilia, varicose veins
Past medical history	Most have a clear history of peripheral, coronary and cerebrovascular disease	More than 20% have a clear history of DVT; many more have a history suggestive of occult DVT, i.e. leg swelling after childbirth, hip/knee replacement or long bone fracture
Symptoms	Severe pain is present unless there is (diabetic) neuropathy; pain may be relieved by dependency	About a third have pain, but it is not usually severe and may be relieved on elevation
Site	Normal and abnormal (diabetics) pressure areas (malleoli, heel, metatarsal heads, 5th metatarsal base)	Medial (70%), lateral (20%) or both malleoli and gaiter area
Edge	Regular, 'punched-out', indolent	Irregular, with neo epithelium (whiter than mature skin)
Base	Deep, green (sloughy) or black (necrotic) with no granulation tissue; may involve tendon, bone and joint	Pink and granulating but may be covered in yellow-green slough
Surrounding skin	Features of severe limb ischaemia	Lipodermatosclerosis, varicose eczema, atrophe blanche
Veins	Empty, 'guttering' on elevation	Full, usually varicose
Swelling	Usually absent	Often present

25

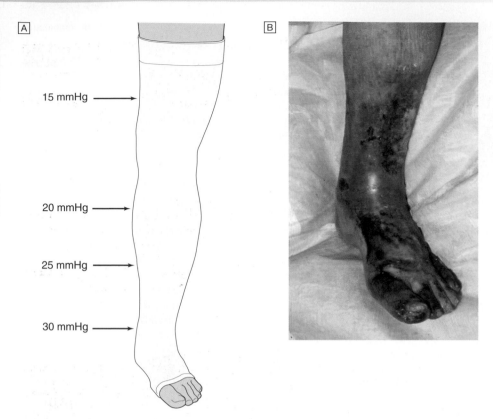

Fig. 25.39
Graduated elastic compression for venous ulcer.
A Compression from the base of the toes to the tibial tuberosity usually suffices. B Extensive necrosis in a patient treated with compression for a venous ulcer in the presence of significant arterial disease. Above-knee amputation was required.

determined as described above, and gait, particularly ankle mobility, assessed.

Investigations

Patients may require a full blood count, standard biochemistry, thyroid function tests, blood glucose determination, lipid profile and rheumatoid serology. Duplex ultrasound can be performed to define the nature and distribution of superficial and deep venous disease, as this has a bearing on both treatment and prognosis. In patients with absent pulses and/or a low ABPI, it can also provide valuable information about the pattern of arterial disease.

MANAGEMENT

Medical therapy

Patients with leg ulcers often have multiple medical comorbidity, the treatment of which must be optimal if the chances of ulcer healing are to be maximized. There are no drugs that have been proved to increase ulcer healing or reduce recurrence. Most ulcers are colonized with bacteria rather than infected, and antibiotics are not usually indicated.

Dressings

There are many different types of dressing on the market but none has been proved to increase ulcer healing. Leg ulcer patients are notorious for developing contact sensitivity to all manner of substances present in ointments and dressings. Thus, the least expensive, simplest and blandest forms of dressing are to be recommended. Topical antibiotics should never be applied.

Compression therapy

Although it is still unclear exactly how compression therapy works, it continues to be the mainstay of treatment and, correctly applied, is highly effective in healing the majority of venous ulcers and preventing recurrence (Fig. 25.39A). To be maximally effective, compression should be:

- *elastic*, as this achieves the best and most durable pressure profile
- *multilayer*, as using many layers evens out the high- and low-pressure areas found under any bandage; the 'four-layer bandage' is a popular system
- *graduated*, with the pressure greatest at the ankle (*c.* 30–40 mmHg) and least at the knee (*c.* 15–20 mmHg).

Of course, it is vitally important to exclude arterial disease before compression is applied (Fig. 25.39B). If pulses are not easily palpable, the ABPI should be measured (see above). Any patient with an ABPI of < 0.8 should be referred to a vascular surgeon. Such patients will have to be treated with modified compression or undergo revascularization to allow compression to be applied. Oedema is frequently present and significantly reduces the

EBM 25.5   SURGERY FOR CHRONIC VENOUS ULCERATION

'Eradication of superficial venous reflux in patients with chronic venous ulceration reduces recurrence at 2 years by over 50%.'
Barwell JR, et al. Lancet 2004; 363(9424):1854–1859.

chances of healing. Even expertly applied graduated compression may fail to control severe oedema while the patient is still ambulant, and a period of bed rest for leg elevation may be required.

Elastic compression hosiery

Once the ulcer has been healed with compression bandaging, compression stockings will reduce the chance of recurrence and should be prescribed to all patients for life (assuming the arterial circulation is adequate).

Surgical therapy

There are now data from a randomized controlled trial (EBM 25.5) to show that, in patients with chronic venous ulceration due to superficial venous reflux, the addition of VV surgery to compression therapy reduces ulcer recurrence rates. Although the trial did not show that such surgery leads to a statistically significant increase in ulcer healing rates, most surgeons believe that it does and would offer it to this group of patients, provided they were surgically fit. The problem is that many of these patients are elderly with multiple comorbidity and are not fit for and/or do not want surgery. Furthermore, many of them have combined superficial and deep venous reflux and, in the presence of the latter, there is much less certainty that surgical eradication of the former is of any benefit, especially if the deep venous disease is post-thrombotic in aetiology. There is continuing controversy as to the benefit of ligating medial calf perforating veins. This can be performed at open operation or endoscopically: so-called subfascial endoscopic perforator surgery (SEPS). The available data suggest that it adds little, if anything, to standard VV surgery in patients with superficial venous reflux, and that it is as ineffective as VV surgery in patients with deep, post-thrombotic, venous disease. Some surgeons believe that performing split-skin or 'pinch' grafting speeds up ulcer healing. This is only likely to be the case if one has successfully corrected the underlying venous abnormality. Patients with arterial disease may require angioplasty or bypass surgery to relieve pain and allow compression therapy to be applied.

New treatments

Several companies are undertaking clinical trials of various artificial skin substitutes for the treatment of leg ulcers, including those due to venous disease. If these trials show these skin substitutes to be clinically effective, then they may enter mainstream clinical practice over the next few years. However, as they are likely to be extremely expensive, one can envisage cost-effectiveness being an issue in the UK.

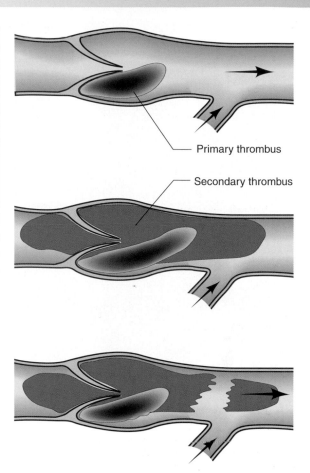

Fig. 25.40   Mechanism of embolus formation from thrombus in a deep vein.

Labels: Primary thrombus; Secondary thrombus

VENOUS THROMBOEMBOLISM (VTE)

EPIDEMIOLOGY

DVT is a common condition in medical and surgical patients and pulmonary embolism (PE) is consistently cited as the most common cause of potentially preventable death in the surgical patient. DVT also renders the leg prone to CVI and ulceration (the so-called post-phlebitic limb or syndrome).

PATHOPHYSIOLOGY

DVT probably begins in the calf in most cases (Fig. 25.40). Clot may extend into the popliteal, femoral or iliac veins, and even the inferior vena cava. In some cases, DVT originates in the pelvic veins.

At first, the clot is free-floating within a column of flowing blood. The risk of PE is highest at this point. Later, when thrombus has completely occluded the vein and incited an inflammatory reaction in the vein wall, the clot becomes densely adherent and is unlikely to embolize. The classic features of the 'medical' DVT are due to this occlusion (leg swelling, dilated superficial veins) and throm-

25

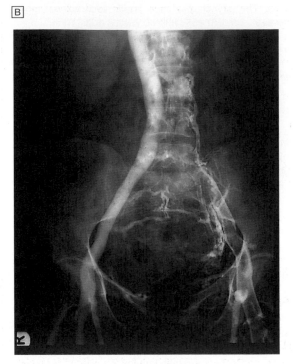

Fig. 25.41 Ascending phlebography.
A Deep venous thrombosis in the left popliteal vein. B Thrombus in left iliac veins.

bophlebitis (redness, pain and tenderness, heat). The important point is that most surgical patients developing a post-operative PE do so on about the 10th day and have clinically normal legs. By the time a clinically apparent DVT has developed, the danger period for PE has largely passed.

AETIOLOGY

Three factors are traditionally associated with thrombogenesis (Virchow's triad): namely, venous stasis, intimal damage and hypercoagulability of the blood. Many of the recognized clinical risk factors for DVT relate to venous stasis: for example, immobility, obesity, pregnancy, paralysis, operation and trauma. In most instances of DVT, no evidence of direct intimal damage can be detected. However, external trauma to a vein—for example, during a hip replacement operation—can provide a starting point for thrombogenesis. There is increasing interest in hypercoagulable states, also known as thrombophilia, which can be congenital (primary) or acquired (secondary). These include antithrombin III, protein C and protein S deficiency, as well as factor V Leiden (activated protein C resistance, APCR). These should be suspected if thrombosis occurs in a young patient (< 45 years), if there is a family history, or if thrombosis is recurrent or at an unusual site. Secondary hypercoagulable states include pregnancy and the puerperium, and malignancy.

DIAGNOSIS

Clinical examination alone is poor at confirming or excluding the presence of DVT. This means that the diagnosis of DVT cannot be made on clinical grounds alone, and that some form of investigation is required.

Ascending venography

This involves injecting contrast media into a pedal or a digital vein and directing flow into the deep veins by applying superficial tourniquets above the ankle. The aim is to delineate fully any thrombus in the deep veins of the calf, thigh and pelvis (Fig. 25.41).

Colour flow duplex ultrasound

Colour duplex ultrasound imaging has largely replaced venography in the diagnosis of DVT. It is non-invasive, avoids ionizing radiation and contrast, and is as accurate as venography in most cases.

VENOUS GANGRENE

In certain circumstances—notably where there is underlying malignancy—DVT may propagate to involve not only the main venous trunks, but also the venous collaterals and/or microcirculation. The former leads to an intensely swollen, cyanosed limb (phlegmasia caerula dolens), whereas the latter can lead to obstruction of the arterial inflow and the development of a swollen white leg (phlegmasia alba dolens). The patient may then go on to develop venous gangrene.

PREVENTION

Rationale

Because of our inability to diagnose DVT easily in its early asymptomatic but dangerous phase, prevention is very important. In this respect, it is helpful to determine which patients are at the highest risk and thus have the most to gain from prophylactic measures. The most important risk factors are a history of previous DVT or embolism, advanced age, malignant disease, obesity, and congenital or acquired thrombophilia. However, even patients at apparently low risk do sometimes develop DVT and PE. This fact, together with increasing concerns about litigation, has led many surgeons to institute active thromboembolic prophylaxis in almost all their patients.

General measures

Aspects of modern surgical care that help to reduce the likelihood of post-operative DVT include regional anaesthesia, accurate fluid replacement to avoid dehydration, effective pain control to facilitate early ambulation and, perhaps above all, the use of outpatient- or day-case-based minimally invasive alternatives to traditional open surgery.

Physical methods

Graduated compression (thromboembolic deterrent, TED) stockings, which exert a pressure of about 20 mmHg at the ankle, augment flow in the deep veins and reduce the risk of thrombosis.

Pharmacological methods

Low-dose subcutaneous unfractionated heparin or, more commonly nowadays, low molecular weight heparin (LMWH) protects against DVT and PE. The first dose may be given with the premedication (if an epidural is not being planned), and treatment is continued until the patient is fully ambulant. In high-risk patients, it can be continued following discharge.

MANAGEMENT

Overview

Before treatment is instituted, the diagnosis of DVT should normally have been established by means of ultrasound or venography. However, where the clinical suspicion of DVT and/or PE is high and there is no contraindication to heparin, then the potential benefits of 'blind' treatment may out-weigh the risks. The aims of treatment are to relieve the acute symptoms, protect against PE, and minimize the risk of recurrent thrombosis and post-thrombotic sequelae to the limb.

Uncomplicated DVT

If thrombus is confined to the calf, the patient is fully mobile and other risk factors are reversible, then an elastic stocking and physical exercise may be all that is required. However, the 'surgical' patient does not usually fulfil these criteria post-operatively and there is often thrombus extension into the femoropopliteal segment. In these cases, specific treatment is indicated. Traditionally:

- The patient was confined to bed.
- The foot of the bed was elevated to reduce swelling.
- The patient received a continuous intravenous infusion of heparin.
- Once the swelling had subsided, the patient was mobilized, with graduated compression stockings.
- After 5 days of heparin, the patient was changed to warfarin, which was continued for 3–6 months.

For most uncomplicated DVT, it is now clear that:

- Bed rest is unnecessary and the patient can be mobilized almost immediately, wearing a stocking.
- LMWH given by intermittent subcutaneous injection is just as, if not more, effective.

DVT is thus increasingly treated this way, often entirely on an outpatient basis. Even some PEs are treated like this.

Complicated DVT

In a proportion of patients, however, treatment is more complicated because of one or more of the following:

- The DVT is more extensive (iliofemoral, vena cava, phlegmasia).
- The DVT is recurrent.
- The patient has (probably) had a PE.
- The patient has one or more major irreversible congenital and/or acquired thrombophilias.
- Heparinization is contraindicated (heparin-induced thrombocytopenia, trauma—especially intracranial, recent haemorrhage).

In these circumstances, treatment must be tailored to the individual patient, and in selected cases it may be appropriate to use thrombolysis, insert a caval filter or consider thrombectomy. It is important to remember that a high proportion of patients with extensive DVT have an underlying malignancy, and reasonable steps should be taken to ensure that is diagnosed and appropriately treated in order, hopefully, to reduce the thrombotic risk.

Thrombolysis

Catheter-directed intraclot thrombolytic therapy has been advocated as a means of rapidly clearing the iliofemoral segment in patients with extensive proximal DVT. It is hoped that this will reduce the incidence of PE and post-phlebitic syndrome. Although the rate and extent of clot clearance is certainly greater than with heparin alone in the short term, it is not clear whether this results in improved patency and clinical outcome in the long term. The clinical benefit of thrombolysis in DVT may be in the facilitation of the development of venous collaterals and the prevention of valvular damage. The other potential

25

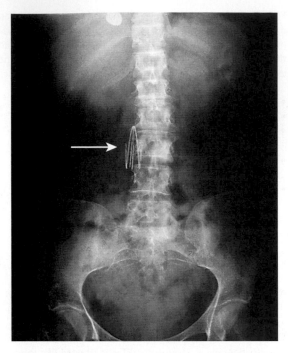

Fig. 25.42 Filter (arrow) placed in the inferior vena cava to prevent pulmonary embolism.

role for thrombolysis is in phlegmasia with venous gangrene. In this situation, not only is the lytic agent given into the clot, it is also administered into the arterial circulation to try to clear the microcirculation. Again, although clot can be lysed in the short term, it is unclear whether this confers long-term benefit. Many of these patients have underlying malignancy and, unless the hypercoagulable state can be corrected, re-thrombosis is likely. Furthermore, thrombolysis is associated with a significant incidence of serious haemorrhagic complications in these patients.

Thrombectomy

In the UK, surgical thrombectomy to clear iliofemoral thrombus is rarely performed nowadays. Percutaneous mechanical venous thrombectomy is still under evaluation.

Caval filters

The rationale behind inserting a caval filter is that it will trap embolus that would otherwise have been destined for the lungs (Fig. 25.42). The most widely accepted indication for a filter is the patient in whom it can be proved that PE is still occurring despite adequate anticoagulation, or where anticoagulation is contraindicated or has had to be discontinued owing to a complication of therapy. However, there are many other scenarios where the use of caval filters has been advocated: for example, in a patient with severely impaired cardiorespiratory function in whom even a small embolus might be fatal, and in the patient who cannot be heparinized. Filters are usually inserted percutaneously under local anesthesia by interventional radiologists via the jugular or femoral veins. Some of the newer filters can also be removed percutaneously.

OTHER FORMS OF VENOUS THROMBOSIS

Superior vena caval thrombosis

Mediastinal tumours or enlarged lymph nodes (e.g. from breast or bronchial carcinoma) may obstruct the superior vena cava and induce thrombosis. Central venous catheters for parenteral nutrition, pressure monitoring or haemodialysis may cause thrombosis of the vena cava, or of the subclavian or axillary veins. The patient experiences an unpleasant bursting feeling in the head, neck and upper limbs. There is oedema, cyanosis and venous distension.

The obstruction is defined by bilateral upper limb venography. In occlusion secondary to malignancy, percutaneous stenting, radiotherapy or chemotherapy may relieve malignant obstruction, and whilst the outlook remains poor, symptoms may be significantly relieved.

Subclavian and axillary vein thrombosis

Spontaneous axillary thrombosis is relatively common and usually occurs in otherwise healthy young adults following exercise, when it is termed 'effort thrombosis'. There may be a previous history of intermittent venous obstruction in the limb due to a mechanical cause at the thoracic outlet. A cervical rib, abnormal muscle or ligamentous band at the inner border of the first rib, or a narrow interval between the clavicle and the first rib, may constrict the vein and lead to thrombosis.

The patient complains of an uncomfortable, heavy, cyanosed arm with venous engorgement. Venous collaterals develop over the shoulder and anterior chest wall. Upper limb venous duplex scanning and/or venography define the occlusion. The arm should be elevated, e.g. in a towel suspended from a drip stand. Heparin therapy followed by oral anticoagulants is standard treatment. Thrombolytic therapy can be very effective in early cases. Many surgeons believe that after the axillary thrombosis has been

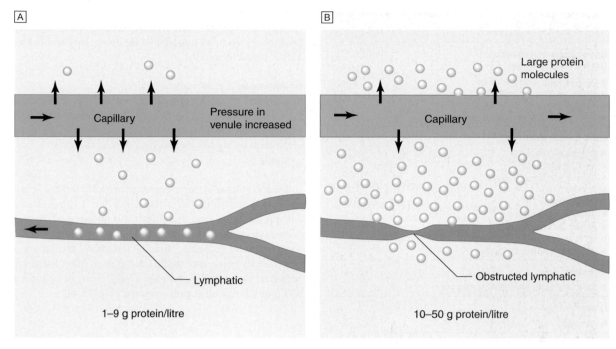

25

Fig. 25.43 Types of oedema.
A Low-protein oedema due to abnormally high net fluid filtration. B High-protein oedema due to failure of lymphatics to remove interstitial protein.

cleared, the thoracic outlet should be explored and the first rib or other obstructing element removed. Once the rib is out, stenting of any underlying venous stenosis may be of value.

LYMPHOEDEMA

PATHOPHYSIOLOGY

The lymphatic system removes excess water and protein from the interstitial space. Flow is directed centrally by intrinsic lymphatic contractions and endothelial valves, and is increased by muscle contraction. Lymph passes through lymph nodes before it re-enters the venous system, mainly through the thoracic duct. The total daily lymph flow is only 2–4 litres. Failure of this mechanism leads to the accumulation of protein-rich oedema fluid in the tissues (lymphoedema) (Fig. 25.43). Lymphoedema may be primary or secondary, and must be differentiated from other causes of leg swelling (Table 25.7).

PRIMARY LYMPHOEDEMA

This often familial condition is estimated to affect 2% of the adult population and is caused by a developmental failure in which the lymphatics may be absent, hypoplastic, or varicose and dilated. It is usually categorized by the age of onset:

- *Lymphoedema congenita*. Swelling is present at birth or develops within the first year of life.

- *Lymphoedema praecox*. Swelling develops between 1 and 35 years, usually during adolescence. It affects predominantly females, and may be unilateral or bilateral.
- *Lymphoedema tarda*. In patients developing lymphoedema after the age of 35, an underlying pelvic tumour (benign or malignant) compressing the proximal lymphatic (and venous) systems must be excluded.

SECONDARY LYMPHOEDEMA

This develops when the lymphatic system is obstructed by tumour, recurrent infection or infestation (filariasis), or obliterated by surgery or radiotherapy.

CLINICAL FEATURES

Symptoms
The patient usually complains of gradual painless swelling of one or both legs. At first, lymphoedema is like other forms of oedema, in that it is present only upon dependency; that is, worse at the end of the day and absent in the morning. However, as the oedema fluid becomes more protein-rich, it is less and less affected by position. Lymphoedema nearly always commences distally on the foot and extends proximally, usually only to the knee.

Thus, there may be a complex interplay between nature and nurture; that is, many patients with apparently primary lymphoedema also have a secondary component. Some patients first present to medical attention because

25

Table 25.7 DIFFERENTIAL DIAGNOSIS OF THE SWOLLEN LIMB
Non-vascular or lymphatic **General disease states** • Cardiac, renal and liver failure • Hyperthyroidism (myxoedema) • Allergic disorders • Immobility and lower limb dependency
Local disease processes • Ruptured Baker's cyst • Myositis ossificans • Bony or soft tissue tumours • Arthritis • Haemarthrosis • Calf muscle haematoma • Achilles tendon rupture • Other trauma • Reflex sympathetic dystrophy
Gigantism • Rare; all tissues are uniformly enlarged
Drugs • Steroids
Obesity • Lipodystrophy, lipoidosis
Venous **Deep venous thrombosis** • The classic signs of pain and redness may be absent
Post-thrombotic syndrome • Venous skin changes, secondary varicose veins on the leg and collateral veins on the lower abdominal wall • Venous claudication may be present
Varicose veins • Do not usually cause significant swelling
Venous malformations • Most common is Klippel–Trenaunay syndrome • Abnormal lateral venous complex, capillary naevus, hypo(a)plasia of deep veins and limb lengthening • Lymphatic abnormalities often coexist
External venous compression • Pelvic or abdominal tumour including the gravid uterus • Retroperitoneal fibrosis
Arterial **Ischaemia–reperfusion** • Following lower limb revascularization for chronic and particularly acute ischaemia
Arteriovenous malformation • May be associated with local or generalized swelling
Aneurysm • Popliteal • Femoral • False aneurysm following (iatrogenic) trauma

Signs

Unlike other types of oedema, lymphoedema characteristically involves the foot, as opposed to the lower calf and ankle. This is characterized by:

- infilling of the submalleolar depressions
- a 'hump' on the dorsum of the foot
- 'square' toes due to confinement by footwear; also, the skin on the dorsum of the toes cannot be pinched owing to subcutaneous fibrosis (Stemmer's sign).

Lymphoedema usually spreads proximally to knee level, and less commonly affects the whole leg. Lymphoedema will pit easily at first, but with time fibrosis and dermal thickening prevent pitting, except following prolonged pressure. Chronic eczema, fungal infection of the skin (dermatophytosis) and nails (onychomycosis), fissuring, verrucae and papillae are frequently seen in advanced conditions. Frank ulceration is unusual (Fig. 25.44).

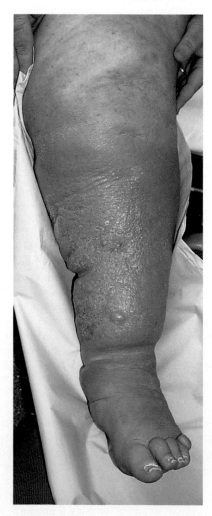

Fig. 25.44 Lymphoedema.

of acute cellulitis. Such patients are prone to recurrent episodes, each one of which damages the lymphatic system still further, leading to a vicious circle.

INVESTIGATIONS

Lymphoedema is essentially a clinical diagnosis and most patients require no further investigation.

MANAGEMENT

Physical methods

The patient should elevate the foot above the level of the hip when sitting, elevate the foot of the bed when sleeping, and avoid prolonged standing. Various forms of massage are effective at reducing oedema. Intermittent pneumatic compression devices are also useful. The mainstay of therapy is graduated compression hosiery. Pressures exceeding 50 mmHg at the ankle may be required. Below-knee stockings are usually sufficient.

Drugs

Diuretics are of no value and are associated with side-effects, including electrolyte disturbance. No other drugs are of proven benefit.

Antibiotics

These should be prescribed promptly for cellulitis. Patients who suffer recurrent spontaneous episodes of cellulitis should be considered for long-term prophylactic antibiotic therapy. Fungal infection must also be treated aggressively. The feet must be dried after washing and the skin kept clean and supple with water-based emollients to prevent entry of bacteria.

Surgery

Only a small minority of patients will benefit from surgery. Operations fall into two categories: bypass procedures and reduction procedures. They are only rarely performed. The details of these procedures are beyond the scope of this book.

25

26

W.S. WALKER

Cardiothoracic surgery

BASIC CONSIDERATIONS

PATHOPHYSIOLOGICAL ASSESSMENT

The history and examination suggest the presence of probable cardiac pathology. The initial clinical assessment is then refined and pathology quantified using specific investigations (Table 26.1).

ASSESSMENT OF RISK

The risks of perioperative mortality and stroke are significantly higher with cardiac than with many other forms of surgery. A frank discussion of these risks is an essential element of the pre-operative consultations between the surgeon and the patient.

Mortality

The risk of operative mortality is estimated by means of a scoring system (Parsonnet, Euroscore), where a variable number of points are given for specific clinical features. The sum of these, calculated either directly or via a correction graph, indicates the percentage operative mortality, which ranges from 2% for routine and relatively straightforward procedures to over 50% for complex emergency procedures.

Stroke

Stroke risk varies from 1% to over 10%, and is associated with intracardiac thrombus and severe atheromatous disease of the proximal aorta and carotids. Patients with high-grade symptomatic carotid disease may benefit from carotid endarterectomy prior to cardiac surgery (Ch. 25).

SPECIFIC ASPECTS OF SURGICAL TECHNIQUE

Cardiopulmonary bypass

Modern cardiac and great vessel surgery became feasible with the development of cardiopulmonary bypass. Venous blood is extracted via cannulae inserted into the right atrium or venae cavae and drained to a reservoir. It is

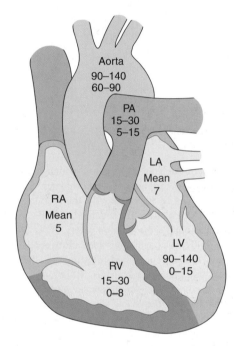

Fig. 26.1 Normal cardiac chamber pressures.
(Ao = aorta; LA = left atrium; LV = left ventricle; RA = right atrium; RV = right ventricle; PA = pulmonary artery)

Table 26.1 SPECIFIC ASSESSMENTS OF CARDIAC PATHOPHYSIOLOGICAL STATUS	
Investigation	**Potential yield**
ECG Resting Exercise	 Rhythm; conduction abnormalities; atrial and ventricular hypertrophy; established ischaemic changes; evidence of previous myocardial infarction Exercise-induced ischaemic changes or arrhythmias
Chest X-ray	Cardiac enlargement; valvular calcification; evidence of pulmonary oedema (Kerley B lines, pleural effusion, interstitial marking, hilar flare); absent or enlarged cardiac or great vessel structures
Thallium isotope scan	Areas of low radio-uptake indicative of impaired myocardial perfusion
Echocardiography Precordial Transoesophageal	 Ventricular contractility; valvular stenoses, regurgitation or leaflet abnormalities; intracardiac morphology, including septal defects and intracardiac masses; pericardial effusion Enhanced views of posterior cardiac structures (aortic and mitral valves, ascending aorta, great veins and posterior septae); posterior pericardial fluid collections
Cardiac catheterization Chamber pressures Angiography O_2 saturations Cardiac output	 Assess left and right ventricular function via determination of left ventricular end-diastolic pressure; atrial pressures in valve disease; transvalvular gradients (Fig. 26.1) Coronary arterial anatomy; intracardiac anatomy; trans-septal flow Intracardiac shunts Cardiac function and determination of secondary derived parameters, including peripheral and pulmonary vascular resistance

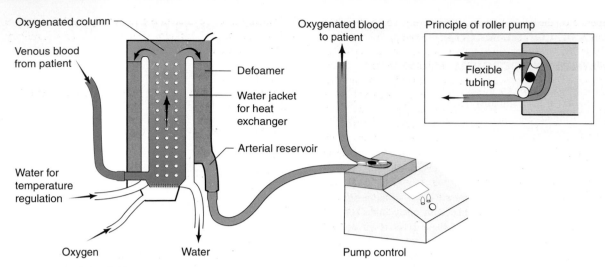

Fig. 26.2 Schematic of a bypass circuit.

then pumped through an oxygenator, which adds O_2 and removes CO_2, and through a heat exchanger coil so that its temperature can be varied. Finally, the blood is returned to the arterial circulation via a cannula in the ascending aorta or, occasionally, the femoral artery (Figs 26.1, 26.2 and 26.3). Full anticoagulation with intravenous heparin is required to prevent blood clotting in the tubing, oxygenator and pump mechanisms. Roller or centrifugal pumps are used, as these minimize haemolysis related to red cell trauma. Semipermeable sheet membranes, or more commonly hollow fibres, form the blood–gas interfaces within the oxygenator. A trained perfusion technician (perfusionist) controls the bypass machine.

Cardiopulmonary bypass carries several risks. Cerebral damage occurs in about 1% of cases due to intracerebral bleeding, embolization of microbubbles or arterial debris, or inadequate cerebral perfusion. Subtle deterioration in cerebral function, as detected by psychological testing, is more frequent. There is also significant activation of

systemic inflammatory mechanisms, with cytokine release, complement activation and white cell stimulation. These changes do not generally cause clinical problems but may occasionally be implicated in post-bypass pulmonary and renal dysfunction. Coagulopathy and haemolysis are associated with prolonged bypass.

Myocardial preservation

Cardioplegia

Intracardiac surgery requires a still and bloodless heart. This is achieved by the use of cardioplegic arrest. A clamp is applied across the ascending aorta proximal to the point of insertion of the bypass arterial inflow cannula. This prevents blood flow into the coronary arteries. The heart is then arrested by perfusing the coronary circulation with a cardioplegic solution, either progradely via the aortic root or coronary artery ostia, or retrogradely via a catheter placed in the coronary sinus. The essential component of a cardioplegic solution is a high potassium concentration (circa 18 mmol/l), which causes the heart to arrest in diastole. Cardioplegia is typically delivered at a temperature of 4–6° C and via either a crystalloid solution or one derived from the patient's own blood. Blood-based solutions are believed to have buffering characteristics that are helpful in reducing the deleterious effects of ischaemic metabolites generated by the arrested myocardium. Local anaesthetic agents may be added to stabilize the myocardial cell membranes. In principle, therefore, cardioplegia solutions minimize myocardial energy requirements by abolishing energy expenditure on contraction and by reducing basal cellular metabolism by local tissue cooling. Reducing the core temperature to 26–34° C may enhance cardiac cooling. Cardioplegia combined with mild systemic hypothermia (32° C) will provide the surgeon with a safe period of cardiac arrest (of up to 120 minutes) within which to carry out surgery without the risk of myocardial damage.

In some circumstances, the surgeon may elect to leave the coronary arteries perfused while on bypass and to

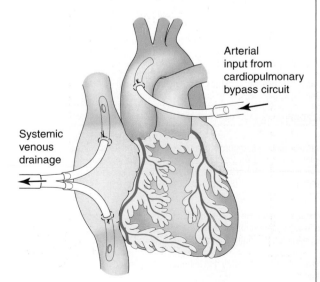

Fig. 26.3 Cannulation for cardiopulmonary bypass.

operate on the beating heart. Alternatively, coronary bypass surgery can be performed using a technique in which an aortic clamp is intermittently applied to cut coronary flow while the heart is electrically fibrillated so as to reduce movement. The resulting ischaemic episodes are tolerated because they are brief and activate mechanisms within the myocardial cells that reduce damage caused by subsequent ischaemia—a phenomenon known as 'pre-conditioning'.

Recently, there has been considerable interest in the use of specific stabilizer instruments that allow the surgeon to perform coronary artery surgery on suitable patients without the use of cardiopulmonary bypass. Proponents of 'off-pump' surgery claim that the risks of artificial perfusion (particularly transient cognitive impairment) are avoided and that recovery may be quicker. Many surgeons, however, feel that the bloodless, still operative field provided by cardioplegic arrest may facilitate more accurate anastomoses.

POST-OPERATIVE CARE

Intensive care

Post-operatively, patients are routinely ventilated for several hours until they are fully rewarmed and have satisfactory haemodynamics, pulmonary gas exchange and acid–base status. Urine output is copious and potassium levels are, therefore, checked frequently and potassium administered intravenously to correct urinary losses. Invasive measurement of arterial and central venous pressure is standard.

Pulmonary artery catheters are frequently used to measure pulmonary artery pressure, pulmonary artery capillary wedge pressure and cardiac output.

Complications

Other than the catastrophes of death or stroke, established complications include:

- low cardiac output
- arrhythmias
- fluid accumulation
- short-term memory impairment
- wound infection
- pulmonary infection.

Recovery time

Patients undergoing routine elective coronary or valve surgery will usually leave acute hospital care within 1 week. Those requiring more extensive surgery or emergency procedures may take longer to recover. Most patients will have undergone a median sternotomy (Fig. 26.4). This wound heals quickly and well and, as the sternal edges are approximated securely by wire or heavy sutures, chest discomfort eases rapidly. Leg vein donor sites may take longer to heal, particularly around the knee. By 2 weeks the patient should be able to walk a few hundred metres, and by 3 months should have returned to full activity, including work.

26

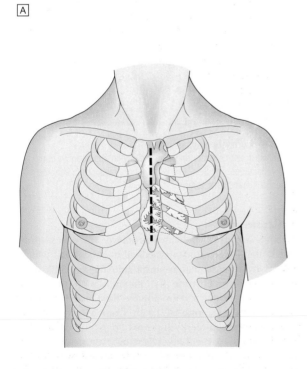

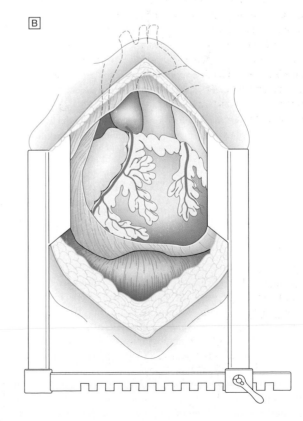

Fig. 26.4 Surgical approach to the heart.
A Vertical sternotomy incision. B Right atrium and ascending aorta exposed.

26

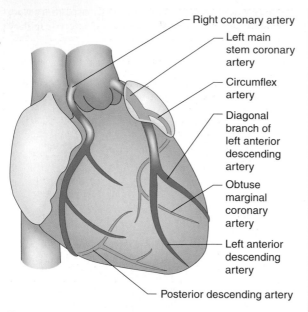

Right coronary artery

Left main stem coronary artery

Circumflex artery

Diagonal branch of left anterior descending artery

Obtuse marginal coronary artery

Left anterior descending artery

Posterior descending artery

Fig. 26.5   Coronary circulation.

ACQUIRED CARDIAC DISEASE

Surgical intervention may be required in the management of:

- ischaemic heart disease
- cardiac valvular disease
- aortic aneurysm
- pericardial pathology
- cardiac trauma.

ISCHAEMIC HEART DISEASE

Ischaemic heart disease encompasses coronary artery disease and its complications, principally acute mitral regurgitation, ventricular septal defect and left ventricular aneurysm.

CORONARY ARTERY DISEASE

This is caused by coronary artery atheroma (Ch. 25). Most patients will present for surgery because of angina or previous myocardial infarction (MI).

Assessment

Exercise electrocardiography (ECG) is often used as an initial screening test for patients with suspected stable angina. Those with confirmed ischaemia then undergo coronary angiography and assessment of left ventricular function by means of angiography or echocardiography. Contrast medium is injected into the coronary circulation (Fig. 26.5) via a catheter that is usually inserted through the femoral artery (Fig. 26.6). Images are obtained in several different planes so as to minimize the risk of missing eccentric lesions. Bypass surgery is usually only advised for stenoses that exceed a 70% reduction in vessel diameter.

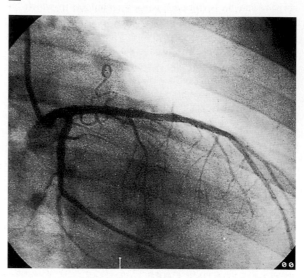

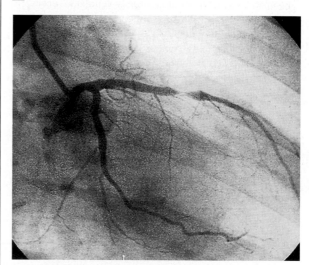

Fig. 26.6   Coronary angiography.
A Selective left coronary angiogram showing appearances after balloon dilatation. B Selective left coronary angiogram, showing stenosis of descending artery.

Indications

Elective surgery is indicated primarily for the control of angina that is refractory to medical treatment and which is caused by disease that is unsuitable for angioplasty and stent insertion. Historically, patients with three-vessel disease or left main stem disease have exhibited a high (c. 8% per year) risk of death from MI with medical therapy alone. Surgery improves long-term survival for such patients, particularly when left ventricular function is also impaired. Some patients requiring other cardiac procedures may be shown to have significant coronary disease during cardiological assessment. In these cases, coronary surgery may be added to the primary procedure in order to improve perioperative survival and prevent future ischaemic problems. Emergency coronary surgery is rare. Patients with incipient or established MI usually fare better with supportive medical therapy, as the mortality of surgery in this setting is much increased. Emergency surgery is required mainly for failed interventional procedures that have caused coronary occlusion.

Coronary bypass

A coronary artery bypass graft (CABG) delivers blood to the distal coronary artery beyond a stenosis. If the distal artery is obliterated by atheroma, an endarterectomy procedure may be performed to restore the lumen. Originally, nearly all grafts comprised reversed segments of the long saphenous vein anastomosed proximally to the anterior ascending aorta and distally to the coronary artery. Such grafts have patency rates of around 70% at 5 years and 40% at 10 years. Venous graft failure occurs as a result of intimal hyperplasia, which is thought to be, in part at least, a response to arterial pressure. The relatively high rate of vein graft failure stimulated interest in arterial grafts and led to the almost universal use of the internal mammary artery (IMA). This is usually employed as a pedicled graft when it is left attached to the subclavian artery proximally, but can also be used as a free graft in the same manner as vein. IMA graft patency exceeds 90% at 5 years and 70% at 10 years. The IMA's relatively short length restricts its use to the front of the heart. A common combination (Fig. 26.7) is to use the left IMA for the left anterior descending artery and vein grafts for the other vessels. The radial artery is becoming an increasingly popular option as a free graft for use in people with poor-quality saphenous vein, and may be used together with mammary grafts to achieve 'total arterial revascularization'. Occasionally, when there is a shortage of good conduit (e.g. in a 'redo' operation), the surgeon may consider using the

BOX 26.1 CORONARY ANATOMY

- There are two coronary arteries
- The left coronary arises from the left posterior aspect of the aortic root and passes behind the pulmonary trunk before dividing into two large branches: the left anterior descending coronary, which supplies the anterior left ventricle and anterior two-thirds of the interventricular septum, and the circumflex coronary, which supplies the posterior and lateral left ventricles
- The right coronary artery arises at the front of the aorta and passes down anteriorly between the right atrium and right ventricle, which it supplies via anterior right ventricle and acute marginal branches
- Either the right or circumflex may terminate as the posterior descending artery, which supplies the inferior surface of both ventricles and the lower septum
- The right, left anterior descending and circumflex are each considered to be a 'vessel system'. Disease within any one of these three vessels or its branches is termed single-vessel disease. Similarly, two- and three-vessel disease indicates involvement of two and three systems, respectively

inferior epigastric artery, the right gastro-epiploic artery, the short saphenous vein and the cephalic vein. Prosthetic grafts occlude early and are not used.

Results

Uncomplicated coronary surgery should carry a 2–3% risk of mortality and a 1–2% risk of stroke. Angina is relieved completely in about 70% of cases, is significantly improved in the remainder, and recurs with a frequency of about 10% per year. Successful revascularization may also improve breathlessness if it is related to myocardial ischaemia, and survival is probably enhanced in patients with three-vessel disease. Logically, increased use of arterial conduits should be associated with better graft patency

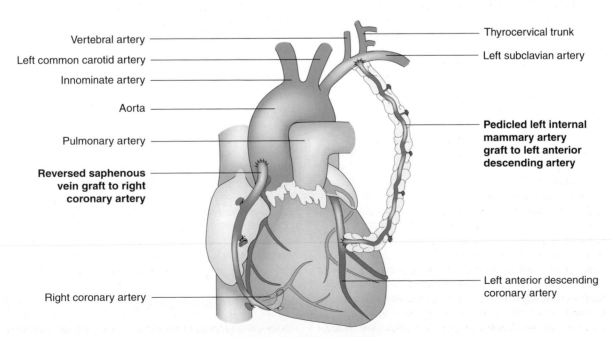

Vertebral artery
Left common carotid artery
Innominate artery
Aorta
Pulmonary artery
Reversed saphenous vein graft to right coronary artery
Right coronary artery

Thyrocervical trunk
Left subclavian artery
Pedicled left internal mammary artery graft to left anterior descending artery
Left anterior descending coronary artery

Fig. 26.7 Completed coronary bypass procedure with venous and left internal mammary artery grafts in situ.

EBM 26.1   CORONARY BYPASS SURGERY

'Coronary bypass surgery significantly improves anginal symptoms compared with medical therapy. Survival is enhanced in patients with triple vessel disease, left main stem disease and two-vessel disease, including severe proximal left anterior descending coronary artery disease. Long-term graft survival is enhanced with the use of low-dose aspirin.'

SIGN. Coronary revascularisation in the management of stable angina pectoris; Scottish Intercollegiate Guideline 32;15–18; Nov 1998.

---

and improved survival. There does appear to be a trend in that direction for patients with multiple arterial grafts followed up beyond 10 years, but the added benefit over one IMA graft placed to the left anterior descending coronary is small. This may reflect the progression of native coronary disease. All patients must receive antiplatelet medication (aspirin) and appropriate secondary prevention advice and medication in order to reduce this risk (EBM 26.1).

SURGERY FOR THE COMPLICATIONS OF CORONARY ARTERY DISEASE

Mitral valve reflux

Chronic

Chronic ischaemia may cause reflux, owing to papillary muscle fibrosis. Surgery may be indicated to replace the valve as an elective procedure, usually concurrently with CABG. The operative mortality is around 8–11%.

Acute

An infarcted papillary muscle may rupture, causing gross reflux. The patient is usually very ill, with pulmonary oedema and low cardiac output, and often requires emergency ventilation. Emergency mitral valve replacement and CABG is associated with a mortality of 15–40%, mainly because of poor myocardial function and secondary multiorgan failure.

Post-myocardial infarction ventricular septal defect

Necrosis of the intraventricular septum due to MI may lead to a ventricular septal defect. Blood flows from the high-pressure left to the low-pressure right ventricle (left-to-right 'shunt'). This increases right ventricular work and pulmonary blood flow and decreases cardiac output. Typically, the patient complains of sudden, severe breathlessness 3–8 days after an MI and is noted to have developed a pansystolic murmur. Cardiac chamber oximetry is used to calculate the shunt magnitude, which is expressed as the ratio between the pulmonary (Qp) and systemic (Qs) blood flows. Coronary arteriography and assessment of right and left ventricular function are also performed. In general, if the shunt is below 1.5:1 the patient will tolerate the defect reasonably well. A shunt ratio of 2 or more will usually cause death from right ventricular failure, pulmonary oedema, renal failure and cardiogenic shock.

Emergency repair is technically difficult because it can be impossible to find sound tissue to which a patch may be sutured. In addition, these patients are in the aftermath of an acute MI and consequently have impaired cardiac function. Surgical mortality ranges from 20 to 50%. Patients with lesser shunts are managed medically and considered for surgery some weeks later. By this stage, cardiac function has stabilized and the margins of the defect have healed by fibrosis, making patch repair relatively straightforward. Operative mortality is below 10%.

Left ventricular aneurysm

This occurs when a large left ventricular free-wall MI scar becomes aneurysmal as a result of intraventricular pressure and complicates about 8% of infarcts. A large aneurysm impairs cardiac contraction and increases myocardial work. Clot forms within the aneurysm and may embolize. Arrhythmias may be generated within the zone of ischaemic myocardium around the periphery of the aneurysm. The aneurysm is excised, the clot removed and the resulting defect usually closed by direct suture, reinforced by buttressing strips of Teflon felt or vascular graft. Occasionally, a small patch repair is performed to preserve the shape of the left ventricle. Surgery is performed electively, with a mortality of 6–10% and an increased risk of stroke.

CARDIAC VALVULAR DISEASE

Valve disease may obstruct forward flow (stenosis) or permit reverse flow (incompetence/reflux/regurgitation), or both. The aortic and/or mitral valves are primarily affected. Primary tricuspid pathology is rare and pulmonary valve disease is virtually unknown. Formerly, rheumatic fever following streptococcal infection was the most common aetiological factor. This remains the case in many developing countries, but in the UK it is rare except in the elderly or in overseas patients.

ASSESSMENT

Precordial echocardiography provides useful data on forward gradients using Doppler techniques and can indicate regurgitation. Transoesophageal echocardiography can be particularly helpful, as this allows the valves and intracardiac anatomy to be imaged more effectively. Coronary arteriography is indicated in patients of middle age or older. Left ventricular angiography and aortic root angiography may allow the quantification of mitral and aortic reflux. A full catheterization study should include measurement of cardiac output and chamber and pulmonary artery pressures. Formulae exist that allow the effective orifice areas of stenotic mitral and aortic valves to be calculated.

SURGICAL MANAGEMENT

Options include valve replacement or repair. Replacement utilizes either a mechanical or a biological prosthesis.

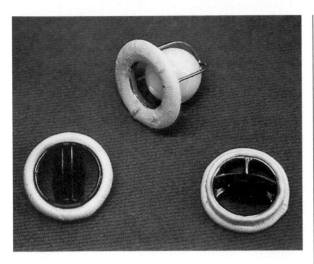

Fig. 26.8 Mechanical valve prosthesis.

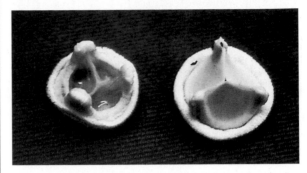

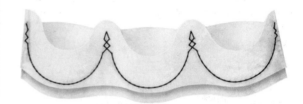

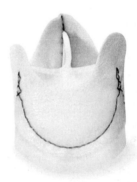

Fig. 26.9 Biological valve prostheses.
A Stented. B Unstented.

Mechanical valves have developed from the original ball-in-cage design through single disc designs to the current range of carbon bileaflet devices (Fig. 26.8). These devices should last indefinitely, but patients require lifelong warfarin to prevent thrombotic occlusion or embolism. Embolism risk is about 1–6% per year and is influenced by how accurately the INR is controlled. Mechanical valves produce audible clicks. Biological valves are derived from:

- glutaraldehyde-preserved porcine aortic valves mounted on a frame (stent)
- glutaraldehyde-preserved bovine pericardium formed into a three-leaflet valve and mounted on a stent
- human aortic root homografts removed from cadaveric hearts and preserved in antibiotic solution (Fig. 26.9A).

Recently, interest has developed in the use of unstented aortic bioprosthetic valves (Fig. 26.9B) derived from either a porcine aortic valve or pericardial tissue; these are sewn into the aortic root as a direct replacement for the aortic leaflets. Unstented valves offer the advantage of a larger effective orifice area and, therefore, minimize the residual pressure gradient. Warfarin is not required with biological valves provided the patient remains in sinus rhythm, and the valves are silent. However, such valves deteriorate over time and after 10–20 years will need to be replaced. Unless there is a contraindication to anticoagulation, mechanical valves are commonly used in those under the age of 70. In young women intending to have children it is usual to advise a biological valve, with the intention of replacing it with a mechanical device when the valve fails. This avoids problems with warfarin during pregnancy (placental separation and abortion, and teratogenicity).

Repair is relatively uncommon and is largely restricted to the mitral and tricuspid valves. When possible, it is preferable to valve replacement, as the problems associated with a prosthesis are avoided. Mostly, the surgeon is concerned with the correction of valvular incompetence. The techniques utilized for mitral incompetence include repositioning of the cordae, excision of portions of redundant leaflet and tightening of the annulus (annuloplasty). Generally, only annuloplasty is applicable to the tricuspid valve. Very rarely, isolated mitral stenosis without calcification may be found, in which case separation of the fused leaflets under direct vision on bypass (commisurotomy) is performed.

ENDOCARDITIS

Abnormal native heart valves and artificial valves are prone to subacute bacterial endocarditis and prosthetic valve endocarditis, respectively. Antibiotic prophylaxis is required to cover any surgical or dental procedure. If infection does develop, prolonged parenteral antibiotic therapy may be effective. However, surgery may be required if the infection does not respond or if the valve develops a large paravalvular leak or annular abscess. Surgery is a high-risk venture as the patient is systemically septic, the perivalvular tissues are of poor quality and the newly implanted prosthesis may itself become infected. Post-operative recovery is usually slow, with renal and ventilatory failure being common sequelae.

26

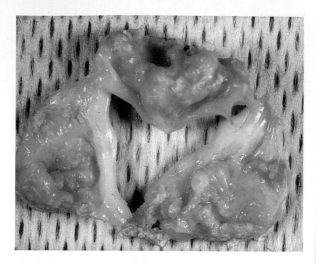

Fig. 26.10   Calcified aortic valve.

AORTIC VALVE DISEASE

Stenosis

This is the most frequent indication for valve surgery in the UK. Although stenosis can be due to rheumatic disease, it usually results from a congenital bicuspid aortic valve. Such valves function normally in early adult life but develop progressive leaflet calcification from the sixth decade onwards (Fig. 26.10). Aortic stenosis causes left ventricular hypertrophy, effort angina, episodes of arrhythmia with syncope or even sudden death, and left ventricular failure. There is a slow rising pulse, a forceful apex beat and an ejection systolic murmur in the right upper parasternal area that may radiate to the root of the neck. Echocardiography and catheterization will confirm a valvular gradient, which is typically greater than 60 mmHg. If the patient is well, an observational course is pursued; the onset of symptoms, however, should trigger referral for surgery. Patients with cardiac failure have a low output and consequently a low gradient. In these cases, the decision to operate may be a difficult judgement, based on the absence of any other likely cause of poor left ventricular function and echocardiographic evidence of severe aortic valve disease.

Reflux

Native aortic reflux may be due to primary valve pathology (rheumatic fever, endocarditic valve destruction or, rarely, a bicuspid valve) or secondary to aortic root pathology (see below). Prosthetic valve reflux can occur as a result of deterioration of a biological prosthesis, partial obstruction of a mechanical device, or paraprosthetic leakage. Chronic aortic reflux causes progressive left ventricular dilatation and hypertrophy. There is a wide pulse pressure, lateral displacement of the apex beat and a diastolic murmur in the left parasternal area. Chronic aortic reflux is well tolerated and often asymptomatic. In severe cases, the patient may complain of dyspnoea and angina, and may exhibit features of congestive cardiac failure. Surgery is advised to forestall the onset of cardiac failure and

irreversible myocardial damage when serial echocardiography indicates that the left ventricle is starting to dilate. Acute aortic reflux produces severe dyspnoea, with rapid onset of left ventricular failure and pulmonary oedema. The patient may require emergency ventilation and very urgent surgery.

Surgical outcomes

Elective aortic valve replacement is a relatively straightforward procedure, with a mortality of about 3% and stroke rate of 1%. The risk is increased several-fold in cases that have progressed to cardiac failure, and in emergency cases with acute severe reflux.

MITRAL VALVE DISEASE

Stenosis

This is usually the end result of rheumatic disease and is becoming less common. Elderly women in their sixth or seventh decade are usually affected. Mitral stenosis restricts the flow of blood into the left ventricle, which is consequently small and thin-walled, and cardiac output is considerably reduced. The left atrium is dilated and left atrial and pulmonary artery pressures are raised. Chronic pulmonary hypertension causes right ventricular hypertrophy and dilatation, and in advanced cases tricuspid incompetence may develop (see below). Patients complain of shortness of breath on exertion and may experience palpitations. Most will have been on warfarin therapy for chronic atrial fibrillation for many years, and diuretic therapy for pulmonary congestion. Examination reveals atrial fibrillation, a left parasternal heave due to right ventricular enlargement, and a diastolic murmur best heard at the lower left sternal edge, accompanied by a loud second heart sound. Chest X-ray shows right ventricular and atrial enlargement and the pulmonary artery is prominent. A progressive increase in heart size is often evident on serial yearly films. Renal function is frequently impaired.

The timing of surgery is a matter of judgement but an echocardiographic calculated mitral valve area below 1 cm^2 is indicative of severe stenosis and suggests that surgery should be advised. Very occasionally, the patient may have echocardiographic evidence of leaflet fusion only, in which case percutaneous balloon valvuloplasty may be effective. Conservative surgery with separation of the fused leaflets and reconstruction of the valve is possible in some younger patients. Usually, however, there is extensive leaflet calcification, with involvement of the papillary muscles and chordae tendinae, which become grossly thickened and shortened, tethering the leaflets to the tips of the papillary muscles (Fig. 26.11). Valve replacement is, therefore, the only practical option.

Rarely, patients with a mechanical mitral prosthesis may develop thrombotic occlusion of their valve secondary to inadequate control of anticoagulation or to fibrous tissue (pannus) ingrowth from the sewing ring. This acute emergency causes catastrophic pulmonary oedema and a severe reduction in cardiac output. Emergency salvage valve replacement or debridement is required.

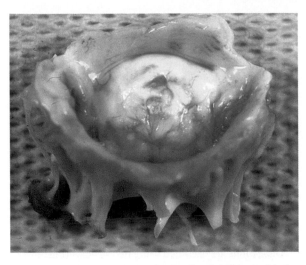

Fig. 26.11 Excised mitral valve showing the shortening and fusion of the papillary muscles and chordae tendinae in advanced mitral stenosis.

Reflux

Chronic mitral reflux occurs with rheumatic disease, ischaemic papillary muscle dysfunction, myxomatous degeneration of the mitral valve, a variety of systemic connective tissue disorders and chronic paraprosthetic valvular leakage. Acute reflux is much less common and follows acute MI involving a papillary muscle, as noted above, but can also result from spontaneous rupture of a chorda tendina, sudden failure of a bioprosthetic valve leaflet or perforation of an infected native valve. Chronic mitral reflux presents a volume load to the left ventricle, which ejects blood preferentially backwards through the incompetent mitral valve. This situation is often well tolerated for years, with patients typically complaining of shortness of breath on exertion and of occasional episodes of palpitation. Clinical examination is often relatively unremarkable, apart from a pansystolic murmur radiating from the lower left sternal edge to the axilla and leftward displacement of the apex beat. Surgery is indicated where there is chest X-ray and echocardiographic evidence of left ventricular dilatation, as this process correlates with declining left ventricular function consequent upon the continued volume overload. Acute reflux causes pulmonary oedema and emergency surgery is necessary. Mitral valves that reflux are often replaced with a prosthesis, but some can be repaired.

Surgical outcomes

Elective mitral valve surgery for reflux is generally a low-risk procedure, with a mortality rate of 4–6% and a stroke rate of about 2%. The risk is much greater (10–15%) for patients with ischaemic regurgitation, owing to the concomitant coronary disease and previous myocardial damage. Valve replacement for mitral stenosis also carries a significant mortality (8–12%) due to established pulmonary hypertension, right ventricular failure and poor renal function. The stroke rate is increased to 3–4%.

Emergency valve replacement for acute obstruction or reflux carries a mortality of the order of 20%.

TRICUSPID VALVE DISEASE

Stenosis is very rare. Tricuspid endocarditis is occasionally encountered in intravenous drug abusers. Tricuspid incompetence secondary to enlargement of the tricuspid annulus is the most common pathology and occurs when the right ventricle is dilated, as in advanced mitral valve disease. Typically, the patient will have the features of the underlying mitral valve disease, an elevated jugular venous pressure with 'v' waves, an enlarged pulsatile liver, peripheral oedema and, occasionally, ascites. Liver function tests are deranged and clotting is impaired. The preferred surgical option is to restore the normal dimensions of the valve through annuloplasty. It is uncommon to replace the tricuspid valve, except in rare cases of organic stenosis. If replacement is performed, a biological prosthesis is preferable, as the risk of mechanical valve thrombosis is increased in this position.

MULTIPLE AND REPEAT VALVE PROCEDURES

Some patients require multiple valve procedures, typically aortic and mitral valve replacement, or mitral replacement and tricuspid annuloplasty. Such operations attract a higher operative mortality (10% and 35%), as patients are often in poor condition. They may require prolonged periods of intensive care following surgery. Similarly, revisional valve surgery to replace a valve for a second time is technically more difficult and will involve a prolonged procedure against a background of impaired cardiac function or sepsis related to the defective prosthesis. Mortality is increased by two to three times the primary procedure risk, and the ICU stay is likely to be prolonged.

AORTIC ANEURYSM

TUBULOSACCULAR ANEURYSMS

These are 'true' aneurysms that form either a fusiform (tubular) or a focal (saccular) type of swelling (Fig. 26.12). They are lined by layered thrombus and most are due to medial degeneration secondary to smoking and hypertension (Ch. 25).

FALSE 'ANEURYSMS'

These result when bleeding from an aortic injury is contained within the mediastinum, so that the aneurysm wall is formed only by fibrous tissue and organized thrombus. There is usually a history of a road traffic accident or fall, which may have occurred many years previously.

Both true and false aneurysms may rupture and present as an acute emergency, with chest pain and catastrophic intrathoracic bleeding. However, they are often noted as incidental chest X-ray findings. Occasionally, an aneurysm

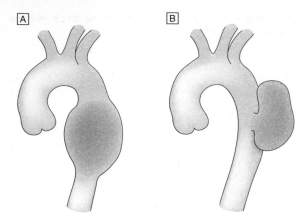

Fig. 26.12 Thoracic aortic aneurysm.
A Tubular. B Saccular.

may present with symptoms due to secondary pressure effects, such as dysphagia (oesophagus), stridor (left bronchus), chest wall pain (erosion of ribs), back pain (erosion of the vertebrae) or hoarseness (stretching of the left recurrent laryngeal nerve).

AORTIC DISSECTION

This is caused when blood enters into the wall of the aorta through a split in the intima, creating a false lumen that spirals along the vessel within the medial layer. The entry point is usually either just above the aortic valve or immediately beyond the left subclavian artery. However, the dissection process may extend along the entire length of the aorta into the iliac vessels. The false lumen may rupture through the adventitia into the mediastinum or pleural cavity, causing massive and frequently fatal

haemorrhage, or into the pericardium, causing fatal tamponade. The origins of aortic side branches, which are encountered by the false lumen, tend to be encircled and occluded. This process can lead to widespread ischaemic damage to the heart (coronaries), brain (branches of the aortic arch), spinal cord (spinal arteries), kidneys (renal arteries), abdominal viscera (coeliac and mesenteric arteries) and the limbs. A dissection that involves the aortic root tends to lift the aortic valve leaflets away from the wall, leading to reflux. Finally, a dissected aorta may dilate over months to years, causing a progressive aneurysmal process. Acute dissection is often fatal prior to arrival at hospital. There may be severe interscapular pain, collapse, shock aortic incompetence, unequal peripheral pulses, features of a left haemothorax, stroke, paraplegia and abdominal discomfort, and lower limb ischaemia.

Dissections are classified using two systems (Fig. 26.13). Dissections that originate distal to the left subclavian, do not spread retrogradely to involve the aortic arch or ascending aorta, and are clinically stable, are usually managed conservatively by control of blood pressure, as the results of medical and surgical treatment are not different. The decision to operate on such patients is based on the development of rupture and organ/limb ischaemia. In contrast, most patients with dissections that involve the ascending aorta or arch are offered emergency surgery to prevent rupture, stroke, MI and aortic valve incompetence. Surgery involves excising and replacing the portion of the aorta containing the entry point. This prevents more blood entering the false lumen and reapposes the layers of the aortic wall. Additional surgery to repair the aortic valve or to replace the aortic arch or descending aorta will be determined by individual circumstances.

AORTO-ANNULO ECTASIA

This is characterized by a flask-shaped aneurysmal dilatation of the aortic root and ascending aorta. This

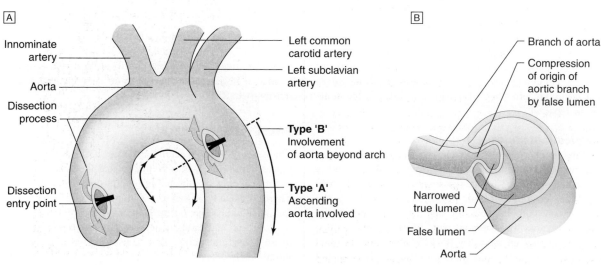

Fig. 26.13 Aortic dissection.

expanding aneurysm may rupture, initiate a dissection and lead to severe aortic reflux, with all the potential sequelae of these conditions. Aorto-annulo ectasia is most frequently associated with Marfan's disease.

ASSESSMENT

A patient with an incidentally discovered aneurysm should be thoroughly investigated, including tests of respiratory function and coronary angiography and contrast CT to determine whether the magnitude of surgery required could be sustained. Aneurysms that extend from the chest into the abdomen (thoracoabdominal aneurysm) require further investigations to clarify the relationship of the aneurysm to the renal and visceral vessels. Larger aneurysms (6 cm or greater) are more likely to rupture, and several review appointments will confirm whether or not an aneurysm is enlarging. Based on these considerations, a decision can then be taken regarding the potential benefit of surgery. Patients presenting with acute rupture of an aneurysm may undergo emergency surgery, if they are potentially salvageable and considered likely to benefit from operative intervention.

SURGERY FOR AORTIC PATHOLOGY

Lesions of the aortic root and ascending aorta are repaired on bypass via a median sternotomy. A woven nylon tube graft is used to replace an ascending aortic aneurysm, but in aortic annulo-ectasia a graft containing an aortic valve prosthesis is used to replace the whole aortic root. The coronary artery ostia are then sewn into side holes cut in the graft. Aneurysms involving the aortic arch require complex surgery. The patient is cooled to 16° C on bypass, the circulation arrested and the patient exsanguinated. Profound hypothermia protects against cerebral damage while the surgeon operates in a bloodless field. The innominate, left carotid and left subclavian arteries are anastomosed to the arch graft. Descending aortic aneurysms can often be repaired using a local bypass system in order to deliver blood to the lower body. Clamps are applied to exclude the aneurysm, which is excised and replaced with a suitable length of graft. If a thoracoabdominal aneurysm is being repaired, the visceral arteries are also anastomosed to the graft.

All thoracic aortic aneurysm surgery is high-risk. Elective procedures carry a 5–15% mortality risk and a risk of stroke of several percent. Procedures involving the descending aorta carry an additional 5–10% risk of paraplegia, owing to interference with spinal arterial supply. Emergency thoracic aneurysm surgery is in most cases a desperate measure. Mortality rates vary between 10% and over 60%, depending upon the extent of surgery required and, very importantly, the degree of pre-existing and acquired morbidity the patient has prior to surgery. It is not uncommon for the primary repair procedure to proceed satisfactorily, only for the patient to die later from multiorgan failure and/or stroke. In some instances, it may be possible to manage a descending thoracic aneurysm or dissection by inserting an endoluminal stent under radiological guidance via the iliac artery (Ch. 25).

PERICARDIAL PATHOLOGY

PERICARDIAL EFFUSION

In chronic pericardial effusion, the pericardial sac will stretch and the clinical effects of the accumulated fluid may be modest. In contrast, a rapidly evolving effusion will prevent the heart from filling in diastole (tamponade) and lead to a low stroke volume. In order to maintain cardiac output and blood pressure, there is a tachycardia and intense peripheral vasoconstriction. The raised intrapericardial pressure leads to elevation of atrial pressure, and hence the central venous pressure rises in order to maintain a filling gradient. A pericardial effusion can often be drained through a catheter placed under echocardiographic guidance. This may help clarify the diagnosis, but surgical drainage is likely to be required in infection, malignancy with reasonable life expectancy, and in chronic effusions. Chronic effusions are often drained into the left pleural cavity. This is achieved by creating a window in the left lateral pericardium either via an open left lateral thoracotomy or, more recently, as a minimal-access videothoracoscopic procedure. Acute and malignant effusions can be drained relatively simply into the peritoneal cavity via a short epigastric incision. Whichever approach is used, specimens of fluid and pericardium are sent for culture and histology.

PERICARDIAL CONSTRICTION

Chronic pericardial inflammation, often from tuberculosis, may heal by intense fibrosis and calcification (Fig. 26.14).

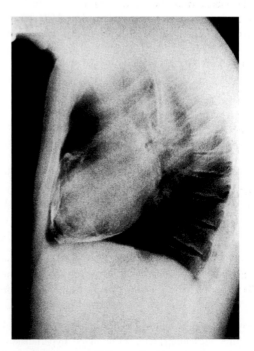

Fig. 26.14 Calcified constrictive pericardium.

This leads to chronic tamponade. Surgery is undertaken via a median sternotomy to remove the parietal pericardium and any fibrotic visceral pericardium. The results of surgery are frequently disappointing because the patient has developed irreversible hepatic cirrhosis and myocardial function is poor.

CONGENITAL CARDIAC DISEASE

This may be classified as cyanotic or acyanotic, depending on the presence of central cyanosis. Those with cyanosis will have a right-to-left shunt, preventing complete oxygenation of systemic arterial blood. Some patients with high-flow left-to-right shunts develop severe pulmonary hypertension as a consequence of the massive pulmonary blood flow. This can result in pressures in the right heart chambers that are greater than those in the left heart and, consequently, in reversal of the shunt direction to right to left, causing cyanosis. This situation is called Eisenmenger's syndrome. Primary repair is usually advised for congenital defects, but in some instances it may be helpful to delay definitive repair until the child is older, larger and fitter. In this situation, a temporizing palliative procedure is performed. This is usually designed to augment or restrict pulmonary artery blood flow.

ATRIAL SEPTAL DEFECT

This is the most common abnormality, causing a left-to-right atrial shunt and hence an increase in right heart and pulmonary blood flow. Patients may be asymptomatic or may present with frequent chest infections. There is a fixed split second heart sound and a pulmonary ejection systolic murmur. Small defects are of little haemodynamic significance, but if the pulmonary to systemic flow ratio exceeds 2:1, closure is necessary. ECG frequently demonstrates right ventricular hypertrophy and echocardiography is diagnostic. Three anatomical types exist, named after the developmental area giving rise to the defect:

- *Sinus venosus defects* arise in the upper atrium adjacent to the superior vena cava. They are repaired with a Dacron or pericardial patch, which must be placed with care, as the right upper pulmonary vein can be abnormally located within the apparent right atrial area.
- *Ostium secundum defects* are the most common lesions and are located at mid-atrial septal level. Closure by patch or simple suture is straightforward, but may also be achieved by an interventional cardiologist using a catheter-inserted closure device.
- *Ostium primum defects* are usually associated with clefts in the anterior mitral leaflet and septal tricuspid leaflet, which are repaired at the same time as closure of the atrial septal defect with a patch. Left axis deviation is common.

Surgical repair in children carries a low mortality (< 1%), but adults presenting with pulmonary hypertension are at greater risk (10%).

VENTRICULAR SEPTAL DEFECT

Many ventricular septal defects are small and close within the first year of life. Larger lesions cause a left-to-right shunt and pulmonary congestion. Defects may again be subdivided according to their embryological origins, but most (85%) occur in the membranous septum. Infants with large defects may present with frequent respiratory infections but patients are often asymptomatic. A pansystolic murmur is audible, maximal at the left sternal edge. The second heart sound may be loud. Biventricular hypertrophy is present on ECG and pulmonary plethora may be noted on chest X-ray. Echocardiography is diagnostic. Asymptomatic defects are observed, but early operation is preferred for larger defects to prevent irreversible pulmonary hypertension. Repair is undertaken using a patch, with an operative mortality of 3–5%.

PATENT DUCTUS ARTERIOSUS

If the ductus arteriosus fails to close after birth, pulmonary blood flow is abnormally high, producing pulmonary congestion and hypertension. Infants have retarded growth and a continuous 'machinery' murmur is audible over the precordium and back. The chest X-ray shows pulmonary congestion, and echocardiography can exclude concurrent intracardiac defect(s). In premature children, the duct may close with an indometacin infusion (prostaglandin E_1 inhibition), but clipping or division at left thoracotomy is likely to be needed. Endovascular closure is an option in older children. The operative mortality is low in older children (< 1%) but high (25%) in preterm infants, who are generally very unwell.

COARCTATION OF THE AORTA

This condition is caused by a narrowing of the thoracic aorta, usually at the level of the ligamentum arteriosum. The lower body is perfused via extensive chest wall collaterals. Upper body hypertension develops, partly due to relative renal hypoperfusion, and may lead to heart failure in infancy. Untreated adults develop hypertensive cerebrovascular and renal problems and accelerated coronary atheroma. Most children and young adults are asymptomatic and present with high blood pressure or an abnormal chest X-ray. The femoral pulses may be impalpable or weak and delayed, and a systolic murmur may be audible over the back. Left ventricular hypertrophy is seen on the ECG and the chest X-ray shows an enlarged heart, reduced aortic knuckle and characteristic rib 'notching', caused by enlarged and tortuous intercostal arteries eroding the ribs near the posterior angles (Fig. 26.15). Balloon angioplasty has been used to dilate some coarctations in infants, but surgical correction is usually required. In infants, an onlay patch graft created from the left subclavian artery is used. This has the advantage of growing with the child, although left arm growth is slightly decreased. Older children and adults are usually managed with a Dacron bypass graft. Surgical correction tends

26

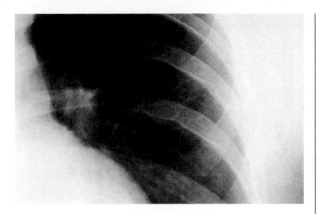

Fig. 26.15 Rib notching in coarctation.

to reduce upper body hypertension in children. It is less effective in adults but pharmacological control of hypertension becomes more reliable. The operative risk is about 5%.

TETRALOGY OF FALLOT

This is the most common cause of cyanotic congenital heart disease; it comprises a high ventricular septal defect, an aorta that tends to overlie the interventricular septum, pulmonary valvular and subvalvular stenosis, and right ventricular hypertrophy. Right ventricular outflow obstruction causes cyanosis as a result of right-to-left shunting across the ventricular septal defect. Clinical features depend upon the severity of the obstruction. This may not be significant when the child is at rest but it may be precipitated by adrenergic events, as these increase the subvalvular obstructive effect of hypertrophied right ventricular muscle. Consequently, the child may become blue and faint during feeding or crying. Right ventricular hypertrophy is found on ECG and the pulmonary artery shadow is small on chest X-ray. Echocardiography is diagnostic but complemented by right ventricular angiography, which demonstrates the pulmonary arterial tree. Correction entails closing the ventricular septal defect with a patch, resecting muscle bands contributing to right ventricular outflow obstruction, and enlarging the

26

Table 26.2 COMMON THORACIC SURGICAL INVESTIGATIONS	
Investigation	**Yield**
ECG Resting	Rhythm; conduction abnormalities; atrial and ventricular hypertrophy; established ischaemic changes; evidence of previous myocardial infarction
Chest X-ray Posterior–anterior and lateral	Preliminary assessment of location of lesion; malignant involvement of phrenic nerve or ribs; presence of additional lesions or effusion; presence of pneumothorax or mediastinal air
Thoracic CT scan	Further refine radiological assessment of mass lesions as above; review mediastinum for enlarged nodes in bronchogenic carcinoma; inspect bronchi for dilatations in suspected bronchiectasis; determine exact location of mediastinal mass lesions; determine areas of greatest disease in interstitial lung disease; locate intrathoracic collections; map out distribution of bullous/emphysematous lung disease
Upper abdominal CT scan	Exclude or confirm liver abnormalities; identify adrenal metastases
Upper abdominal ultrasound	Determine probable nature of cystic hepatic lesions; provide guidance for biopsy of hepatic or adrenal lesions; review diaphragm motion in cases of suspected diaphragmatic rupture or phrenic nerve paralysis
MRI	Useful for assessing relationships of tumours to adjacent neural structures, e.g. detecting possible intraspinal extension of paravertebral neurogenic tumours or involvement of brachial plexus by superior sulcus (Pancoast) tumours
Isotope scans Bone Lung	Search for skeletal metastases; review chest wall for possible direct invasion by carcinoma Identify areas of low uptake indicative of impaired perfusion ($\dot{Q}$ scan) or ventilation ($\dot{V}$ scan)
Pulmonary function tests FEV_1 FVC CO transfer Walking test Arterial blood gas	Forced expiratory volume in 1 second; provides a measure of airway obstruction Forced vital capacity; indicates presence of restriction of ventilation Measures the diffusion capacity of the patient's lungs Measures distance walked by the patient in a set time period (4 mins) and the perceived exercise level achieved as assessed by the final heart rate; useful as an indicator of functional status in patients with poor FEV_1, as they may not comply well with the methodology of formal respiratory testing and hence underachieve Useful in demonstrating patients with CO_2 retention who should be excluded from surgical consideration

right ventricular outflow tract with a patch placed across the pulmonary valve annulus and along the pulmonary artery if necessary. In those not fit for this procedure or in those with very small pulmonary vessels, a shunt (usually subclavian artery to pulmonary artery, Blalock–Taussig) is created in order to increase pulmonary blood flow and, hopefully, lead to further pulmonary arterial growth. Definitive correction may then be possible at a later stage. Operative mortality is about 10%.

26

THORACIC SURGERY

ASSESSMENT

This is concerned with confirming the diagnosis, determining in oncological cases whether resection is appropriate, and establishing that the patient is fit for the intended surgical procedure. The principal investigations are summarized in Table 26.2. As noted below, history can be instructive in suggesting advanced malignant disease. It is also helpful in providing evidence of the patient's premorbid functional status.

BRONCHOGENIC CARCINOMA

Aetiology, pathology and presentation

This usually presents from the fifth decade onwards and is now the leading cause of cancer death in the UK for both men and women. The principal risk factor is smoking, particularly cigarettes, but other rare causes include exposure to arsenic, radon gas, bichromates and nickel ore. The combination of asbestos exposure and cigarette smoking produces a many-fold increase in risk. With the exception of alveolar cell carcinomas, which arise from cells lining the alveoli, primary lung cancers arise within the bronchial

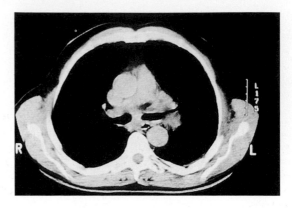

Fig. 26.17 Central bronchogenic carcinoma.
This patient has an advanced carcinoma of the proximal left bronchus visible on CT scan. Extensive mediastinal lymphadenopathy may be seen in front of the bronchi and in the subcarinal area.

epithelium and are hence termed bronchogenic carcinoma. They are described as peripheral or central, according to their location within the lung (Figs 26.16 and 26.17). Peripheral lesions may grow to 8 cm or more before causing local symptoms such as chest wall pain. Many are detected as incidental findings on a chest film taken for unrelated reasons, or for non-specific symptoms such as weight loss. Central lesions tend to occlude the airways, causing varying degrees of pulmonary collapse and consolidation (Fig. 26.18). Nodal spread occurs to the intralobar, hilar and mediastinal nodes, and thence to the scalene nodes. Metastases occur in bone, brain, liver, adrenals and lung. Local direct spread may involve the chest wall, vertebrae, trachea, oesophagus and great vessels.

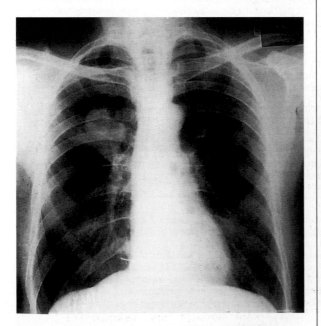

Fig. 26.16 Chest X-ray showing cancer in the right upper lobe.

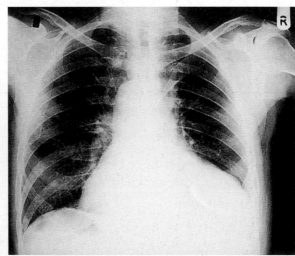

Fig. 26.18 Consolidation/collapse of the right middle and lower lobes associated with a bronchogenic carcinoma.
Resection of these lobes would not alter respiratory function in the same way as resection of the tumour in Figure 26.16, as they are non-functional.

Cell types and approximate frequencies are as follows:

- squamous 35%
- adenocarcinoma 25%
- undifferentiated 15%
- small cell 20%
- alveolar cell 5%.

Patients with small cell lung cancer are not usually referred for surgery as this condition is regarded as a systemic disease at presentation and is, therefore, treated with chemotherapy. All other varieties are resected if possible, and bronchogenic carcinoma is, therefore, frequently split into two functional categories: small cell and non-small-cell.

There may be no clinical features, but haemoptysis, pulmonary infection and weight loss are common presenting symptoms. Paraneoplastic syndromes are infrequent but well described, including ectopic hormone production (adrenocorticotrophic hormone (ACTH), parathyroid hormone (PTH), antidiuretic hormone (ADH)) and a painful periosteal reaction affecting the joints and long bones, termed hypertrophic pulmonary osteoarthropathy (Fig. 26.19). Patients frequently have finger clubbing.

ASSESSMENT FOR PULMONARY RESECTION

Prior to referral to the surgeon, the diagnosis will often have been confirmed by sputum cytology, bronchoscopy or CT-guided needle biopsy, but approximately 30% of cases will be undiagnosed at this stage. Surgical assessment addresses two questions:

- Would the patient be fit for pulmonary resection?
- If so, is the disease potentially curable?

Fitness for resection

Fitness is determined by cardiorespiratory investigations. A history of angina or myocardial infarction does not preclude surgery, provided the symptoms are stable. However, patients with poor left ventricular function and/or unstable angina are not suitable for pulmonary resection. Respiratory investigations are orientated towards confirming that pulmonary reserve will be adequate following the intended resection. The forced expiratory volume in 1 second (FEV_1) and carbon monoxide (CO) transfer data are most helpful in this regard. Patients with an FEV_1 < 50% predicted, prior to resection, are likely to be significantly breathless following surgery and may not be suitable candidates for surgical management. If the CO transfer value is low, implying poor alveolar gas exchange, the minimum FEV_1 figure would have to be revised upwards. However, resection of consolidated or collapsed lung does not affect residual respiratory capability.

Staging

Assessment of the potential for curative resection is determined by staging. Initial clinical assessment will normally filter out advanced disease and provide evidence of incurability because of local irresectability or disseminated disease (Table 26.3). Simple chest X-ray may reveal an elevated diaphragm, indicating phrenic nerve involvement, bone metastases or direct invasion of the rib cage. If an effusion is present, this should be aspirated; if malignant cells are noted on cytology, this would preclude resection. A contrast-enhanced thoracic and upper abdominal CT scan will clarify the nature and position of the pulmonary mass and should exclude other pulmonary lesions that might represent metastases or synchronous tumours. Mediastinal nodes < 1 cm in long axis are generally considered to be

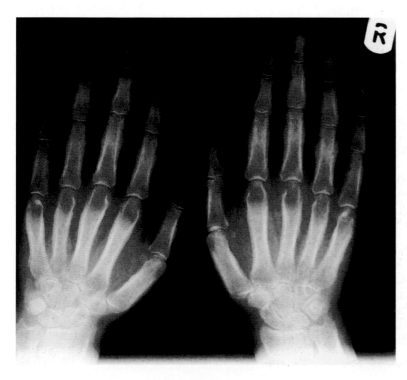

Fig. 26.19 Hypertrophic pulmonary osteoarthropathy.

Table 26.3   CLINICAL INDICATORS OF LOCALLY IRRESECTABLE OR INCURABLE LUNG CANCER

Clinical finding	Pathological implication
Local inoperability	
Horner's syndrome	Involvement of upper sympathetic chain
Hoarseness	Involvement of left recurrent laryngeal nerve
Upper body venous congestion	Involvement of superior vena cava
Severe shoulder/inner arm pain	Involvement of brachial plexus (Pancoast tumour)
Disseminated disease	
Scalene node enlargement	Nodal spread out of operative field
Hepatomegaly	Hepatic metastases
Focal bone pain	Bone metastases
Skin deposits	Cutaneous metastases
Behavioural/balance disturbance	Cerebral/cerebellar metastases
Headache	

26

benign, but surgical sampling is necessary to confirm this. Where available, a combined thoracic CT/positron emission tomography (PET) scan is helpful in both locating and characterizing mediastinal lymph nodes. A negative PET scan is highly accurate in predicting the absence of tumour involvement; a positive scan may indicate tumour but can also arise with inflammatory conditions, and, therefore, the positive glands must be sampled by mediastinoscopy. The liver and adrenals are common sites for metastases. Suspicious areas can be sampled by means of ultrasound-guided biopsy. Further investigations, such as bone or brain scans, will depend upon the clinical suspicion.

Surgical staging is concerned with further refining the intrathoracic assessment so as to ensure that thoracotomy will be associated with a reasonable chance of cure. In practical terms, this means excluding those with involved mediastinal lymph nodes and, where possible, confirming the diagnosis and local operability. Three techniques are employed:

- *Mediastinoscopy* is used to sample the paratracheal and subcarinal lymph nodes. A low anterior cervical incision is made just above the jugular notch and the mediastinoscope used to create a passage in the pretracheal region. The lymph nodes are dissected and biopsied.
- *Mediastinotomy* is used mainly to assess lymph nodes within the concavity of the aortic arch or anterior to the aorta, as these areas cannot be reached at mediastinoscopy. Access is gained via a short left anterior second interspace incision.
- *Videothoracoscopy* is a relatively new technique that allows the surgeon to inspect the pleural cavity, biopsy the primary lesion and sample the lower mediastinal and aortic arch lymph nodes. The extent of resection likely to be required can also be assessed in relation to the patient's lung function. Videothoracoscopy may also reveal unforeseen causes of irresectability, such as pleural seedlings.

Table 26.4   LUNG CANCER STAGING

Stage category	TNM classification
0	Carcinoma in situ (Tis)
IA	$T_1 N_0 M_0$
IB	$T_2 N_0 M_0$
IIA	$T_1 N_1 M_0$
IIB	$T_2 N_1, M_0$
	$T_3 N_0 M_0$
IIIA	$T_3 N_1 M_0$
	$T_1/T_2/T_3 N_2 M_0$
IIIB	Any T_4, Any N_3, M_0
IV	Any M_1

Abbreviated definitions:

T_1	Peripheral tumour < 3 cm not involving pleura
T_2	Tumour > 3 cm or involves main bronchus beyond 2 cm from carina/parietal pleura
T_3	Tumour involves chest wall/mediastinal pleura/pericardium/diaphragm or main bronchus within 2 cm of carina
T_4	Tumour involves mediastinal structures/vertebral column/carina; tumour is associated with pericardial or pleural malignant effusion; satellite tumour deposits are present within lobe containing primary tumour
N_0	No lymph nodes involved by tumour
N_1	Ipsilateral peribronchial or intrapulmonary nodes involved
N_2	Ipsilateral mediastinal or subcarinal nodes involved
N_3	Contralateral mediastinal nodes involved; involvement of scalene nodes on either side
M_0	No distant metastases
M_1	Distant metastases present

Resection

Lung tumours are normally removed en bloc with the surrounding parenchyma and local draining lymphatics. This involves either lobectomy or pneumonectomy. Occasionally, in unfit patients, small cancers are excised within a wedge or segment of lung. The risk of local recurrence is greater in these lung-sparing cases. An area of anterior chest wall directly invaded by tumour can be excised and replaced with an acrylic patch, provided it is lateral to the posterior rib angles. Following assessment and surgical resection, a final pathological TNM stage (Table 26.4) is allocated. This is helpful in indicating prognosis and determining whether a patient might benefit from adjuvant therapy or be suitable for inclusion in a trial. Patients who are found to have positive mediastinal nodes following resection are routinely referred for adjuvant radiotherapy to the mediastinum in view of the high risk of recurrence in that area. Post-surgical chemotherapy may improve 5-year survival across all resected stages by approximately 5%. Although still controversial, this form of adjuvant therapy is likely to become an increasingly common option for suitable fit patients. Operative mortality is about 2% for lobectomy and 6% for pneumonectomy.

Survival

Long-term survival depends on tumour stage at the time of resection. Reported 5-year survival data are of the order of 60% for stage I, 35% for stage II and < 20% for stage IIIa disease. Relatively few patients (< 20%) with non-small-cell bronchogenic carcinoma are suitable for resection at presentation. One strategy to address this problem is the use of neoadjuvant pre-operative induction chemotherapy to downstage tumours, although there are as yet no data to support the widespread use of this approach. The other obvious possibility for improving resection rates would be to detect lung cancers at an earlier stage. Previous mass chest X-ray screening studies did not appear to show an improvement in long-term survival, but there is currently renewed interest in screening high-risk individuals (smoking history, > 50 years old) using CT as a more sensitive test.

METASTATIC DISEASE

Pulmonary metastases (Fig. 26.20) are the most common form of intrathoracic malignancy. A confirmatory diagnostic lung biopsy may be helpful for patients with no evident primary. A palliative pleurodesis in patients with associated pleural effusion can be achieved by instilling an irritant such as aluminium silicate powder (kaolin) into the pleural cavity. Rarely, a solitary metastasis or limited pulmonary metastases (e.g. in osteogenic sarcoma) may be found in patients without any other evidence of disseminated disease. In these rare situations, surgery may be advised to remove the metastatic lesion(s).

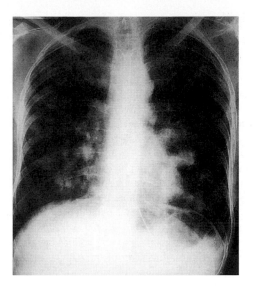

Fig. 26.20   Multiple pulmonary metastases.

OTHER LUNG TUMOURS

These tend to present either as an incidental chest X-ray finding, in which case the concern is that they may in fact be malignant tumours, or as a cause of bronchial obstruction and infection. True benign lung tumours are rare and can arise from all tissue elements within the lung architecture. If the lesion can be shown to be benign by transthoracic biopsy, no treatment is required. Where there is doubt, local excision will be required. If a main bronchus is obstructed, lobectomy will be necessary to remove the tumour and the damaged portion of lung. Carcinoid tumours arise from argentaffin-containing cells within the bronchial epithelium. They are divided on histological grounds into 'typical' tumours, which grow slowly locally, and 'atypical' tumours, which grow more quickly and can metastasize. Resection is by lobectomy. As local recurrence may occur up to 15 years following resection, good local clearance is essential. Unlike abdominal carcinoids, thoracic carcinoids do not secrete vasoactive substances.

An adenochondroma is a hamartoma, a tumour that develops from residual embryological tissue within the lung parenchyma. It presents as an incidental chest X-ray finding and is typically partly calcified and has a very smooth outline. CT-guided needle biopsy should provide the diagnosis, and surgery is only undertaken when the diagnosis is in doubt.

MESOTHELIOMA

This causes progressive thickening of the parietal and visceral pleura, with subsequent encasement of the lung and the formation of a large pleural effusion. In the later stages, the growth penetrates the chest wall, causing pain, and involves the mediastinal structures and abdominal cavity. Metastatic spread is rare until an advanced stage is reached. Mesothelioma is strongly related to a history of asbestos exposure, but there is usually a latent period of 20–40 years before the onset of symptoms. The patient commonly presents with shortness of breath, owing to a large pleural effusion. In many cases, the diagnosis is made by a percutaneous pleural biopsy but, if this is not successful, thoracoscopy or open pleural biopsy will provide the diagnosis. The main differential diagnosis is disseminated adenocarcinoma involving the pleural cavity. It can be difficult to distinguish these two pathologies on light microscopy, and diagnosis may be delayed while immunohistochemistry and electron microscopy studies are performed. Surgical resection by excision of the parietal pleura, lung, diaphragm and pericardium (pleuropneumonectomy) is not generally reported to offer a survival benefit, except possibly in very early lesions. Radiotherapy and chemotherapy have no curative value. Therapy is, therefore, usually directed towards controlling symptoms as they occur. If the lung re-expands after drainage of the effusion, kaolin may be instilled in order to promote pleurodesis and so prevent recurrence. Life expectancy varies between 1 and 4 years from initial presentation, depending on age, the rate of tumour growth and the stage at presentation.

MEDIASTINUM

Mass lesions

Benign and malignant masses may arise in the mediastinum. Some clue to the likely diagnosis is provided by the location of the lesion (Fig. 26.21) within the mediastinum. Where the diagnosis is in doubt, tissue may be obtained by CT-guided needle biopsy. If this is either not feasible or is unsuccessful, a surgical biopsy can be obtained using mediastinotomy, mediastinoscopy or videothoracoscopy. The clinical features vary considerably, with some quite large masses being asymptomatic and identified on routine chest films. Non-specific symptoms include vague chest pain, cough, weight loss, fever and general malaise. Other lesions may cause direct pressure effects, such as tracheal compression by a retrosternal thyroid goitre or oesophageal compression by malignant lymphadenopathy. Small thymic tumours may be identified during the evaluation of patients with myasthenia gravis.

Wherever possible, primary mediastinal tumours are resected, although in many cases this is precluded because the growth encircles or invades the great vessels and mediastinal viscera. Benign cysts are usually resected or, less commonly, marsupialized in order to prevent pressure effects or the development of infection. Surgery is generally undertaken via a median sternotomy for anterior lesions and via a thoracotomy for mid- and posterior lesions.

Infection

Mediastinal infection is an uncommon but serious condition that is associated with a rapid onset of septicaemia and

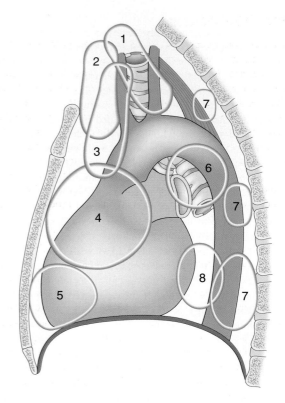

1 Goitre
2 Lymph node tumours, primary and metastases
3 Thymoma
4 Dermoid/teratoma
5 Pleuropericardial cyst
6 Bronchogenic cyst
7 Neurogenic tumour
8 Enterogenous cyst

Fig. 26.21 Topography of mediastinal lesions.

septic shock. It is almost always a consequence of oesophageal or pharyngeal leakage, which may follow perforation or breakdown of an oesophageal anastomosis. Perforation usually occurs after attempted dilatation of a stricture but can result from swallowing sharp objects or caustic substances, and rarely with external trauma. The diagnosis may be suggested by the history. A chest film will usually show mediastinal widening, gas streaks from mediastinal emphysema together with pleural fluid, and possibly a hydropneumothorax. Surgical management requires broad-spectrum parenteral antibiotics, adequate mechanical drainage, and correction of the cause if possible. Mechanical drainage may be achieved by pleural drainage alone if the lesion is low in the mediastinum and has burst directly into the pleural cavity, as may be the situation with a leaking oesophagogastric anastomosis. It is often necessary to perform a thoracotomy so that the pleura can be widely opened and the mediastinum fully drained and debrided. Further surgery to attend to the underlying cause—for example, by repairing the oesophagus—may be necessary either immediately or subsequently when the patient is more stable.

PNEUMOTHORAX

Pneumothorax occurs when air enters the potential space between the visceral and parietal pleura through either an external chest wound or an internal air leak. External air entry occurs with a traumatic chest wall defect, and the resulting open pneumothorax is often associated with a 'sucking wound', where air moves in and out of a chest wound with respiration. Internal air leakage may follow oesophageal perforation or anastomotic breakdown, as air can enter the pleural cavity via the mouth.

However, by far the most common cause of pneumothorax is leakage of air from the lung, due either to a traumatic puncture wound or to spontaneous leakage from a large (bulla) or small (< 1 cm, 'bleb') air sac (Fig. 26.22) on the lung surface. Occasionally, the pulmonary leak point may have a flap valve mechanism that allows air out of but not back into the lung, causing a rapid build-up of pressure within the pleural cavity and 'tension' pneumothorax (Fig. 26.23). This can be fatal, as the high intrapleural pressure completely flattens the ipsilateral lung while deviating the mediastinum to the opposite side, impeding venous return. Spontaneous pneumothorax is described as primary or secondary. Primary pneumothorax typically occurs in young (15–35 years) individuals with essentially normal lungs apart from a few apical bullae or blebs. Secondary pneumothorax develops in elderly patients (55–75 years) with a background of emphysema and chronic obstructive pulmonary disease. It is caused by rupture of a large bulla.

Management

Initial management involves inserting a chest drain connected to an underwater seal drain into the pleural space (Fig. 26.24). This allows the lung to re-expand. In most cases of primary pneumothorax, air leakage stops within 48 hours or so, after which the drain can be removed. If the pneumothorax recurs or the air leakage does not

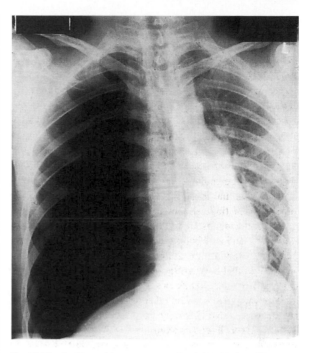

Fig. 26.23 Radiographic appearance of a right-sided tension pneumothorax (note the mediastinal shift to opposite side).

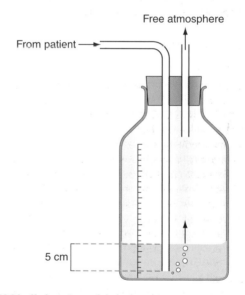

Fig. 26.24 Underwater seal drain.
The water acts as a hydraulic valve. This allows air to escape from the pleural cavity with ease but the pressure required to cause reverse air flow is much greater, being increased by the ratio of the surface areas inside and outside the tube that enter the water.

stop, surgery is indicated. This is now undertaken as a thoracoscopic procedure. The lung is inspected and any blebs or bullae are stapled. These are usually found at the apices of the upper or lower lobes. Pleurodesis is then performed either by using an abrasion technique to scarify the parietal pleura, or a pleural strip (pleurectomy), or by insufflation of kaolin. Bullectomy and abrasion or pleurectomy carry about an 8% risk of further recurrent

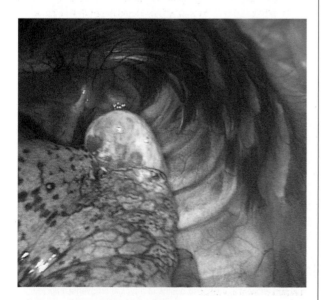

Fig. 26.22 Typical blebs/microbullae.

pneumothorax. This is reduced to 1–2% with kaolin insufflation, but as this technique involves leaving foreign material in the chest of a young person, it is usually kept in reserve for recurrent pneumothorax or for patients with no obvious culprit bulla or bleb.

Secondary pneumothorax may not settle rapidly, owing to the poor quality of the underlying lung tissue. However, it occurs in individuals who are clearly poor candidates for general anaesthesia and major thoracic surgery. It is customary, therefore, to wait for 1–2 weeks to see if the air leak will stop spontaneously. If not, videothoracoscopy is undertaken in better-risk patients to inspect the lung for a leaking bulla, which can be closed by stapling. Alternatively, kaolin mixed with local anaesthetic can be inserted as a slurry up the drain. This option avoids general anaesthesia but results in significant pain. Either treatment is associated with an appreciable mortality of 5–10%, owing to respiratory and cardiovascular complications.

EMPHYSEMA

Emphysema causes progressive loss of respiratory function, culminating in respiratory failure and death. Recurrent infection and pneumothorax are common. Emphysema is characterized by progressive loss of interalveolar septae. Large air spaces form throughout the lung, which become grossly enlarged, and areas of severely diseased lung develop that are neither ventilated nor perfused. This is typically a smoking-related disease affecting patients from the fourth or fifth decade onwards, with a tendency towards an upper lobar distribution. In less than 10% of cases, however, it can also result from a deficiency of α_1-antitrypsin, affecting younger patients from the third decade and having a lower lobar distribution. Medical treatment with bronchodilators and steroids may improve symptoms but transplantation is the only definitive cure. This is only an option for younger patients, and even in these it should be put off as long as possible. A surgical procedure called lung volume reduction has been developed, which aims to improve lung function by excising the worst-affected areas. This removes the space-occupying effect of these non-functional areas and allows the overall lung volume to return towards normal, thereby improving diaphragmatic and chest wall function. The improvement in respiratory function is modest in absolute terms, being in the order of 0.5 litres for FEV_1. However, patients eligible for this surgery typically have FEV_1 values of less than 1 litre, so that the percentage improvement and hence the perceived benefit can be significant. The procedure may be performed either as a videothoracoscopic operation or through a median sternotomy. The clinical improvement only lasts for a few years, as lung function continues to fall, reflecting the progressive nature of emphysema. The operative mortality is high (6–12%), reflecting the generally very poor condition of these patients.

INTERSTITIAL LUNG DISEASE

This can arise from many causes and correct treatment depends on an accurate diagnosis. Transbronchial biopsy can be effective in some instances, particularly sarcoidosis, but provides only a small tissue sample, which may not be diagnostic. It is usually preferable to use videothoracoscopic techniques to excise a wedge of affected lung. The patient is typically allowed home on the first post-operative day.

PLEUROPULMONARY INFECTION

Empyema

This is a collection of pus within the pleural cavity; it commonly follows a pneumonia due to secondary infection of a reactive parapneumonic effusion. In the initial phase, the infected fluid is thin and may be completely evacuated by a low intercostal drain. The empyema quickly becomes thick and loculated as a result of the deposition of fibrin, and at this stage formal surgical drainage is required. The collection is typically placed posteriorly towards the base of the pleural cavity and causes a D-shaped shadow on the chest film (Fig. 26.25). Drainage is achieved by excising a 2 cm segment of rib over the lowest part of the empyema and suctioning and curetting the cavity clean. Dense fibrosis surrounds an empyema, so that drainage creates a fixed cavity. In elderly or unfit patients, a simple open tube drain is left in situ for many months, during which the cavity gradually shrinks and finally obliterates. In younger patients, open thoracotomy allows the fibrous cavity to be excised and any cortex over the lung removed. This returns more lung function to the patient and avoids open drainage, so that recovery is more rapid. Other causes of empyema include post-surgical bronchial or oesophageal suture line leakage, oesophageal rupture or perforation, repeat aspiration of pleural effusion, secondary infection of a clotted haemothorax and, rarely, a subphrenic abscess.

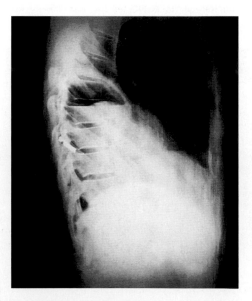

Fig. 26.25 Lateral X-ray of empyema.
This film shows the D-shaped outline of a typical empyema. Infected fluid collections can, however, occur anywhere within the chest.

Bronchiectasis

Dilatation of bronchi and bronchioles can follow childhood infections. The stagnant pools of secretions that collect are subject to continued infection, resulting in episodes of acute pulmonary infection or pneumonia and, more rarely, in haemoptysis. Management is by antibiotic therapy, physiotherapy and daily postural drainage. Evaluation by CT scan usually demonstrates that the condition is fairly widespread throughout the lungs, but occasionally one lobe may be particularly badly affected. This is more likely when the bronchiectasis is secondary to chronic bronchial obstruction by an inhaled object or, more rarely, from external glandular compression. In this relatively uncommon situation, lobectomy may result in a gratifying decrease in chronic sputum production and in the frequency of recurrent infection. Resection can be technically difficult, as dense vascular adhesions surround the affected lobe.

CHEST WALL DEFORMITIES

Sternal protuberance (pectus carinatum) or retraction (pectus excavatum) may be detected and corrected in early childhood. Pectus excavatum can be associated with connective tissue disorders such as Marfan's syndrome, and with unilateral breast hypoplasia. There is often a mild degree of scoliosis present and patients characteristically stand with a hunched posture. Often, however, patients with these deformities present in their early teenage years. At this time, the deformity is exacerbated by accelerated growth and the individual becomes extremely sensitive about his or her appearance. Neither deformity is of physiological significance, and correction is only indicated when the patient's quality of life is clearly impaired because of appearance. Correction involves major surgery, with resection of the costal cartilages from the third rib downwards bilaterally in order to mobilize the sternum so that it can be repositioned. In addition, a steel bar is implanted behind the elevated sternum for excavatum cases so as to maintain the new sternal position. The patient and family must be advised that, as with all major thoracic surgery, this procedure can be associated with serious post-operative complications, including death. Also, the sternum must be given time to fuse in the corrected position, and so contact or vigorous sports are not permitted for about 9 months after surgery. In general, if repair is to be undertaken, it is best delayed until the patient is at least 17 years old, as major growth has stopped by this time, thereby reducing the chance that further deformation could follow repair.

POST-OPERATIVE CARE

The majority of major thoracic surgery is performed through a lateral thoracotomy incision, which is inherently much more painful than a median sternotomy. However, patients are not usually electively ventilated, as this is not helpful to healing lung or to lung function. Patients undergoing major thoracic surgery are therefore usually cared for in a high-dependency unit (HDU) for the first 24–48 hours following surgery. The key objectives are to enable the patient to breathe effectively and to clear secretions properly.

Pain control

Pain management during the HDU phase is achieved in two ways. An epidural catheter can be placed prior to surgery. This provides very effective pain control in the immediate post-operative period but can have disadvantages related to increased fluid requirement, nursing care, and marked pain appreciation when the epidural infusion is stopped. Many units prefer not to place an epidural catheter and to rely instead on a combination of patient-controlled morphine infusion supplemented by parenteral non-steroidal analgesics and local intercostal nerve blocks. These can be conveniently given via a paravertebral catheter inserted at surgery.

Management of secretions

It is vital that patients cough and clear secretions. This requires humidification of oxygen to prevent the secretions becoming excessively viscous, effective pain control, and considerable input from physiotherapy. Many patients undergoing thoracic surgery have been chronic heavy smokers and have impaired lung function. They have heavy production of secretions and in some cases these accumulate, threatening to cause pneumonia and respiratory failure. In this situation, a suction bronchoscopy is performed under light general anaesthesia to remove the secretions, and a mini-tracheostomy tube may be inserted via the cricothyroid membrane so that secretions can be aspirated. In severe cases, ventilation and formal tracheostomy may be required.

Fluid management

Following major thoracic surgery, the pulmonary alveolar–capillary membrane becomes relatively leaky, so that fluid tends to accumulate within the pulmonary interstitial spaces. This decreases lung compliance and increases the work of breathing. A degree of post-operative fluid restriction for the first 48 hours ensures that the left atrial pressure is kept low, thereby decreasing pulmonary venous pressure and the transcapillary gradient.

Late management

All patients receive subcutaneous heparin as prophylaxis for deep venous thrombosis until fully mobile, because the risk of thrombosis is high in thoracic surgery and the consequences of pulmonary embolism are that much worse when lung has been resected. Drains are withdrawn when air leakage stops, and patients are mobilized as rapidly as possible. In an uneventful recovery, discharge home should occur about 6–9 days after major open resection, and after 1–5 days following a videothoracoscopic minimal-access procedure. The patient's age, general health and social circumstances will influence these estimates.

CARDIAC AND PULMONARY TRANSPLANTATION

Transplantation for end-stage cardiac and pulmonary disease is discussed in Chapter 29.

26

L.H. STEWART
P. MARIAPPAN

Urological surgery

ASSESSMENT

GENERAL POINTS

Many patients presenting to a urological clinic require further investigation. Blood in the urine (haematuria) always requires a full urological assessment. Seemingly unrelated symptoms may also be urological: backache from metastatic prostatic carcinoma; fever of unknown origin from renal carcinoma; lethargy and anaemia from obstructive renal failure. However, common things being common, an elderly male complaining of difficulty in passing urine probably has outflow tract obstruction due to benign prostatic enlargement.

URINARY TRACT SYMPTOMS

Pain

Renal pain occurs in the angle between the 12th rib and the sacrospinalis muscles. Ureteric pain (or colic) typically radiates forwards and downwards into the groin, testes or labia. Acute bladder obstruction usually causes central lower abdominal pain. By contrast, chronic bladder obstruction may be virtually asymptomatic. Disease of the bladder and prostate causes ill-defined perineal or penile pains. A prostate that is grossly enlarged can cause rectal symptoms, including tenesmus. Recognition of penile and testicular pain is usually easy.

Disorders of micturition

The history aims to distinguish obstruction (e.g. poor stream), detrusor contraction (e.g. urgency), infection (e.g. frequency, dysuria) and malignancy (e.g. dark, discoloured or brown urine). Frequency is recorded numerically: D/N 6/3 (by day, six times; by night, three). Poor stream and dribbling are characteristic of urinary outflow tract obstruction. Urgency, a sudden uncontrollable urge to empty the bladder, may be associated with incontinence (urge incontinence). Stress incontinence indicates the involuntary loss of urine due to raised intra-abdominal pressure. Dysuria describes painful micturition.

EXAMINATION

Examination should not be confined to the urinary system, as cardiological, neurological and gynaecological problems may be associated with urological symptoms and signs. Many urological patients are elderly and require an assessment of their fitness for further investigations and operative treatment. Furthermore, the patient's cardiovascular status may be relevant to subsequent treatment: for example, administration of oestrogens for carcinoma of the prostate. If the patient relaxes the abdominal muscles, the kidney can be lifted with one hand placed behind the loin and compressed by the other hand pressing downwards (Fig. 27.1). The ureter cannot be palpated. An enlarged bladder rises centrally out of the pelvis, is dull to percussion and may even be visible. In men, the hernial orifices, cords, testes and epididymes are examined with the patient

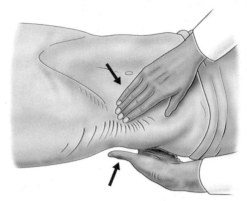

Fig. 27.1 Bimanual palpation of the right kidney.

27

standing and lying. If the foreskin is uncircumcised, it must be confirmed that it retracts and that the glans and meatus are normal. In women, the vulva, urethra and vagina must also be examined. A speculum examination should be carried out if there is any suspicion of vaginal or cervical abnormality. A full pelvic bimanual examination, whether in males or females, is best carried out under general anaesthesia with a muscle relaxant. A rectal examination is mandatory, not only to examine the prostate but also to detect abnormalities of the anal margin (haemorrhoids, fissures) and lower rectum (carcinoma).

INVESTIGATIONS

Urine

In the absence of infection, urine is normally almost protein-free. Proteinuria of more than 150 mg/24 hrs mandates further investigation. Glycosuria suggests the presence of diabetes. Screening for urinary tract infection may also be done by dipstix. Microscopic examination may detect casts or tubular epithelial cells associated with renal parenchymal disease, crystals in patients with renal calculi, or ova in schistosomiasis. Urine cytology is useful in the diagnosis and follow-up of bladder (urothelial) cancers. For micro-biological examination, the patient is asked to pass some urine into the toilet. Then, without interrupting the flow, the next part is directed into a special container, and the remainder into the toilet; hence the term midstream specimen of urine (MSU). If it is necessary to store the specimen, it should be kept at 4°C. To exclude contamination, fine-needle suprapubic aspiration of a full bladder may be required.

Blood tests

Creatinine does not begin to rise until the glomerular filtration rate (GFR) is halved. Creatinine clearance can be used to estimate GFR. Patients with chronic renal disease often have a normocytic, normochromic anaemia. The erythrocyte sedimentation rate (ESR) can be markedly raised in idiopathic retroperitoneal fibrosis, a cause of ureteric obstruction. Human chorionic gonadotrophin (HCG), α-fetoprotein (AFP) and prostate-specific antigen (PSA) are useful tumour markers.

27

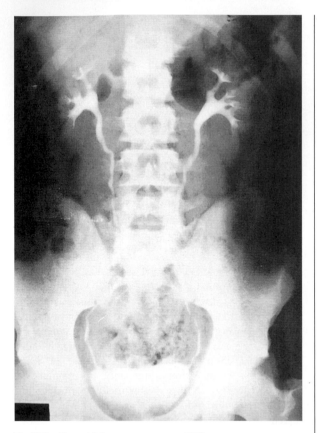

Fig. 27.2 Normal intravenous urogram (IVU).

Intravenous urography (IVU)

A plain X-ray of the abdomen and pelvis is obtained to outline the kidneys, ureters and bladder (KUB film). The lumbar spine and pelvis, as well as stones in the region of the urinary tract, will be shown. An intravenous urogram (IVU) involves injecting iodine-containing contrast material intravenously and taking serial X-rays (Fig. 27.2) to demonstrate the renal pelvis and calyces, the rate of kidney emptying, the calibre of the ureters and the bladder outline. Once the bladder has filled, a 'post-micturition' film will demonstrate bladder emptying and the amount of residual urine.

Ultrasonography

This now rivals IVU as a means of first-line imaging (Fig. 27.3). It tends to give superior information about the renal parenchyma but less about the collecting system. It also allows visualization of other related organs, such as the liver, spleen and gynaecological organs.

Special radiological investigations

To define the ureter, pelvis and calyces more clearly, a retrograde ureteropyelogram may be necessary. This involves retrograde injection of contrast material through a catheter placed in the lower ureter (Fig. 27.4). A ureteroscope can also be used to examine the ureter directly. Abnormalities of the renal vessels can be demonstrated by renal angiography. Computed tomography (CT) is now the preferred method for imaging renal tumours. A mic-

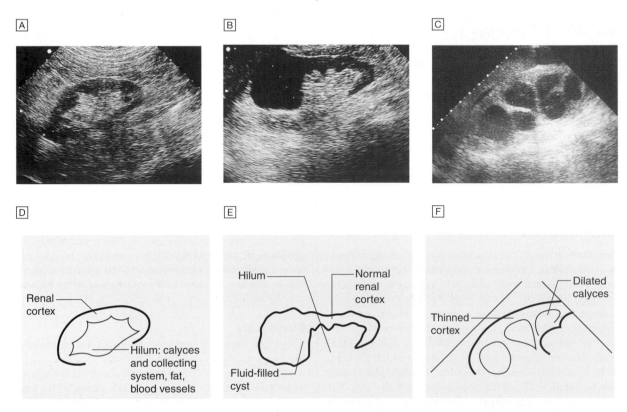

Fig. 27.3 Renal ultrasound.
A Normal kidney. B A simple cyst occupies the upper pole of an otherwise normal kidney. C The renal pelvis and calyces are dilated by a chronic obstruction to urinary outflow. The thinness of the remaining renal cortex indicates chronicity. D, E and F The diagrams beneath show the anatomical features.

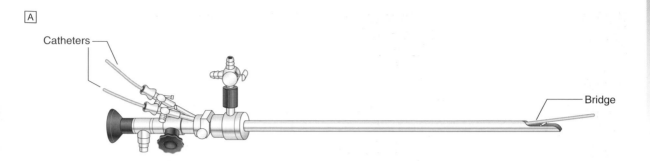

Catheters

Bridge

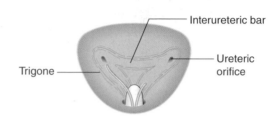

Interureteric bar

Ureteric orifice

Trigone

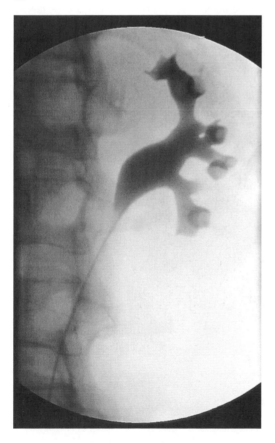

Fig. 27.4 Retrograde ureteropyelography.
A Cystoscope and ureteric catheterization. B The best views of the normal collecting system are shown by pyelography. A catheter has been passed into the left renal pelvis at cystoscopy. The anemone-like calyces are sharp-edged and normal.

turating cystourethrogram (MCU) will outline the bladder, detect ureterovesical reflux and examine the bladder neck and urethra. The bladder is filled with contrast material (via a catheter) and emptying is then studied by X-ray screening. An ascending urethrogram, in which contrast medium is injected into the urethra, can be used to define strictures but is less useful than an MCU, which provides a descending urethrogram.

Nuclear imaging

Radiolabelled substances are used for two main purposes:

1. *Detecting bony metastases from carcinoma of the prostate.* ^{99m}Tc-labelled methylene diphosphonate (MDP) is the most reliable method.
2. *Measurement of renal function.* MAG3 is now used extensively, as it is excreted by the proximal tubules

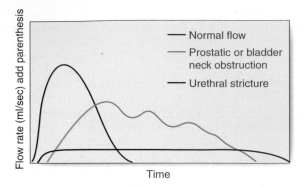

Fig. 27.5   Urinary flow rates.
The normal flow rate shows a rapid rise to maximum high-peak flow. In a typical bladder outflow obstruction due to benign prostatic hyperplasia, there is a slow rise to poor maximum flow rate and prolonged variable flow. In a typical urethral stricture, there is prolonged flow with little variability, giving a plateau- or box-shaped curve.

and in the glomerular filtration. Diethylenetetramine penta-acetic acid (DTPA) is reserved for patients in whom there is renal failure. Dimercaptosuccinic acid (DMSA) is concentrated in the renal tubule. As only 5% is excreted, static imaging can be carried out some 2–3 hours after injection. Parenchymal defects such as scars, haematomas, lacerations or ischaemia may be demonstrated. Differential renal function can be quantified from measuring the DMSA concentration in each kidney.

Urodynamic studies

The maximum urinary flow rate during micturition can be measured using a flow meter. The norm in males is 15–30 ml/s and in females 20–40 ml/s. It is important to measure flow rate when the voided volume is at least 150 ml; otherwise, the values may be misleadingly low. A flow rate of less than 10 ml/s is abnormal. The flow rate pattern can help to determine the cause of obstruction (Fig. 27.5). Measurements of flow rate can be combined with cystometry to provide a measure of residual urine, bladder capacity, the capacity at which a desire to void occurs, and the detrusor pressures when the bladder is full and during maximum flow. Spontaneous detrusor contractions during bladder filling may indicate an unstable bladder, a cause of urgency and urge incontinence. Pressures along the urethra may also be measured (urethral pressure profile). These may distinguish between bladder and urethral abnormalities in an incontinent patient, as well as neurological, pharmacological and mechanical causes of outflow tract symptoms.

Semen analysis

Microscopic examination of the semen is a basic investigation in infertile males. The specimen is collected 3 days after the last ejaculation and is examined within 2 hours. Normal semen has a volume of 2–6 ml and a sperm concentration of 20–120×10^6/ml. More than 60% of the sperm should be motile at 2 hours. The morphology, biochemistry and viability of the sperm may also be studied. In selected cases, immunological tests may help to determine the cause of infertility.

Biochemical screening for stones

All patients with recurrent urinary tract calculi should be screened for hyperparathyroidism, idiopathic hypercalciuria, hyperoxaluria and cystinuria. Serum calcium, phosphate, oxalate and uric acid are measured. More detailed investigation requires 24-hour collection of urine for determination of calcium, phosphate, oxalate and uric acid excretion. The composition of passed or removed stones should be analysed to determine their metabolic type.

UPPER URINARY TRACT (KIDNEY AND URETER)

ANATOMY

The two kidneys lie retroperitoneally on the posterior abdominal wall. Each is approximately 12 cm long, 6 cm wide and 3 cm thick. The upper pole of the kidney lies on the diaphragm, which separates it from the pleura and the 11th and 12th ribs. Below this, it lies on the psoas, quadratus lumborum and transversus abdominis muscles from medial to lateral (Fig. 27.6). Anteriorly, the right kidney is covered by the liver, the second part of the duodenum and the ascending colon. The spleen, stomach, tail of pancreas, left colon and small bowel overlie the left kidney. The renal hilum lies medially and transmits from front to back the renal vein, renal artery and renal pelvis. The ureter begins at the renal pelvis and runs for 25 cm to the bladder. The abdominal ureter lies on the medial edge of the psoas muscle, which separates it from the tips of the transverse processes. It then crosses the bifurcation of the common

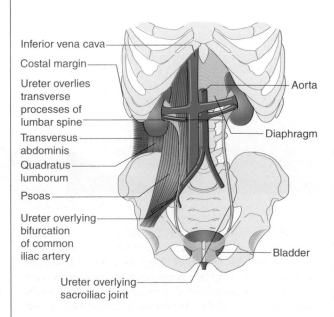

Fig. 27.6   Anatomy of kidneys and ureters.

iliac artery, which separates it from the sacroiliac joint, to enter the pelvis. The pelvic ureter runs on the lateral pelvic wall to just in front of the ischial spine, when it then turns medially and forward to enter the bladder. In the male, it is crossed by the vas deferens. In the female, it lies close to the lateral fornix of the vagina and is crossed by the uterine vessels, where it is vulnerable to damage during hysterectomy. The section of ureter that lies within the bladder wall functions as a flap valve to prevent reflux. Stones tend to impact at the three points where the ureter narrows: namely, the pelviureteric junction, the pelvic brim and the ureteric orifice.

PHYSIOLOGY

The healthy kidney can produce between 0.3 and 17 ml of urine per minute, depending on the state of hydration, but on average produces 1 ml of urine per minute. This is transported down the ureter by 4–5 peristaltic waves per minute to reach the bladder, where it is stored without reflux up the ureters.

TRAUMA

Kidney and renal pedicle

Penetrating injuries
Gunshot or stab wounds may injure the kidney and renal pedicle. Inadvertent damage during percutaneous access surgery or needle biopsy can cause severe bleeding and, rarely, an arteriovenous fistula. Open lacerations of the parenchyma, collecting system or pedicle are usually associated with other injuries within the abdomen.

Blunt injury
This may be caused by a fall against a hard object or by a blow to the loin. These injuries are commonly associated with fractured ribs and occasionally damage to the spleen (left) or liver (right).

Deceleration injury
Rapid deceleration—for example, during a road traffic accident—tends to damage the renal pedicle rather than the parenchyma, often through the development of intimal tears, resulting in thrombosis of the renal artery.

Late effects
These include perirenal collection of urine (urinoma), scarring of the kidney or renal artery stenosis (hypertension). Hydronephrosis may be an early or a late complication.

Clinical features
Whereas a gunshot wound is obvious, a penetrating knife wound may appear trivial, even if it involves several important deep structures. Commonly, the patient presents with a history of injury to the loin followed by haematuria. Gross haematuria is usually, but not always, associated with more severe injuries. Severe injuries are characterized by a mass in the loin that is increasing in size, and by signs of shock. These patients often have other serious injuries. Damage to the renal pedicle may cause few signs, or the patient may be severely shocked.

Investigations
Urgent intravenous urography is indicated to determine the extent of renal damage. Urographic information about the other kidney must be obtained prior to emergency surgery. With mild contusion, the urogram may be normal. With increasing damage, there is distortion of the renal outline and calyces, and extravasation of contrast. A CT scan will more accurately determine the extent of the injury. Non-visualization of the kidney implies serious damage to the pedicle and is an indication for angiography. Angiography is also helpful in assessing parenchymal/vascular damage in patients who are likely to need surgical exploration. Ultrasonography and isotope scanning are of more help in the follow-up of an injured kidney than in immediate care.

Management
A shocked patient must be resuscitated. Renal contusion is managed conservatively by bed rest and observation. Lacerations that are part of an open injury are explored to determine the extent of the damage. Those due to closed injury may be treated conservatively at first, but should be explored if haematuria persists or loin swelling increases. Severe lacerations with fragmentation of the kidney must be explored if the patient is shocked. The extent of operation depends on the severity of the laceration. Whenever possible, partial rather than total nephrectomy is carried out; this is, in fact, rarely possible.

Ureter

Mechanism of injury
The ureter is occasionally damaged by a knife or a bullet, but always in association with other injuries. The principal cause of open injury to a ureter is inadvertent damage during an operation: most commonly, hysterectomy. Injury may lead to complete or partial obstruction, with subsequent hydronephrosis, or to a urinary fistula. A fistula may occur immediately (if the damage is not recognized at operation) or later (if the injury to the ureter causes late necrosis). Urine may leak to the skin (cutaneous fistula), form a 'urinoma' or, after a gynaecological operation, leak through the vagina (ureterovaginal fistula). The ureter is occasionally damaged in major road traffic accidents and during endoscopic procedures to treat stones.

Clinical features
The patient may complain of renal pain, but even a completely obstructed kidney may cause few symptoms. If there is infection in the obstructed kidney, the patient may be extremely ill, with pain, fever and rigors. Any excessive 'watery' discharge from a wound is suspicious.

Investigations
A rapid way to determine whether a watery discharge is urine or serum is to measure its concentration of urea. Alternatively, intravenous methylene blue quickly appears in a urinary leak. An IVU will show the site of the damage. Occasionally, cystoscopy and ureteric catheterization are indicated.

Management

A percutaneous nephrostomy tube should be placed to drain the kidney on the affected side and minimize further leakage from the distal ureter. It may now be possible to pass a stent up or down the ureter if there is only a partial injury; this may lead to complete recovery. If conservative management fails, surgical exploration and repair is required.

RENAL CYSTS

Simple cysts

These are usually single, almost always asymptomatic, and often found incidentally on IVU or ultrasound. A cyst is easily differentiated from carcinoma by ultrasound. Malignant change is only seen in complex cysts containing multiple septa.

Polycystic kidney disease

This is an autosomal dominant congenital anomaly that affects both kidneys and often leads to chronic renal failure in middle life. Despite their very large size, the cystic kidneys cause few symptoms. Infection or bleeding into a cyst can occur and may require exploration to relieve symptoms. The condition may cause haematuria.

BENIGN TUMOURS

Renal adenomas are small and are usually an incidental finding. Haemangiomas are a rare cause of dramatic haematuria.

NEPHROBLASTOMAS

Epidemiology

This tumour usually occurs in children under 4 years of age, and is the most common childhood urological malignancy, with an incidence of 7 per million children per year. The tumour is probably derived from embryonic mesodermal tissue, and microscopically has a mixed appearance of spindle cells, epithelial cells and muscle fibres. Growth is rapid and there is early local spread, including invasion of the renal vein. Invasion of the renal pelvis occurs late, and so haematuria is seen in only 15% of cases. Distant metastases most commonly appear in the lungs, liver and bones. Tumours presenting in the first year of life have a better prognosis.

Clinical features

The cardinal sign is a large abdominal mass. Some of the unusual clinical features associated with a renal carcinoma in adults, such as fever or hypertension, may be present.

Investigations

A CT scan of the abdomen and chest is essential for diagnosis and staging. The main differential diagnosis is from neuroblastoma affecting the adrenal, but other causes of a large kidney, such as hydronephrosis and cystic disease, must also be considered. The tumour is bilateral in 5–10% of cases.

Management

Transabdominal nephrectomy with wide excision of the mass is carried out after preliminary ligation of the renal pedicle. This is followed by chemotherapy using actinomycin D and vincristine. Radiotherapy is reserved for residual disease. In some centres, pre-operative chemotherapy is used to downsize the tumour prior to resection. As a result of this treatment, the 5-year survival rate has improved from 10% to 80%.

RENAL ADENOCARCINOMA

Epidemiology

This is the most common malignant tumour of the kidney. The incidence is 16 cases per 100 000 and it is twice as common in males. It is uncommon before the age of 40 years and has a peak incidence between 65 and 75 years of age. The tumour arises from renal tubules. There is early spread into the renal pelvis, causing haematuria. Invasion of the renal vein, often extending into the inferior vena cava, also occurs early. Direct spread into perinephric tissues is common, so that the whole fascial envelope and kidney should be removed en bloc. Lymphatic spread occurs to para-aortic nodes, but blood-borne metastases (which may be solitary) may develop almost anywhere.

Clinical features

The triad of pain, haematuria and a mass is an important but late feature, occurring in only 15% of cases; 60% present with haematuria, 40% with loin pain and only 25% with

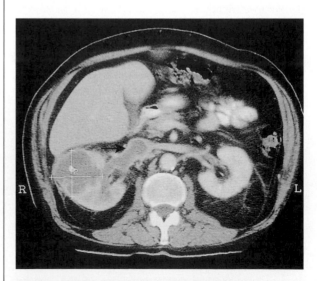

Fig. 27.7   Contrast-enhanced CT scan of renal cancer.
The right kidney is expanded by a low-density cancer that fails to take up the contrast. Tumour is seen extending into the renal vein and inferior vena cava (arrow).

BOX 27.1 RENAL CARCINOMA

- Renal carcinoma is by far the most common malignant renal tumour and is twice as common in males
- The carcinoma arises in the renal tubules and spreads early to the renal pelvis, producing haematuria. Later spread involves the renal vein (with blood-stream dissemination), perinephric invasion and lymphatic spread
- The clinical presentation is very varied. The triad of pain, haematuria and a mass may be late features, and early systemic effects include fever, polycythaemia, disordered coagulation and pyrexia of unknown origin
- The key investigations are ultrasonography, chest X-ray and contrast CT
- Treatment consists of radical nephrectomy; the tumour is not radiosensitive. The natural history of renal carcinoma is very variable and excision of solitary metastases may be worth while

a mass. Patients may also present with pyrexia of unknown origin (PUO), raised ESR, polycythaemia, disorders of coagulation, and abnormalities of plasma proteins and liver function tests, or with neuromyopathy due to secretion of renin, erythropoietin, parathormone and gonadotrophins.

Investigations

The initial investigation is ultrasound, followed by a staging contrast CT scan of the abdomen and chest (Fig. 27.7).

Management

Radical nephrectomy, including the perirenal fascial envelope and ipsilateral para-aortic lymph nodes, is performed whenever possible, as it may abolish systemic effects and lead to regression of a solitary metastasis; the tumour is resistant to radiotherapy and chemotherapy. Immunotherapy using interferon and interleukin-2 may be of benefit.

TRANSITIONAL CELL CARCINOMA (TCC) OF THE UPPER TRACTS

This arises from the urothelium that lines the whole of the urinary tract from collecting system to urethra. These tumours are common in the bladder (see below) but uncommon in the upper tracts. They tend to present with haematuria and/or obstruction of the upper tract, and are diagnosed on IVU. Treatment is by nephroureterectomy and regular surveillance of the bladder. If the tumour is solitary and low-grade, it may be treated endoscopically; however, surveillance remains problematic.

RENAL AND URETERIC CALCULI

Types of stone

Stones that form in the kidney are of two main types: infective and metabolic.

An infective stone is whitish and chalky; crumbles or breaks easily; is composed mainly of calcium, ammonia and magnesium phosphates; develops wherever drainage is impaired; and is usually associated with an anatomical abnormality such as a diverticulum or with long-term recumbency or paraplegia. The formation of infective stones indicates an established infection that cannot be eradicated by antibiotics alone. As the stone enlarges, drainage is further impaired and there is progressive damage to the kidney.

A metabolic stone, commonly of calcium oxalate, is usually hard and dark with an irregular sharp surface. It develops as a result of an abnormality of the composition of the urine. There may be abnormal concentration of normal constituents (e.g. due to dehydration); excess excretion of normal constituents (e.g. calcium in hyperparathyroidism or uric acid in gout); or the urine may contain abnormal constituents (as in cystinuria). It is likely that several aetiological factors must occur together or in sequence for a stone to form. All patients with recurrent urinary calculi should be screened for metabolic abnormalities as described above. Up to 80% of the stones seen in the UK are mixed calcium oxalate/phosphate stones. Some 10% are magnesium ammonium phosphate stones with a variable proportion of calcium. Most of the remainder are uric acid stones. Cystine and xanthine stones are rare.

Clinical features

Renal pain, renal colic or ureteric colic is characteristically unilateral. Renal pain is dull and aching, whereas ureteric colic is acute and severe, and occurs in waves that pass down the line of the ureter. A stone may cause bleeding or there may be symptoms of urinary tract infection. However, a stone in the kidney may remain silent, even one large enough to fill the pelvis and calyces (a 'staghorn' calculus).

Investigations

An IVU usually provides all the necessary information on the position of the stone (Fig. 27.8). Routine haematological and biochemical tests are needed to assess renal function and to exclude metabolic causes. A urine sample is cultured to determine whether there is infection. If obstruction is acute, its relief is the prime clinical need; if it is chronic and has caused renal damage, the surgical approach depends on the function of the affected kidney. This is best determined by radioisotope methods.

Management

Symptomatic treatment should be instituted as soon as the diagnosis is confirmed. Intramuscular diclofenac, a non-steroidal anti-inflammatory, is the most effective analgesic; pethidine is an alternative. The likelihood of spontaneous passage depends on the size of the stone and on its smoothness. A stone less than 0.5 cm in diameter should pass down the ureter. If it becomes fixed (causing increasing hydroureter and hydronephrosis), if the urine is infected or if the patient has increasing pain and fever, treatment is necessary. Extracorporeal shock-wave lithotripsy (ESWL), the technique of focusing external shock waves to break up stones, has revolutionized the

27

27

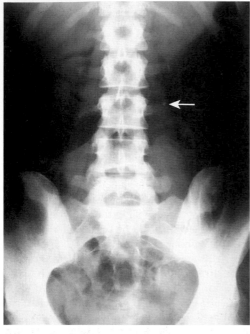

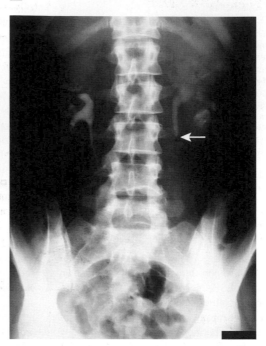

Fig. 27.8   IVU showing ureteric stone.

A Eighty per cent of stones are visible on a plain X-ray (arrow). B The contrast excreted by the kidney in an IVU clearly shows the obstruction caused by the stone in the ureter (arrow).

treatment of renal and ureteric stones (Fig. 27.9). If a stone can be visualized on X-ray or ultrasound, then it can be treated by ESWL. Other stones can be visualized directly by passing a fine telescope up the ureter (ureteroscope) and the stones may be either broken up or removed intact. Some stones in the kidney that are unlikely to pass even if broken up are best treated by direct puncture of the kidney, insertion of a sheath and removal under vision with a nephroscope (percutaneous nephrolithotomy, PCNL). Stones within a kidney can be the cause of renal destruction, especially if the urine is infected. If the damage is so severe that the kidney contributes less than 10% of total

renal function, then a nephrectomy is recommended. It is now very rare to remove stones from the renal tract at open operation.

UPPER TRACT OBSTRUCTION

Obstruction may be due to extrinsic, intrinsic or intraluminal causes (Table 27.1). In the kidney, stones within the pelvi-calyceal system and a congenital abnormality of the pelviureteric junction (see below) are the main causes of obstruction leading to hydronephrosis. More rarely, a sloughed renal papilla, blood clot or tumour may be the cause.

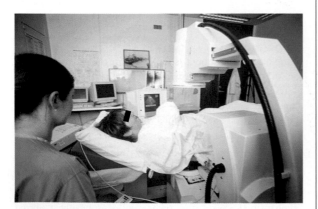

Fig. 27.9   Extracorporeal shock-wave lithotriptor.

Table 27.1   CAUSES OF URINARY TRACT OBSTRUCTION
Extrinsic • Retroperitoneal fibrosis • External pressure (e.g. carcinoma of the cervix, prostate)
Intrinsic • Transitional cell tumours • Tuberculosis/schistosomiasis • Ureterocoele • Ectopic ureter
Intraluminal • Calculi

BOX 27.2 URINARY TRACT OBSTRUCTION

Common causes of obstruction of the lower outflow tract

- Benign prostatic hyperplasia
- Prostatic cancer
- Bladder cancer involving the bladder neck
- Bladder-neck obstruction (dyssynergia, infection, neurological disorders)
- Urethral obstruction (congenital posterior urethral valves, blocked urinary catheter, trauma, infection, stricture)

Common causes of obstruction of the upper urinary tract

- Renal and ureteric calculi (80% are calcium oxalate/phosphate stones)
- Pelviureteric junction obstruction (idiopathic hydronephrosis)
- Retroperitoneal fibrosis (idiopathic/malignant infiltration/radiotherapy)
- Transitional cell carcinoma (with or without bleeding and clot)
- Congenital abnormalities (e.g. ectopic ureter, ureterocoele)
- Infections (notably schistosomiasis and tuberculosis)

PELVIURETERIC JUNCTION OBSTRUCTION (IDIOPATHIC HYDRONEPHROSIS)

Narrowing of the junction between the renal pelvis and the ureter is a common cause of hydronephrosis. As the aetiology is obscure, the term 'idiopathic' hydronephrosis is appropriate. This condition is seen in very young children. It is likely to be congenital and is often bilateral, but gross hydronephrosis may present at any age.

Clinical features

Idiopathic hydronephrosis may produce a large painless mass in the loin; in its grossest form, the volume of urine in the hydronephrotic sac may simulate free fluid in the peritoneal cavity. The more usual moderate hydronephrosis causes ill-defined renal pain or ache that may be exacerbated by drinking large volumes of liquid. The patient may regard these symptoms as 'indigestion'. Rarely, there may be no symptoms.

Investigations

An IVU, with or without delayed films, provides sufficient information in many cases. The calibre of the ureter is normal. There are a few patients in whom there is doubt as to whether the dilatation of the pelvis and calyces is truly obstructive in nature. Methods to resolve this include urography and renography during induced diuresis, and antegrade pressure–flow measurements.

Management

Operation (pyeloplasty) is designed to remove the obstructing tissue and refashion the pelviureteric junction (PUJ) so that the lower part of the renal pelvis drains freely into the ureter (Fig. 27.10). Endoscopic alternatives to pyeloplasty have been developed and give as good results in most cases.

Outcome

It is not possible to predict the degree of recovery of renal function after the relief of obstruction, but it is generally felt that a kidney contributing less than 10% of total renal function should be removed.

RETROPERITONEAL FIBROSIS

Pathology

Fibrosis of the retroperitoneal connective tissues may encircle and compress the ureter(s), causing hydroureter and hydronephrosis. Fibrosis occurs in three groups of conditions:

- *Idiopathic*. In this, the largest group, the fibrosis extends across the pelvic brim to involve the ureters, the vena cava and even the aorta. The aetiology is unknown, although it may be associated with methysergide or analgesic abuse. Mediastinal fibrosis and Dupuytren's contracture may coexist.
- *Malignant infiltration*. The fibrosis contains malignant cells that have metastasized from primary sites such as the breast, stomach, pancreas and colon.
- *Reactive fibrosis*. Radiotherapy to the pelvic organs, resolving blood clot after major vascular or other surgical procedures, or extravasation of sclerosants (e.g. phenol for a nerve block) can lead to fibrotic change in the retroperitoneum.

As the gross appearance of fibrosis in all three groups may be similar, biopsy of the tissue is essential for diagnosis.

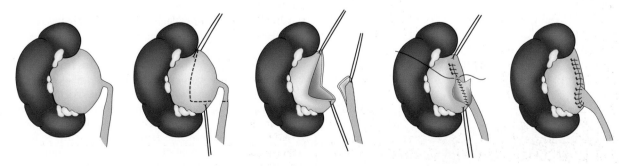

Fig. 27.10   Anderson–Hynes pyeloplasty.

Clinical features

Ureteric obstruction may cause symptoms similar to idiopathic hydronephrosis: namely, ill-defined renal pain or ache. Some patients complain of low backache.

Investigations

An IVU shows hydronephrosis and usually hydroureter down to the level of the obstruction. The anatomy of the ureter is often difficult to define, but it is usually pulled medially. It is rarely necessary to pass a ureteric catheter up to the kidney, although it is characteristic of retroperitoneal fibrosis that a ureteric catheter will pass easily through what appears to be a severe obstruction. A markedly raised ESR is found in more than 50% of cases with idiopathic fibrosis.

Management

Relief of obstruction may be difficult. The ureter is dissected out of the fibrous sheet of tissue (ureterolysis) and wrapped in omentum to prevent further involvement. Although obstruction may regress with steroids, these agents are reserved for recurrent obstruction.

MISCELLANEOUS CAUSES OF OBSTRUCTION

Congenital abnormalities

All microbiologically proven urinary tract infections (UTIs) in boys and recurrent proven UTIs in girls should be investigated for evidence of underlying structural urinary tract abnormalities that may cause mechanical or functional obstruction. These include ectopic ureter with a duplex kidney (Fig. 27.11) and associated vesicoureteric reflux (VUR), PUJ obstruction causing hydronephrosis, and ureterocele causing vesicoureteric junction obstruction. Initial imaging investigations should include a urinary tract ultrasound scan and a DMSA radioisotope study. Where reflux is suspected on the basis of these two initial investigations, a micturating cystogram or a DTPA reflux study (in toilet-trained children) should be undertaken. VUR is graded from I (mild reflux into the lower ureter) to V (severe reflux with dilatation of the ureter, renal pelvis and calyces). The milder grades of reflux (I and II) are managed with prophylactic antibiotics to prevent renal injury and scarring. More severe grades require a surgical procedure to prevent the reflux if breakthrough infection persists.

Unusual infections

Tuberculosis of the urinary tract is a rare cause of stricture of the ureter and even of complete obstruction. This process may be silent and 'autonephrectomy' may be detected at a later date. Schistosomiasis affecting the urinary tract is common in parts of Africa and the Middle East. Ureteric fibrosis and obstruction are part of the process that can affect the whole of the urinary tract. Many patients present in such an advanced state of disease that surgical treatment is not feasible. Both infections require specific drug treatment. When the ureters are involved and obstructed, a variety of reconstructive surgical procedures may be used to conserve renal function and correct obstruction and/or reflux.

LOWER URINARY TRACT (BLADDER, PROSTATE AND URETHRA)

ANATOMY

The bladder is a muscular reservoir that receives urine via the ureters and expels it via the urethra. In children up to 4 years of age, it lies predominantly in the abdomen; in the adult it is a pelvic organ, well protected in the bony pelvis. Superiorly, the bladder is covered with peritoneum, which separates it from coils of small bowel, the sigmoid colon and, in the female, the body of the uterus. Posteriorly lie the rectum, the vas deferens and seminal vesicles in the male, and the vagina and supravaginal cervix in the female. Inferiorly, the neck of the bladder transmits the urethra and fuses with the prostate in the male and with the pelvic fascia in the female.

The bladder is composed of whorls of detrusor muscle, which in the male become circular at the bladder neck. They are richly supplied with sympathetic nerves that cause contraction during ejaculation, thereby preventing semen from entering the bladder (retrograde ejaculation). There is no such sphincter in the female. The bladder is lined with specialized waterproof epithelium, the urothelium. This is thrown into folds over most of the bladder, except the trigone where it is smooth.

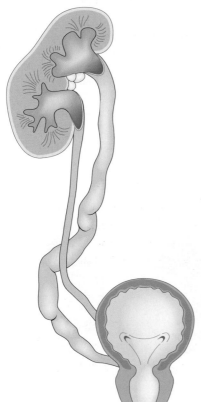

Fig. 27.11 Duplex kidney.

The male urethra is 20 cm long; the prostatic urethra descends for 3 cm through the prostate gland, and the membranous urethra is 1–2 cm long and intimately associated with the main urethral sphincter, the rhabdosphincter. The spongy urethra is 15 cm long and is surrounded by the corpus spongiosus throughout its complete length, opening on the tip of the glans penis as the external meatus. The spongy urethra is further subdivided into the proximal bulbar urethra and the distal penile urethra. The female urethra is 3–4 cm long, descending through the pelvic floor surrounded by the urethral sphincter and embedded in the anterior vaginal wall to open between the clitoris and the vagina.

In the male, the prostate is pyramidal, with its base uppermost. It resembles the size and shape of a chestnut and surrounds the prostatic urethra. Traditionally described as having a median and two lateral lobes, it is better considered as being composed of a small central and a larger peripheral zone (Fig. 27.12).

PHYSIOLOGY

Neurological control of micturition

Parasympathetic fibres arising as pre-ganglionic axons from S2 to S4 relay through ganglia, mostly within the detrusor muscle. Post-ganglionic nerves supply the detrusor muscle. These (cholinergic) nerves stimulate detrusor contraction.

Sympathetic nerves arise from T10 to L2 and relay in the pelvic ganglia. Their exact role in the control of micturition is unclear. It is known that α-adrenergic receptors and their nerve terminals are found mainly in the smooth muscle of the bladder neck and proximal urethra, whereas β-receptors are found in the fundus of the bladder. The α-receptors respond to noradrenaline (norepinephrine) by stimulating contraction, whereas the β-receptors relax the smooth muscle. It is possible that the sympathetic neurons play a role in both urethral closure and detrusor relaxation during the filling phase of the micturition cycle.

27

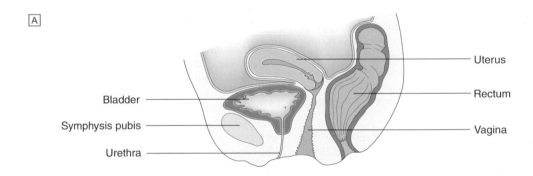

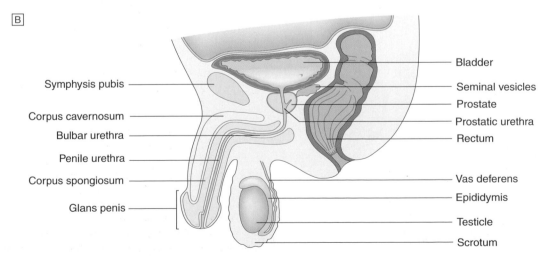

Fig. 27.12 Anatomy of the lower urinary tracts.
A Female. B Male.

27

The distal sphincter mechanism is innervated from the sacral segments S2–S4 by somatic motor fibres that reach the sphincter either by the pelvic plexus or via the pudendal nerves. Afferent nerves are carried in both the parasympathetic and pudendal pathways and transmit sensory impulses from the bladder, urethra and pelvic floor. These sensory impulses pass to the cerebral cortex and the micturition centre, where they produce reflex bladder relaxation and increased tone in the distal sphincter, so helping maintain continence. Cortical control is a basic part of the micturition cycle described below. The higher centres suppress detrusor contractions and their main function is to inhibit micturition until an appropriate time. Afferent impulses pass to the brain via the posterior columns. The higher centres are situated in the pons, the periaqueductal grey, the anterior cingulate gyrus and the pre-optic area of the hypothalamus.

The micturition cycle

The micturition cycle has two phases.

Storage (or filling) phase

Due to the high compliance (elasticity) of the detrusor muscle, the bladder fills steadily without a rise in intravesical pressure. As the volume of urine increases, stretch receptors in the bladder wall are stimulated, resulting in reflex bladder relaxation and reflex increased sphincter tone. At approximately three-quarters of bladder capacity, sensation produces a desire to void. Voluntary control is now exerted over the desire to void, which temporarily disappears. Compliance of the detrusor allows further increase in capacity until the next desire to void. Just how often this desire needs to be inhibited depends on many factors, not the least of which is finding a suitable place in which to void.

Emptying (or micturition) phase

The act of micturition is initiated first by voluntary and then by reflex relaxation of the pelvic floor and distal sphincter mechanisms, followed by reflex detrusor contraction. These actions are coordinated by the pontine mic-

turition centre. Intravesical pressure remains greater than urethral pressure until the bladder is empty.

The normal control of micturition requires coordinated reflex activity of autonomic and somatic nerves, as described above. These responses depend on normal anatomical structures and normal innervation. There are thus two main types of disorders of micturition: structural and neurogenic. Examples are extensive carcinoma of the prostate that has damaged the sphincter mechanism (structural), and spinal cord injury that has damaged the innervation (neurogenic).

TRAUMA

Bladder

Open injuries

The bladder may rupture as a result of a penetrating injury to the lower abdomen, in which case the bladder, urethra and rectum are all likely to be damaged. The bladder may also be injured in the course of extensive cancer surgery in the pelvis. Occasionally, a large inguinal or femoral hernia may include the bladder in the medial wall of the sac and it may be damaged during repair of the hernia. Unrecognized damage during surgical procedures may lead to a wound fistula, a vesicovaginal fistula or a vesicocolic fistula.

Closed injuries

Intraperitoneal rupture typically occurs in a patient who has been drinking alcohol, has a full bladder and is assaulted and kicked in the abdomen. The dome of the bladder ruptures and urine extravasates into the peritoneum, causing intestinal ileus and abdominal distension. Extraperitoneal rupture is usually due to a major road traffic accident in which the pelvis has also been fractured when the bladder is not full, but may follow endoscopic resection of the prostate or a bladder tumour (Fig. 27.13).

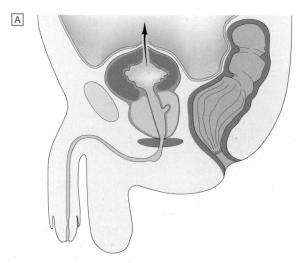 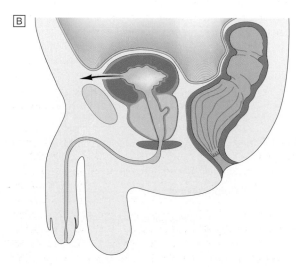

Fig. 27.13 Rupture of the bladder.
Ⓐ Intraperitoneal. Ⓑ Extraperitoneal.

Clinical features

The ileus and distension that occur with intraperitoneal rupture of the bladder are often detected late because of the circumstances surrounding the injury. However, the patient will soon note that he is not passing urine and seek advice. Extraperitoneal extravasation of urine, if part of a major accident, adds to what already are severe pelvic injuries. When the leak occurs during an endoscopic procedure, the patient later complains of suprapubic pain with varying degrees of lower abdominal tenderness.

Investigations

Generally, the circumstances of the bladder injury establish the diagnosis. If confirmation of injury is required, water-soluble contrast is injected via a urethral catheter and the bladder examined on the X-ray screen (cystogram).

Management

Intraperitoneal rupture demands laparotomy. The bladder rupture is oversewn, the viscera are examined for other injuries, and drainage by a suprapubic catheter is established. Extraperitoneal rupture of the bladder may require surgical exploration to remove blood and serum, correct bony injuries, close the tear and establish bladder drainage. However, if a small extraperitoneal rupture is recognized during any pelvic operation, a urethral catheter to keep the bladder empty is usually all that is needed. Very rarely, a suprapubic drain is required.

Urethra

Open injuries

Penetrating injuries resulting in damage to the anterior or posterior urethra are rare.

Closed injuries

Damage to the anterior urethra is typically due to falling astride a hard object, although a kick can cause a similar injury. There may be contusion or laceration, and a laceration may be partial or complete. The mechanism of injury to the posterior urethra is similar to that of extraperitoneal rupture of the bladder: for example, a road traffic accident. For such an injury to damage the urethra, a fracture of the pubis or fracture–dislocation of the pelvis must occur. Both the posterior urethra and bladder are damaged in 10% of cases. The urethral rupture may be partial or complete. Injury to the posterior urethra may also be iatrogenic. Inexpert instrumentation can tear the mucosa and cause a false passage, with subsequent stricture formation (Fig. 27.14).

Clinical features

Anterior urethral injuries are usually located at the bulb, so that the patient presents with a perineal haematoma. If this becomes infected, there may be sloughing of the skin, urethra and even the scrotal tissues. Because of the mechanism of injury, patients with posterior urethral tears are usually shocked and require resuscitation before a detailed assessment can be made. If the patient has passed clear urine, the bladder and urethra are probably intact. If there is blood at the external meatus, urethral injury must be suspected. A distended bladder can occur

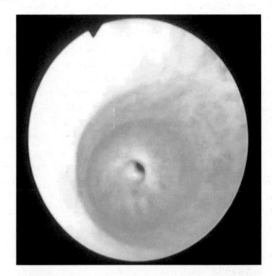

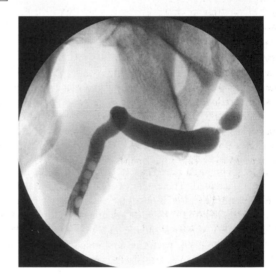

Fig. 27.14 Stricture of posterior urethra.
A Endoscopic view. B Urethrogram.

because of spasm of the urethral sphincter or because of a torn posterior urethra.

Investigations

If the physical signs suggest an anterior urethral injury and the patient has passed clear urine, no further steps need be taken. If there is blood at the external meatus or the urine is blood-stained, a urethrogram using water-soluble contrast material may demonstrate the extravasation (Fig. 27.15) and may worsen the injury. A catheter should never be passed in the emergency room 'just to see'. If the patient passes clear urine, nothing further should be done. If the urine is blood-stained, retrograde urethrography may be carried out. The radiological distinction between a rupture of the membranous urethra and an extraperitoneal bladder rupture may be difficult.

27

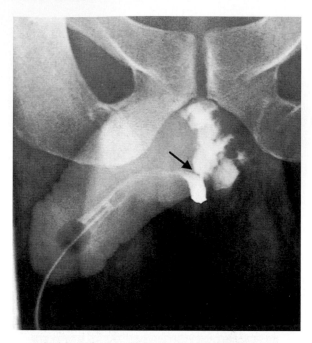

Fig. 27.15   Ascending ureterogram in urethral rupture.
Contrast is seen extravasating at the site of the disrupted urethra (arrow).

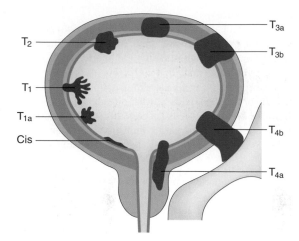

Fig. 27.16   T categories of bladder tumour.
(Cis = carcinoma in situ)

Management

All patients with an injury to the bulb of the urethra have a perineal haematoma. If the injury is only a contusion, this will resolve, but prophylactic antibiotics are indicated. A large haematoma may need to be drained if the urethra has been lacerated. The extent of injury should be defined and the urethra repaired if possible. A urethral or suprapubic catheter drains the bladder. Treatment of a posterior urethral injury depends on the expertise available. It is quite acceptable to perform a suprapubic cystostomy and deal with the injury to the urethra at a later date. If laparotomy is necessary for other reasons, this may give an opportunity to pass a catheter. If the rupture is incomplete, the catheter will act as a splint. If the rupture is complete, the ends of the urethra can be approximated and splinted by the catheter. The late complications of these injuries are stricture and impotence.

BLADDER TUMOURS

Pathology

The vast majority of bladder tumours arise from the urothelium or transitional cell lining, which it shares in continuum with the renal pelvis and the proximal urethra. The urothelium is exposed to chemical carcinogens excreted in the urine, such as naphthylamines and benzidine, which were extensively used in the chemical and dye industries until their carcinogenic properties were recognized. The bladder is more susceptible to urinary carcinogens, as urine is stored in the bladder for relatively long periods of time.

Almost all tumours are transitional cell carcinomas. Squamous carcinoma may occur in urothelium that has undergone metaplasia, usually due to chronic inflammation or irritation caused by a stone or schistosomiasis. An adeno-carcinoma is a rarity but may occur in a urachal remnant in the dome of the bladder, or from local infiltration, e.g. bowel cancer. The prevalence of transitional cell carcinoma in the bladder is 45 cases per 100 000, and it is three times more common in men than women. The appearance of a transitional cell tumour ranges from a delicate papillary structure to a solid ulcerating mass. The appearance correlates well with subsequent behaviour, in that papillary tumours are relatively benign cancers, whereas those that ulcerate are much more aggressive.

Staging

A biopsy is essential to confirm the diagnosis, determine the degree of cell differentiation (i.e. the grade), and assess the depth to which the tumour has penetrated the bladder wall (i.e the stage). The TNM system of tumour classification is also applicable to bladder tumours. Assessment of the primary tumour (T) is of prime clinical importance and requires bimanual examination under anaesthesia to judge the degree of penetration through the bladder wall. This is especially important for T_2 and T_3 tumours (Fig. 27.16). Clinical examination, urography and CT are used to assess the involvement of regional and juxtaregional lymph nodes (N). Assessment of distant metastases (M) requires clinical examination and radiography. Histopathological examination allows a much more accurate assessment of the tumour and guides the choice of treatment. Biopsy gives accurate information on superficial tumours, but invasive tumours cannot be assessed precisely without examining the full thickness of the bladder wall.

Clinical features

More than 80% of patients have haematuria, which is usually painless (Fig. 27.17). It should be assumed that

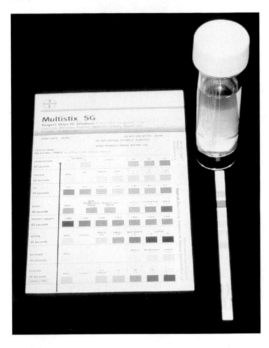

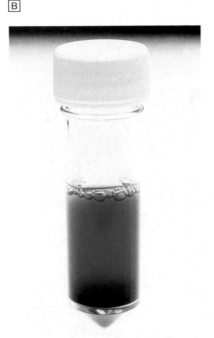

Fig. 27.17 Haematuria.
A Microscopic. B
Macroscopic.

such bleeding is from a tumour until proved otherwise. In women, symptoms of cystitis are so common that occasional bleeding may be thought to be part of an infective problem. In men, symptoms of bladder outflow obstruction are common and may include bleeding. Bleeding at the end of micturition, and especially the passage of pink/red urine, suggests that the bladder is the site of bleeding. Uniformly dark-coloured urine suggests that the source is in the upper tract. A tumour at the lower end of a ureter or a bladder tumour involving the ureteric orifice may cause obstructive symptoms, but there are often few symptoms apart from discolouration of the urine. Examination is usually unhelpful. Rectal examination detects only advanced tumours.

Investigations

Because upper tract tumours are much less common, they may be overlooked in the presence of an obvious bladder tumour. Both may occur together, and the whole of the urothelium must be examined on the IVU (Fig. 27.18). If there is any suspicious filling defect in the ureter, a retrograde ureteropyelogram is necessary. Cystourethroscopy and examination under anaesthesia are the basic investigations for all suspected bladder tumours (Fig. 27.19). With the patient relaxed under general anaesthesia, the bladder and tumour are examined bimanually to determine the depth of spread. The physical features of the tumour(s) are noted, the normal bladder mucosa is inspected and the tumour is fully resected if possible. If not, biopsies are taken from the tumour and any other suspicious areas.

Management

Superficial bladder tumours (T_a, T_1)

These can be treated by endoscopic diathermy but, whenever possible, biopsy followed by formal transurethral resection of the tumour (TURT) is recommended. Intravesical chemotherapy (epirubicin, mitomycin C) is useful to treat multiple low-grade bladder tumours and to reduce the recurrence rate (EBM 27.1). Regular check cystoscopies are required. Recurrences are mostly treated

Fig. 27.18 Filling defect on IVU due to bladder tumour.

27

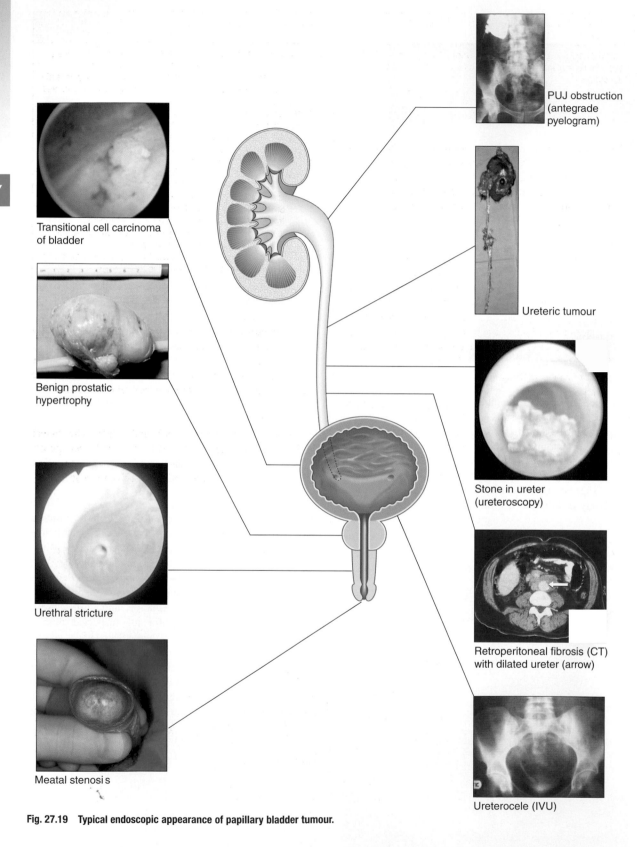

Transitional cell carcinoma
of bladder

Benign prostatic
hypertrophy

Urethral stricture

Meatal stenosis

PUJ obstruction
(antegrade
pyelogram)

Ureteric tumour

Stone in ureter
(ureteroscopy)

Retroperitoneal fibrosis (CT)
with dilated ureter (arrow)

Ureterocele (IVU)

Fig. 27.19   Typical endoscopic appearance of papillary bladder tumour.

by repeat diathermy or resection but, if they become very frequent and excessive, cystectomy may be advisable. Carcinoma in situ (Cis) may be present in mucosa that appears normal or in association with a proliferative tumour. Cis can also exist as a separate entity, when there may be only a generalized redness (malignant cystitis). Untreated

EBM 27.1 ROLE OF INTRAVESICAL CHEMOTHERAPY IN
SUPERFICIAL BLADDER CANCER

'A single dose of intravesical mitomycin C following transurethral
resection of a bladder tumour reduces the risk of subsequent
recurrence.'

Tolley DA, et al. J Urol 1996; 155(4):1233–1237.

BOX 27.3 UROTHELIAL TUMOURS

- The urothelium or transitional cell epithelial lining of the urinary
  tract extends from the renal papilla to the distal urethra
- The incidence of urothelial cancer is increasing, possibly because
  of increasing exposure to occupational carcinogens, smoking and
  analgesic abuse
- Almost all urothelial cancers are transitional cell tumours and the
  vast majority occur in the bladder. Squamous cancers are rarer
  and are associated with chronic irritation or inflammation (e.g.
  calculi and schistosomiasis). Adenocarcinomas are extremely rare
- Frank haematuria is present in 80% of cases
- Transitional cell cancers of the bladder are treated as follows:
  Carcinoma in situ (Cis) may respond to intravesical BCG but
  is unpredictable and may require more aggressive treatment
  Superficial tumours (T_a, T_1) are usually treated by
  transurethral resection ± intravesical chemotherapy
  Invasive tumours (T_2, T_3) may be best dealt with by radical
  cystectomy (or by radical radiotherapy)
  Invasive T_4 tumours with fixation to the pelvis or surrounding
  organs are dealt with by palliative radiotherapy

patients with Cis have a high risk of progression to invasive
cancer. The tumour responds well to intravesical bacille
Calmette–Guérin (BCG) treatment. However, if there
is any doubt about the response, and especially if there
is any pathological evidence of progression, more
aggressive treatment is warranted.

Invasive bladder tumour (T_2–T_{3s})

Management is controversial. For patients under 70 years
of age, radical cystectomy is recommended. In older
patients, radiotherapy may be a better option. Unfortunately,
this may not always cure the tumour and 'salvage'
cystectomy may be needed. Cystectomy always necessitates
urinary diversion. Where the urethra can be retained, it
may be possible to construct a new bladder from colon or
small bowel (orthotopic bladder replacement), so achieving
normal continence. Alternatively, the urine is collected in
an internal reservoir that is connected to the body surface
via a continent conduit (ileum or appendix), through which
the patient drains the urine at regular intervals with a
catheter. In less favourable circumstances, an ileal conduit
should be performed (Fig. 27.20). In some countries where
an 'ostomy' is not acceptable, the ureters can be implanted
into the sigmoid colon (ureterosigmoidostomy). However,

renal infection and metabolic disturbances are potentially
serious complications of this procedure. An invasive T_4
tumour, fixed to the pelvis or surrounding organs, is
inoperable and only palliative treatment can be given. The
place of adjuvant chemotherapy is not yet established.

Prognosis

This depends on tumour stage and grade. The 5-year
survival rate varies, from 20–30% in those with deep muscle
invasion, to 50–60% in those with mucosal tumours.
Overall, about one-third of patients survive for 5 years.

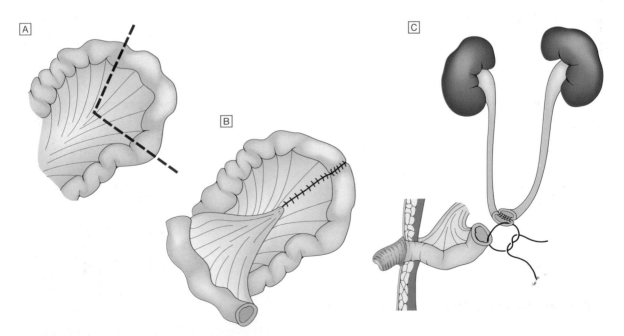

Fig. 27.20 Ileal conduit urinary diversion.

[A] and [B] Isolation of segment of terminal ileum. [C] Fashioning of uretero-ileal anastomosis. The stoma is made to protrude from the skin to
minimize skin contact with urine and so reduce irritation.

CARCINOMA OF THE PROSTATE

Epidemiology

In the UK, this is the second most common malignancy in males, with a prevalence of 50 cases per 100 000 population, and is increasing in frequency. It is the second most common cause of cancer death in men in the UK. The tumour is common in northern Europe and the USA (particularly in the black population), but rare in China and Japan. It rarely occurs before the age of 50 and is uncommon before the age of 60. The mean age at presentation is approximately 70 years. The aetiology is unknown, but genetic, hormonal and possibly viral factors are implicated.

Pathology

Almost all malignant tumours of the prostate are carcinomas. If a prostate is examined by serial section, a small malignant focus is detected in almost all men over the age of 80. Thus, there is a very high prevalence of histological prostate cancer and many men will die with a cancer of the prostate—but not *from* that cancer. It is estimated that the prevalence of focal histological cancer in men aged 50–75 is approximately 40%, whereas the prevalence of clinical prostate cancer is approximately 8%, one-quarter of whom will die from that cancer. The TNM system is used in classification (Table 27.2).

Metastatic spread to pelvic lymph nodes occurs early. One-third of clinically localized tumours at the time of presentation will have spread to regional nodes. Metastases to bone, mainly the lumbar spine and pelvis, occur in some 10–15% of cases.

Clinical features

The presentation of patients with prostatic carcinoma is usually indistinguishable from benign prostatic hyperplasia (BPH); one-quarter present with acute retention (Fig. 27.21). Occasionally, the tumour extends posteriorly around the rectum and causes alteration in bowel habit. Presenting symptoms and signs due to metastases are much less common, but include back pain, weight loss, anaemia and ureteric obstruction. On rectal examination, the prostate feels nodular and stony hard. The diagnosis must never be made on clinical grounds alone; many irregular prostates, even those with nodules, are not malignant. Conversely, 50–60% of malignant prostates are not palpably abnormal on rectal examination.

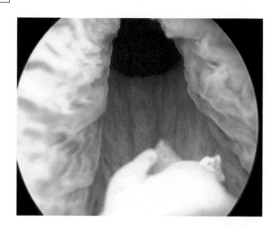

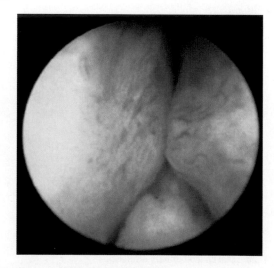

Fig. 27.21 Endoscopic view of prostate.
A Normal. B Obstructed.

Table 27.2 TNM CLASSIFICATION OF PROSTATE CANCER*

T (Tumour)
- T_0 No evidence of primary tumour
- T_x Primary tumour cannot be assessed
- T_1 Tumour clinically inapparent and not palpable
- T_{1a} Incidental finding following TURP in ≤ 5% prostate chips
- T_{1b} Incidental finding following TURP in > 5% prostate chips
- T_{1c} Prostate cancer detected by prostate biopsy
- T_{2a} Palpable nodule involving half of one lobe
- T_{2b} Palpable nodule involving one lobe
- T_{2c} Palpable nodule involving both lobes
- T_{3a} Extracapsular extension of prostate cancer
- T_{3b} Prostate cancer involving the seminal vesicles
- T_{4a} Prostate cancer involving the bladder neck and/or external sphincter and/or rectum
- T_{4b} Prostate cancer involving the lateral pelvic wall

N (Nodes)
- N_0 No regional lymph node metastasis
- N_x Regional lymph nodes cannot be assessed
- N_1 Regional lymph node metastasis

M (Metastases)
- M_0 No distant metastasis detected
- M_x Distant metastasis cannot be assessed
- M_{1a} Metastasis to non-regional lymph nodes
- M_{1b} Skeletal metastasis present
- M_{1c} Metastasis to other sites

* Sobin LH, Wittekind C, eds. TNM classification of malignant tumours, 6th edn. Chichester: John Wiley; 2002.
(TURP = transurethral resection of the prostate)

27

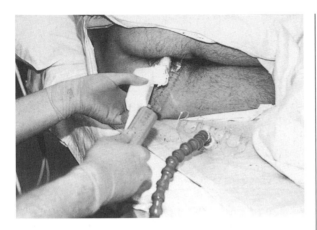

Fig. 27.22 Transrectal ultrasound of the prostate (TRUS) and needle biopsy.
Scanning alone will miss 40% of cancers and biopsy is mandatory.

BOX 27.4 PROSTATIC CANCER

- In the UK this is the second most common cancer in men, presents at a mean age of 70, and is increasing in incidence
- The carcinoma may be incidental (i.e. found on histological examination), clinically apparent (bladder outflow obstruction and a hard craggy prostate) or occult (metastatic disease)
- Metastatic spread may occur early; one-third of clinically confined cancers have spread to lymph nodes, and 10–15% of all new cases have bony spread (to lumbar spine and pelvis)
- Treatment of prostatic cancer varies:
  Incidental or focal cancer. If well differentiated, then life expectancy can be normal with a watch-and-wait policy. If the cancer contains undifferentiated cells, then either radical surgery or radiotherapy is considered
  Localized cancer with no evidence of bony metastases. Treated by either radical surgery or radiotherapy, keeping endocrine therapy in reserve
  Metastatic cancer. Treated by androgen depletion (orchiectomy) or androgen suppression (gonadotroph in releasing hormone analogues)
- Tumours localized to the prostate and amenable to radical curative treatment have a 10-year survival rate of 60–75%

Investigations

As most patients present with outflow tract obstruction, ultrasound and serum creatinine determinations are performed to assess the urinary tract. An X-ray of the pelvis or lumbar spine (to investigate backache) may show osteosclerotic metastases as the first evidence of prostatic malignancy. Whenever possible, the diagnosis is confirmed by needle biopsy, usually performed under transrectal ultrasound (TRUS) guidance (Fig. 27.22), or by histological examination of tissue removed at endoscopic resection if this is needed to relieve outflow obstruction. The patient is assessed for distant metastases by a radioisotope scan. Prostate-specific antigen (PSA) is now the main serum marker for the detection of prostate cancer. High levels (> 100 ng/ml) almost always indicate distant bone metastases. PSA is also the main test for monitoring response to treatment and disease progression. A bone scan may be carried out at follow-up to localize and define the extent of metastases.

Management

Prostatic cancer, like breast cancer, is sensitive to endocrine influences (EBM 27.2). Management is best considered in three clinical groups, as follows.

Incidental or focal cancer

Such patients will usually have had a prostatectomy and the diagnosis of cancer is made incidentally on histological examination. With increasing use of PSA, a raised value

---

EBM 27.2 HORMONE MANIPULATION IN PROSTATE CANCER

'Reducing circulating testosterone levels (either by castration or by medication) results in a 70% initial response rate. Additional androgen blockade produces a small increase in survival but with poorer quality of life.'

Huggins C, et al. Cancer Res 1941; 1:293–297.
Schmitt B, et al. Cochrane Library, issue 3, 2005. Oxford: Update Software.

---

may be the only abnormality that leads to the diagnosis of cancer confirmed by a needle biopsy. A patient with a small focus of well-differentiated carcinoma may be managed by a watch-and-wait policy because treatment is rarely required for these tumours and the patient has a normal life expectancy. A large tumour with a less well-differentiated cell pattern may progress; either radical surgery or radiotherapy is recommended for a man with a life expectancy of more than 10 years.

Organ-confined cancer; no evidence of bone metastases

If the general health of the patient is good, then either radical surgery or radiotherapy should be considered. Endocrine treatment is kept in reserve until there is evidence of tumour progression.

Metastatic prostate cancer

Approximately half of the men diagnosed with prostate cancer will have metastatic disease. The basis of treatment is androgen depletion (orchiectomy) or androgen suppression (gonadotrophin-releasing hormone analogues with or without an anti-androgen). A small number of patients fail to respond to endocrine treatment; a larger number respond for a year or two, but then suffer disease progression. Other oestrogens or progestogens are of limited value, but chemotherapy with mitoxantrone and taxanes may be effective. Radiotherapy is an effective treatment for localized bone pain. For severe generalized bone pain, hemibody radiotherapy or [89]strontium may give effective palliation, but the basis of treatment remains pain control by analgesia.

Prognosis

The life expectancy of a patient with an incidental finding of focal carcinoma of the prostate is that of the normal population. With tumours localized to the prostate, a 10-year survival rate of 50% can be expected; if metastases are present, this falls to 10%.

27

URETHRAL CANCER

Transitional cell tumours, which may be associated with bladder tumour, and squamous carcinoma of the distal urethra are uncommon. They may cause obstructive symptoms, urethral bleeding, or haematuria confined to the initial stream. The external meatus must always be examined and, if the foreskin is present, it should be retracted for full inspection. The urethra should be palpated, but usually the diagnosis can only be made at cystoscopy and biopsy. As the urothelium of the urethra is attached directly to vascular corpus spongiosum, these tumours spread early, and should be treated aggressively by cystourethrectomy.

BENIGN PROSTATIC HYPERPLASIA

Pathology

From about the age of 40 years, the prostate undergoes enlargement as the result of hyperplasia of periurethral tissue, which forms adenomas in the transitional zone of the prostate, characteristically lateral 'lobes' and often a 'middle lobe'. Normal prostatic tissue is compressed to form a surrounding shell or capsule. There is considerable variation in the growth rates of the adenomas and in the proportions of stromal and epithelial tissue. A prostate that has been previously infected or has a preponderance of stromal tissue is firm and fibrous on rectal examination. Adenomas with an epithelial preponderance can grow to form large discrete masses weighing more than 100 g, and on examination have a characteristic rubbery consistency. These changes are generally referred to as benign prostatic hyperplasia (BPH). Enlarging adenomas lengthen and obstruct the prostatic urethra, causing outflow obstruction and detrusor muscle hypertrophy. The muscle bands form trabeculae, between which saccules form diverticula (Fig. 27.23). Occasionally, a diverticulum may become quite large, even larger than the bladder. Bladder diverticula empty poorly and are liable to the three main complications of urinary stasis: infection, stones and tumour. With progressive inability to empty the bladder completely (chronic retention), the risk of urinary infection and stone formation increases. Eventually, the residual urine volume may exceed 1 litre, leading to progressive obstruction and dilatation of the ureters (hydroureter) and pelvicalyceal system (hydronephrosis). This ultimately leads to obstructive renal failure.

Clinical features

Signs and symptoms correlate poorly with the size of the prostate. Frequency, nocturia, urgency, dysuria and poor stream are common. Straining may cause vessels at the bladder neck to bleed. These clinical features may be separated into two main groups: those that are due to obstruction (slow stream and hesitancy) and those that are due to detrusor instability (urgency and urge incontinence). The latter in isolation is not an indication for prostatectomy. Increasing frequency may deceive the patient into thinking that he is passing an adequate amount

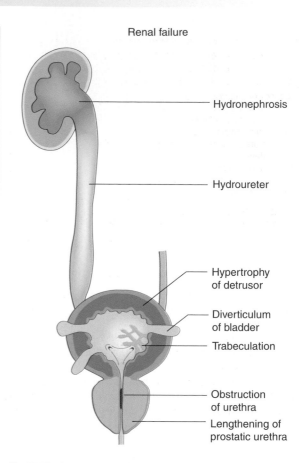

Renal failure

Hydronephrosis

Hydroureter

Hypertrophy of detrusor

Diverticulum of bladder

Trabeculation

Obstruction of urethra

Lengthening of prostatic urethra

Fig. 27.23 Late sequelae of prostatic obstruction.

of urine, whereas the bladder may be almost full all of the time (chronic retention); that is, it has a small functional capacity. Frequency may progress to continual dribbling incontinence. Such patients are liable to develop the signs and symptoms of obstructive uraemia, including drowsiness, anorexia and personality changes. Urinary infection, cold weather, anticholinergic drugs or excessive alcohol intake can cause sufficient congestion of the bladder neck to provoke acute or acute-on-chronic retention. If the patient has a bladder stone, he may have obstructive symptoms during micturition, and there may also be bladder pain at the end of micturition. Examination reveals little except rubbery, symmetrical and smooth prostatic enlargement, with a median groove between the two lateral 'lobes'. Asymmetry or a hard consistency raises the suspicion of malignancy. In a patient with acute painful retention of urine, the size of the prostate is more difficult to determine. In patients with chronic retention, the painless, enlarged bladder rises out of the pelvis, almost to the umbilicus. Even if it is not visible, the overlying area will be dull on percussion. In addition, the patient with chronic retention may be ill from obstructive uraemia.

Investigations

Assessment of renal function, haemoglobin and electrolytes, urine culture and PSA is mandatory. Prostatic cancer can occur with normal PSA values (0–4 ng/ml) while BPH

Table 27.3 FACTORS AFFECTING THE LEVEL OF PROSTATE-SPECIFIC ANTIGEN (PSA)

Causes of increase in PSA
- Increase in age
- Acute retention of urine
- Urethral catheterization
- Transurethral resection of the prostate (TURP)
- Prostatitis
- Prostate cancer
- Large benign prostatic hyperplasia
- Prostatic biopsy

Cause of decrease in PSA
- Patient taking a 5-α reductase inhibitor (finasteride, dutasteride)

EBM 27.3 BENIGN PROSTATIC HYPERPLASIA: α-BLOCKERS IN PATIENTS WITH ACUTE URINARY RETENTION

'Alfuzosin 10 mg/day increases the likelihood of successful trial without catheter (TWOC) in men with a first episode of spontaneous urinary retention.'

McNeill SA, et al. Urology 2005; 65(1):83–90.

---

can cause elevated values, so careful interpretation is required (Table 27.3). If the digital rectal examination raises suspicion, then needle biopsy is indicated. Ultrasound will detect bladder diverticula and stones as well as measure residual urine volume. A urine flow rate will quantify a reduction in urinary stream. A symptom score sheet will quantify the degree of inconvenience and bother. In some patients, especially the elderly, neurological or pharmacological causes for the changes in micturition must be considered. A pressure–flow urodynamic assessment may be necessary.

Management

Patients can be divided into three clinical groups, each requiring a different approach to management.

Symptomatic only

The patient's assessment of the severity of symptoms is influenced by his age, the social inconvenience caused, and the symptoms' frequency and progression. A young man may be greatly inconvenienced by symptoms that are quite acceptable to one who is elderly. If the exact role of the prostate in causing symptoms is difficult to determine, urodynamic studies may be helpful, especially if the symptoms appear to be irritative rather than obstructive. Once sinister pathology has been excluded (prostate carcinoma, renal failure) and it is established that the prostate is the principal problem, initial management should be medical. Alpha-blockers can relax the smooth muscle of the bladder neck and prostatic capsule, and are useful in small prostates; 5α-reductase inhibitors block the intraprostatic conversion of testosterone to dihydrotestosterone, resulting in shrinking of the prostate, and are useful in large glands. Prostatectomy (transurethral or open) is reserved for medical failures. Few patients are unfit for this operation; only if there is a history of myocardial infarction within the last 3 months should operation be delayed.

Acute retention

This is an emergency that usually requires admission to hospital. If there is a history of bladder outflow obstruction, conservative measures aimed at encouraging micturition (sedation, a warm bath) only delay the inevitable require-

ment for catheterization. A self-retaining Foley catheter (size 16 Fr) is passed using strict asepsis and connected to a closed drainage system. If it is not possible to pass a urethral catheter, the bladder is entered directly by puncture with a trocar/cannula (suprapubic cystostomy). A specimen of urine is cultured and, if there is microbiological evidence of an infection, antibiotics are given. If the history of urinary symptoms is short, the catheter can be removed after 12 hours (trial without catheter), following which normal voiding may occur. This is more likely if the patient is also given α-blockers (EBM 27.3). If retention recurs, then definitive treatment is carried out.

Chronic retention

It is essential to determine whether the patient has any complications of obstruction, especially renal damage. Although the upper urinary tracts may be dilated, renal function is not necessarily impaired. If the patient is well, with no haematological or biochemical disturbance, there is no indication for preliminary bladder drainage and prostatectomy may be planned in the usual way. If the patient is uraemic, his general fitness for operation must be assessed. Uraemia alone is not a contraindication, but hyperkalaemia, dehydration or other evidence of fluid and electrolyte disturbance must be corrected. The bladder is catheterized and prostatectomy is carried out as soon as the patient is fit. Relief of chronic obstruction is almost always followed by a diuresis, due partly to an osmotic (urea) diuresis and partly to renal tubular changes resulting from back pressure. Accurate intake/output fluid charts can detect these losses. The blood pressure should be monitored and intravenous fluid replacement may be necessary.

Open prostatectomy

Earlier open procedures used a transvesical approach, during which the bladder was opened and the adenomatous obstruction enucleated from the capsule. Later, a retropubic approach was used in which the adenoma was enucleated through a transverse incision in the prostatic capsule (Fig. 27.24). These open procedures are now reserved for very large adenomas. Apart from the length of hospitalization (7–10 days) and the presence of an abdominal wound, enucleation of smaller adenomas may damage the external sphincter and cause incontinence. This is a particular problem with more fibrous glands and those that contain a focus of cancer.

Closed (endoscopic) prostatectomy

During transurethral resection of the prostate (TURP), the prostate is removed piecemeal by electroresection using

27

a resectoscope (Fig. 27.25). The advantages of this approach are patient acceptance, short hospitalization (3–5 days) and the precision of removal of the obstructing tissue. However, serious damage can be inflicted on the prostatic sphincter mechanism by inexpert use of the resectoscope. Also, a prolonged resection can result in excessive absorption of irrigating fluid and electrolyte imbalance (TURP syndrome). Retrograde ejaculation is a common sequel to any operative procedure on the prostate (and bladder neck), and all patients should be advised pre-operatively of this effect. If the patient has a bladder stone, this may be crushed with a lithotriptor or removed by suprapubic lithotomy.

After either form of prostatectomy, the bladder must be allowed to drain freely via a urethral catheter while the prostatic bed heals and bleeding stops. After TURP, the catheter is normally removed on the second post-operative day. After an open procedure, because of the bladder or prostatic incision, it is usually left in place until the fifth post-operative day. The main post-operative hazard is bleeding. In an open procedure, blood vessels at the bladder neck are sutured but bleeding within the capsule is less easy to control. With TURP, coagulation of the blood vessels is more precise but not always complete. If post-operative bleeding is excessive, clot may lead to obstruction (clot retention). This hazard can be minimized by continuous irrigation through a three-way urethral catheter. The results of all forms of prostatectomy continue to improve, but TURP has the lowest morbidity and mortality (< 1%) and requires a shorter hospital stay (50% less) than other procedures.

BLADDER NECK OBSTRUCTION

Occasionally, the obstruction to the outflow tract appears to be at the bladder neck. The prostate is often quite small. The cause may be an infective condition such as prostatitis or schistosomiasis, or a neurological disorder such as diabetes or a prolapsed intervertebral disc. More commonly, the obstruction is due to failure of the bladder neck to open when the detrusor contracts (dyssynergia). Characteristically, bladder neck dyssynergia is found in younger middle-aged men: that is, at an age when benign prostatic hyperplasia is not expected. The urinary stream is poor, although the patient may have thought it normal, and there may be frequency and urgency. Alpha-adrenergic blocking drugs may improve the muscular dysfunction that causes dyssynergia. Endoscopic incision or excision of the bladder neck is preferable to long-term drug treatment, but surgery is contraindicated if the risk of retrograde ejaculation and hence infertility is of concern to the patient.

EXTERNAL SPHINCTER OBSTRUCTION

In cases of spinal injury, spina bifida and multiple sclerosis, the external sphincter may have high resting tone (isolated distal sphincter obstruction) or lose its normal coordination with the detrusor muscle. This results in the sphincter closing when the detrusor contracts (detrusosphincter dyssynergia). In both cases the result is a functional obstruction. Specialized urodynamics is required to make the diagnosis accurately and treatment may require endoscopic sphincterotomy.

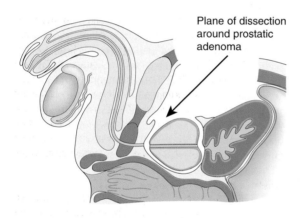

Plane of dissection around prostatic adenoma

Fig. 27.24 Retropubic prostatectomy.

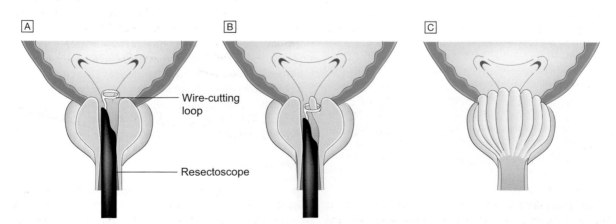

Wire-cutting loop

Resectoscope

Fig. 27.25 Transurethral resection of the prostate (TURP).
A Wire-cutting loop and resectoscope. B The wire-cutting loop is drawn back along the sheath of the resectoscope and is shown cutting into the hypertrophied prostate. C Completed resection with only the prostate capsule remaining.

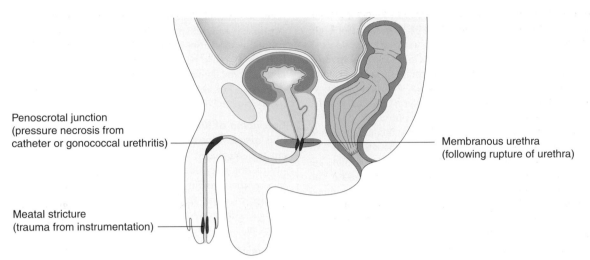

Penoscrotal junction
(pressure necrosis from
catheter or gonococcal urethritis)

Membranous urethra
(following rupture of urethra)

Meatal stricture
(trauma from instrumentation)

Fig. 27.26 Common sites and causes of urethral stricture.

URETHRAL OBSTRUCTION
Pathology
Obstruction of the urethra may be congenital, or due to a stricture or malignancy (Fig. 27.26). Foreign bodies, including urinary stones, may also be responsible. The complications include infection with periurethral abscess, fistulation and stone formation. Congenital valves in the posterior urethra occur only in boys. They lie at the level of the verumontanum and may cause gross obstructive changes in the bladder and upper urinary tracts at birth. Increasingly, this diagnosis is being established during pregnancy by ultrasound examination. If the diagnosis is established after birth, it is confirmed by micturating cystourethrography. Treatment consists of endoscopic incision of the valves. Urethral diverticulum is a rare cause of obstruction. More commonly, it is secondary to obstruction and infection in women. An important late sequel of urethral trauma or infection is a stricture, the severity of which is related to both the site and the extent of the insult. Thus, a posterior urethral stricture that follows major trauma to the pelvis may be surrounded by dense fibrous tissue, whereas healthy tissues may surround a stricture of the bulb of the urethra. The former requires major reconstructive surgery; urethral dilation or incision can readily manage the latter. It must be remembered that rough inexpert use of any instrument (including a catheter) in the urethra can be followed by stricture formation. The principal organism responsible for inflammatory scarring and stricture of the urethra is *Neisseria gonorrhoeae*. Long-term use of a self-retaining catheter, although not necessarily associated with infection, can also cause an inflammatory reaction in the urethra. This may result in a stricture, most commonly at the external meatus.

Clinical features
A change in micturition due to urethral narrowing may be indistinguishable from that which occurs with BPH and bladder neck obstruction. However, the diagnosis should be considered if there is a history of urethral infection, instrumentation or trauma. The external meatus must always be examined and, if the foreskin is present, it should be retracted for full inspection. The urethra is palpated. It is still possible for a patient to pass urine, albeit with difficulty, in the presence of a urethral stone.

Investigations
Urinary flow rate will help differentiate urethral strictures from bladder neck and prostatic obstruction, the former giving a uniformly low and prolonged (box-like) pattern (Fig. 27.5). Post-micturition ultrasound is more useful than an IVU in assessing bladder emptying and residual volume. An ascending and descending urethrogram will adequately demonstrate the urethral anatomy. Urodynamic assessment of the urethra and bladder may be helpful, especially when neurological and mechanical problems coexist. The final investigation to assess a urethral lesion is cystourethroscopy.

Management
Many simple strictures are easily treated by repeated dilatation with metal bougies, or may be incised under direct vision using a urethrotome. Most simple short strictures in the region of the bulb respond well, but recurrence is common (50%) and may require operative reconstruction (urethroplasty). Short strictures can be excised and the healthy urethra reanastomosed. Longer strictures can be patched with full-thickness skin flaps or buccal mucosal grafts, to restore normal calibre.

DISORDERS OF MICTURITION—INCONTINENCE

OVERVIEW
Incontinence may be due either to problems in storage, resulting in urge and stress incontinence or continual incontinence with fistulae, or to problems in emptying, resulting in chronic retention with overflow incontinence. In stress incontinence, leakage occurs because passive bladder pressure exceeds normal urethral pressure. This may be

because of poor pelvic floor support or because of a weak urethral sphincter; most often there is an element of both. In urge incontinence, leakage usually occurs because detrusor overactivity produces an increase in bladder pressure that overcomes the urethral sphincter (motor urgency). A hypersensitive bladder (sensory urgency) resulting from urinary tract infection (UTI) or bladder stone may also drive urgency. Incontinence in these circumstances is less common. Stress incontinence and urge incontinence may coexist (mixed incontinence). All of the above terms, with the exception of a fistula, are descriptive only and do not accurately diagnose the underlying pathophysiology, which can only be determined by urodynamic testing.

STRUCTURAL DISORDERS

Clinical assessment

Abnormalities of function of the lower urinary tract are notoriously difficult to assess because there is frequently dual underlying pathology. For example, incontinence in an elderly man may be due to cerebral cortical degeneration, but could also be due to chronic outflow tract obstruction resulting from prostatic hyperplasia. The history is important but may be deceptive, mainly because different abnormalities can produce similar symptoms. The exact character of the urinary abnormality must be determined so that structural causes can be separated from neurological ones. Details of drug treatment are noted. Diuretics and drugs with anticholinergic side-effects may tip the balance when there is already dysfunction. Urine is tested for glycosuria and infection. In addition to intravenous urography, there is now a range of more specific methods for assessing micturition, but not all are required for a diagnosis. Their value lies in resolving specific clinical questions relating to management. They include radiology (cystourethrography), urodynamic studies (uroflowmetry, cystometrography and urethral pressure measurement) and direct inspection (cystourethroscopy and pelvic examination under anaesthesia). A full history and physical examination, with cystourethroscopy and bimanual examination, remain the basic initial investigation of structural disorders.

Structural causes of incontinence in males

Post-prostatectomy

Disordered control of micturition occurs in 3–5% patients after prostatectomy. In this operation the bladder neck sphincter is deliberately excised posteriorly but the external sphincter is carefully preserved. However, any inadvertent damage to the external sphincter can lead to difficulties with continence. Stress incontinence may occur, but as the damage to the sphincter is usually incomplete, it usually responds to physiotherapy.

Chronic outflow obstruction

Chronic obstruction commonly leads to involuntary contractions or unstable bladder. Relief of obstruction alone is usually sufficient to correct the associated urgency and urge incontinence, but in about 10% of cases the instability is primary and antispasmodics may be necessary. Chronic retention may also lead to overflow or dribbling incontinence. It must be emphasized that continence requires normal cortical control, and in an elderly patient this may be impaired. Possible abnormalities of both structure and innervation need to be considered in these patients.

Carcinoma of the prostate

This may involve the external sphincter, preventing it from closing. Repeated transurethral resections for recurring obstruction may convert the posterior urethra into a rigid tube so that dribbling incontinence occurs; that is, there is leakage of urine during the storage phase. An indwelling catheter or condom incontinence appliance may be necessary.

Post-micturition dribble incontinence

This is very common, even in relatively young men, and is caused by a small amount of urine becoming trapped in the 'U-bend' of the bulbar urethra. This then leaks out passively when the patient moves. The condition is more pronounced if associated with a urethral diverticulum or urethral stricture.

Chronic illness and debility

Especially in the elderly, this may lead to incontinence because of poor tone in the periurethral striated muscle of the pelvic floor and difficulty in getting to the toilet. This may be worsened by loss of cortical inhibition of micturition.

Structural causes of incontinence in females

Incontinence is more prevalent than generally suspected; approximately 14% of all women have been incontinent at some time, half of them within the last 2 months. This figure rises rapidly in older patients, and reaches 50–70% in geriatric units. Only a proportion of younger women seek advice, either because of embarrassment or because of stoical acceptance of some incontinence as being normal.

Childbirth and operations

Multiparous women commonly lose some of the tone in the pelvic floor muscles with each pregnancy. Symptoms may range from occasional stress incontinence to almost continual dribbling incontinence. Examination shows weakening of the pelvic floor muscles and anterior vaginal wall (cystocoele). It is important to distinguish stress incontinence from urge incontinence. The former responds well to pelvic floor exercises and to surgical procedures designed to support the bladder neck, but the latter should be treated by bladder retraining and drug therapy. Stress incontinence is characterized by an involuntary loss of urine during coughing, laughing, sneezing or any other activity that suddenly raises the intra-abdominal pressure. A cough, however, may stimulate involuntary detrusor contractions (cough-induced detrusor instability), which cause motor urge incontinence. This differential diagnosis can be made only by urodynamic assessment. In parts of the world where obstetric services are poor, prolonged labour may lead to a vesicovaginal fistula, which presents as continuous dribbling incontinence. The association with delivery is usually clear, but a small fistula may be missed. Investigation of dribbling incontinence must distinguish between urethral damage and a fistula. Treatment consists of closing the fistula through a vaginal or suprapubic approach.

Hysterectomy may also be followed by urinary incontinence, suggesting either vesicovaginal fistula or damage to the ureter(s) at operation, which have resulted in ureterovaginal fistula. Investigations are directed at establishing whether the bladder or the ureters are involved, and which ureter has been damaged. Treatment consists of reimplanting the ureter into the bladder.

Cystitis

Cystitis is common in women and, in addition to causing frequency, urgency and dysuria, sometimes causes sensory urge incontinence. Treatment of both the infection and the bladder spasm is required. Interstitial cystitis (painful bladder syndrome) is a chronic inflammatory condition that, in addition to causing frequency and dysuria, may also cause urgency and urge incontinence. Treatment is often unsatisfactory. Hydrostatic dilatation may be effective. The urethral syndrome is characterized by symptoms of cystitis in the absence of infection. There may be some incontinence. The urethral syndrome usually responds to regulation of micturition habits and careful perineal hygiene. Resistant cases may benefit from urethral dilatation, although they are seldom, if ever, strictured.

Ectopic ureter

Dribbling incontinence in a child should raise the suspicion of an ectopic ureter, in which the lower of the two ureters opens outside the control of the urethral mechanism. The abnormal ureter must be relocated in the bladder.

Cervical cancer

Carcinoma of the cervix or its treatment by radiotherapy may cause vesicovaginal fistula and incontinence.

NEUROGENIC DISORDERS

Clinical assessment

A full history, including an interview with relatives, is required. Examination must include assessment of the plantar reflexes and the sensation and tone of the anal canal. Glycosuria and urinary infection should be excluded. Urodynamic, radiological and electromyographic studies may all be required.

Aetiology of abnormal micturition

Impaired cortical control

Diseases affecting the frontal lobe can alter the pattern of micturition by increasing or decreasing its frequency, or by affecting the social awareness of incontinence. There may also be failure to inhibit initiation of micturition. The paracentral lobule controls the activity of skeletal muscle, so that lesions in this area may cause sustained pelvic and perineal muscular contraction. It must be remembered that a disorder of micturition may be accentuated by, or may even be due to, the physical inability to prepare for micturition.

Emotional state

This may affect the postponement of micturition, giving rise to 'giggle' incontinence and possibly to enuresis in some patients. Incontinence with epilepsy is also due to a loss of inhibitory control. Excessive sensory stimuli, as with the pain of cystourethritis in women, may cause 'sensory urge incontinence'.

Drugs

Drugs, including alcohol, may alter cortical control of micturition. Sedatives can affect the postponement phase and precipitate incontinence, especially at night. The intoxicated patient may lack the mental alertness to maintain continence, or may continually suppress the desire to void, leading to prostatic congestion and retention.

Damage to the spinal cord

Two aspects of disease or injury to the spinal cord influence disordered micturition: namely, the level of the disease and the completeness of the damage.

Injury at or below the sacral outflow (S2, 3, 4) may be due to a fracture of the spine at the level of T12 and L1, which damages the conus medullaris, a central prolapsed intervertebral disc, leading to cauda equina injury, or to spinal stenosis. The bladder distends without sensation, the external sphincter is weak and the cystometrogram is flat. The patient develops retention with overflow, but emptying is possible with abdominal straining or hand pressure.

Injury between the sacral segment and the pontine micturition centres (upper motor neuron lesions) may be due to fractures of the spine; tumours that compress the cord; surgical removal of such a tumour; and diseases of the cord itself, such as multiple sclerosis, transverse myelitis and cervical cord stenosis. If these central connections are disrupted, the patient develops a reflex bladder with impaired or absent cortical control; that is, the bladder loses the coordination imposed by the pontine micturition centre. The detrusor becomes overactive and attempted voiding results in detrusor contraction occurring synchronously with that of the external sphincter (detrusor–sphincter dyssynergia). The net result is poor bladder emptying and the development of a thick, trabeculated bladder wall. The resultant high-pressure bladder will, over time, lead to renal impairment. Usually the central connections are not completely disrupted and there may be some sensation and some cortical inhibition.

Damage to pelvic nerves may occur in the course of surgery, especially when dissection involves the side walls of the pelvis, as in radical dissection of the rectum or the uterus. Similarly, aneurysm surgery may disrupt neural pathways in the pelvis. Diseases affecting the autonomic system, principally diabetes mellitus, also affect the control of micturition. With the loss of sensation and contraction, the bladder becomes an atonic sac, prone to the complication of stasis infection. The external sphincter remains closed by uninhibited tonic contractions, but the internal sphincter is partly open as it partly depends on detrusor activity.

Abnormalities within the bladder itself may also be responsible. Primary failure of the detrusor has been described, but is usually secondary to chronic overdis-

27

tension. Atonic myogenic bladder is caused by prolonged outlet obstruction and is found in the late stages of bladder decompensation. The most common cause is silent prostatic obstruction, where progressive loss of the desire to void results in overflow incontinence. In women, conscious postponement can lead to a large, atonic bladder.

PRINCIPLES OF MANAGEMENT

The diagnosis must be as complete as possible. More than one mechanism may account for disordered micturition. A urodynamic assessment is mandatory in all patients with a suspected or proven neuropathic bladder.

Neurologically intact patients

Patients with congenital defects or fistulae should have these repaired surgically if possible. If the fistula is malignant or the surrounding tissues are poor because of radiation, urinary diversion is preferable. Stress incontinence in both males and females should be treated initially with pelvic floor exercises. If it persists in males, it is best treated by the insertion of an artificial urinary sphincter. In females, the urethra and bladder neck should be returned to their natural positions and supported by means of colposuspension or a pubovaginal sling. The injection of bulking agents at the bladder neck can improve continence, but remains under evaluation. Urge incontinence should be treated initially by bladder retraining, supplemented by anticholinergic drugs. If this fails, good results can be obtained by surgery, either by stripping off a substantial proportion of the detrusor muscle (myectomy) or by splitting the bladder in half and suturing a strip of small bowel to augment the bladder (clam ileocystoplasty). Patients with atonic bladders are best managed by regular intermittent self-catheterization (ISC).

Neuropathic patients

These patients are prone to urinary infection and renal impairment, and the preservation of renal function takes

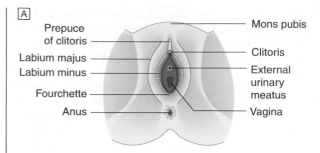

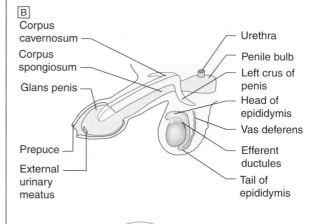

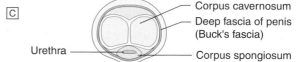

Fig. 27.27 Anatomy of the external genitalia.
A Female. B Male. C Cross-section through the penis.

priority. Management depends as much on the patient's overall condition as on their specific urological problem. Regardless of pathology, poorly motivated immobile patients with poor cognition and hand function are best managed by suprapubic catheterization or urinary diversion. Highly motivated intelligent patients should be treated in much the same way as the neurologically intact, although the results are often less good.

EXTERNAL GENITALIA

ANATOMY

In the male, these comprise the penis, testicles and scrotum; in the female, the mons pubis, labia majora, labia minora and the clitoris (Fig. 27.27).

The penis consists of three cylinders of erectile tissue. The ventral corpus spongiosum is expanded proximally as the bulb and distally as the glans penis, and transmits the urethra. Two dorsolateral corpora cavernosa attach to each side of the inferior pubic arch as the crura. They form the body of the penis and become embedded in the glans.

The penile skin is hairless, free of fat, and extends over the glans as the prepuce or foreskin. Blood is supplied from the internal pudendal arteries. The scrotum is a thin rugose pouch of skin containing the two testicles. Each testicle is contained within a tough capsule (tunica albuginea) and has the epididymis attached to it posteriorly. This highly coiled tubular structure arises from the rete testis, where some 20 small tubules enter it. This head of epididymis is considerably larger than the lower tail, from which the vas deferens arises to traverse the spermatic cord and finally to open into the prostatic urethra as the ejaculatory duct. The testicle and epididymis are invaginated into the tunica vaginalis, which lies anteriorly, so providing a potential space where a hydrocoele may form. The testicular arteries supply the testes. Venous blood drains along the spermatic cord as the pampiniform plexus. The scrotum drains lymph to the inguinal lymph nodes, and the contents of the scrotum drain along the spermatic cord to nodes in the pelvis and abdomen.

In the female, the mons pubis is the fatty elevation over the pubis from which the labia run backwards, enclosing between them the vestibule into which open the vagina and urethra. The clitoris lies above the urethral opening and is a smaller replica of the penis, with the same erectile tissues.

PHYSIOLOGY

Parasympathetic stimulation leads to erection through the release of nitric oxide, with resultant vasodilatation of the arterioles, increased penile blood flow and passive closure of the venules. After sufficient stimulation, sperm from the epididymis and seminal fluid from the seminal vesicles are emptied into the prostatic urethra. Sympathetic stimulation is responsible for this emission, and also closes the bladder neck to prevent leakage of semen into the bladder. Ejaculation proper is due to rhythmic contraction of the bulbospongiosus muscles expelling the semen out through the urethra.

CIRCUMCISION

The foreskin is normally non-retractile for the first few months of life. By the end of the first year, half will retract, but it may be 3–4 years before all do so. Provided the parents are reassured, there is no reason, apart from religious grounds, to remove the foreskin within the first few years of life. In some children, the foreskin remains non-retractile and has to be treated by division of preputial adhesions or by circumcision. Otherwise, secretions collect under the foreskin, leading to infection (balanitis) and narrowing of the orifice (phimosis).

Severe phimosis may obstruct urinary flow (Fig. 27.28). In those whose foreskin retracts only with difficulty, pain during intercourse may be a problem. Keeping the glans and coronal sulcus clean can also be difficult; accumulated secretions may predispose to carcinoma of the penis. If a poorly retracting foreskin remains retracted, it can act as a tight band and cause engorgement and oedema of the glans (paraphimosis). This demands urgent treatment. It

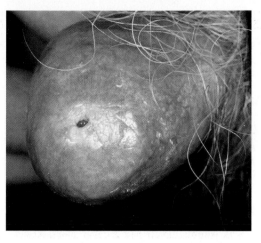

Fig. 27.28   Severe phimosis.

may be possible to compress the glans and draw the foreskin forwards, but if this fails, the tight band must be incised under general anaesthesia. Later, elective circumcision is advocated.

CONGENITAL ABNORMALITIES OF THE PENIS

Hypospadias
Failure of the embryonic folds to fuse results in abnormal placing of the external urinary meatus on the ventral surface of the penis. The opening may be coronal, penile, scrotal or even perineal. The corpus spongiosum may be scarred and fibrosed, leading to a ventral curvature or chordee of the penis. The aim of treatment is to correct the chordee by excising the fibrosis, and then to construct a new urethral opening in the normal position on the glans. This procedure should be completed before the boy goes to school.

Epispadias
In this condition the external urinary meatus opens on the dorsal surface of the penis. The extent of the malformation varies from an isolated penile abnormality to gross malformation of the bladder and urethra. The mucosa of the bladder and the ureteric orifices may be exposed and form the infra-umbilical part of the abdominal wall (exstrophy). The urethra then lies opened out like a gutter. Other abnormalities include separation of the symphysis pubis and rectal prolapse. Reconstruction of these deformities is not always successful, and urinary incontinence may remain a major problem and require urinary diversion.

DISORDERS OF ERECTION (IMPOTENCE)

Impotence may be psychogenic, organic or drug-induced. Psychogenic problems, the most common cause, can usually be established from a careful history that includes details of sexual habits. Organic impotence is associated with diabetes mellitus, neurogenic disorders, major pelvic injury or operations, vascular disease of the pelvic vessels (Leriche's syndrome), priapism and Peyronie's disease. Most of these conditions constitute irreversible impotence. Drug-induced impotence occurs with hormonal manipulation for prostatic cancer; some antihypertensive drugs may cause loss of erection or inability to ejaculate, and barbiturates, benzodiazepines, corticosteroids, phenothiazines and spironolactone may affect libido. Medical treatment is by oral sildenafil (Viagra), intracavernosal (self)-injection of papaverine, or prostaglandin E. Vacuum suction devices or a prosthesis implanted into the corpora cavernosa are effective alternatives.

PRIAPISM

This is a painful maintained erection unassociated with sexual desire. It is associated with intracavernosal self-injection for impotence (the most common cause), leukaemia, disorders of coagulation, renal dialysis and sickle-cell trait, and is believed to be due to venous sludging in the corpora cavernosa. (The corpus spongiosum and glans are unaffected.) Aspiration and intracavernosal injections of vasoconstrictors (phenylephrine) may be effective, especially in self-injection cases. If these fail, the creation of a venous shunt within 6–12 hours gives satisfactory results, and the patient can achieve normal erections subsequently. If treatment is delayed or incomplete, the erectile tissue is damaged and the patient will be impotent.

PEYRONIE'S DISEASE

This is the occurrence of a hard fibrous plaque (or plaques) in the wall of a corpus cavernosum, causing curvature of the penis. The cause is obscure but is possibly related to trauma, leading to the formation of hard scar tissue. In addition to the deformity, the patient complains of pain during intercourse. Various treatments, including cortisone injections, vitamins and radiotherapy, have met with little success. Excision of the plaque and replacement by a dermal patch graft, or excision of a wedge of tissue on the convex (opposite) border of the penis, may be effective.

CARCINOMA OF THE PENIS

This uncommon tumour has a prevalence of 1.5 cases per 100 000 and is generally attributed to poor hygiene associated with a non-retractile foreskin (Fig. 27.29). It is very rare in circumcised men and almost always occurs in the elderly. The cancer may be a papillary or an ulcerating squamous cell carcinoma. Local spread occurs early and the tumour may ulcerate and fungate. Lymphatic spread to inguinal lymph nodes is common; associated infection may also lead to lymphadenopathy. The patient may present with a purulent or blood-stained discharge. Unfortunately, many patients do not seek help until the lesion is advanced—some only when much of the penis is already destroyed and the inguinal lymph nodes are involved. The diagnosis must be confirmed by biopsy. Circumcision may cure early tumours confined to the prepuce. Early tumours confined to the glans

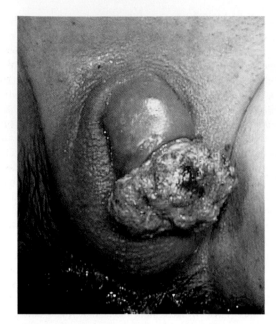

Fig. 27.29 Penile carcinoma.

may be treated by excision of the glans and skin grafting. Advanced tumours will require partial or total penile amputation, and often bilateral block dissection of the inguinal lymph nodes. Inoperable tumours are treated by radiotherapy.

INFLAMMATION OF THE PENIS

Inflammation of the glans penis (balanitis) usually also involves the prepuce (posthitis) and is common in children with poorly retractile foreskins. Circumcision usually cures recurrent non-specific balanitis. Balanitis xerotica obliterans (BXO) is the local manifestation of lichen sclerosus et atrophicus of the glans and prepuce. It causes typical white scarring of the prepuce and glans, and may involve the urethral meatus and distal urethra. Meatal stenosis occurs as a result of either recurrent infection, trauma or BXO. It may respond to removal of the inflammation (by circumcision) and meatal dilatation; alternatively, it may require meatotomy or meatoplasty.

UNDESCENDED TESTES (CRYPTORCHIDISM)

Retractile testis

Normally, both testes are in the scrotum by 6 months of age. However, they may be excessively mobile and readily retract towards the external inguinal ring, even into the inguinal canal, especially when the patient is examined in a cold room. Such retractile testes may easily be misdiagnosed as being incompletely descended. Care must be taken to examine the baby in a warm room or after a bath. True undescended testes are of two types:

1. *Incomplete.* Such a testis is arrested in its normal pathway to the scrotum. Usually this is within the inguinal canal, more rarely within the abdomen. The

testis is smaller than normal and cannot be palpated. Its ability to produce sperm is doubtful. As the spermatic cord is short, such testes are difficult to bring down into the scrotum by operation (orchidopexy). If this can be carried out before the age of 2–4 years, the testis may be of some use; otherwise, it should be removed. Occasionally, an incompletely descended testis is situated just inside the external inguinal ring, through which it can be coaxed (emergent testis). Testes that remain incompletely descended have a 3–4% chance of becoming malignant; the risk is greater if the testis is retained in the abdomen. Laparoscopy is increasingly used to locate and remove an intra-abdominal testis.

2. *Ectopic.* An ectopic testis has developed normally, but after passing through the external inguinal ring its further descent is impeded. It either remains in the superficial inguinal pouch (common) or is transposed to perineal, femoral or pre-pubic sites (rare). Because an ectopic testis is normal in size, it is palpable and its cord is normal. Orchidopexy is achieved without difficulty. Provided this is done early, preferably before the age of 6 years, spermatogenesis is believed to occur normally. However, even if the diagnosis is not made until later (frequently just before puberty), orchidopexy should still be performed. This consists of mobilizing the testis and its cord and placing the testis in the scrotum. Various methods are used to stop the testis from retracting towards the inguinal canal. The simplest is to place the testis in a pouch between the dartos muscle and the scrotal skin.

TORSION OF THE TESTIS

Torsion of the cord can occur where the visceral layer of the tunica vaginalis completely covers the testis so that it lies suspended within the parietal layer. The patient, usually a teenager, presents with sudden onset of testicular pain and swelling. There may be a history of minor trauma, or previous episodes of pain due to partial torsion. On examination there is a red, swollen hemiscrotum that is usually too tender to palpate. Misdiagnosis of the swelling as epididymo-orchitis, which is rare in teenagers, is a serious error. Torsion of the testis is a surgical emergency; if the blood supply is not restored within 12 hours, the testis infarcts and must then be excised. If at operation the testis is found to be viable, it is sutured to the parietal tunica to prevent recurrence. As the underlying abnormality of the tunica is bilateral, the other testis must be fixed at the same time.

TESTICULAR TUMOURS

Pathology

Tumours of the testes are uncommon, with a prevalence of 5 cases per 100 000. They most commonly affect men between 20 and 40 years of age. Seminoma and teratoma account for 85%; malignant lymphoma, yolk-sac tumours, interstitial cell tumours and Sertoli cell/mesenchyme tumours make up the remainder. Seminomas arise from seminiferous tubules and are of relatively low-grade malignancy. Metastases occur mainly via the lymphatics and may involve the lungs. Teratoma (non-seminomatous tumour) arises from primitive germinal cells. It may contain cartilage, bone, muscle, fat and a variety of other tissues, and is classified according to the degree of differentiation. Well-differentiated tumours are the least aggressive; at the other extreme, trophoblastic teratoma is highly malignant. Occasionally, teratoma and seminoma occur in the same testis.

Clinical features

The most common presentation is the incidental discovery of a painless testicular lump. The history is often vague, however, and symptoms may be attributed to an injury, or there may be pain and swelling suggesting inflammation. The patient may have wrongly received treatment for 'acute epididymitis'. Very rarely, patients with teratoma may complain of gynaecomastia. Irrespective of the history, any new painless testicular lump in a young man must be regarded with suspicion. A hydrocoele in a young man also demands investigation, as testicular tumours may be accompanied by blood-stained effusion in the tunica vaginalis.

Investigations

All suspicious scrotal lumps should be imaged by ultrasound, which provides a high degree of accuracy. As soon as a tumour is suspected, and before orchiectomy, serum levels of AFP and the β-subunit of HCG should be determined. The levels of these 'tumour markers' are increased in extensive disease. Accurate staging is based on CT scans of the lungs, liver and retroperitoneal area, and an assessment of renal and pulmonary function (Table 27.4).

Management

Through an inguinal incision the spermatic cord is divided at the internal ring; only then is the testis removed. Radiotherapy is the treatment of choice for early-stage seminoma, as this tumour is very radiosensitive. The management of a teratoma depends on the stage of the disease. Early disease confined to the testes may be managed without further treatment, provided that there is close surveillance for at least 2 years; tumour progression is treated by chemotherapy. More advanced cancers are

Table 27.4 ROYAL MARSDEN CLASSIFICATION FOR TESTICULAR CANCER	
• Stage 1	Tumour confined to testis
• Stage 2	Tumour spread only to lymph nodes below diaphragm
• Stage 3	Tumour spread only to lymph nodes above and below diaphragm
• Stage 4	Tumour spread to inguinal lymph nodes or distant metastases

27

27

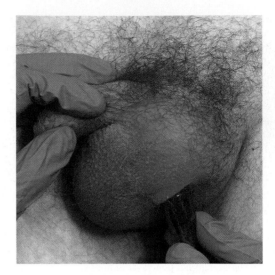

Fig. 27.30 Hydrocoele demonstrating trans-illumination.

managed initially by chemotherapy, usually with a combination of bleomycin, etoposide and cisplatin. Retroperitoneal lymph node dissection is now only performed for residual or recurrent nodal masses. AFP and β-HCG each offer a valuable means of monitoring response to treatment and detecting recurrent disease. Both markers should be monitored in all patients with testicular tumours for at least 2 years after they are considered to be tumour-free. CT is used to follow the response of enlarged lymph nodes to treatment.

Prognosis

The 5-year survival rate for patients with seminoma is 90–95%. The more variable prognosis of teratomas depends on tumour type, stage and volume. With more favourable tumours the 5-year survival rate may be as high as 95%, but in more advanced cases 60–70% is more usual.

EPIDIDYMO-ORCHITIS

Acute epididymo-orchitis is usually the appropriate term, as both testis and epididymides are involved in the acute inflammatory reaction. The spermatic cord is also often thickened (funiculitis). After infection has subsided, the epididymis alone may remain thickened and irregular, so that chronic epididymitis may be diagnosed. Thus a late effect of tuberculosis is an irregularly hard (craggy) epididymis. Apparent involvement of the testis alone may be a feature of viral infections such as mumps orchitis. The usual cause of epididymo-orchitis is bacterial spread, either from infected urine or from gonococcal urethritis. The affected side of the scrotum is swollen, inflamed and very tender. In all cases, the urine or urethral discharge must be cultured. Sometimes there is no evidence of a bacterial cause and a viral aetiology is then likely. Treatment consists of antibiotics, analgesia, bed rest and a scrotal support. The choice of antibiotic depends on the results of culture and sensitivity determination of

the organism responsible. If there is any doubt about the diagnosis, the testis should be explored. Abscess formation is now rare, but if signs of localization or fluctuation develop, the pus should be drained. Infertility is an important late complication of epididymo-orchitis.

HYDROCOELE

This is a common condition, especially in older men, in which fluid collects in the tunica vaginalis, resulting in an enlarged but painless scrotum. The inconvenience of its size usually leads the patient to seek advice. The cause of most hydrocoeles is unknown (idiopathic). The fluid is straw-coloured and protein-rich. In some patients, a hydrocoele develops as a reaction to epididymo-orchitis. Rarely, it may develop with a malignant testis (secondary hydrocoele) and the fluid may then be blood-stained. On examination of the scrotum, a normal spermatic cord can be palpated above a smooth oval swelling. Typically, an idiopathic hydrocoele transilluminates (Fig. 27.30), but where it is long-standing this may be difficult to elicit, owing to fibrosis and thickening of its wall. It is important always to seek this physical sign and also to examine the neck of the scrotum carefully to exclude an inguinal hernia as the cause of the swelling. It may be possible to palpate the testis and confirm that it is normal, but this is unusual as it lies behind and is enveloped by the hydrocoele. If there is any doubt about the diagnosis, then an ultrasound should be performed. Injury to the scrotum may result in a swelling that resembles a hydrocoele but does not transilluminate because the tunica has filled with blood (haematocoele). Aspiration alone does not cure an idiopathic hydrocoele and the tunica soon refills. It is possible to obliterate the sac by injecting a sclerosant after aspiration, but surgical excision and eversion is associated with a much lower recurrence rate. If the hydrocoele fluid becomes infected, incision and drainage of the pus are necessary. Similarly, a haematocoele may require treatment by incision and drainage.

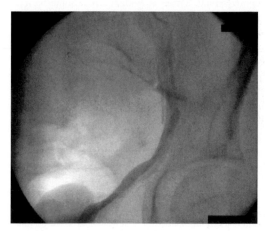

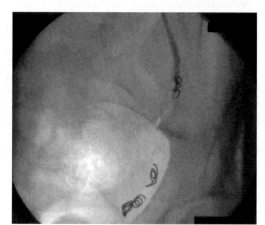

Fig. 27.31 Varicocoele.
A Before treatment. B After radiological coil embolization.

Hydrocoele is a common abnormality in children. It is due to failure of closure of the processus vaginalis after descent of the testis. This patent processus vaginalis (PPV) allows fluid to drain into the scrotum around the testis. Most congenital hydrocoeles of this sort resolve before the first birthday. Those that persist require surgical treatment comprising ligation of the PPV through a small groin incision.

CYST OF THE EPIDIDYMIS

Cysts in the epididymis arise from diverticula of the vasa efferentia. The distinction between a cyst of the epididymis and a hydrocoele is easy. Epididymal cysts are almost always multiple and, therefore, nodular on palpation; they are located above and behind the testis, which is palpably separate from the cysts, and always transilluminate brightly. A solitary epididymal cyst may even resemble a testis, so giving rise to fables of three testes and the term 'pawnbroker's sign'. Sometimes the fluid within an epididymal cyst is opalescent and contains sperm (spermatocoele). Usually the fluid is clear. It is best to leave these cysts alone unless increasing size warrants excision. Careful dissection is needed to remove the cyst completely. Often several other little cysts are present which, if not removed, will eventually increase in size and produce a so-called recurrence. If all the cysts are removed, the pathway for sperm will almost certainly be damaged. Bilateral operations can result in sterility.

VARICOCOELE

The veins of the pampiniform plexus are dilated and tortuous, producing a swelling in the line of the spermatic cord that resembles a 'bag of worms'. It is more common on the left side, possibly because the right-angled drainage of the left testicular vein into the renal vein renders it more liable to stasis. In some men, varicocoele is associated with infertility. A dragging sensation in the scrotum may cause concern. Treatment is by ligation of the spermatic vein, which may be done surgically (laparoscopically) at the internal inguinal ring. Alternatively, the feeding veins can be obliterated radiologically by means of coil embolization (Fig. 27.31).

INFERTILITY

Assessment
Although, only the causes of male infertility are discussed here, the investigation and management of infertility does, of course, require the assessment of both partners. A detailed history is essential, particularly with regard to factors that may contribute to an abnormal sperm count. These include operations (e.g. for hernia), infections (mumps, tuberculosis and gonorrhoea) and certain drugs (nitrofurazone, cyclophosphamides and possibly some tranquillizers). Excessive smoking, alcohol intake, obesity and working in a hot environment may all suppress spermatogenesis. The patient should be asked about any psychosexual problems, including impotence or premature ejaculation. Physical examination may be entirely normal. Physical build and hair distribution are noted. Testicular size is a crude but useful guide to spermatogenic potential. For example, a tall male with female hair distribution and pea-sized testes almost certainly has Klinefelter's syndrome. Examination of the scrotum may reveal dilated spermatic veins (varicocoele).

Investigations
The principal investigation is the analysis of seminal fluid. Values given as 'normal' are only a guide, as pregnancy can occur even with low sperm concentrations (oligozoospermia). However, the lower the concentration of sperm, the less the chance of pregnancy. If a patient has no sperm (azoospermia), it is necessary to distinguish between obstruction and primary failure of spermatogenesis. This may be possible by measuring

27

27

plasma gonadotrophins (follicle-stimulating hormone, FSH). A normal value indicates obstruction, which is usually in the epididymis. In these patients, the testes are also normal in size. More detailed tests, such as immunological compatibility and chromosome analysis, may be necessary.

Management

There is no treatment for a patient with azoospermia due to primary spermatogenic failure. Testicular biopsy to confirm the diagnosis is all that is possible. Azoospermia due to obstruction may be treated by bypass (epididymovasostomy). This may be successful if the obstruction is in the tail of the epididymis. However, if it is elsewhere in the epididymis or the vasa efferentia, the results are generally poor. In these cases, aspiration or biopsy can usually recover sperm. The introduction of intracytoplasmic sperm injection (ICSI), which requires only a single sperm for fertilization, has greatly increased the pregnancy rate in those circumstances. Patients with oligozoospermia are initially advised to reduce their weight, improve dietary and smoking habits, and (if possible) adjust their occupation or working environment. It is important to ensure that the patient understands the basis of reproductive biology, especially the timing of intercourse in relation to the menstrual cycle. These measures alone often lead to a successful pregnancy. The role of a varicocoele as a cause of infertility remains controversial. There is evidence that some varicocoeles affect testicular temperature and, therefore, spermatogenesis. Most series have shown improvements in seminal quality following the ligation, but none of these studies is controlled. Drug treatment for oligozoospermia is disappointing; clinical trials are in progress but no one treatment can at present be recommended. If infertility is due to antisperm antibodies, courses of high-dose steroids may be of use.

VASECTOMY AND VASECTOMY REVERSAL

Bilateral ligation of the vasa deferentia, in the neck of the scrotum, is now widely practised as a form of permanent contraception. This is usually done as an outpatient procedure under local anaesthesia. Each vas is divided and ligated, and the ends are separated in order to avoid recanalization. It is essential to repeat the semen analysis 3 months post-operatively to confirm azoospermia. Two negative tests are required for assurance that fertilization cannot occur, but the patient is still warned of the very rare risk of recanalization. Reversal of a vasectomy may be requested, usually because of remarriage. Reported pregnancy rates vary from 50% to 80% following microsurgical repair.

28

I.R. WHITTLE

L. MYLES

Neurosurgery

INTRODUCTION

Although surgery has been performed on the brain since antiquity, neurosurgery as we would recognize it today dates back no more than 120 years. Over the last 50 years, there have been major advances in imaging, anaesthesia, instrumentation, pharmacology, microsurgery and, most recently, computer-assisted surgery. In particular, the application of computerized neuroimaging with frameless image-guided surgery has facilitated many operations. These advances have considerably reduced mortality and morbidity for many conditions.

28

SURGICAL ANATOMY AND PHYSIOLOGY

THE SKULL

The skull is made up of the skull base and the calvarial skeleton, which comprises the frontal bone, the paired parietal and temporal bones and the occipital bone. The frontal and parietal bones are joined by the coronal suture, the parietal bones by the sagittal (midline) suture, and the parietal and occipital bones by the squamosal sutures. These sutures close at about 18 months, and thereafter the brain is enclosed in a rigid container. The skull base comprises the orbital roof, cribriform plates and sphenoid bones (anterior cranial fossa); sphenoid wings and petrous temporal bone (middle cranial fossa); and the squamous occipital bones, the clivus and petrous temporal regions (posterior cranial fossa). The cranial cavity is subdivided by thick folds of dura. The falx separates the two cerebral hemispheres and the tentorium separates the middle from the posterior cranial fossa. At the base of the posterior cranial fossa is the foramen magnum, through which the medulla projects inferiorly towards the spinal cord.

THE SPINE

The bony axial spinal skeleton comprises 7 cervical, 12 thoracic and 5 lumbar vertebrae, as well as the sacrum and coccyx. Although vertebral structure varies between regions, the vertebrae are basically comprised of a body, pedicles, lamina and a posterior spine. The bony spinal canal is formed by the body (anteriorly), the pedicles (laterally) and the lamina (posteriorly). The canal contains the spinal dura, the spinal cord and, inferiorly, the cauda equina. The vertebral bodies are joined by fibroelastic discs and articulate via facet joints.

THE BRAIN

The brain is a gelatinous structure that, in adults, weighs about 1.4 kg. It comprises the paired cerebral hemispheres, the brain stem and the cerebellum. Primary fissures divide the brain into lobes (frontal, parietal, occipital, temporal and limbic). The temporal lobe is separated from the frontal and parietal lobes by the sylvian fissure, and the rolandic (central) sulcus separates the frontal from the parietal

lobes. Commissural fibres, the largest of which is the corpus callosum, connect the cerebral hemispheres. Cortical grey matter lies on the surface of the brain and comprises laminae of neurons that project into the white matter (tracts). Important deep cortical nuclear regions include the basal ganglia, thalamus and hypothalamus. The brain stem comprises the midbrain, pons and medulla. The cerebellum attaches to the back of the pons and is responsible for movement, coordination, balance and posture.

THE MENINGES AND CEREBROSPINAL FLUID

The brain and spinal cord are encased by the meninges. The outer layer is like leather and is called the dura. The two inner layers are much finer: a spider's web-like tissue, the arachnoid, and a very thin layer over the surface of the brain called the pia. Between arachnoid and pia lies the cerebrospinal fluid (CSF) space. The CSF is made up of fluid secreted from the choroid plexus and extracellular fluid from the brain that passes across the ependyma. The paired lateral ventricles, which are lined by ependyma, are the large CSF-containing spaces within the hemispheres. They communicate via the foramina of Munro with the third ventricle, which in turn communicates via the aqueduct with the fourth ventricle in the pons and medulla. Outflow foramina (Luschka and Magendie) connect with the basal and spinal subarachnoid spaces. There are several large CSF cisterns around the base of the brain (e.g. cisterna magna, cerebellopontine cistern). CSF flows over the hemisphere to be reabsorbed in the arachnoid granulations.

THE CRANIAL NERVES

The 12 paired cranial nuclei arise from the base of the brain. The olfactory nerve (cranial nerve (CN) I) transmits the sense of smell via the olfactory bulbs and tracts to the rhinencephalon ('old smell brain') in the temporal lobes. Vision is conveyed from the retina by the optic nerves (CN II) that connect through the optic tracts to the lateral geniculate body of the thalamus. The oculomotor (CN III) and trochlear (CN IV) nerves project from the midbrain and control ocular motility. The trigeminal nerve (CN V) provides sensation to the face, as well as innervating the muscles of mastication. The abducens nerve (CN VI) controls abduction of the eye. The facial nerve (CN VII) arises from the pontomedullary junction and controls the facial musculature, conveys taste from the anterior two-thirds of the tongue, and is secretomotor to the lacrimal and submandibular glands. The vestibulocochlear nerve (CN VIII) conveys hearing from the cochlea and balance from the labyrinth. Nerves IX (glossopharyngeal), X (vagus), XI (accessory) and XII (hypoglossal) project from the medulla to innervate the tongue, pharynx, larynx, bronchus and intestines.

THE SPINAL CORD

The spinal cord consists of central grey (neurons) and white (tracts) matter, and gives off 8 cervical, 12 thoracic,

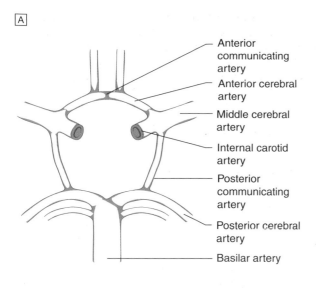

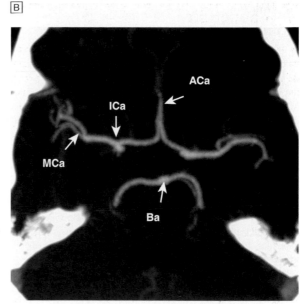

Fig. 28.1 Circle of Willis.
A Diagram outlining the major arteries. B View on a CT angiogram. The basilar artery (Ba) bifurcation, carotid bifurcation (ICa), anterior cerebral arteries (ACa) and middle cerebral arteries (MCa) can all be clearly seen.

5 lumbar and 4 sacral paired spinal roots. Each root comprises a ventral and a dorsal rootlet. The spinal cord is enlarged in the lower cervical region and at the thoracolumbar (conus), and terminates at about L1–L2 level. It continues as the cauda equina in the lower spinal canal to innervate the lower limbs, bladder and genitalia.

BLOOD SUPPLY

The brain requires a large blood flow (800 ml/min, 16% of cardiac output) to satisfy its oxygen and glucose requirements. The cortex receives about 50 ml/100 g/min, and white matter about 20 ml/100 g/min. Cerebral blood flow (CBF) is largely pressure-autoregulated (i.e. for mean arterial pressures between 60 to 140 mmHg, CBF remains constant), but is directly related to $PaCO_2$. Other compounds, such as nitric oxide and endothelin, also regulate local CBF. The anterior and posterior circulations of the brain communicate with each other and across the midline through the circle of Willis (Fig. 28.1). In some circumstances, occlusion of a major artery can be compensated for by collateral flow.

ANTERIOR CIRCULATION

The major vessels supplying the anterior circulation of the brain are the paired internal carotid arteries. These arise from the common carotid artery, pass through the skull base and cavernous sinus, and then divide into the anterior and middle cerebral arteries. Smaller but important branches include the posterior communicating artery, which interconnects the anterior and posterior circulations, the anterior choroidal arteries, and fine perforating vessels to the inferior

part of the brain. The anterior cerebral arteries supply large parts of the frontal and medial parts of the parietal lobes. The middle cerebral artery supplies the posterior frontal region and most of the temporal and parietal regions.

POSTERIOR CIRCULATION

The posterior cerebral circulation arises from paired vertebral arteries that pass through the cervical foramina, enter the skull and join to form a single midline basilar artery. This divides terminally into the paired posterior cerebral arteries. The posterior cerebral arteries communicate with the anterior circulation through the posterior communicating arteries. The posterior circulation supplies the brain stem, cerebellum, occipital lobes and inferior parts of the temporal lobes. Because many of these are 'end-arteries', occlusion often leads to a well-defined stroke syndrome.

INTRACRANIAL PRESSURE

The brain is enclosed within a rigid bony container. Intracranial pressure (ICP) therefore depends on the relative volumes of intracranial blood, CSF and brain parenchyma. ICP also fluctuates in response to changes in intrathoracic pressure (e.g. increased by coughing, defaecation) and cardiac pulsation. These transient increases do no harm. In a normal supine adult, ICP is the same as the CSF pressure obtained at lumbar puncture (5–15 cm H_2O, 4–10 mmHg). In patients with intracranial mass lesions (tumour, haemorrhage), oedema or CSF obstruction, the extra volume is at first compensated for by a reduction in cerebral blood volume and CSF volume. However, a critical point is soon

511

28

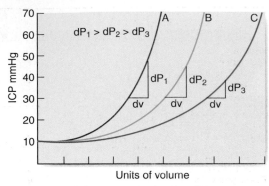

Fig. 28.2 Diagrammatic representation of the effects of a mass lesion on intracranial pressure (ICP).
Generally, ICP increases exponentially with the mass lesion. However, the shape of the pressure–volume curves varies depending on the brain. Thus curve A would represent a mass lesion in a young healthy brain (limited compensation), curve B the brain of a middle-aged patient, and curve C a patient with brain atrophy who is thus enable to compensate for a large intracranial mass lesion before ICP rises.

reached where no further compensation is possible, and any additional volume insult will lead to exponential rises in ICP (Fig. 28.2).

Generalized or localized increases in ICP may lead to marked displacement of intracranial structures (brain herniation syndromes) and can compromise brain perfusion. The cerebral perfusion pressure (CPP) equals mean arterial pressure (MAP) less the ICP (CPP = MAP | ICP). Progressive rises in ICP lead to increases in MAP and reflex bradycardia. However, if there is a severe and sustained elevation of ICP, autoregulation will be ineffective and cerebral perfusion may be focally or generally compromised, leading to cerebral ischaemia and infarction. A CPP of > 60 mmHg is generally required to sustain adequate cerebral perfusion. Although children and young adults can tolerate lower levels, the consequences of a profound, prolonged lowering of CPP are often devastating (e.g. following severe head injury with raised ICP, or after cardiac arrest). The rate of increase in the volume of intracranial mass is crucial to the shape of the ICP

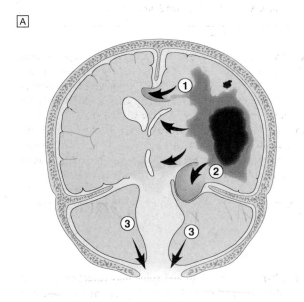

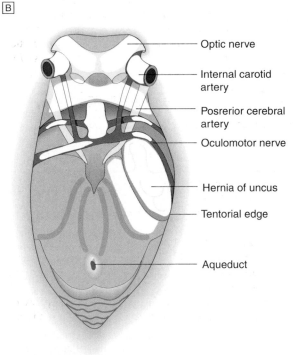

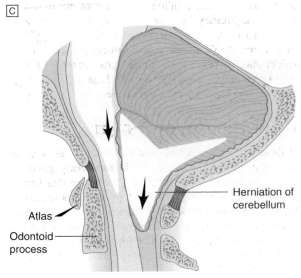

Fig. 28.3 Herniation syndromes.
A Coronal diagram of the dynamics of an intracranial mass lesion. Tumour (T) causes mass effect that compresses the midline and the ventricles (unnumbered arrows), provoking subfalcine or cingulated herniation (arrow 1), and transtentorial herniation (arrow 2). If the mass effect is uncontrolled, tonsillar herniation may also occur (arrows 3). B Transtentorial herniation in the axial plane (plane of dotted line in Fig. 28.3A). C Foraminal herniation.

pressure–volume curve (Fig. 28.2). With more chronic, slow-growing lesions such as brain tumours, abscesses or congenital abnormalities, extraordinary degrees of compensation can occur. In some situations, even massive lesions can lead to minimal symptoms and signs, despite brain herniation.

BRAIN HERNIATION SYNDROMES

Transfalcine (cingulate gyral) herniation

With a parasagittal mass, the ipsilateral cingulate gyrus may herniate beneath the free edge of the falx (Fig. 28.3A). The anterior cerebral artery may be compressed sufficiently to cause medial hemispheric infarction, but otherwise there are no obvious clinical signs except deteriorating conscious level.

Transtentorial (uncal) herniation

With large ipsilateral brain lesions, the medial part of the temporal lobe is pushed down through the tentorial notch to become wedged between the tentorial edge and the midbrain (Fig. 28.3B). The opposite cerebral peduncle is pushed against the sharp tentorial edge, and the midbrain and uncus become wedged at the tentorium. The aqueduct is compressed, obstructing CSF flow, and venous obstruction leads to midbrain haemorrhage. The clinical features of an uncal herniation, most often due to a traumatic intracranial haematoma, are:

- The Glasgow Coma Score (GCS) falls (Table 28.1).
- The motor component of the GCS becomes asymmetrical.
- The ipsilateral pupil dilates and becomes non-reactive to light.
- The blood pressure rises.
- The pulse slows.
- The respiratory rate falls and the patient become apnoeic.

Foraminal (tonsillar) herniation

With mass lesions of the posterior cranial fossa, the cerebellar tonsils and medulla are displaced downwards through the foramen magnum (Fig. 28.3A and C). Cerebellar impaction leads to medullary compression. Following traumatic or spontaneous haematomas, this can

---

Table 28.1 GLASGOW COMA SCALE

Eyes open	
● Spontaneously	4
● To verbal command	3
● To pain	2
● No response	1
Best motor response	
To verbal command	
● Obeys verbal command	6
To painful stimulus	
● Localizes pain	5
● Flexion withdrawal	4
● Abnormal flexion (decorticate rigidity)	3
● Extension (decerebrate rigidity)	2
● No responses	1
Best verbal response	
● Orientated and converses	5
● Disorientated and converses	4
● Inappropriate words	3
● Incomprehensible sounds	2
● No response	1

Total number of points (minimum 3, maximum 15)

---

lead to a dramatic decrease in the GCS, acute hypertension, bilateral extensor responses and bilateral fixed dilated pupils, followed by sudden respiratory arrest. A similar syndrome may occur following the removal of CSF at lumbar puncture in patients with raised ICP due to a posterior fossa tumour, and is also known as 'coning'. There is a rapid deterioration in conscious level, with decerebration. Lumbar puncture must not be performed in patients suspected of having raised ICP due to a mass lesion.

INVESTIGATIONS

PLAIN X-RAY

Plain X-rays of the skull and spine may reveal evidence of metastatic tumour spread, narrowing of the intervertebral discs, congenital abnormalities, bony erosion due to tumour (e.g. of the pituitary fossa) or abnormal vascular markings. Calcification of the pineal gland or choroid plexus may allow displacement to be detected, and abnormal calcification can develop in certain cysts and tumours. This investigation has, however, largely been superseded by computed tomography and magnetic resonance imaging.

COMPUTED TOMOGRAPHY (CT)

Although CT does not image brain tissue as well as magnetic resonance imaging, it is particularly good for visualizing bony tissue and has the advantage that images can be acquired more simply and rapidly. It is the investigation of choice following trauma and for imaging spontaneous intracerebral haematomas. Modern spiral CT scanners allow the craniofacial skeleton and blood vessels (CT-angiography, or CT-A) to be reconstructed in remarkable detail.

BOX 28.1 INTRACRANIAL PRESSURE

- The rigid bony framework enclosing the central nervous system means that any increase in mass content increases intracranial pressure (ICP)
- Acute increases in ICP lower perfusion pressure and, if unrelieved, lead progressively to decreased coma score, herniation syndromes, bradycardia, hypertension, respiratory abnormalities (e.g. apnoea), vasoparalysis and death
- The principal symptoms of chronic raised ICP are headache, vomiting and visual disturbance (blurring of vision). Papilloedema may be apparent
- If ICP is due to a unilateral mass lesion, intracranial structures may be displaced. There are three major forms of herniation: transfalcine, transtentorial and foraminal

28

MAGNETIC RESONANCE IMAGING (MRI)

Magnetic resonance images can be reconstructed in axial, coronal or sagittal planes. As the water in bony tissue is tightly bound, the cranium is not as well visualized as it is with CT. However, as the cortical grey matter comprises approximately 78% water and white matter approximately 68% water, these two areas, as well as subnuclei within the brain, can be clearly distinguished. CSF is also well imaged. By using different magnetic pulse sequencing techniques, the anatomy of the normal and abnormal brain can be imaged in millimetre detail. With both CT and MRI, an intravenous enhancing agent can be administered (iodine-based compounds with CT and gadolinium-based for MRI). Both of these compounds are normally excluded from the brain parenchyma by the blood–brain barrier (BBB). However, with either neoplastic, inflammatory or ischaemic breakdown of BBB integrity or the development of tumour neovascularity, enhancement will be seen in areas involved with the pathological process. MRI is limited by certain conditions (cardiac pacemakers, early pregnancy, some metallic aneurysm clips).

CT AND MR ANGIOGRAPHY

By employing certain contrast agents and rapid sequence imaging, both MRI and CT can be used to perform angiography (MRA, CT-A). In some circumstances, these non-invasive techniques are replacing conventional intra-arterial digital subtraction angiography (IA-DSA). More complex imaging sequences can be used to show white matter disorders, subtle changes in brain water (diffusion tensor imaging) and chemical signals from the brain (magnetic resonance spectroscopy). The function of brain tissues can also be evaluated, since active areas of the brain will have increased blood flow (functional MRI).

CEREBROVASCULAR DISEASE

Stroke is a common major clinical disorder in clinical neuroscience practice. Occlusive disease often affects the extracranial vessels and is a common cause of stroke and transient ischaemic attack, usually managed by vascular surgeons (Ch. 25). Most forms of embolic and ischaemic stroke are dealt with by medical neurologists, whereas many large primary intracerebral haemorrhages and, more importantly, subarachnoid haemorrhage (SAH) are dealt with by the neurosurgeon. Brain tissue metabolism is vitally dependent on a consistent delivery of oxygen and glucose substrates for energy. If there is cessation of substrate delivery, the brain tissue will either die (if CBF is below a threshold of 12–15 ml/100 g/min) or stop functioning (if CBF is between 15 and 25 ml/100 g/min). These ischaemic thresholds are very important in terms of the extent of stroke (i.e. the amount of tissue that will die) and the penumbra (i.e. tissue that is damaged but still able to recover from these acute events).

SUBARACHNOID HAEMORRHAGE

Spontaneous SAH affects 100 persons per million per year and most frequently (70%) results from the rupture of an intracranial 'berry' aneurysm. Other causes include arteriovenous malformation (AVM), cavernoma, tumour, infection and trauma. Typically, the patient complains of a sudden onset of severe headache that peaks in intensity within 1 minute. Patients often describe it as like being 'hit on the head with a hammer' or as 'the worst headache they have ever had'. There is usually associated neck stiffness and photophobia. A positive Kernig's sign denotes meningism. In some cases, a small 'herald' bleed may go unnoticed, or is only remembered when a major bleed occurs. Nausea and vomiting are common. The patient's conscious level is variably affected, ranging from mild disorientation to coma to rapid death.

Grading of SAH depends on the coma score of the patient at time of presentation. The most widely used system, and also the easiest to use, is the World Federation of Neurosurgical Societies' (WFNS) grading, which goes from grade 1 to grade 5 (Table 28.2). When the SAH has produced a syndrome of grade 2–5, it is quite apparent that some neurological catastrophe has occurred. However, when the syndrome is of a grade 1 haemorrhage, differential diagnosis is quite extensive and not infrequently the primary event is overlooked. SAH can mimic atypical migraines, thunderclap headache, coital cephalgia, pituitary apoplexy and meningitic-like syndromes. Sudden death is not uncommon when an aneurysm ruptures into the brain substance rather than the subarachnoid space. The focal signs depend upon the vessel affected. When symptoms and signs are mild, the differential diagnosis is quite extensive and diagnosis depends on having a high index of suspicion.

Saccular intracranial aneurysms

Risk factors include smoking, hypertension, polycystic disease of the kidney and female gender. The median age of affected patients is 47 years, although familial aneurysms may rupture earlier. Most aneurysms (85%) affect the anterior circulation and 15% of patients have more than one. The majority have no symptoms until rupture occurs, although a few may suffer compressive symptoms, and ectatic aneurysms may not rupture at all but cause symptoms by embolic phenomena. The most common compressive clinical signs are features of an oculomotor nerve (CN III) palsy due to an aneurysm of the posterior communicating

Table 28.2 WORLD FEDERATION OF NEUROSURGICAL SOCIETIES' (WFNS) GRADING SYSTEM FOR SUBARACHNOID HAEMORRHAGE

WFNS grade	Glasgow Coma Score	Focal neurological deficits
1	15	No
2	13–14	No
3	13–14	Yes
4	9–12	–
5	3–8	–

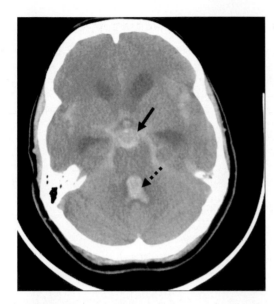

Fig. 28.4 Axial CT scan of a patient following subarachnoid haemorrhage.
Blood is seen in the basal cisterns as a white lesion (solid arrow), and also in the fourth ventricle (broken arrow). There is early enlargement of all ventricles. Courtesy of Dr R Gibson.

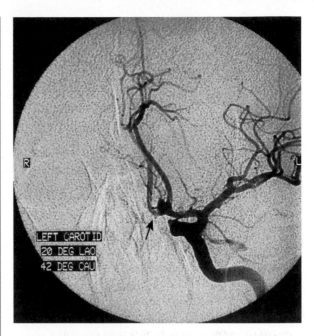

Fig. 28.5 Intra-arterial digital subtraction angiogram outlining the cerebral vasculature and showing an aneurysm of the anterior communicating artery (arrow).

28

artery. Many intracranial aneurysms are now discovered as incidental findings when the brain is imaged.

Investigations

The standard investigation is a CT scan, which characteristically shows blood in the CSF basal cisterns in the acute phase (Fig. 28.4). As CSF blood is broken down, the CT detection rate falls after the first 72 hours. If the diagnosis is in doubt, then a lumbar puncture should be performed, but only in patients whose clinical condition is good and in whom CT has excluded an intracranial mass lesion or midline shift. If this is performed early, the CSF will be uniformly blood-stained; later it will contain haem pigments that will be apparent on naked-eye inspection (xanthochromia) or can be detected by spectrophotometry.

Next, a search must be made for the site of the bleeding. About 80% of aneurysms involve the anterior circulation. Conventionally, carotid or vertebral angiography has been performed (Fig. 28.5). However, CT and MR angiography are equally good at revealing aneurysms greater than 5 mm, and are non-invasive and so associated with less morbidity. As the consequences of missing a diagnosis of SAH are serious, there is a tendency to perform angiography in patients in whom the diagnosis is equivocal. For that reason, a source of bleeding will be identified in only 70% of angiograms. This is usually an aneurysm, less commonly an AVM or a cavernoma. In 30% of cases, no source is found. In the majority, this is a 'true' negative, and many of these patients will have a condition called perimesencephalic SAH, which is of unknown aetiology.

Management of aneurysmal SAH

The medical management of SAH includes intravenous fluids; the calcium antagonist, nimodipine (EBM 28.1);

> **EBM 28.1 NIMODIPINE AND SUBARACHNOID HAEMORRHAGE (SAH)**
>
> 'Nimodipine, a calcium channel antagonist, significantly reduces both death and stroke following SAH.'
> Pickard JD, et al. BMJ 1989; 298:636–642.

---

analgesia; and antiemetics. Patients in coma will usually be intubated and managed in a neuro-intensive care unit. Having initially been quite well, many patients begin to exhibit signs of focal or global cerebral ischaemia 4–10 days following an SAH. This has been attributed primarily to vasospasm and can be ameliorated by the prophylactic use of nimodipine; however, clinical deterioration may occur due to hydrocephalus, seizures, metabolic abnormalities and systemic infections.

Rebleeding is a major cause of morbidity and mortality following aneurysm rupture. Until recently, standard management was occlusion of the aneurysm from the cerebral circulation by surgically clipping its neck (Fig. 28.6 and EBM 28.2). However, it is now possible to place detachable coils within the aneurysm via a catheter passed from the femoral artery into the cerebral circulation (Fig. 28.7). The coils unwind in the aneurysm and induce thrombosis. Coiling is a much less invasive procedure than open surgery and a recent prospective randomized controlled trial showed that, when an aneurysm can be treated by surgery or coiling, the latter is safer (EBM 28.3). Previously, only a proportion of aneurysms were suitable for coiling. However, improvements in coil, stent and basket technology mean most aneurysms can now be coiled.

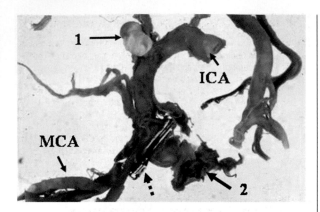

Fig. 28.6   Cerebral arteries at post-mortem showing a surgical clip (broken arrow) on a ruptured middle cerebral artery aneurysm (MCA).
There is also a non-ruptured carotid bifurcation aneurysm (arrow). (ICA = internal carotid artery)

EBM 28.2   ANEURYSM CLIPPING AFTER SUBARACHNOID HAEMORRHAGE (SAH)

'The timing of aneurysm clipping after SAH made little difference to outcome.'
Kassell NF, et al. J Neurosurg 1990; 73:37–47.

Even when an aneurysm has been successfully excluded by means of coiling or surgery, the patient can still suffer stroke. Although nimodipine has significantly decreased the risk of stroke (to 23%) and death (to 22%), there is still no effective treatment for delayed cerebral ischaemia following SAH. Clinical practice has included induced hypertension and plasma volume loading (to keep up CPP), as well as haemodilution (to reduce blood viscosity in the hope of increasing flow), but this triple therapy has its own problems, such as heart failure. The outcome following aneurysmal SAH is heavily dependent upon the condition of the patient on admission and the CSF blood load (the more blood, the worse the outcome). Patients admitted in good condition (grade 1) enjoy a complete recovery in about 90% of cases. By contrast, about 50% of those admitted in coma (grade 5) die or are severely disabled. The outcome of intermediate patients is unpredictable and not necessarily dependent on the clinical excellence of either the attending surgeon or interventional neuroradiologists. Hypotension and fever are also associated with poorer outcome.

PRIMARY INTRACEREBRAL HAEMORRHAGE (ICH)

Primary ICH is becoming an increasing problem as the population of many developed countries ages. It is four times more common than SAH and, in about 30% of cases, is associated with amyloid angiopathy. Most cases are caused by hypertensive rupture of small arterioles in the basal ganglia or cerebellum. Many haemorrhages are small and deep; others may be very large and cause death by

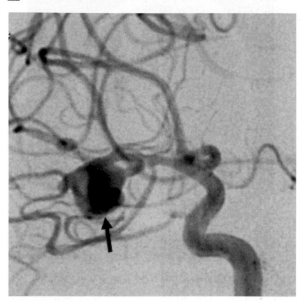

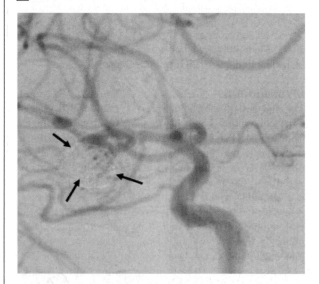

Fig. 28.7   Middle cerebral artery aneurysm.
A Digital subtraction angiogram showing the aneurysm (arrow). B Its occlusion from the cerebral circulation after coiling (arrows).

EBM 28.3   COILING FOR RUPTURED INTRACRANIAL ANEURYSMS

'Coiling ruptured intracranial aneurysms is superior to clipping (the ISAT trial).'
Molyneux AJ, et al. Lancet 2005; 366:809–817.

---

raising ICP and provoking uncal or tonsillar herniation syndromes. Other causes of primary ICH include the rupture of a saccular aneurysm or AVM. The onset is usually abrupt, with many patients developing a flaccid hemiparesis or brain stem–cerebellar syndrome. One-third of patients

---

EBM 28.4   SURGICAL EVACUATION OF INTRACEREBRAL HAEMORRHAGE

'Surgical evacuation of intracerebral haemorrhage is not superior to medical management (the STICH trial).'

Mendelow AD, et al. Lancet 2005; 365:387–397.

BOX 28.2   VASCULAR DISORDERS AND THE CENTRAL NERVOUS SYSTEM

- Symptoms due to occlusive vascular disease most often originate from blockage of extracranial vessels by atherosclerosis. Intracranial occlusion can be thrombotic or embolic
- Transient ischaemic attacks are associated with a high risk of major stroke within 5 years unless treatment is instituted (e.g. by carotid endarterectomy or aspirin therapy)
- Intracranial haemorrhage may be extradural, subdural, subarachnoid or intracerebral. Extradural and subdural haemorrhage are usually the result of trauma; subarachnoid bleeding is due to rupture of an aneurysm in around 70% of cases; and intracerebral bleeding is frequently associated with hypertension and amyloid angiopathy
- Patients with subarachnoid haemorrhage from an aneurysm should be considered for either clipping or coiling of the aneurysm to avoid recurrent bleeding

---

28

die within a few weeks and many of those who survive are permanently disabled. Emergency removal of the haematoma was not uncommon neurosurgical practice in an effort to save life. However, the results of a recent prospective multicentre international randomized controlled trial of surgery for ICH (STICH) have shown that there are no significant differences in outcome with either medical or surgical management of spontaneous, non-aneurysmal, supratentorial ICH (EBM 28.4).

ARTERIOVENOUS MALFORMATIONS

Cerebral AVMs are congenital abnormalities of the capillary system that lead to a direct arteriovenous communication (fistula). This leads to gross dilatation of the draining cerebral veins, as well as ectasia and occasionally aneurysmal dilatation of the feeding artery. AVMs can lead to cerebral ischaemia (because blood preferentially enters the venous system, bypassing the tissues), focal seizures and haemorrhage. Rupture of an AVM typically causes a spontaneous intracerebral haemorrhage rather than an SAH. As the haematoma is under less pressure, the overall prognosis is better than for aneurysmal SAH. The diagnosis is confirmed on CT or MRI and angiography (Fig. 28.8). If the AVM can be excised, then the risk of further haemorrhage is removed, and the incidence and frequency of seizures is considerably reduced. Sometimes, however, the AVM is large and in an important or inaccessible location. In these cases, endovascular 'glueing' or stereo-

tactic radiosurgical treatment is appropriate. The latter is a focused form of X-ray therapy that leads to fibrosis over a 2-year period. AVMs may also affect the spine and lead to cord ischaemia. Symptoms are often progressive and include pain, weakness and, ultimately, paraplegia. Nowadays, the treatment is usually occlusion by interventional neuroradiology.

CAVERNOMAS

These are well-circumscribed collections of small vascular channels (usually capillaries). Patients typically present with headaches, focal neurological deficits or epilepsy, owing to small, recurrent focal haemorrhages. The haemorrhages are usually small in volume and cause a clinical syndrome less dramatic than that associated with SAH or AVM rupture. CT and angiography often miss these lesions, but the lesions have a characteristic appearance on MRI and may be much more common than was previously

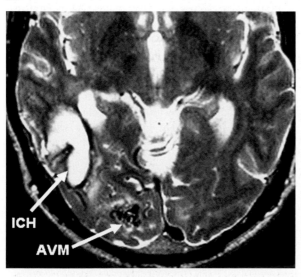

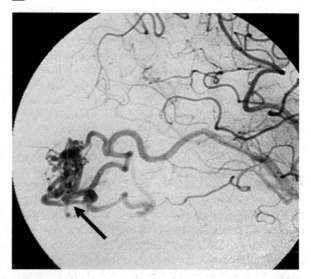

Fig. 28.8   Arteriovenous malformation (AVM).
A MRI scan showing an AVM (arrow) that has bled, causing an intracerebral haematoma (ICH, arrow). B Angiogram of the same AVM.

appreciated. Those causing epilepsy or haemorrhage are usually excised, unless they are in a vital and/or inaccessible place (e.g. brain stem). The risk of rebleeding from cavernomas and AVMs is poorly documented, and prospective natural history studies are under way so that the risks and benefits of intervention can be better defined.

NEUROTRAUMA

Head injury comprises a large proportion of emergency neurosurgical practice. Severity can range from a minor concussive injury through to severe craniocerebral trauma associated with high-velocity motor vehicle accidents. The head injury may be associated with direct injury to scalp or face, and may be penetrating (open) or non-penetrating (closed). From the neurosurgical perspective, the important thing in the management of head injury is to minimize the events that can occur secondary to the primary head injury. Primary brain injury occurs as a direct result of trauma. It may be diffuse or focal and of varying severity, and is essentially irreversible. Secondary brain injury occurs after the primary trauma as a result of hypotension, ischaemia, hypoxia, pyrexia, infection and raised ICP. Secondary brain damage can have a devastating effect on what may initially have been a relatively minor injury and amenable to prevention and treatment.

ASSESSMENT

Glasgow Coma Score

The GCS is a measure of conscious level that has greatly facilitated the classification and objective management of head-injured patients. It is used internationally and records the best verbal response, best motor response and eye opening. The maximum score is 15 and the minimum is 3. Change in GCS over time is much more informative than an absolute reading at any one point in time. The Glasgow Coma Scale can be used in children of all ages, although the 'best verbal' component of the scale needs to be modified to take into account the age of the child, particularly in children under the age of 4 years. The best post-resuscitation GCS is used to classify severity of head injury. Mild injury is GCS from 15 to 13; moderate is from 12 to 9; and less than 8 is classified as severe. Coma is also defined as a GCS of 8 or less.

Neurological examination

This should routinely include an assessment of pupil size and reaction; a search for CSF leaks from nose, mouth and ears; a survey of the scalp for penetrating injuries; signs of a basal skull fracture (Battle's sign, raccoon eyes); and an assessment of the maxillofacial skeleton. Peripheral neurological examination will give a guide to focal brain injury, spinal injury or peripheral nerve injury.

Other systems

Patients with head injury often have extracranial injury. It is important to remember that head injury alone never causes hypovolaemic shock. The management of systemic complications such as severe chest injury, intra-abdominal haemorrhage or major volume loss is a priority in treatment, since these phenomena will lead to secondary cerebral ischaemia and hypoxia and thus secondary brain damage.

MANAGEMENT

As with all injured patients, management commences with airway, breathing and circulation. The neck should be immobilized until a cervical spine injury has been excluded. The GCS should be documented on arrival and following resuscitation, and the findings of a neurological survey recorded. Many patients with head injury are under the effects of alcohol and other drugs that affect conscious level. If in doubt, assume that depressed consciousness is due to brain injury. Continued monitoring of conscious level over time by means of GCS is a key aspect of management, and sedatives must be avoided.

In general, patients with a GCS of 8 or less are intubated and ventilated. This is to prevent hypoxia and aspiration pneumonitis, and to allow hyperventilation, which reduces the $PaCO_2$ and so lowers ICP through cerebral vasoconstriction. Following resuscitation, stabilization and prioritization of injuries, a head CT scan is performed. This will visualize intracranial haematoma, brain contusions (bruises), depressed bone fragments, intracranial air and associated maxillofacial fractures (Fig. 28.8). Mass lesions such as extradural haematoma, subdural haematoma and haemorrhagic contusions may cause brain swelling and shift, and are often surgically evacuated. In many cases, an ICP monitor is inserted for post-operative or elective ICP monitoring. Indications for clot evacuation are > 5 mm midline shift, significant impairment of GCS, or protracted headache or vomiting. Compound cranial wounds need to be surgically explored, dead tissue and foreign bodies removed, depressed bone fragments elevated, haemostasis secured and the dura closed in a watertight fashion. Depending of the age of the wound, bone fragments may be either cleaned and replaced or discarded.

Brain injury evolves over several days and the principal aim of management is to limit secondary damage due to ischaemia and brain herniation caused by raised ICP, hypoxia and hypotension. ICP is often severely elevated following neurotrauma because of oedema, haematoma, contusions, engorgement of the brain vasculature, hydrocephalus or even infection. A sustained ICP that exceeds 25 mmHg is associated with a poorer outcome. Severely brain-injured patients are therefore kept sedated and ventilated and their ICP is monitored. Hyperventilation, mannitol and barbiturates are used to reduce ICP, and the systemic blood pressure may be raised using fluids and inotropes (EBM 28.5). CBF is often directly related to MAP after head injury due to loss of autoregulation, and

---

EBM 28.5 DEXAMETHASONE AFTER HEAD INJURY

'Dexamethasone after head injury is harmful (the CRASH trial).'
Edwards P, et al. Lancet. 2005; 365:1957–1959.

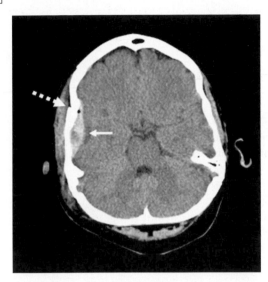

A

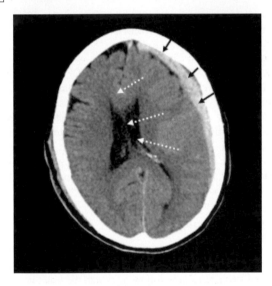

B

Fig. 28.9 Extradural and subdural haematoma.
A Axial CT scan showing an acute extradural haematoma. The extradural clot is lens-shaped (solid arrow), and is associated with a skull fracture and a small amount of intracranial air (broken arrow).
B Axial CT scan showing a subdural haematoma. The subdural clot (black arrows) is compressing the brain and causing significant midline shift and subfalcine herniation (white arrows).

a CPP of > 60 mmHg is generally required to sustain adequate cerebral perfusion. Although children and young adults can tolerate lower levels, the functional consequences of profound and prolonged lowering of CPP are often devastating. Prolonged rehabilitation is required for many neurotrauma patients.

SKULL FRACTURE

The presence of a skull fracture is an important pointer to the likelihood of significant primary and/or secondary brain

injury, especially if accompanied by a depressed GCS. However, the absence of a fracture does not exclude life-threatening brain injury, particularly in young children. A patient without a fracture who has a GCS of 15 has a risk of intracranial haematoma of 1:6000. If a fracture is present, this figure rises to 1:30; if the GCS is 14 or less, the figure is 1:4. Plain X-ray will miss many fractures, particularly of the skull base. CT is the investigation of choice after head injury, and certainly should be performed if there is a skull fracture.

EXTRADURAL HAEMATOMA

This is usually the result of a skull fracture with tearing of a meningeal artery (Fig. 28.9A). It is most common in the middle fossa after a temporal fracture and middle meningeal artery tear. The primary brain injury is often minimal, with a typical 'lucid' interval followed by rapid deterioration as the haematoma enlarges. The prognosis after treatment is usually good.

SUBDURAL HAEMATOMA

This is more common than extradural haematoma and is due to laceration of vessels (especially small cerebral veins) on the brain surface, or 'bursting' of the brain. CT shows a haematoma that is concave on its inner surface (Fig. 28.9B). Craniotomy is performed to remove the haematoma and arrest the bleeding. Morbidity and mortality are often high because of the severity of the primary brain injury. An increasingly common problem with the ageing population is chronic subdural haematoma (CSDH). This is a collection that varies in viscosity from breaking-down clot to blood-stained CSF-like fluid, and which can collect after relatively minor head trauma. Patients with cerebral atrophy who are on aspirin or anticoagulants are predisposed to CSDH. Because the collection can occur slowly, there may be significant midline shift and sometimes very few signs and symptoms. Indeed, CSDH can mimic just about any neurological syndrome in its presentation. Treatment is drainage of the collection. This can be done through burr holes or mini-craniotomy, with or without drainage of the subdural space.

INTRACEREBRAL HAEMATOMA AND CONTUSIONS

Trauma can cause focal intracerebral haematoma or, more commonly, foci of contusions or small areas of brain bruising. Such lesions can cause cognitive and focal deficits in the longer term, but acutely can be associated with severe peri-contusional brain oedema.

DIFFUSE AXONAL INJURY

This type of injury is caused by rotational head movements. It is common after high-speed motor vehicle accidents. The GCS is usually low. Paradoxically, the CT scan may appear normal, or there may be only small punctate brain contusions. The ICP is often normal. However, because

BOX 28.3   HEAD INJURY

- Grading (Glasgow Coma Score, GCS): minor, GCS 13–15; moderate, GCS 8–12; severe, GCS < 8
- May cause extradural haematoma, subdural haematoma, intracerebral haematoma, cerebral contusions, diffuse axonal injury
- Avoidance of hypotension, hypoxia, hypercapnia, pyrexia and ICP > 25 mmHg minimizes secondary brain damage

of the diffuse nature of the brain injury, severe neurological deficits are common.

TRAUMATIC SPINAL INJURY

Injury to the spinal cord may arise as a result of sports injury, following accidents with or without severe craniocerebral neurotrauma, or following relatively minor falls in the elderly. The important factors are whether there is spinal axis instability, and whether there has been myeloradicular injury. The latter is invariably a consequence of the former; however, many cases of spinal axis injury are not associated with neural injury. This is particularly the case for odontoid fractures and pedicular fractures of C2, and many burst fractures of L1. Prompt recognition of cases such as these is required to avoid a devastating spinal cord injury.

Cervical spinal injury

This is commonly caused by trauma that produces subluxation of the cervical vertebra, often C5 on C6, a crush fracture of a cervical vertebral body, or hyperextension or hyperflexion injury in a patient with a narrow cervical spinal canal. The resulting neural injury may cause quadriparesis or a complete cord transection syndrome. A common pattern of injury in the elderly is a central cord syndrome, in which the segmental grey matter is contused but the fibre tracts are relatively spared. This produces weakness in the upper limbs, but relative sparing of the lower limbs.

Management consists of prompt recognition of the injury. Patients will have variable neurological deficits. With cord transection, there may be hypotension and bradycardia (due to loss of peripheral sympathetic tone), areflexia, hypotonicity and paresis. Sensory examination provides a clue to the level of spinal injury. Initially, investigations usually consist of cervical spinal X-rays and then MRI. The spine is then immobilized and, if necessary, spinal realignment is obtained with traction. High-dose steroids can also be given. Surgical stabilization of the spine is then usually performed with anterior discectomy, fusion and plates. Neuro-rehabilitation is important.

INTRACRANIAL INFECTIONS

Infection of the central nervous system and its meninges acquires surgical importance if it produces a mass (abscess or oedema), hydrocephalus or osteomyelitis, or if it occurs

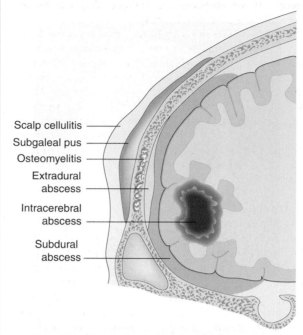

Scalp cellulitis
Subgaleal pus
Osteomyelitis
Extradural abscess
Intracerebral abscess
Subdural abscess

Fig. 28.10   Types of bacterial cranial infection.

as a result of a breach in or absence of the coverings of the brain. In developed countries, intracranial infections are relatively uncommon in immunocompetent patients. However, immunocompromised patients, particularly those affected with HIV, frequently suffer from a range of opportunistic organisms: for example, toxoplasmosis and tuberculosis. Infection may affect the scalp, cranium and meninges, as well as the brain itself (Fig. 28.10).

BACTERIAL INFECTIONS

The brain is relatively resistant to infection but abscesses or subdural empyema (SDE) may form. Initially, there is cerebritis (encephalitis), following which the brain necroses to form pus surrounded by a tough glial capsule. There may be an obvious source of concurrent or contiguous infection (e.g. SDE complicating frontal sinusitis, temporal lobe abscess complicating mastoiditis, brain abscess via haematogenous spread in patients with bronchiectasis), but in many patients the infection appears to arise de novo. Brain abscess and SDE usually present in a subacute or acute manner with headache, seizures and focal neurological deficit. Meningism and pyrexia are common with SDE but are not infrequently absent with brain abscess.

Treatment is a medicosurgical emergency. As well as loculations of pus, the major problems are severe perilesional brain oedema and the propensity to venous sinus thrombophlebitis. CT permits the rapid diagnosis and localization of pus and greatly facilitates surgical drainage. The latter is usually done by image-directed surgery using a frame (stereotactically) or frameless system for an abscess, or craniotomy or burr holes for an SDE. Epidural infections and osteomyelitis of the skull are now very rarely seen in

Europe. If the abscesses are multiple, they can mimic metastatic neoplasia radiologically.

High-dose intravenous antibiotics are necessary and pus is sent for Gram staining, culture and sensitivity. Anaerobic streptococci are the most common agents, although infections due to middle ear disease are often mixed. Dexamethasone can be used to reduce the brain oedema. Although the mortality from brain abscess and subdural empyema has fallen considerably owing to earlier diagnosis, patients frequently have significant neurological sequelae and there is a high incidence (50–60%) of post-infective seizures. Anticonvulsants are prescribed routinely and are often required indefinitely.

Post-surgical infection

Post-craniotomy wound infections occur in less than 1% of procedures and are generally due to staphylococcus. Once the flap is colonized and a nidus of osteomyelitis has developed, the infection will not usually be eradicated by antibiotic therapy. Quite frequently, a sinus will develop along the line of the craniotomy scar and intermittently discharge pus. In most cases, the flap needs to be removed and some form of cranioplastic procedure is performed 9–12 months later. Fortunately, infection of the brain itself following surgery is extremely rare, even following the implantation of prosthetic material.

Meningitis

Although most forms of meningitis are treated by physicians, some involve neurosurgeons. For example, a dural tear following a skull-base fracture leads to the egress of CSF into the paranasal sinuses (cranionasal fistula) or mastoid air cells. From there, the CSF can pass through the Eustachian tube into the nasopharynx (cranio-aural fistula). Under these circumstances, pneumococcal infection can occur, either early or extremely late following injury. Early treatment of post-CSF fistula meningitis is important, as this generally leads to a very satisfactory outcome. Conversely, failure to recognize the disorder can result in death. With post-traumatic CSF fistula, there is no evidence that prophylactic antibiotics reduce the incidence of meningitis. If the CSF leak continues, then the site of leakage needs to be surgically repaired.

INTRACRANIAL TUMOURS

TUMOURS OF THE SKULL

This is an uncommon group of tumours. The differential diagnosis of skull lumps includes osteomas, meningiomas with hyperostosis, metastatic malignancy, fibrous dysplasia, histiocytosis and Paget's disease. Most are painless and diagnosis involves a combination of skull imaging with CT and MRI and systemic investigations.

Gliomas

This group comprises the most common (60%) primary intracranial tumour. Gliomas arise from the brain-supporting cells. Glioma is a generic non-specific term

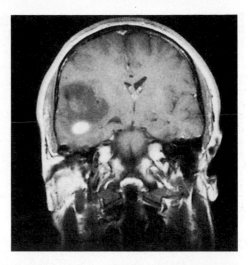

Fig. 28.11 Coronal MRI scan showing a right temporal mass lesion of low signal intensity, with an oval-shaped region of gadolinium enhancement.
The latter suggests malignancy. This tumour was an anaplastic astrocytoma.

applied to such diverse tumours as glioblastoma, astrocytoma, oligodendroglioma and ependymoma. These are infiltrating tumours and are graded using the WHO four-point scale.

- *Grade I tumours* (e.g. pilocytic astrocytoma, dysembryoplastic neuroepithelial, ganglioglioma) are on the borderline between hamartomas and extremely low-grade tumours. They are often cured by surgery.
- *Grade II tumours* (astrocytoma, oligodendroglioma and ependymoma) have variable intrinsic malignancy and survival periods are usually long (median 8.5 years after surgery, radiotherapy and chemotherapy).
- *Grade III tumours* are prefixed anaplastic (e.g. anaplastic astrocytoma, anaplastic oligodendroglioma) and frequently have median survival periods of around 3 years after multimodality treatment (Fig. 28.11). As with grade II tumours, oligodendrogliomas tend to be more responsive to therapies than astrocytomas.
- *Grade IV tumours* are highly malignant and comprise glioblastoma and gliosarcomas.

Grade III and grade IV tumours have features suggestive of malignant transformation (e.g. vascular endothelial proliferation, nuclear pleomorphism, high mitotic rate). Despite multimodality treatment, median survival with glioblastoma is around 9–12 months, depending on age (younger patients do better), performance status (patients in good condition do better) and history of seizures.

Meningiomas

These arise from the dura (Fig. 28.12) and account for 20% of all primary intracranial tumours. They commonly arise from the skull convexity, skull base or sagittal sinus region. They may compress the adjacent brain and cause seizures. They are generally slow-growing (90% are WHO grade I tumours) but may spread widely over the dura ('en plaque'

28

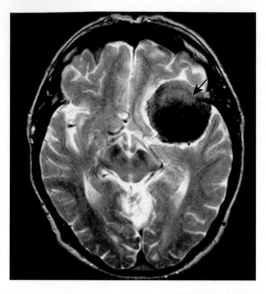

Fig. 28.12 Axial MRI showing a large sphenoid wing meningioma (arrow).
There is no associated brain oedema. This tumour caused troublesome seizures.

tumours), and may invade the skull to form a palpable mass. The treatment is excision and prognosis is usually good. However, recurrences are not infrequent with WHO grade II (atypical) or WHO grade III (anaplastic) meningiomas, or following subtotal excision of a grade I tumour.

Schwannomas

Cranial nerve tumours account for 10% of intracranial tumours and virtually all of them affect the vestibulo-cochlear nerves (acoustic neuroma or vestibular schwannoma) (Fig. 28.13). The tumour grows within, expands and erodes

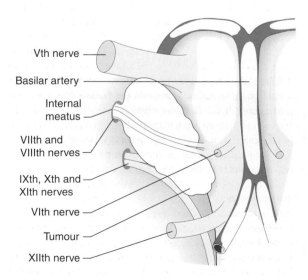

Vth nerve

Basilar artery

Internal meatus

VIIth and VIIIth nerves

IXth, Xth and XIth nerves

VIth nerve

Tumour

XIIth nerve

Fig. 28.13 Right acoustic neuroma.

the internal auditory meatus. The VIIth and VIIIth nerves become stretched over its surface as it grows into the cerebellopontine angle. Early VIIIth nerve symptoms include progressive nerve deafness, tinnitus and vertigo. Larger tumours may involve the trigeminal nerve, leading to diminished facial sensation, as well as the pons and cerebellum, leading to ataxia and nystagmus. Displacement of the fourth ventricle and aqueduct may lead to hydro-cephalus. Patients are often misdiagnosed as having Ménière's disease and the tumour may reach a large size before it is discovered. Treatment options include micro-surgical excision, stereotactic radiosurgery or observation.

Pituitary tumours

These account for 10% of all intracranial tumours. Histologically, most are benign. They produce symptoms through local pressure on the visual apparatus (e.g. distortion of the optic chiasma leads to bitemporal hemianopia) and endocrine effects (by secretion of hormones). They may be treated medically, by trans-sphenoidal hypophysectomy and by radiotherapy.

Brain metastasis

Metastatic tumours are present at post-mortem in 20% of patients dying of cancer, and in 50% they are multiple (Fig. 28.14). They most commonly arise from the lung, breast, kidney, melanoma and colon. Such metastases may be the presenting feature or appear only late in the course of a previously diagnosed primary cancer. Prostate cancer classically spreads to the cranium and never involves the brain parenchyma. Conversely. gliomas very rarely spread beyond the central nervous system.

Clinical features of intracranial tumours

Symptoms of raised ICP

Intracranial tumours commonly present as an intracranial mass lesion, either from tumour volume itself or from surrounding peritumoral oedema. This classically leads to morning headache that is aggravated by bending or straining. If the lesion is large, there may be psychomotor slowing; that is, the patient does everything normally but does it slowly and apathetically. This is a generalized sign of brain hypofunction.

Focal neurological deficit

This refers to any sign or symptom that indicates focal neuronal hypofunction. The most common is hemiparesis due to dysfunction of the motor cortex. Dysphasia occurs in about 50% of dominant hemispheric brain tumours and may be receptive, expressive or mixed. Visual field defects, dyslexia, dysgraphia and dyspraxia are also common.

Seizures

These represent local neuronal hyperfunction. The disorder may be generalized, partial or focal, and the precise nature of the seizures will reflect the anatomical position of the lesion. Seizures are more common with lower-grade tumours and meningiomas, and may respond well to anticonvulsant therapy and excision of the tumour.

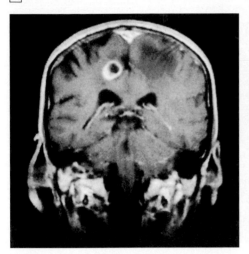
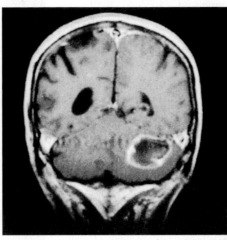

Fig. 28.14 Coronal MRI scans showing two gadolinium-enhancing lesions in the brain. A The smaller lesion is in the cingulate region of the cerebral hemisphere. B The larger lesion is in the cerebellum. Both have low signal intensity centres, suggesting necrosis. The multiplicity of the lesions is highly suggestive of metastatic neoplasia. This MRI appearance can also be seen with multiple brain abscesses.

28

Personality disintegration

There may behavioural disturbances, cognitive decline and problems with insight, judgement, memory and planning abilities. The patient usually has no insight into this progressive decline and may be referred initially to a psychiatrist.

Endocrinopathy

Secondary amenorrhoea, galactorrhoea or (in men) loss of libido caused by a prolactin-secreting pituitary adenoma is the most common example. Acromegaly, Cushing's syndrome, diabetes insipidus and precocious puberty may also occur.

Diagnosis

MRI of the brain parenchyma, before and after the administration of contrast agents, usually clarifies the locality and neuropathology of neoplastic cranial lesions. In most malignant tumours, there is a neovascular capillary bed so that with anaplastic change, tumours will enhance (Fig. 28.11). However, some low-grade tumours (e.g. pilocytic astrocytomas) also enhance, even though these are, in fact, grade I tumours. Meningiomas, which have a mesodermal origin, do not have a BBB and therefore enhance. With the better resolution of MRI, apparently solitary lesions on CT are not infrequently found to be multifocal. A feature of the anaplastic and malignant tumours is peritumoral brain oedema. This fluid occurs in the interstitial white matter due to the neoplastic endothelium not having the integrity of the normal BBB.

Management

The management principles of surgical neuro-oncology generally rely on:

- obtaining tissue diagnosis
- undertaking appropriate surgery to relieve patients' signs and symptoms
- using appropriate radiotherapy and chemotherapy
- providing support services for the patient and family.

The groups of operations that can be performed for brain tumours generally include biopsy, craniotomy and tumour resection. A range of surgical adjuncts, such as awake craniotomy and intra-operative localization techniques, are now employed. The surgical procedure to be undertaken is influenced by the neuroradiological findings (i.e. the likely tumour pathology) and the patient's age, symptomatology and functional status, as well as the accessibility and multiplicity of the lesional pathology.

If peritumoral brain oedema is a feature, the administration of dexamethasone can lead to a dramatic reduction in symptoms and signs over a 12–24-hour period. How steroids work in brain tumours is not well understood, but their pre-operative use has led to a major reduction in surgical morbidity and mortality. If the clinical and radiological parameters suggest only diagnosis is required, then stereotactic or image-guided frameless biopsy is the procedure of choice. This relatively simple procedure involves obtaining special CT or MRI images, entering this detailed information into a computer and then performing the biopsy. The surgery requires a 2.5 cm incision in the head, drilling a burr hole and either affixing a stereotactic frame to the cranium or using a computer image-directed biopsy system. The settings are adjusted so that the biopsy needle is directed at the chosen tumour target. Such systems are accurate to within 1 mm and the tumour diagnostic rate is around 98%. Because this is a minimally invasive procedure, the associated morbidity is generally very low (around 5%) and the 30-day mortality is usually less than 2%. Much of the latter is, however, related to the primary disease process rather direct complications of the surgery.

Excision of the lesion is warranted to reduce mass effect, control seizures and restore lost brain function. If the pre-operative neuroradiology suggests a malignant glioma, then extensive resection may provide optimal symptomatic control, a smoother course during radiotherapy and a reduction in steroid requirement. A recent phase III study has shown survival benefit for patients with malignant gliomas who have had nitrosurea-impregnated biodegrad-

28

able wafers (Gliadel) placed in the resection cavity (EBM 28.6). If the lesion is a meningioma, then a total excision is generally planned, as this is a benign lesion. Similarly, if a posterior fossa lesion looks like a vestibular schwannoma, complete excision may be the treatment of choice. During excisional surgery, a whole variety of adjunctive techniques can be used, ranging from surgical ultrasonic aspirators to intra-operative localization techniques, as well as cortical stimulation of the brain of the awake patient with neurophysiological assessment. The latter technique is extremely useful in operating in areas of eloquent brain, such as the language cortex and motor region.

Outcome after surgical resection is influenced by many factors but, for malignant gliomas, the 30-day mortality is around 5% and neurological morbidity around 10%. Common complications include iatrogenic neurological deficits, cavity and extradural haematomas, and superficial wound infections. Outcome for primary intracranial tumours depends largely on tumour type (see above). Outcome following surgical excision of brain metastases depends on the state of the primary disease, as well as the locality and multiplicity of intracranial disease. Excision plus radiotherapy of a solitary metastasis is typically associated with a median survival of 7 months.

PAEDIATRIC NEURO-ONCOLOGY

Tumours of the central nervous system are the second most common tumours of childhood after leukaemia. The incidence of paediatric central nervous system tumours in the UK is 15 per million of the paediatric population. In children under the age of 2 years, the most common tumours are teratomas, astrocytomas or primitive neuroectodermal tumours (PNET), and these can occur anywhere in the neuraxis. Between the ages of 2 and 15 years, the most common site for tumours is the posterior fossa, and most tumours are PNETs (also known as medulloblastomas (Fig. 28.15) when found in the posterior fossa), astrocytomas and ependymomas.

There may be an insidious onset of symptoms, such as lethargy, nausea and vomiting, with progressive ataxia in posterior fossa tumours. The symptoms of raised ICP (headache, drowsiness, nausea and vomiting) due to hydrocephalus or to the mass effect of the tumour itself may be the factors precipitating admission. Not infrequently, children with posterior fossa tumours present with a torticollis, which is persistent and not related to trauma. General surgeons may be asked to see a child because of persistent vomiting and weight loss, with no other symptoms or signs. Suprasellar tumours, such as craniopharyngioma, may present with visual failure, hydro-

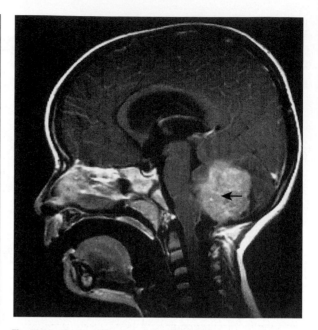

Fig. 28.15   Sagittal MRI of a medulloblastoma.
The tumour (arrow) can be seen filling the fourth ventricle between the pons anteriorly and the cerebellum posteriorly. There is associated obstructive hydrocephalus due to blockage of CSF flow through the fourth ventricle.

cephalus or endocrine dysfunction. Brain-stem gliomas may present with cranial nerve deficits.

One should take seriously the information that a previously well child has lost ground or fallen behind his or her peers. A clumsy child may have ataxia. Endocrine dysfunction may show as short stature, obesity or cachexia. Optic atrophy or papilloedema should always be looked for, as visual problems are difficult to diagnose in small children and visual failure may be profound at the time of presentation. Hemiparesis is occasionally the presenting feature of a hemispheric neoplasm. Spinal cord tumours, although rare in children, may present with back pain, scoliosis, limb weakness or bladder dysfunction. Occasionally, children will present in coma because of a catastrophic bleed into a tumour or the rapid onset of obstructive hydrocephalus. The investigation of choice is MRI, but a CT scan with contrast will often make the diagnosis. MRI should image the spine in order to exclude spinal metastases.

Treatment consists of a combination of surgery, chemotherapy and radiotherapy. Surgical excision remains the mainstay of treatment in most cases, but is usually not curative by itself in malignant tumours, e.g. PNET, ependymoma, malignant astrocytoma. Surgery alone may be curative in the benign tumours (e.g. pilocytic astrocytoma, pineocytoma). Radiotherapy cannot be used in children under the age of 3 because of the risk of damaging the developing brain. Between 3 and 8 years of age, radiotherapy may cause loss of IQ and other neurodevelopmental delays, but to a lesser extent. Some tumours are chemosensitive (e.g. germinomas). Most child-

BOX 28.4 TUMOURS AFFECTING THE SKULL AND ITS CONTENTS

- Common tumours involving the skull are osteomas and metastatic deposits
- Intracranial tumours have a bimodal age distribution (peaks at 6–7 years and the fifth decade). Almost 50% of intracranial tumours are metastatic (the most common primary sources being lung and breast)
- Primary cerebral tumours arise from the supporting cells of the brain (gliomas), from the walls of ventricles (ependymomas) and from the roof of the fourth ventricle (medulloblastomas). They constitute about 60% of intracranial tumours
- Meningiomas account for 20% of intracranial tumours (90% of meningiomas are supratentorial), grow slowly, can cause focal seizures, and are treated by excision
- Pituitary and parapituitary types account for 10% of all intracranial tumours. Pituitary tumours may be functional, both types can cause pressure effects and both types are best removed surgically
- Neurinomas of the cranial nerves account for 10% of all intracranial tumours. Acoustic neurinomas develop in the internal auditory meatus and involve the VIIth and VIIIth cranial nerves, to cause deafness, tinnitus, vertigo and facial weakness. Involvement of the Vth nerve may cause loss of facial sensation

hood brain tumours have a disappointing response to chemotherapy, but it may be used as adjunctive treatment and for recurrent disease. The prognosis for PNET is poor, with only 50% of children surviving for 5 years. In those children who are older than 3 years at the time of presentation, with no CSF seeding or metastatic disease and with a gross total excision of tumour at the time of surgery, the prognosis is better, with 5-year survival as high as 70%. Pilocytic astrocytomas of cerebellum often do well with complete surgical excision alone, and 90% 5-year survival is the norm.

SPINAL DYSRAPHISM

This is a congenital abnormality of the spinal axis, with or without abnormalities of the spinal cord, meninges and nerves, owing to failure of the neural tube to close (Fig. 28.16). Closure usually begins in the mid-dorsal region and extends cranially and caudally. Thus, thoracic defects are rare and cervical defects uncommon, and most affect the lumbar/lumbosacral region. Fortunately, maternal folate supplementation and prenatal screening for raised serum α-fetoprotein at 16 weeks' gestation have reduced the incidence of this condition. There are two categories of dysraphism: open and closed.

OPEN SPINAL DYSRAPHISM

This is known as classic spina bifida aperta or myelomeningocoele. The child has an obvious open spinal defect and lower motor neuron signs below the level of the lesion, with numbness, weakness and a neuropathic bladder. These children often develop hydrocephalus following surgical closure of the spinal lesion and require ventriculo-peritoneal shunting. Around 90% of these children have an associated abnormality of the hindbrain known as a Chiari II malformation, which may cause respiratory or feeding difficulties. They may develop scoliosis as they grow. These children require life-long follow-up in a multidisciplinary clinic, where the renal tract, neurological status and orthopaedic deformities can be regularly reviewed.

A
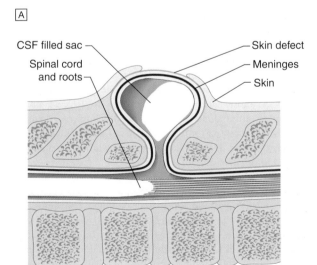

B
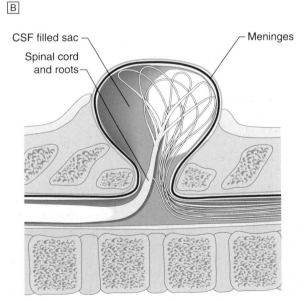

Fig. 28.16 Spinal dysraphism.
A Simple meningocoele. B Meningomyelocoele.

28

CLOSED SPINAL DYSRAPHISM

This is also known as spina bifida occulta and encompasses lesions such as lipomyelomeningocoele, meningocoele, tight filum terminale syndrome, sinus tracts and intradural dermoids, split cord malformations and caudal agenesis. The condition may be apparent at birth owing to the characteristic overlying skin lesions, which include midline lumbar lipomas, hairy patches, dimples and sinuses. However, the diagnosis may not be noted until later in childhood, when the child develops neurological symptoms (often following minor trauma or a growth spurt), pain in the legs and/or recurrent urinary tract infections. Late neurological deterioration and/or bladder dysfunction are due to tethering of the developing spinal cord at the level of the lesion. The treatment is surgical untethering. Other causes include splitting of the cord by a bony projection from the posterior surface of the vertebral body (diastematomyelia), which can be removed, and the presence of intracord lipomas, which are often diffuse and multiple and whose removal is difficult and hazardous. In severe cases, one foot may be smaller than the other. Dural sinus tracts may lead to meningitis. In general, affected individuals do not develop hydrocephalus and there is no association with the Chiari malformation. Low-lying sacral dimples, within the natal cleft, are much more benign and rarely signify serious intradural pathology.

HYDROCEPHALUS

Aetiology and clinical features

Hydrocephalus is the accumulation of CSF within the ventricles or over the surface of the brain. This may rarely be due to over-production of CSF (because of a choroid plexus papilloma), but the vast majority are due to reduced drainage secondary to obstruction of normal CSF flow (Fig. 28.17). Obstruction may be congenital, such as in aqueduct stenosis (Fig. 28.18), or acquired, as a result of tumour or arachnoidal adhesions and fibrosis.

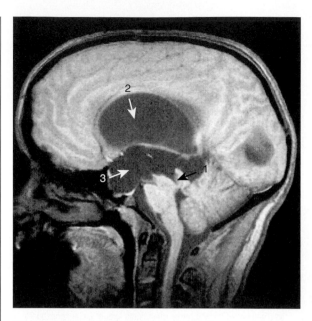

Fig. 28.18   MRI of aqueduct stenosis (arrow 1).
This is an example of an obstructive hydrocephalus. There is gross ventricular enlargement (arrow 2) and herniation of the floor of the third ventricle into the interpeduncular cistern (arrow 3).

Hydrocephalus due to obstruction to flow within the ventricular system, leading to dilatation of the ventricles, is termed 'internal', 'non-communicating' or 'obstructive'. In 'external' or 'communicating' hydrocephalus, the ventricular system is patent but there is reduced flow through the basal cisterns or absorption of CSF by the arachnoid granulations. This is commonly due to fibrosis following meningitis or subarachnoid haemorrhage, or to sagittal sinus thrombosis. In this type, the ventricles and the CSF spaces around the surface of the brain will be enlarged. In adults, chronic hydrocephalus may cause the 'normal pressure hydrocephalus' syndrome of gait ataxia, incontinence and cognitive decline. Diagnosis is often difficult in the elderly because brain atrophy causes ex-vacuo dilatation of the ventricles due to loss of brain substance, mimicking hydrocephalus. Cognitive decline can be associated with Alzheimer-like pathology or cerebrovascular disease, and urinary disturbances may be related to prostate problems.

Congenital hydrocephalus usually presents at birth or in early infancy. The cranial sutures may start to open and the fontanelle will be tense and bulging. The veins of the scalp and the bridge of the nose will be dilated. As the hydrocephalus worsens, the eyes may become downcast (sunsetting). The child may be floppy and develop apnoeic spells and episodes of bradycardia. In older children and children with closed fontanelles, the symptoms are those of raised ICP (headache, vomiting and drowsiness). The eyes may develop a squint owing to a VIth cranial nerve palsy. Papilloedema may be present and, if severe or chronic, may lead to blindness.

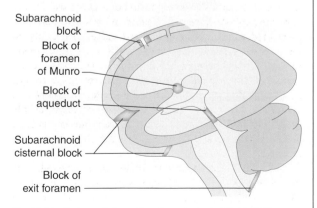

Subarachnoid block

Block of foramen of Munro

Block of aqueduct

Subarachnoid cisternal block

Block of exit foramen

Fig. 28.17   Hydrocephalus: sites of cerebrospinal fluid (CSF) blockage.

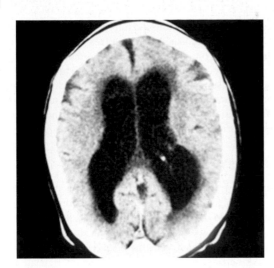

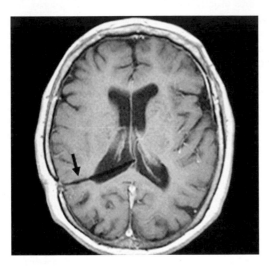

Fig. 28.19 Hydrocephalus.
[A] CT scan showing adult hydrocephalus. [B] MRI after operation (ventriculo-peritoneal shunt, arrow). There has been dramatic resolution of the hydrocephalus.

Management and prognosis

Treatment consists of relieving the pressure by bypassing the block to CSF drainage. In some cases of aqueduct stenosis, this can be done in a minimally invasive way by endoscopic third ventriculostomy. In this procedure, a small hole is formed in the floor of the third ventricle, allowing CSF to flow into the basal cisterns. In most cases, however, a ventriculo-peritoneal (VP) shunt will have to be inserted (Fig. 28.19). This consists of a catheter in the lateral ventricle, which drains CSF through a valve (that sits on the skull under the scalp) into the peritoneal cavity. The risk of bleeding into the ventricular system or brain during the insertion or removal of a VP shunt is of the order of 1–2%. There is also a risk of early infection, usually with skin commensal organisms such as *Staphylococcus epidermidis*.

Shunts can become blocked or malfunction, causing a rapid return of symptoms, and this can be a medical emergency. Shunts can also become infected many months or years after insertion, in which case the shunt has to be removed and reinserted once the infection has cleared. Occasionally, a shunt will over-drain the ventricles, leading to premature closure of the cranial sutures and microcephaly. Over-drainage may be symptomatic, with headache and vomiting. It also predisposes to blockage of the ventricular catheter.

The long-term prognosis depends very much on the underlying cause of the hydrocephalus. In cases of simple aqueduct stenosis treated early, the prognosis for normal IQ and normal neurological function is good. Repeated episodes of raised ICP or ventriculitis can lead to loss of IQ and neurological deficit.

MALFORMATIONS OF THE SKULL

Abnormalities of the scalp and skull are often a source of worry for parents. The common problems are moulding at the time of birth, which is self-limiting, and scalp haematomas caused by ventouse extractions. These usually resolve spontaneously. Subgaleal haematomas in infants, often related to underlying skull fractures, can be extensive and can cause the haemoglobin to drop significantly. Growing skull fractures are peculiar to infancy and are caused when a fracture is associated with an underlying dural tear. The CSF pulsations cause the edges of the bone at the fracture site to absorb, and the child may present some months later with a palpable skull defect in the line of the fracture. The treatment is to repair the dura. The defect can be repaired with bone, but this is not always required.

CRANIOSYNOSTOSIS

This refers to the premature closure or absence of a cranial suture. Several intramembranous ossification centres occur in the skull vault and form plates of bone. Sutures form where these plates of bone meet each other. This is where further bone growth occurs. Overall bone growth is driven by the expanding brain. The brain has reached 85% of its adult size by the age of 2 years but continues to grow slowly after this time. The midline frontal metopic suture fuses at the age of 2 years. Premature fusion of a suture will lead to asymmetrical skull growth. Fusion of a single suture is associated with certain typical head shapes, depending on the particular suture affected (Fig. 28.20). The common ones are scaphocephaly and plagiocephaly (premature fusion of the sagittal and coronal sutures respectively). Plagiocephaly may also be caused by fusion of a lambdoid suture but this is much rarer. Many cases of plagiocephaly are due to head moulding, when the baby lies on its back to sleep. This usually resolves when the child starts to sit and walk.

Sometimes, more than one suture can be affected. This can be syndromal (e.g. Crouzon's or Apert's syndrome). These syndromes are associated with characteristic craniofacial deformities. Craniosynostosis may also lead to a reduction in cranial volume, causing raised ICP. Surgery

28

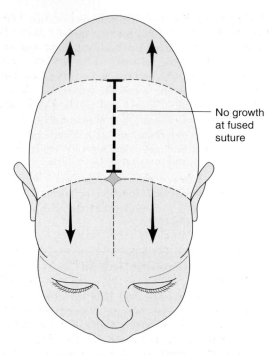

Fig. 28.20 Sagittal suture craniosynostosis.
The sagittal suture is prematurely fused (broken line). Growth normally occurs perpendicular to the suture line. In this case, the skull cannot widen, as there is no growth at the fused suture, which may be palpable as a ridge in the midline. There is compensatory growth at the coronal and lambdoid sutures, leading to an elongated head shape (scaphocephaly), with bulging of the forehead (frontal bossing) in severe cases.

can be undertaken to remodel the skull into a more acceptable shape or to increase the cranial volume.

CRANIAL DERMAL SINUSES AND ANGULAR DERMOIDS

Dermal sinuses are midline tracts lined with squamous epithelium that may communicate with the intracranial cavity and may predispose to meningitis. They are also found in the spine. In the head, most are found in the occipital region; 70–80% are associated with inclusion dermoids and 80% extend subdurally. In the face, because of the complex embryology, dermoids can be found at the tip of the nose and the lateral aspect of the eye.

FUNCTIONAL NEUROSURGERY

A relatively small but highly specialized branch of neurosurgical practice involves the treatment of movement disorders, intractable epilepsy and even certain cases of psychiatric disorder. The aim of surgery in such cases is to modify brain function.

MOVEMENT DISORDERS

Stereotactic surgery for movement disorders such as tremor (Parkinson's disease, essential tremor), dystonia, chorea and

tics involves selecting a target within the central nervous system for either ablation or stimulation. The latter is thought safer and is thus preferred. Neural transplantation is still being evaluated and involves the implantation of neural tissues into the target brain areas in the hope that they will produce missing neurosecretory products. The target nucleus or subnucleus for each disorder is dependent upon the understanding of neuroanatomy and neurophysiology. These various techniques are currently the subject of ongoing trials.

EPILEPSY

The types of seizure disorder that can be helped by neurosurgical intervention are those that, firstly, are intractable to medical therapies; secondly, have a focal onset of seizure disorder; and thirdly, have a structural disorder of the brain associated with the seizure disorder that relates to the seizure focus. The most common indications for neurosurgery are in patients with refractory complex partial seizures usually known as temporal lobe epilepsy. Many of these patients will have either a hamartoma, a low-grade neoplasm or a condition termed hippocampal sclerosis, which leads to chronic seizures. Resection of the involved temporal tissues and hippocampus leads to resolution of the seizure disorder in about 70% of cases. The success rates for surgery in non-temporal epilepsy are lower. However, successful treatment of chronic refractory childhood epilepsy associated with hemispheric dysgenesis is often found following hemispherectomy in young children. Rather surprisingly, resection of the anatomically and physiologically abnormal hemispheric tissues leads to resolution of the seizure disorder and often dramatic improvements in both motor and developmental milestones. Vagal nerve stimulators can also be useful or refractory epilepsy.

VERTEBRAL COLUMN

SPINAL DEGENERATIVE DISEASE

Aetiology and clinical features
Degenerative changes in the intervertebral discs and reactive changes in the vertebral bones are common in the low lumbar and low cervical regions. Disc degeneration is associated with loss of 'disc space' height. This throws abnormal strain on the intervertebral (apophyseal) joints, leading to osteophyte formation and narrowing of the intervertebral foramina. This condition is known as spondylosis and is associated with chronic disc herniation; it may lead to nerve root (lateral recess stenosis), cord (spondylitic myelopathy) or cauda equina (lumbar canal stenosis) compression. These may result in a radiculopathic (i.e. a specific nerve root syndrome), myelopathic or lumbar claudication-type syndrome, with or without low back or neck pain.

In response to acute trauma, the nucleus pulposus may protrude (herniate) through a tear in annulus (Fig. 28.21).

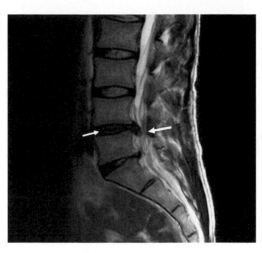

Fig. 28.21 Sagittal MRI scan of the lumbar spine showing bulging and herniation of the L4/5 disc (arrows).

Posterolateral protrusion usually compresses the adjacent nerve root or radicle, causing a sciatica (lumbar) or brachialgic (cervical) syndrome, with or without neurological deficit. Leg pain may be exacerbated by coughing and sneezing, and arm pain by neck movement. There is usually loss of normal lumbar lordosis, and a scoliosis often develops that is concave to the affected side. Straight leg raising is diminished. The neck may have paravertebral spasm. Tendon jerks and muscle power are diminished according to the site of the lesion Thus a L5/S1 prolapse affects the S1 nerve root and produces pain down the back of the thigh, the lateral side of the calf and the lateral border of the foot. There is sensory loss in the latter region. The ankle jerk may be diminished or absent and, as plantar flexion of the ankle is weak, the patient may have difficulty standing on tiptoe. With an L4/L5 disc prolapse, the L5 root is compressed. Pain radiates down the back of the thigh, the lateral aspect of the calf and the dorsum of the foot into the great toe. There may be accompanying sensory loss; the ankle jerk is normal but ankle dorsiflexion is weak.

A surgical emergency occurs if the disc prolapses or herniates directly into the spinal canal (Fig. 28.22). In the cervical region, this will cause a progressive myelopathy, with numb, clumsy hands and spasticity. In the lumbar region, it is usually associated with severe pain in both lower limbs, loss of foot function, urinary retention and numbness up the back of the legs and around the genitalia, anus and buttocks (saddle anaesthesia). A rectal examination should

28

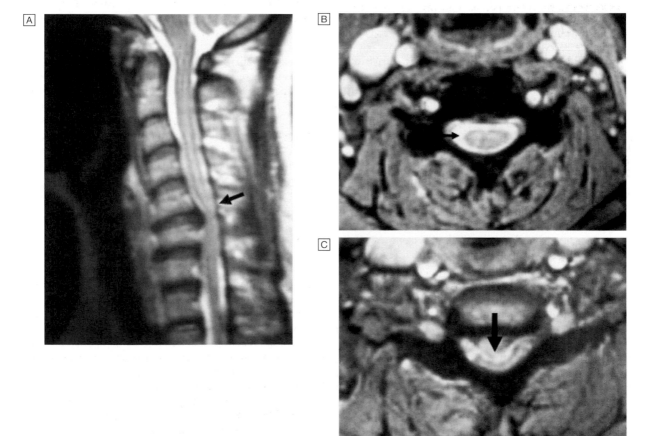

Fig. 28.22 MRI of the cervical spine.
A The sagittal image shows severe spinal cord compression by a central disc prolapse (arrow). **B** Axial image showing the spinal canal, cord and CSF (arrow) at a normal level. **C** Axial image at the level of compression. The posterior disc herniation (arrow) is easily seen.

BOX 28.5   ACUTE LUMBAR DISC PROLAPSE

- The condition is most common in the fourth and fifth decades, and men are most often affected
- The annulus fibrosus ruptures, allowing protrusion of the central nucleus pulposus. The prolapse most commonly occurs posterolaterally, and compresses and angulates the spinal nerve(s) as it leaves the spinal canal. Less commonly, the disc ruptures posteriorly, with compression of the cauda equina
- The most common levels for disc prolapse are L4–5 and L5–S1
- Pain is the predominant symptom and is exacerbated by coughing and sneezing. Tendon jerks and muscle power are diminished, straight leg raising is restricted (e.g. from 80–90° to 30°) and lumbar lordosis is flattened, with scoliosis concave to the side of the lesion
- Most cases settle on conservative therapy, but those with major protrusions or persistence of symptoms beyond 6 weeks should be considered for removal of the prolapsed material
- The cauda equina syndrome (severe back pain, urinary retention and weakness bilaterally below the knees) requires urgent surgical relief

---

be performed to assess anal tone. These features, known as a cauda equina syndrome, may be unilateral if the disc prolapse is asymmetrical.

Management

Degenerative lumbar and cervical spine problems are extremely common, but the majority of problems respond to a cervical collar, bed rest (lumbar), analgesia, physiotherapy and acupuncture. Persistent pain associated with signs of neural compression may require surgical decompression. The investigation of choice is spinal MRI. Flexion and extension X-rays may be useful if there is a spondylolisthesis and any question of spinal instability contributing to the clinical syndrome. In some cases, unusual pathology, such as metastatic tumours, neurofibromas and spinal ependymomas or meningiomas, is discovered.

The type of surgery is determined by the clinical syndrome and radiological investigations. A microdiscectomy may be performed for a simple posterolateral disc prolapse causing a sciatica-radicular syndrome. A posterior foramenotomy or anterior cervical discectomy, with or without fusion and plating, may be performed for a cervical disc prolapse. For multiple-level spinal canal stenosis, a laminectomy may be required in either the cervical or lumbar region. For lumbar spondylolisthesis associated with canal stenosis or radicular signs, decompression and fusion with pedicle screws for stabilization may be necessary. Results depend on many parameters.

PERIPHERAL NERVE LESIONS

Lesions of the peripheral nerves can be classified as: traumatic, compressive, metabolic, inflammatory, autoimmune, neoplastic and genetic. The neurosurgeon will see many compressive lesions, a small amount of trauma and the occasional nerve tumour. The common compressive neuropathies are carpal tunnel syndrome, ulnar nerve compression at the elbow and meralgia paraesthetica.

CARPAL TUNNEL SYNDROME

The syndrome consists of symptoms of pain and numbness in the distribution of the median nerve in the hand. It is more common in patients with diabetes, hypothyroidism, acromegaly and pregnancy. Symptoms may be intermittent, are usually worst at night, and may be relieved by shaking the hand while holding it in a dependent position. The symptoms are often provoked by wrist flexion. On examination, there are usually no signs. Occasionally, there may be wasting of the thenar eminence and weakness of the abductor pollicis brevis, and diminished or altered sensation in the median nerve distribution. Tapping over the nerve in the carpal tunnel may elicit paraesthesia in the median nerve distribution (Tinel's sign). Phalen's test involves acutely flexing the wrist and holding it in this position. This may precipitate paraesthesia or numbness, and this is abnormal if it occurs within 1 minute. The diagnosis can be confirmed using electrophysiology to measure nerve conduction velocity and distal motor latency.

Treatment depends on severity of symptoms. Splinting the wrist or injections of steroid into the carpal tunnel provide relief in a third of cases. If this fails, the transverse carpal ligament can be divided surgically, and in many cases this can be performed as a day case under local anaesthetic.

ULNAR NERVE COMPRESSION AT THE ELBOW

This is usually due to acute and chronic trauma, osteoarthritis or rheumatoid arthritis. The nerve may suffer repeated dislocation over the medial epicondyle on flexion of the elbow. Sometimes, the nerve may be compressed by the aponeurosis between the two heads of flexor carpi ulnaris. There is pain in the forearm and wasting of the small muscles of the hand, leading in the worst cases to an ulnar 'claw' hand. There may be reduced sensation in the ulnar distribution of the hand. The diagnosis may be made clinically, but electrophysiology is recommended to confirm the diagnosis. Treatment consists of surgically releasing and decompressing the nerve.

MERALGIA PARAESTHETICA

This is numbness and painful paraesthesia in the lateral thigh caused by compression or injury of the L2/3 sensory lateral cutaneous nerve. The nerve emerges from the lateral border of the psoas muscle just above the iliac crest and crosses the iliacus to pass beneath or through the inguinal ligament, 1 cm medial to the anterior superior iliac spine, to pass into the thigh. Seat belts, pregnancy, trauma and postsurgical scar tissue, to name but a few, can cause mechanical compression. Diabetes is present in up to 10% of cases. The clinical diagnosis can be confirmed by injecting local anaesthetic into the inguinal region 1 cm medial to the anterior superior iliac spine. Treatment includes weight loss, the removal of constricting clothes and belts, non-steroidal anti-inflammatory drugs, ice packs and injections of corticosteroid. Most cases will settle within 2 years. Surgical decompression is reserved for those that do not.

EVIDENCE-BASED NEUROSURGERY

Much of neurosurgery lacks an evidence base but is performed because the results are considered generally satisfactory. There are, however, many areas of controversy and there is an increasing demand for evidence-based practice. Where randomized controlled trials (RCTs) have been performed, the results have usually led to significant improvements in practice and a softening of entrenched opinion (see the EBM boxes throughout this chapter). There are many other areas, such as the management of low-grade and malignant gliomas, where evidence from RCTs is urgently required in order to optimize patient treatments.

28

L.P. MARSON

J.L.R. FORSYTHE

Transplantation

INTRODUCTION

For many patients, the optimal treatment of their end-stage renal failure (ESRF) is kidney transplantation because it not only improves quality of life but may also confer survival benefits (EBM 29.1). Liver, heart and lung transplantation can be truly life-saving, as often no alternative treatments are available. The two main obstacles to transplantation are overcoming the recipient's immune response and a shortage of donor organs.

TRANSPLANT IMMUNOLOGY

PHASES OF THE RECIPIENT'S IMMUNE RESPONSE TO THE DONOR ORGAN

Early events
Brain-stem death and retrieval of organs, as well as the cold ischaemic time (while the organ is stored on ice) and the warm ischaemic time (while the vascular anastomoses are completed), lead to an early inflammatory response within the donor organ. Next, reperfusion of the donor organ is associated with endothelial activation and the infiltration of inflammatory cells, particularly macrophages. The importance of these early events in shaping the patient's subsequent course is illustrated by the superior outcome observed following living donor transplantation, despite more significant major histocompatibility (MHC) mismatching and the adverse impact of a more prolonged cold ischaemia time on graft outcome.

The afferent arm of the immune response
Donor MHC antigens are recognized as foreign (allo-recognition) by recipient T cells following presentation upon donor (direct) or recipient (indirect) antigen-presenting cells (APCs) (Fig. 29.1). MHC antigen-binding to the T-cell receptor (TCR) in the presence of certain co-stimulatory molecules leads the T cells to undergo clonal expansion and to differentiate into regulatory (CD4-positive) and effector (CD8-positive) cells that are able to secrete cytokines and kill target cells. CD4-positive T (helper) cells play a central role in initiating and amplifying the rejection response.

EBM 29.1   TRANSPLANTATION VERSUS DIALYSIS IN RENAL FAILURE

'Recent studies have demonstrated a significant survival benefit for renal transplantation compared with dialysis for virtually all ages. In addition, long-term dialysis is a major risk factor for graft loss, with best outcomes occurring in those patients transplanted early in the course of end-stage renal failure.'

Wolfe RA, et al. N Engl J Med 1999; 341 (23):1725–1730.
Oniscu GC, Brown H, Forsythe JL. J Am Soc Nephrol 2005; 16(6):1859–1865.
Meier–Kriesche HU, Kaplan B. Transplantation 2002; 74(10):1377–1381.

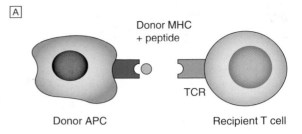

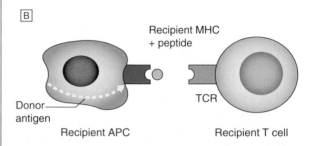

Fig. 29.1   Antigen presentation.
A Direct. B Indirect. (APC = antigen-presenting cell; MHC = major histocompatibility complex; TCR = T-cell receptor)

The efferent arm of the immune response
Donor organ damage can be mediated via cellular or antibody-mediated (humoral) mechanisms. The latter depends on B-lymphocyte maturation and the production of antibodies that activate complement. The former, also known as delayed-type hypersensitivity (DTH), involves cytotoxic T cells, natural killer (NK) cells, macrophages and neutrophils.

PATTERNS OF ALLOGRAFT REJECTION

Hyperacute rejection
This is usually apparent following removal of the vascular clamps as the donor organ becomes swollen and discoloured, leading to graft destruction within 24 hours. It results from the presence of preformed cytotoxic antibodies directed against donor HLA antigens, but has largely been overcome by screening for such antibodies and cross-matching.

Acute rejection
This occurs in up to 50% of grafts, usually in the first 6 months. It may be classified as mild, moderate or severe depending on histological findings from transplant biopsy, and can usually be reversed by treatment with high-dose corticosteroids.

Chronic rejection
This usually occurs after 6 months and often leads to a progressive decline in, and eventually loss of, organ function. The aetiology of chronic rejection is multifactorial: immune-mediated injury, ischaemia–reperfusion injury, toxicity from immunosuppressive agents or viral infections.

29

29

IMMUNOSUPPRESSION

The challenge is to minimize the risk of graft rejection with as few side-effects (such as infection and malignancy) as possible. Prophylactic immunosuppression is commenced immediately following transplantation (induction therapy); it is continued as maintenance therapy and used to treat episodes of rejection. Corticosteroids play an important role in induction and maintenance and are the first-line treatment for acute rejection (Table 29.1).

Antiproliferative agents include azathioprine and mycophenolate mofetil (MMF). Azathioprine was one of the earliest effective immunosuppressive agents to be used and it remains a useful component of many regimes for both induction and maintenance therapy. Side-effects of azathioprine include severe myelosuppression resulting in neutropenia and gastrointestinal symptoms. MMF was developed in the 1990s and is effective in preventing acute rejection episodes when used in conjunction with steroids and a calcineurin inhibitor (CNI) such as ciclosporin. The most common side-effects are gastrointestinal disturbances, leucopenia, thrombocytopenia and anaemia. CNIs, such as ciclosporin and tacrolimus (EBM 29.2), inhibit T-cell activation and commonly provide the mainstay of maintenance therapy. The main side-effects are nephrotoxicity, hypertension, hyperlipidaemia and hyperglycaemia. Monoclonal (e.g. anti-CD25) and polyclonal (e.g. antilymphocyte globulin) therapy is most commonly used as induction therapy and is usually associated with minimal side-effects.

The risk of infection is related to the dose of immunosuppression and patients are therefore at greatest risk early after transplantation. Bacterial infections are most common during the first month. Viral infections are most common

---

BOX 29.1 THE IMMUNE RESPONSE

- The immune response to a transplanted organ is largely mediated by T cells, and these are the target for immunosuppressive therapy
- Acute rejection is seen in up to 50% of grafts and episodes are treated with high-dose steroids
- Chronic rejection has a multifactorial aetiology and results in significant graft loss over the months and years following transplantation

---

between 1 and 6 months and, of these, cytomegalovirus (CMV) is the most clinically relevant; it can be prevented by using antiviral agents. Opportunistic infections with protozoa and fungi are also important and most patients receive up to 6 months' co-trimoxazole prophylaxis against *Pneumocystis jirovecii* (formerly *carinii*).

The risk of developing skin cancer is particularly high following transplantation, with squamous cell carcinoma being 20 times more common in transplant patients than in the normal population. Post-transplant lymphoproliferative disorders (PTLDs) are usually related to infection with Epstein–Barr virus and associated with a high risk of developing B-cell lymphoma. Treatment of PTLD involves reduction in immunosuppression and, in some cases, chemotherapy.

Tolerance can be defined as the coexistence of a transplanted organ or tissue within a recipient without the need for continuous, long-term immunosuppression, whilst maintaining an otherwise intact immune system, and is one of the major goals of transplant research.

ORGAN DONATION

BRAIN-STEM DEATH

The majority of donors are patients who have been diagnosed as brain-stem dead (Table 29.2) following an intracerebral event.

Few absolute contraindications for organ donation exist; those that do are directed against the avoidance of disease transmission from donor to recipient (Table 29.3).

Liaison between staff at the donor hospital and the organ procurement teams is provided by the transplant coordinator who, following the diagnosis of brain-stem death, will meet with the family to discuss organ donation. Current UK legislation is based on an 'opt in' policy, so that lack of objection must be obtained from the family in order to proceed. Other countries adopt an 'opt out' policy of presumed consent. There is a real need to raise public awareness of organ donation and to encourage individuals to carry organ donor cards.

MULTI-ORGAN RETRIEVAL

Organ retrieval begins with opening the abdomen (midline incision) and the chest (sternotomy). Once other pathology has been excluded and the liver mobilized, exposure of

---

Table 29.1 SIDE-EFFECTS OF CORTICOSTEROIDS

- Hypertension
- Diabetes mellitus
- Osteoporosis
- Peptic ulceration
- Cushingoid features
- Pancreatitis
- Poor wound healing
- Psychiatric disorders

EBM 29.2 TACROLIMUS VERSUS CICLOSPORIN IN RENAL AND LIVER TRANSPLANT PATIENTS

'Treatment with the calcineurin inhibitor, tacrolimus, reduces acute and steroid-resistant rejection rates when compared with ciclosporin following renal transplantation, and results in better long-term function. In liver transplant patients, tacrolimus is the agent of choice, with improved outcomes in patient and graft survival.'

Margreiter R, European Tacrolimus vs Ciclosporin Microemulsion Renal Transplantation Study Group. Lancet 2002; 359(9308):741–746.
O'Grady JG, et al. Lancet 2002; 360(9340):1119–1125.

Table 29.2 CRITERIA FOR DIAGNOSIS OF BRAIN-STEM DEATH

Preconditions

- Ventilated and in a coma
- Known diagnosis for coma
- Sufficient length of time on ventilator to determine severity of brain injury
- Optimization of condition, to reverse injury
- Interval of 6–24 hours from latest intervention and testing

Exclusions

- Drug or alcohol intoxication require a delay appropriate to half-life of drug
- Time for clearance of neuromuscular blocking agents
- Primary hypothermia, metabolic and endocrine disturbances
- Coma of unknown aetiology

Investigation

Absent brain-stem reflexes

- No papillary response to light
- Absent corneal reflexes
- Absent vestibulocochlear reflexes: caloric tests
- No motor response in cranial nerve distribution
- No gag reflex

Apnoea testing

- No attempt to breathe despite arterial $P\text{CO}_2 > 6.65$ kPa following pre-oxygenation with 100% oxygen

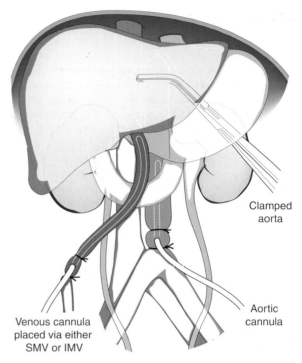

Fig. 29.2 Multi-organ retrieval, showing placement of intra-abdominal cannulae.

(IMV = inferior mesenteric vein; SMV = superior mesenteric vein)

29

Table 29.3 ABSOLUTE CONTRAINDICATIONS TO ORGAN DONATION

- HIV infection
- Presence or history of extracranial malignancy
- Severe systemic sepsis
- Disease of unknown aetiology

the inferior mesenteric vein and the aorta allows insertion of the perfusion cannulae (Fig. 29.2). Cold perfusion is commenced and the vena cava is divided in the mediastinum. The abdomen is also filled with ice-cold saline. The heart and lungs are excised. The pancreas is usually retrieved in conjunction with the liver. The kidneys are excised with ureters and the renal arteries on an aortic patch. A portion of spleen and mesenteric lymph nodes are excised for the purpose of tissue typing and cross-matching, and the iliac vessels are excised and preserved for formation of conduits if necessary.

Organ preservation comprises intravascular flushing with chilled preservation fluid and hypothermic storage by placing the organ in bags and immersing it in crushed ice until transplantation. Although recent improvements in cold preservation fluids allow extended preservation times (e.g. kidneys up to 24 hours and livers up to a maximum of 20 hours, but ideally within 12 hours), prolonged cold ischaemia remains a significant cause of delayed graft function.

STRATEGIES TO INCREASE ORGAN DONATION

Despite extensive publicity for organ donation over recent years, the number of organ donors has remained relatively constant over the last 5 years, while the number of patients on transplant waiting lists has risen inexorably, as shown in Figure 29.3. Strategies to combat the fall in numbers of such organs include the use of non-heart-beating donors, living donors and marginal donors (those would not have previously been accepted, due to age, for example).

The UK has well-developed programmes for living donor renal transplantation. The advantages include transplantation prior to dialysis, reduced incidence of delayed graft function and rejection, and improved patient and graft survival figures. However, this must be balanced against the potential for donor morbidity and mortality. The potential donor will undergo rigorous assessment (Table 29.4), excluding any comorbidity, and will be counselled regarding the risks. The kidney can be removed using open or laparoscopic techniques. The latter is associated with a reduction in post-operative pain, hospital stay and recovery time. In the US, about 30% of these operations are performed laparoscopically, but the technique has yet to be widely adopted in the UK.

Living donor liver transplantation may soon be under way in the UK, as it is in other countries, although the risks to the donor are higher. Lung, small intestine and pancreas transplantation may follow.

It has been suggested that use of non-heart-beating donors (i.e. kidneys obtained from donors declared dead

29

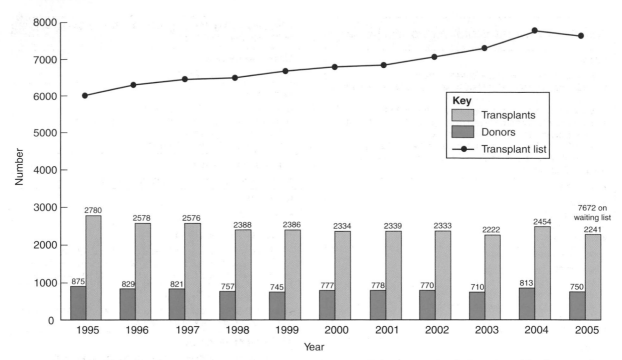

Fig. 29.3 **Number of cadaveric donors and transplants in the UK, 1 April 1995–31 March 2004, and patients on the waiting lists at 31 March each year (UK Transplant statistics).**

on cardiopulmonary criteria) could increase transplant numbers by 30%. Encouragingly, despite concerns about warm ischaemia time, recent case-control studies have demonstrated no significant differences in 5- and 10-year graft survival from donors with and without a heart beat (EBM 29.3). The criteria for non-heart-beating kidney donation are age less than 60 years, warm ischaemic time without effective cardiopulmonary resuscitation less than 40 minutes, and interval between insertion of aortic balloon and procurement less than 2 hours. Contraindications include patients with known renal disease, uncontrolled hypertension, complicated diabetes mellitus, systemic sepsis and malignancy.

In the UK, the majority of non-heart-beating donors are patients in intensive treatment units (ITUs) with near-fatal head injuries, in whom a decision has been made to withdraw treatment, independent of the transplant team ('category III' donors). Following declaration of death, the donor is transferred to the operating theatre and a laparotomy is performed. There is rapid surface cooling

of the kidneys with ice and insertion of a cannula into the distal aorta, allowing rapid perfusion of the kidneys. Kidneys that appear well perfused are harvested and preserved in cold storage.

The number of liver transplants performed from non-heart-beating donors is small due to concern about high primary non-function rates, although this has not been borne out in more recent studies. Biliary complications may be more common, requiring radiological or surgical intervention. In the face of a major donor shortage it is likely that more centres will use such organs in the future.

RENAL TRANSPLANTATION

INDICATIONS AND PATIENT ASSESSMENT

For many patients with ESRF, renal transplantation is the preferred treatment. Absolute contraindications to renal transplantation are active infection and malignancy; relative contraindications include advanced age, severe cardio-vascular disease and likelihood of non-compliance with immunosuppressive therapy. In addition, heed must be paid to the likelihood of the underlying disease (e.g. diabetes mellitus, glomerulosclerosis, amyloidosis and hypertension) giving rise to problems within the transplanted kidney. Potential recipients need to undergo rigorous medical (Table 29.5), psychological and social evaluation. An important component of this is the education of the patient and their family about the benefits and risks of transplantation and of immunosuppression, so that fully informed written consent can be obtained.

BOX 29.2 ORGAN DONATION

- Shortage of organs for donation remains a significant challenge to the transplant community
- Strategies aimed at increasing use of organs for donation include use of marginal donors and donors without a heart beat
- Well-established programmes for living donor kidney transplants exist within the UK, with an increasing drive to establish living donor liver transplantation

---

Table 29.4   ASSESSMENT OF THE POTENTIAL LIVING DONOR

History
- General health: obesity, hypertension, diabetes
- Cardiovascular risk: past medical history, family history, smoking, obesity
- History of thromboembolic events or bleeding disorders
- Respiratory risk (for anaesthetic): past medical history of asthma, chronic obstructive pulmonary disease, smoking
- Risk of renal disease: family history, particularly if disease in recipient is familial; past history of renal infections, haematuria
- Psychiatric history

Examination
- General
- Cardiovascular
- Respiratory
- Abdominal

Investigations
Immunology
- Blood group; HLA type; T- and B-cell flow cytometric cross-matching

Haematology
- Full blood count; coagulation studies

Biochemistry
- Urea and electrolytes; creatinine clearance; liver function tests; blood glucose

Urinalysis
- Protein; blood; sugar culture; sensitivity and microscopy

Cardiovascular
- Serial blood pressure measurements; electrocardiogram

Virus screen
- Hepatitis B and C; human immunodeficiency virus (HIV); cytomegalovirus infection; Epstein–Barr virus; syphilis; *Toxoplasma*

Radiology
- Chest X-ray; isotope glomerular filtration rate; renal ultrasound; angiogram/spiral computerized tomography/magnetic resonance angiography

---

Table 29.5   ASSESSMENT OF THE POTENTIAL RECIPIENT FOR RENAL TRANSPLANTATION

General assessment
- History, clinical examination

Blood tests
- Haematology: full blood count, clotting screen
- Biochemistry: urea and electrolytes, liver function tests
- Virology: HIV, hepatitis B and C
- Immunology: ABO and HLA typing

Urinalysis and culture
- 24-hr urine collection for creatinine clearance

Other tests
- ECG, chest X-ray

Cardiovascular assessment
- Patients > 45 yrs, history of diabetes or of cardiovascular disease: exercise tolerance test, stress echocardiogram or stress radionuclide scan; if abnormal, proceed to coronary angiography

Gastrointestinal assessment
- Abnormal liver function tests, history of peptic ulcer disease: liver ultrasound scan, upper GI endoscopy

Assessment for infection
- Active bacterial infection: contraindication to transplantation
- Viral infections: cytomegalovirus status

Urological assessment
- Urine culture and renal ultrasound; if positive, require assessment of bladder emptying, e.g. post-micturition ultrasound, cystoscopy

Immunological assessment
- Blood group: for ABO compatibility
- HLA typing, anti-HLA antibodies: for HLA matching and organ allocation

---

EBM 29.3   NON-HEART-BEATING VERSUS HEART-BEATING KIDNEY DONORS

'Initial concerns about poorer long-term outcome from non-heart-beating donor kidneys have not been borne out, with recent studies demonstrating no significant differences in 5- and 10-year graft survival. However, one study has demonstrated a significantly higher serum creatinine at 5 and 10 years in the non-heart-beating donor group compared with kidneys from donors with a heart beat, suggesting some irreversible damage has been sustained.'

Metcalfe MS, et al. Transplantation 2001; 71(11):1556–1559.
Weber M, et al. N Engl J Med; 2002; 347(4):248–255.

THE OPERATIVE PROCEDURE

In the UK, kidneys are allocated via a national scheme that is based primarily on HLA matching. Once the kidney has been allocated, a final cross-match test is undertaken for anti-HLA antibodies that may have developed in response to blood transfusion, pregnancy or a previous transplant. This is crucial to avoid hyperacute rejection.

Final preparation of the donor kidney is undertaken at the recipient centre. The iliac vessels are exposed by retroperitoneal dissection and a space developed in the iliac fossa to accommodate the transplant, as illustrated in Figure 29.4. The anastomosis between the renal and the external iliac vein is performed first, followed by the arterial anastomosis. Once the kidney is reperfused, the urinary tract is reconstructed.

POST-OPERATIVE MANAGEMENT AND COMPLICATIONS

Post-operatively, a brisk diuresis is common and careful assessment and maintenance of volume status, blood pressure and serum electrolytes is crucial to optimize renal function. Delayed graft function is defined as the need for dialysis in the first post-operative week and occurs in approximately 30% of cadaveric transplants. Once an ultrasound scan has excluded urinary leakage or obstruction and inadequate renal blood flow, a renal biopsy is performed

29

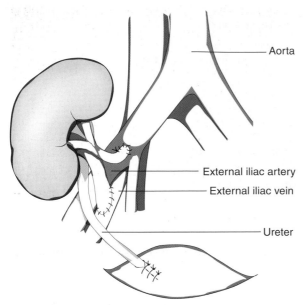

- Aorta
- External iliac artery
- External iliac vein
- Ureter

Fig. 29.4 Renal transplantation.
The renal transplant is placed retroperitoneally on to the iliac vessels with the ureteric anastomosis as shown.

Table 29.6	INDICATIONS FOR LIVER TRANSPLANTATION
Type of liver disease	**Examples**
Chronic liver failure	Primary biliary cirrhosis, alcoholic cirrhosis, viral hepatitis (e.g. HBV, HCV), autoimmune chronic active hepatitis, sclerosing cholangitis
Acute liver failure	Drug-induced (e.g. paracetamol), viral hepatitis
Metabolic disease	Haemochromatosis, Wilson's disease, oxalosis
Tumours	Hepatoma, secondary endocrine tumours

BOX 29.3 RENAL TRANSPLANTATION

- Renal transplant is the optimal treatment for patients with end-stage renal failure, improving quality of life and survival compared with dialysis
- Renal transplantation is associated with 90% 1-year and 70% 5-year survival
- Chronic rejection remains a significant cause of late graft loss

---

to look for rejection or acute tubular necrosis (ATN). Surgical re-exploration offers the only chance of graft salvage in the presence of acute renal artery (c. 1% incidence) and/or venous (c. 6%) thrombosis. Renal artery stenosis occurs in about 10% of patients and usually presents several months post-transplantation with hypertension and deteriorating graft function. The diagnosis is confirmed by angiography and the treatment of choice is angioplasty. Fluid collections (lymphocoeles) around the transplant are a common finding on ultrasound scan but are only relevant if they become symptomatic or are causing urinary obstruction. Percutaneous drainage gives temporary symptomatic relief. Definitive management involves drainage of the cyst into the peritoneal cavity, which can be achieved laparoscopically. Urinary leaks are usually obvious clinically, with pain and reduction in urine output. They usually close spontaneously with prolonged urinary catheterization, but if they are clinically significant, will be best managed by surgical exploration. Urinary tract obstruction can occur early or late. The diagnosis is confirmed by a percutaneous antegrade nephrostogram, during which a nephrostomy tube may be placed for temporary decompression. Subsequent percutaneous dilatation and insertion of a double J stent will often treat the stricture, with open surgery reserved for cases in which percutaneous management has failed.

OUTCOME

The 1-year renal graft survival is approximately 90% and patient survival exceeds this. However, there remains 2–5% perioperative mortality, as many renal patients have severe comorbidity, a relative but not an absolute contraindication to transplantation. The 5-year graft survival is around 70%, and at this time graft losses are commonly due to chronic

rejection or to cardiovascular death in a patient with a functioning graft.

LIVER TRANSPLANTATION

INDICATIONS AND PATIENT ASSESSMENT

Patients with acute or chronic liver failure who show signs of hepatic decompensation despite optimal medical management, patients with certain metabolic diseases that are correctable by liver transplant, and patients with tumours may be considered (Table 29.6).

Patient assessment must be undertaken by a multidisciplinary team comprising hepatologists, surgeons, anaesthetists and, where appropriate, psychiatrists. Patients with alcoholic liver disease must demonstrate evidence of at least 6 months' abstinence prior to assessment and a low risk of recidivism. Patients should be expected to have at least a 50% chance of surviving 5 years. Table 29.7 sets out UK-specific criteria for urgent transplantation in patients with acute liver failure not otherwise expected to survive beyond 3 days and Table 29.8 lists the contraindications to liver transplantation.

THE OPERATIVE PROCEDURE

The operation begins with preparation of the donor liver. The recipient's abdomen is opened via a 'Mercedes–Benz' incision (Fig. 29.5) and the liver removed by dividing the blood supply and the bile duct. The new liver is secured in place by completion of the caval anastomosis, followed by the portal venous and hepatic arterial anastomoses (Fig. 29.6). The liver is reperfused following completion

Table 29.7 CRITERIA FOR LISTING PATIENTS FOR SUPER-URGENT TRANSPLANT IN FULMINANT HEPATIC FAILURE

Paracetamol-induced

- Arterial pH < 7.3 on admission after rehydration *or* all of the following:
- Prothrombin time > 100 s
- Creatinine > 300 μmol/l
- Encephalopathy

Non-paracetamol-induced

- Prothrombin time > 100 s *or* three of the following:
- Age < 10 or > 40 years
- Non-A, non-B, halothane hepatitis or idiosyncratic drug reaction
- Duration of jaundice before encephalopathy > 1 week
- Prothrombin time > 50 s
- Serum bilirubin > 300 μmol/l

Table 29.8 CONTRAINDICATIONS TO LIVER TRANSPLANTATION

Absolute

- Active substance abuse
- Systemic sepsis
- Significant comorbidity, e.g. cardiac/respiratory disease
- Uncontrolled psychiatric disorder
- Extrahepatic malignancy
- Likely failure of compliance with immunosuppressive therapy

Relative

- Late primary hepatic malignancy
- Age > 75 years
- HIV-positive
- Patients with acute liver failure must be assessed on a daily basis for evidence of severe haemodynamic compromise

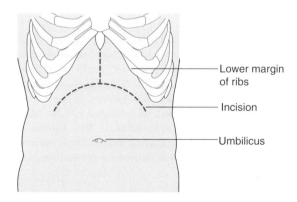

Fig. 29.5 The Mercedes–Benz incision for orthotopic liver transplantation.

29

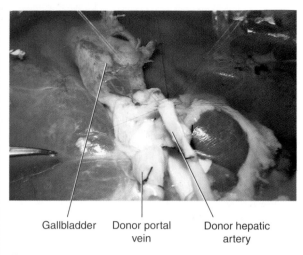

Gallbladder   Donor portal vein   Donor hepatic artery

Fig. 29.6 Hepatic artery anastomosis prior to reperfusion of liver.

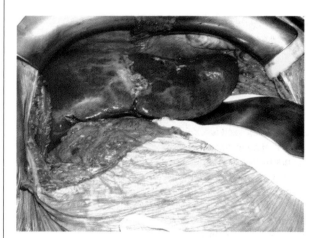

Fig. 29.7 Liver transplant post-perfusion.

POST-OPERATIVE MANAGEMENT AND COMPLICATIONS

Post-operatively, in the ITU, evidence of a functioning graft is based initially on blood biochemistry. A Doppler ultrasound scan is performed within the first 24 hours to evaluate the hepatic artery and portal vein. Primary non-function occurs in approximately 5% of patients and requires urgent retransplantation. Haemorrhage in the early post-operative period is not uncommon; it should be treated with clotting factors in the first instance but, if there is evidence of ongoing bleeding, re-exploration is indicated. Vascular

of the portal vein anastomosis. The donor gallbladder is excised and an end-to-end bile duct anastomosis is fashioned. Figure 29.7 illustrates a well-perfused liver on completion of the transplant operation.

BOX 29.4 LIVER TRANSPLANTATION

- Liver transplantation is a potentially life-saving treatment for patients with acute or chronic liver failure
- Patients must undergo rigorous medical and psychosocial assessment prior to being listed for this major operation
- Outcome for patients following liver transplantation is excellent

29

thrombosis can be detected on ultrasound or arteriography and necessitates re-exploration. Failure of the biliary anastomosis requires conversion to a Roux-en-Y hepatico-jejunostomy. Early rejection typically occurs at 7 and 10 days, manifests as deteriorating liver function tests, is confirmed by liver biopsy and can be treated with methylprednisolone.

OUTCOME

The 1- and 3-year survival rates for liver transplantation are 80% and 70% respectively. One-year survival for elective liver transplant is 90% and close to 70% for patients with fulminant hepatic failure. The 5-year survival exceeds 70% with a relatively low incidence of late rejection in this immunologically privileged organ.

PANCREAS TRANSPLANTATION

INDICATIONS AND PATIENT ASSESSMENT

Despite recent advances in the treatment of diabetes mellitus, patients still experience a suboptimal quality of life with dietary restrictions, need for glucose monitoring and insulin injections. Some cannot achieve glycaemic stability and live with the potentially fatal consequences of hypoglycaemia or the chronic consequences of hyper-glycaemia, such as retinopathy, nephropathy and neuro-pathy. Pancreas transplantation can vastly improve quality of life by normalizing blood sugar, thereby reducing the risk of secondary complications. The generally accepted indications are inadequate glucose control by medical management alone, hypoglycaemic unawareness and 'brittle diabetes', where extremely high or low blood glucose levels are precipitated by minor dietary

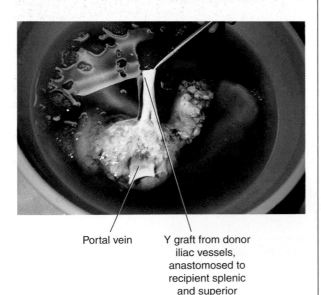

Portal vein   Y graft from donor
iliac vessels,
anastomosed to
recipient splenic
and superior
mesenteric arteries

Fig. 29.8   Pancreas graft showing interposition Y graft prior to implantation.

> **BOX 29.5   PANCREAS TRANSPLANTATION**
>
> - Combined kidney and pancreas transplantation is an excellent treatment for a carefully selected group of patients with type 1 diabetes mellitus
> - Patients must undergo rigorous medical evaluation prior to being listed, as they have complicated diabetic disease
> - Pancreas rejection is difficult to diagnose and this may lead to delay in initiating therapy for such episodes
> - Despite this, combined kidney-pancreas transplant is associated with a 5-year survival of 70%

modifications. The contraindications are systemic sepsis, malignancy and significant medical comorbidity. Insulin resistance is a relative contraindication and should be suspected in obese patients, those with late-onset diabetes or those requiring high insulin doses. Thorough assessment of these patients is essential as the majority have ESRF.

It is important to counsel patients and relatives that a pancreas transplant is a major undertaking and one that is life-enhancing rather than life-saving, as in the case of a liver transplant. Most patients will require a simultaneous renal transplant and the results for such combined trans-plants are better than for solitary pancreas. Cardiovascular assessment is important as patients have a high prevalence of coronary, carotid and lower limb arterial disease. Significant aorto-iliac disease is a relative contraindication.

THE OPERATIVE PROCEDURE

Figure 29.8 illustrates a pancreas graft just before implan-tation and shows the vascular reconstruction that is performed on the back table.

OUTCOME

Rejection of a pancreas transplant alone has been notoriously difficult to diagnose, whereas renal function and renal biopsy can be usefully employed as a surrogate marker of pancreas rejection if a combined kidney–pancreas procedure has been carried out. This, coupled with better immunosuppression, has enabled 5-year combined kidney–pancreas graft survival to exceed 70%. In addition, some recent evidence has indicated that diabetics who receive a renal transplant alone have a worse patient and graft survival than those who receive a combined kidney and pancreas.

HEART AND LUNG TRANSPLANTATION

INDICATIONS AND PATIENT ASSESSMENT

Ischaemic heart disease and cardiomyopathy account for more than 80% of the heart transplants performed today. Children can be treated as successfully as adults, although the shortage of suitable paediatric donors is limiting. A bilateral lung and heart bloc is often advocated for the treatment of patients with congenital heart disease, pulmonary hypertension and secondary respiratory failure. However, if the heart is healthy, as in cystic fibrosis, bilateral lung transplantation can be carried out to remove all potential sources of sepsis. It is also possible to perform single lung transplants in selected patients with emphysema or fibrosing lung disease.

The aetiologies that cause congestive cardiac failure requiring transplantation are primary cardiomyopathy, coronary artery disease with resultant ischaemic cardiomyopathy, and inoperable ischaemic coronary disease with refractory chest discomfort. Potential candidates for heart transplant are patients with advanced heart failure who are on maximal medical therapy, including vasodilators, digoxin, diuretics and β-blockers. Patients should be considered if they have increasing medication requirements, frequent hospitalizations or overall deterioration in clinical status. Exclusion criteria were outlined in 1992 by United Network for Organ Sharing (UNOS) as age > 65 years, significant systemic or multisystem disease, active or extrapulmonary infection, significant hepatic or renal disease, cachexia or obesity, severe osteoporosis, current cigarette smoking, psychiatric illness, and recent (< 2 years) drug or alcohol abuse.

THE OPERATIVE PROCEDURE

With cardiac transplantation, the cold ischaemic time is kept to a minimum, and certainly under 6 hours. To facilitate this, the recipient procedure is normally well under way before the heart reaches the recipient centre. The recipient is fully heparinized and placed on cardiopulmonary bypass with systemic cooling to 28°C. Following removal of the diseased heart and implantation of the donor heart, the patient is rewarmed and the heart is reperfused. Cardioversion and temporary pacing may be required.

Lung transplantation similarly requires a short cold ischaemic time. A lateral thoracotomy is used for single lung transplants, and cardiopulmonary bypass may be required if the patient becomes unstable. With a bilateral procedure, a median sternotomy can be used, although improved access is gained by using a submammary incision.

POST-OPERATIVE MANAGEMENT AND COMPLICATIONS

A complication common to all types of lung transplantation is dehiscence of the tracheal or bronchial anastomosis, which is life-threatening, with prolonged air leak and

---

BOX 29.6   HEART–LUNG TRANSPLANTATION

- Ischaemic heart disease and cardiomyopathy are the most common indications for heart transplant
- Both heart and lung transplantation require short cold ischaemic times in comparison with intra-abdominal organs
- Outcomes following heart and lung transplantation are similar to those seen following transplantation of intra-abdominal organs

---

29

mediastinitis. Routine endocardial biopsies are taken from the right ventricle of heart transplant recipients using X-ray screening and right internal jugular venous access. If rejection is confirmed, augmentation of immunosuppression is carried out. Rejection can also cause rapidly progressive coronary artery disease, with thickening and narrowing of the coronary arteries. Because the donor heart is denervated, the patient will not experience angina, and therefore coronary angiography is performed annually from 2 years onwards.

OUTCOME

Overall, 85% of cardiac recipients are alive and well at 1 year, and 75% 5-year survival has been reported. Recipients are able to lead a very normal life although, like other transplant patients, they do require life-long immunosuppression, with its attendant complications. Sadly, demand outstrips organ supply and the death rate on the cardiac transplant waiting list is high. The 5-year survival of lung transplant recipients is close to 50% or better in some series, chronic rejection causing obliterative bronchiolitis being quoted as a major cause of both graft and patient loss.

SUMMARY

Solid organ transplantation provides excellent treatment for patients with end-stage organ failure, with 1-year graft survival exceeding 80% for most organs. The advantage of transplantation must be weighed against the price of immunosuppression and it is important that potential recipients are fully counselled. One of the greatest challenges facing transplantation is the shortage of organs for donation and this chapter has described specific strategies aimed at combating this: namely, use of marginal donors, living donors and donors without a heart beat.

30

R.P. MILLS

Ear, nose and throat surgery

EAR

ANATOMY

External ear

The pinna (Fig. 30.1) is made of fibroelastic cartilage. Post-auricular muscles are attached posteriorly and allow limited movement in some individuals. The external auditory meatus consists of an outer portion made of cartilage and an inner part formed by the tympanic bone (Fig. 30.2). It is lined by squamous epithelium and contains ceruminous glands that produce wax. There is very little subcutaneous tissue and soft tissue swelling is very painful.

Middle ear

The tympanic membrane is a conical vibrating membrane that is attached to the margin of the bony ear canal peripherally and to the handle of the malleus, the first of the three ossicles, centrally (Fig. 30.2). The head of the malleus is attached to the body of the incus in the space superior to the middle ear known as the attic. The long process of the incus attaches to the head of the stapes via its lenticular process. The stapes occupies the oval window and is surrounded by the annular ligament that attaches to its bony margin. The middle ear is mostly lined by a simple cuboidal epithelium, but there are tracts of mucus-secreting cells within it. The middle ear space is connected to the nasopharynx by the Eustachian tube, which is responsible for maintaining the middle ear at atmospheric pressure.

The inner ear

The inner ear consists of a series of spaces, the membranous labyrinth, surrounded by a bony shell, the otic capsule. The interior of the membranous labyrinth is filled by a fluid called endolymph; the bony labyrinth is filled with perilymph. The cochlea is a coiled tube with an oval window at one end and a round window at the other. The vestibular portion of the inner ear consists of three semicircular canals and the saccule and utricle. The saccule and utricle are situated in a space called the vestibule, medial to the stapes footplate. The acoustic nerve and the three vestibular nerves combine in the internal auditory meatus and pass medially to the brain stem. The facial nerve enters the temporal bone through the internal auditory meatus and passes laterally to the geniculate ganglion, where it turns posteriorly (the first genu). It passes through the middle space superior to the oval window and turns inferiorly (the second genu) to exit at the stylomastoid foramen.

PHYSIOLOGY

The pinna collects sound and funnels it into the ear canal. The tympanic membrane and ossicular chain combine to act as an impedance-matching transformer, so that vibrations in air are transferred to the cochlear fluids without excessive loss of energy. This is achieved through three mechanisms: the drum lever mechanism, the ossicular lever mechanism and the relative sizes of the tympanic membrane and the stapes footplate. The cochlea converts vibrations in endolymph into electrical impulses in the auditory nerve. This is achieved by stimulation of hair cells in the organ of Corti. The maximum response to high frequencies occurs in the basal turn of the cochlea, while low frequencies produce maximal stimulation at its apex. Auditory neurons connect via the brain stem to the auditory cortex. Different groups of cells within the cortex are stimulated by nerve impulses coded for different frequencies. The semicircular canals have ampullae that contain hair cells, and that are stimulated by angular acceleration. The saccule and utricle are stimulated by linear acceleration. Information for the labyrinths, eyes and limbs is combined within the brain stem. Connections from the vestibular nuclei pass to the cortex and the cerebellum (Fig. 30.3).

ASSESSMENT

Clinical features

Conductive deafness is due to disorders of the external or middle ear and results from impairment of the transmission of sound to the inner ear. Sensorineural deafness results from lesions of the cochlea or acoustic nerve. Deafness is often associated with a noise in the ear (tinnitus). Ear pain (otalgia) may be due to ear disease but may also be referred

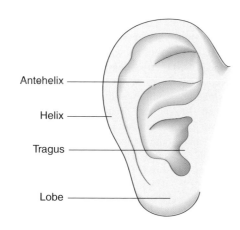

Antehelix

Helix

Tragus

Lobe

Fig. 30.1 Anatomy of the pinna.

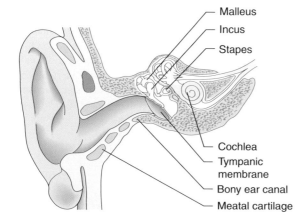

Malleus

Incus

Stapes

Cochlea

Tympanic membrane

Bony ear canal

Meatal cartilage

Fig. 30.2 Anatomy of the ear.

30

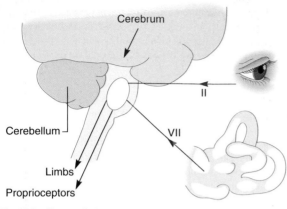

Fig. 30.3 The vestibular system.

from other sites (Table 30.1). Ear-related disorders of balance usually cause a sensation of movement, most often rotation (vertigo). Some patients describe unsteadiness, but this symptom often has a non-otological cause. Patients with ear disease occasionally fall to the ground but never lose consciousness.

Examination

Inspection of the ear canal and tympanic membrane is carried out using an otoscope. A rigid telescope can also be used and is particularly useful for photography. A more detailed examination of the ear can be made using a binocular microscope. This method is also useful when there is a need to remove wax or discharge from the ear. Tuning fork tests can be used to differentiate between conductive and sensorineural hearing loss. Sensorineural hearing loss is due to an abnormality of the cochlea or higher hearing pathways, while conductive hearing loss is due to abnormalities that interfere with the transmission of sound to the inner ear. In practice, this means disease processes affecting the outer and middle ears. In normal individuals and in

Table 30.1   CAUSES OF REFERRED OTALGIA
Pharynx and larynx
• Tonsillitis
• Tonsillectomy
• Tumours
Mouth
• Dental disease
• Tumour
Temporomandibular joints (TMJ)
• TMJ dysfunction
• Arthritis
Neck
• Cervical spondylosis
• Tumour
Paranasal sinuses
• Maxillary sinusitis

sensorineural deafness, a tuning fork is heard better via the ear canal (air conduction) than via the mastoid process (bone conduction). When there is a conductive hearing loss, the tuning fork is heard better by bone conduction (Rinne's test). When there is a symmetrical hearing loss of either type or normal hearing in both ears, a tuning fork placed in the centre of the forehead is heard equally well in both ears. If a conductive hearing loss is present in one ear, the tuning fork is heard better in the deaf ear (Weber's test). If there is a unilateral sensorineural deafness, sound is heard better in the good ear.

Audiometry

Hearing by air conduction can be assessed by pure tone audiometry, in which sounds of known pitch and loudness are presented to each ear in turn via headphones. Air conduction measures the overall hearing loss. Bone conduction can be tested via a bone conductor applied to the mastoid process and gives an indication of cochlear function. Ideally, a masking tone should be used in the opposite ear to prevent sound transmission around the skull giving the impression that a conductive hearing loss is present when this is not the case. The difference between the hearing thresholds measured by these two methods indicates the degree of conductive hearing loss that is present. Examples of audiograms showing conductive and sensorineural deafness are shown in Figures 30.4 and 30.5. The patient's ability to hear speech can be tested by presenting lists of words of known loudness via headphones. The percentage correctly identified at different levels of amplification allows a speech reception threshold (50% of words correctly identified) and a discrimination score to be determined. Middle ear function can be assessed by tympanometry. The amount of sound reflected back from the tympanic membrane is measured while the pressure in the ear canal is varied. This allows the compliance of the drum to be measured. Compliance is maximal when the pressure in the ear canal is the same as the pressure in the middle ear. The test is particularly useful for confirming the presence of fluid in the middle ear.

Imaging

In patients with unilateral sensorineural hearing loss, MRI scans are of value in confirming or excluding the presence of an acoustic neuroma (Fig. 30.6). MRI is also a valuable means of demonstrating the presence of fluid in the cochlea in patients being assessed for possible cochlear implantation. CT scans can be used to demonstrate temporal bone anatomy, congenital abnormalities and some unusual pathology in the temporal bone. They can also be used to demonstrate temporal bone fractures.

DISEASES OF THE PINNA

Bat ears

A developmental abnormality results in absence of the antihelical fold (Fig. 30.1). This produces prominent ears that cause embarrassment. The abnormality can be corrected surgically.

30

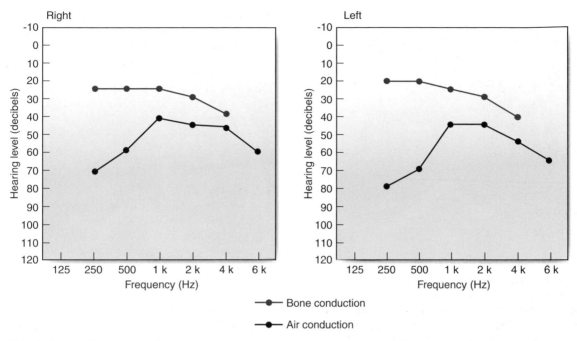

Fig. 30.4   Audiogram showing conductive deafness.

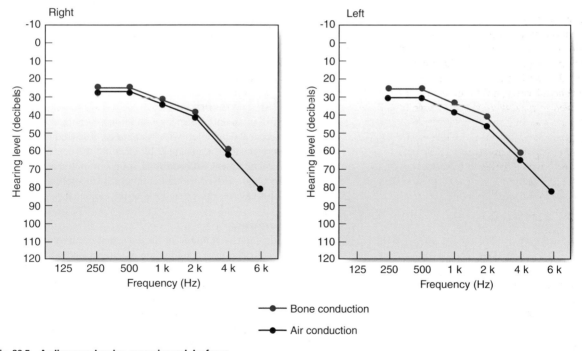

Fig. 30.5   Audiogram showing sensorineural deafness.

Trauma

Trauma to the ear may result in a haematoma, which strips the perichondrium off the underlying cartilage. Secondary infection may lead to loss of cartilage, resulting in a 'cauliflower ear'. Haematomas should be drained to avoid this.

Tumours

Basal cell and squamous carcinomas may occur on the pinna and require excision (Fig. 30.7).

DISEASES OF THE EXTERNAL AUDITORY MEATUS

Wax

Wax (cerumen) is normally found in the ear canal. The ear canal has a migratory epithelium that carries wax to the opening of the external auditory meatus. Wax seldom causes deafness, but can impair hearing if it becomes packed against the eardrum.

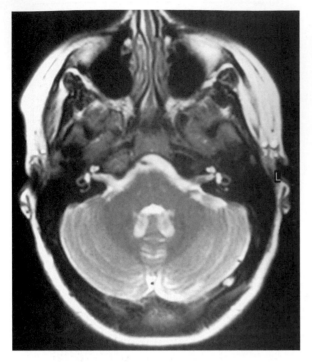

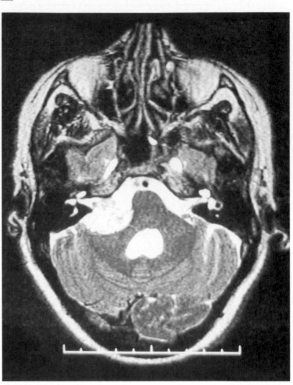

Fig. 30.6   Magnetic resonance imaging (MRI) of the cerebellopontine angle.
A Normal MRI scan of cerebellopontine angle. B MRI showing an acoustic neuroma.

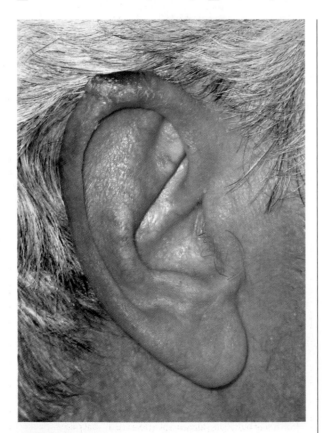

Otitis externa

This is an inflammatory condition of the ear canal skin. Secondary infection with bacteria or, less frequently, fungi may occur. It is managed by cleaning the ear, followed by local treatment with eardrops, sprays or ointment containing a steroid, with or without antibiotics. Uncommonly, chronic otitis externa causes stenosis of the ear canal.

Tumours

Squamous carcinoma of the ear canal occurs uncommonly. It is treated by a combination of surgery and radiotherapy.

DISEASES OF THE MIDDLE EAR

Acute suppurative otitis media

This is a bacterial infection of the middle ear space, usually caused by *Streptococcus pneumoniae* or *Haemophilus influenzae,* most commonly occurring in young children (3 years of age and under). Children present with a combination of ear pain (otalgia), fever and malaise. On examination, dilated blood vessels are seen on the drum surface in the early stages. The drum then becomes red and begins to bulge. Perforation with discharge frequently occurs, but most of these perforations heal spontaneously. Antibiotic therapy shortens the episodes and provides protection against the development of complications (EBM 30.1). In the pre-antibiotic era, infection commonly spread to the mastoid process, causing bone destruction and

Fig. 30.7   Squamous carcinoma of the pinna.

EBM 30.1   ANTIBIOTICS FOR ACUTE OTITIS MEDIA IN CHILDREN

'*Antibiotics provide small benefit for acute otitis media in children. This benefit must be weighed against possible adverse reactions. Antibiotic treatment may have an important role in reducing the risk of mastoiditis.*'

Glasziou PP, et al. (Cochrane Review). Cochrane Library, issue 1, 2006. Oxford: Update Software.

For further information: 🖥 www.cochrane.org

the development of a subperiosteal abscess (mastoiditis). This is now only seen infrequently. Occasionally, facial palsy or meningitis may complicate middle ear infection.

Otitis media with effusion (OME), or 'glue ear'

In this condition, fluid accumulates in the middle ear space. It is much more common in children than adults. Most cases are idiopathic but a minority of adult cases are caused by nasopharyngeal tumours and systemic disease. Childhood OME causes hearing loss and may interfere with the acquisition of language and performance at school. Virtually all cases resolve spontaneously, but this can take as long as 10 years to happen. Initial management involves documentation of the presence of effusion and the degree of hearing loss during a period of watchful waiting. If the effusions persist, hearing may be improved by drainage of the effusion (myringotomy) and insertion of a ventilation tube (Fig. 30.8). In children, removal of the adenoids leads to resolution in a proportion of cases. Spontaneous resolution may also occur in adults, but often effusions persist. Ventilation tubes can also be of value, but some cases are better managed with a hearing aid.

Chronic suppurative otitis media

This causes aural discharge and deafness.

Tubo-tympanic or mucosal disease

This is characterized by the presence of a perforation of the tympanic membrane. Discharge is common but not universal. Swimming and other activities that involve water entering the ear may precipitate discharge. Greater degrees of hearing loss occur when there is erosion of the ossicular chain, most commonly the incus long process. Discharge can be controlled by cleaning the ear and introducing eardrops. Recently, there has been concern about possible ototoxic effects of aminoglycoside drops when used in this way. This has led to the restriction of courses of eardrops to a maximum of 2 weeks. Surgery is indicated to prevent discharge, improve hearing and allow the patient to swim. An operation designed to repair a perforation is called a myringoplasty. Defects of the ossicular chain can be repaired by removing the incus and repositioning it to bridge the gap between the malleus and stapes or by using a prosthesis (ossiculoplasty).

Attico-antral or squamous disease

This is associated with the development of cholesteatoma, which consists of a retracted area of the drum in which

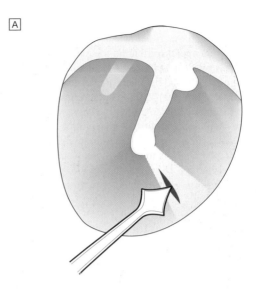

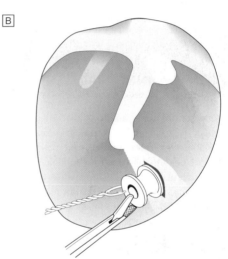

Fig. 30.8   Surgical treatment of otitis media with effusion.
A Myringotomy. B Grommet insertion.

BOX 30.1   OTITIS MEDIA

- Acute otitis media is extremely common in children under the age of 3 years
- The child typically awakes crying at night with a painful ear, and the diagnosis is confirmed by finding a red, inflamed bulging tympanic membrane on otoscopy
- Pain relief is important. Antibiotics should be given to prevent the development of complications
- Otitis media with effusion (glue ear) occurs transiently in many children and is manifested by temporary hearing impairment. Most cases settle spontaneously, but bilateral hearing impairment may demand surgery (adenoidectomy, myringotomy or insertion of a grommet)
- Chronic otitis media involves the middle ear and mastoid mucosa and is associated with permanent perforation of the tympanic membrane, hearing impairment and a mucopurulent discharge. Inactive ears require closure of the perforated membrane (myringoplasty) and rebuilding of the ossicular chain. Ears with cholesteatoma may require surgical removal of the posterior canal wall to create an open mastoid cavity and so reduce the risk of meningitis, intracranial abscess and facial palsy

keratin accumulates. The drum tissue around the periphery of the cholesteatoma is known as matrix. It produces a number of chemical mediators that stimulate osteoclast activity. This means that cholesteatoma is capable of eroding surrounding bone and is therefore associated with complications such as facial palsy and intracranial sepsis. Surgical treatment is mandatory in all but the very elderly and those who are medically unfit. The operation employed to eradicate cholesteatoma is called a mastoidectomy. Erosion of the ossicular chain is more likely to occur in association with cholesteatoma. However, the priority of surgery is to eliminate the disease rather than to improve hearing.

Otosclerosis

This is a condition in which the stapes becomes fixed by new bone formation. It is more common in females and sometimes runs in families. It can be treated by an operation called stapedectomy, in which the stapes is replaced by a piston attached to the incus. This produces excellent hearing improvement in the majority of patients, but in a minority their hearing is made worse by inner ear damage. The hearing loss can also be managed with a hearing aid.

DISEASES OF THE INNER EAR

Deafness

Deafness is most commonly due to changes in the cochlea. Ageing produces a gradual deterioration in hearing acuity known as presbycusis. The cochlea may be damaged by chronic noise exposure, blast injuries and temporal bone fractures. Significant noise exposure may occur in heavy industry and agriculture, and also results from playing in rock bands and shooting. Deafness may also be inherited or be a manifestation of systemic disease. Some drugs, such as aminoglycosides and cytotoxic agents like cisplatinum, can damage the cochlea. Viral infections such as mumps and rubella can also cause sensorineural deafness. Unilateral hearing loss occurs in acoustic neuroma (Fig. 30.6B).

Most cases of inner ear deafness are managed with a hearing aid, but in cases of profound deafness, hearing may be restored by a cochlear implant. This consists of a series of electrodes that are introduced into the cochlea surgically. A speech processor converts sound into electrical energy, which stimulates the cochlear nerve.

Vertigo

In some cases, balance disorders are due to abnormalities of the vestibular portion of the inner ear. Abnormal fluctuations of fluid pressure within the inner ear (endolymphatic hydrops) produce a combination of fluctuating deafness, tinnitus and vertigo known as Ménière's disease. This is initially treated medically, using either a vasodilator agent (e.g. betahistine) or a diuretic. If medical treatment fails, an operation may be required to facilitate the drainage of endolymph (endolymphatic sac decompression) or destruction of the vestibular portion of the labyrinth using a vestibulotoxic agent such as gentamicin introduced via the middle ear. If this fails, destruction of the surgical labyrinthectomy or section of the vestibular nerve produces symptomatic improvement.

Benign positional vertigo is a condition in which debris floating in the posterior semicircular canal stimulates the hair cells in its ampulla, producing vertigo. This happens when the affected ear is downmost and the episodes typically occur when the patient turns over in bed. Debris can be displaced from the posterior canal by positioning the head so that it floats out of the canal into the vestibule (Epley's manoeuvre). If this fails, division of the ampullary (singular) nerve or occlusion of the posterior semicircular canal is beneficial.

Vestibular neuronitis is a condition that causes severe vertigo lasting for as long as several weeks. The hearing remains normal. It is due to severe temporary reduction of vestibular function in the affected ear. Patients are managed by bed rest and vestibular sedatives, such as prochlorperazine.

DISORDERS OF THE FACIAL NERVE

Facial palsy may result from temporal bone fractures or surgical trauma. When the nerve is divided, it may be repaired by end-to-end anastomosis or a cable graft derived from a sensory nerve of the right size, such as the sural nerve. Bell's palsy is an idiopathic facial palsy that usually improves spontaneously. There is some evidence that it is caused by viral infection. Steroid therapy given soon after the onset may be beneficial. Herpes zoster infection of the geniculate ganglion causes facial palsy, often associated with deafness and vertigo (Ramsay–Hunt syndrome). Vesicles may be seen on the palate and on the tympanic membrane. Antiviral treatment appears to influence the course in a favourable manner. Intracranial tumours and malignant tumours in the neck can also cause facial palsy.

NOSE

ANATOMY

The nasal skeleton consists of two nasal bones superiorly and two paired cartilages inferiorly (Fig. 30.9). The nasal cavity is divided into two by a partition composed of cartilage anteriorly and bone posteriorly (the nasal septum). Three turbinate bones protrude from the lateral wall of the nose (Fig. 30.10). Between the inferior and middle turbinates is the middle meatus of the nose. Most of the paranasal sinuses open into this area under cover of a soft tissue flap known as the uncinate process. Obstruction of the sinus ostia in this area can cause sinus pain and may lead to sinus infection. Superior to the superior turbinate is an area of olfactory epithelium from which arise the nerve fibres of the olfactory nerve. The anterior portion of the nasal septum is called Little's area. Here prominent veins are often found, and nose bleeds most often arise from this part of the nose.

PHYSIOLOGY

The functions of the nose are to filter, warm and moisten inspired air. Olfaction is important in its own right and as an adjunct to taste.

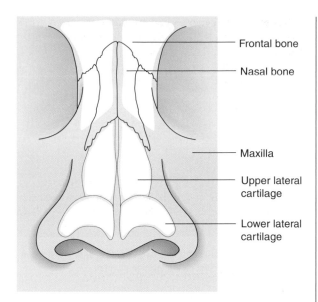

Fig. 30.9   Anatomy of the nasal skeleton.

- Frontal bone
- Nasal bone
- Maxilla
- Upper lateral cartilage
- Lower lateral cartilage

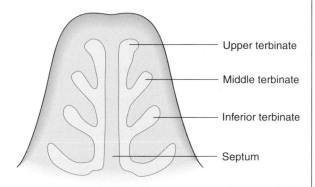

Fig. 30.10   Anatomy of the nasal cavity.

- Upper terbinate
- Middle terbinate
- Inferior terbinate
- Septum

ASSESSMENT

Clinical features

Nasal obstruction is a common symptom with a number of causes. Sneezing and rhinorrhoea are generally due to chronic rhinitis. Purulent nasal discharge and facial pain occur in sinusitis. Loss of smell may be due either to nasal blockage that prevents odours reaching the olfactory epithelium or to damage to the olfactory nerves. Smell is an important part of taste and reduced taste is therefore usually also reported by patients with anosmia.

Examination

The nasal cavity can be inspected using a nasal speculum or an otoscope. More detailed examination, particularly of the posterior part of the nose, can be carried out with a rigid telescope.

Imaging

Computed tomography (CT) is the best means of imaging the paranasal sinuses and also gives information about the middle meatus of the nose, where the sinus ostia are situated, and about variations in the anatomical relationships between the sinuses and the orbit and skull base (Fig. 30.11). This information helps to prevent complications during endoscopic sinus surgery. The sinuses can also be visualized by magnetic resonance imaging (MRI), but the bony anatomy is not shown and mucosal disease is exaggerated.

DISEASES OF THE NOSE

Trauma

This may result in fracture and displacement of the nasal bones. Such fractures should be reduced within 14 days, as after this it becomes difficult to mobilize the nasal bones. There may also be displacement and fracture of the septal cartilage and bone, leading to a deviated nasal septum (Fig. 30.12). Treatment consists of resection (submucous resection, SMR) or repositioning (septoplasty) of cartilage, and should be carried out at a later date when the results of trauma to the soft tissues have settled. Bleeding into the septum causes a septal haematoma, resulting in severe nasal obstruction. This should be drained under aseptic conditions, as infection may cause loss of cartilage and collapse of the nasal bridge.

Chronic rhinitis

In some cases, this condition is a manifestation of sensitivity to inhaled allergens such as pollen or dust. In others, no allergies can be demonstrated and it appears to be a reaction to environmental conditions such as temperature and humidity. It may be seasonal (usually summer) or perennial. Patients complain of nasal blockage that often switches from side to side, sneezing and rhinorrhoea. Most cases are best managed medically with a steroid nasal spray. In severe

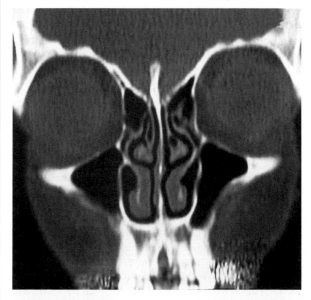

Fig. 30.11   Normal CT scan of the paranasal sinuses (coronal view).

30

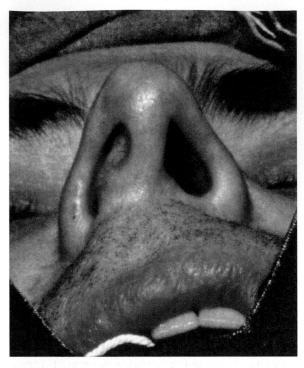

Fig. 30.12 Deviated nasal septum.

cases with nasal obstruction, reduction of the inferior or middle turbinates may provide relief.

Nasal polyps

Oedematous paranasal sinus mucosa extrudes through sinus ostia to produce nasal polyps. When they arise from the ethmoid labyrinth, the polyps are multiple, but when the origin is the maxillary antrum, a large single polyp protruding posteriorly into the nasopharynx is produced (antrochoanal polyp). The extent of sinus involvement is best determined by CT (Fig. 30.13). Temporary improvement in the resulting nasal obstruction can be produced by topical or systemic steroids, but definitive treatment consists of surgical excision, with or without clearance of the

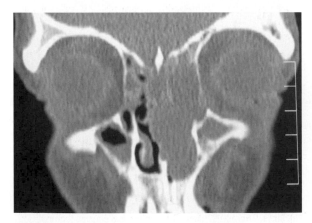

Fig. 30.13 CT scan showing gross nasal polyposis.

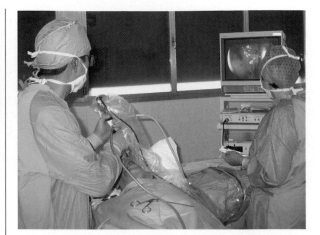

Fig. 30.14 Set-up for endoscopic sinus surgery, with the surgeon viewing the surgical field on a television monitor.

Table 30.2 DISEASES ASSOCIATED WITH EPISTAXIS
Bleeding disorders
• Haemophilia
• Thrombocytopenia
• Von Willebrand's disease
• Excessive anticoagulation (e.g. with warfarin)
Systemic disease
• Liver disease
• Renal disease
• Hypertension
• Hereditary telangiectasia

BOX 30.2 EPISTAXIS

- Epistaxis in young patients usually arises from a small blood vessel in Little's area; in older individuals, it arises from an arteriosclerotic vessel located more posteriorly
- Pressure on Little's area by compressing the anterior septum usually stops the bleeding, and topical applications of 1 in 1000 adrenaline (epinephrine) may be helpful
- Bleeding arising more posteriorly may require balloon compression or packing
- Coagulation defects should always be excluded in patients with troublesome bleeding. In a proportion of patients, these can be caused by alcohol or non-steroidal analgesics
- In persistent epistaxis, it may be necessary to ligate one of the arteries supplying the nose: for example, the maxillary artery

sinus(es) of origin. Nowadays, this is usually carried out using a rigid telescope and camera (Fig. 30.14). Recurrence is common.

Epistaxis

Nose bleeds may be associated with a number of disease processes (Table 30.2). They are common in healthy children and young adults. Bleeding usually arises from Little's area and can be controlled by squeezing the nose

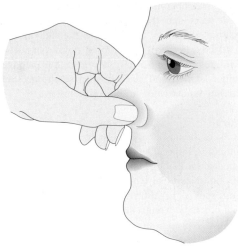

Fig. 30.15   Stopping epistaxis by squeezing the nose.

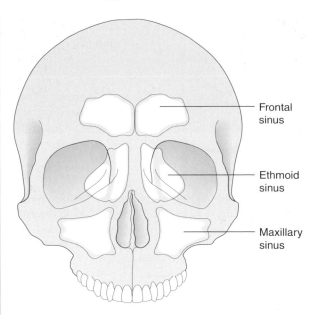

Fig. 30.17   Anatomy of the paranasal sinuses.

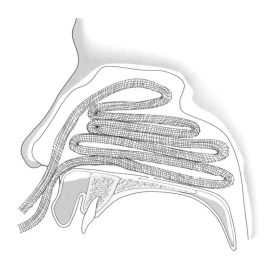

Fig. 30.16   Nasal packing.

(Fig. 30.15). In the elderly, more severe bleeding from further back in the nose may occur. In these cases, a nasal pack may be required to arrest the bleeding (Fig. 30.16). Bleeding may be associated with the use of non-steroidal anti-inflammatory drugs (NSAIDs) in this group. Severe bleeding not controlled by a pack can be arrested by clipping either the sphenopalatine or maxillary artery.

PARANASAL SINUSES

ANATOMY

The paranasal sinuses are air-filled cavities that open into the nasal cavity, mostly into the middle meatus of the nose. The maxillary sinuses occupy the cheeks (Fig. 30.17) and have ostia that are situated closer to the roof of the sinus than to the floor. The ethmoid labyrinth consists of a number of air cells lying between the orbit and the lateral wall of the nose. The frontal sinus is an ethmoid air cell that has migrated into the frontal bone, and it is connected to the nose via the frontonasal duct, which passes down to the middle meatus. The sphenoid sinus is posterior to the ethmoid labyrinth, inferior to the pituitary fossa.

DISEASES OF THE PARANASAL SINUSES

Sinusitis

Any of the sinuses may become infected, but the most commonly involved is the maxillary sinus. The site of the pain caused by sinusitis depends on which sinus it arises from. Pain arising from maxillary sinus is felt in the cheek, that from the ethmoid labyrinth over the nasal bridge, that from the frontal sinus in the forehead, and that from the sphenoid sinus over the occipital region. Acute sinusitis is most commonly caused by *Strep. pneumoniae* or *Haemophilus influenzae* and typically follows an upper respiratory infection. When the origin of the infection is a dental abscess, Gram-negative organisms may be isolated. Uncommonly, fungal infection may occur.

Acute sinusitis is usually managed medically. Chronic sinusitis may result from failure of resolution of acute infection or may arise insidiously. Surgical treatment is frequently required and consists of enlargement of the natural ostium of the maxillary sinus. Chronic infection of other paranasal sinuses also usually calls for surgical intervention. Infection may spread from the sinuses, usually the ethmoid or frontal sinuses, to involve other areas such as the cranial cavity or orbit (Fig. 30.18).

Tumours

The most common neoplasm found in the paranasal sinuses is squamous carcinoma, but adenocarcinomas are seen in workers in the furniture industry. The most common sites

551

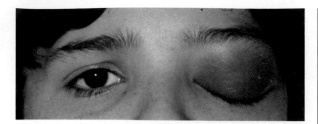

Fig. 30.18   Orbital cellulitis.

30

of origin are the maxillary and ethmoid sinuses. Spread outside the primary site is usually evident at presentation (Fig. 30.19). These relatively uncommon tumours are managed by a combination of surgery and radiotherapy, or by local surgery and topical chemotherapy.

NASOPHARYNX

ANATOMY

The nasopharynx lies posterior to the nasal cavity and superior to the oropharynx. The skull base lies superiorly and the Eustachian tubes open into its lateral walls. Diseases of the nasopharynx

DISEASES OF THE NASOPHARYNX

Adenoids

The adenoids consist of lymphoid tissue and in young children they occupy a significant proportion of the space within the nasopharynx. They increase in size until the age of 4 years and then become progressively smaller, disappearing altogether by the time the individual is an adult. Adenoid hypertrophy causes nasal obstruction in some children. They also have a role in the pathogenesis of childhood OME and sleep apnoea syndrome. Surgical removal may be indicated in these circumstances.

Tumours

Carcinoma of the nasopharynx is common in the inhabitants of southern China. The Epstein–Barr virus has been implicated in its pathogenesis. It may present with middle ear effusion or cervical lymphadenopathy, as well as local symptoms such as nasal obstruction or epistaxis. Treatment is by radiotherapy. Young boys may develop a benign but locally invasive tumour called an angiofibroma. This presents with nasal obstruction and epistaxis and is treated by surgical excision.

MOUTH

ANATOMY

The floor of the mouth is mainly occupied by the tongue. The ducts of the submandibular salivary glands open antero-lateral to it. The roof of the mouth is formed by the hard and soft palates. Its lateral walls are the medial aspects of the cheeks. The parotid ducts open just above the second upper molar teeth.

A

B

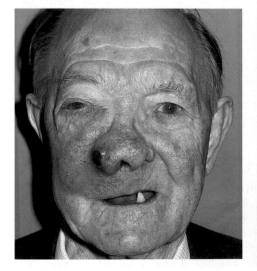

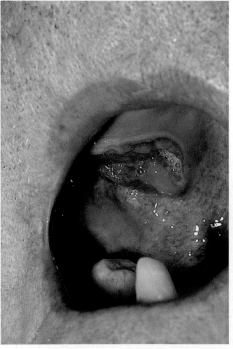

Fig. 30.19   Spread of sinus cancer.
[A] There is evidence of spread into the cheek and orbit, with displacement of the eye. [B] There is ulceration of the hard palate, indicating spread into the mouth.

DISEASES OF THE MOUTH

Stomatitis and gingivitis

Inflammation of the oral mucosa and gums is often associated with poor oral hygiene. It may also be a manifestation of a systemic disorder, such as anaemia (e.g. Paterson Brown–Kelly syndrome, also known as Plummer–Vinson syndrome). Candida is an opportunist infection that may affect the oral cavity. It is characterized by white spots on the mucous membrane. Removal of the white material causes bleeding. Infection in the floor of the mouth may develop secondary to dental sepsis (Ludwig's angina). Pain, dysphagia, trismus and even airway infection may occur.

Mouth ulcers

Aphthous ulcers are the most common type. These have a punched-out appearance and are painful. They are thought to be due to a local failure of the mechanisms that protect the oral mucosa from damage. They resolve spontaneously, but this process can be speeded by the use of local treatment with steroid pellets. Oral ulceration is also seen in systemic disorders such as pemphigus and mucous membrane pemphigoid. Rarely, oral ulceration may be due to tuberculosis or syphilis.

Retention cysts

Mucous retention cysts may occur anywhere in the oral cavity. Those inferior to the tongue are called ranulas. They result from blockage of the openings into mucus and minor salivary glands. This may clear spontaneously, but otherwise excision may be required.

Leucoplakia

Leucoplakia (white patches) may develop on the oral mucosa. It is due to chronic irritation—for example, by tobacco and alcohol—causing hyperkeratosis (Fig. 30.20). Leucoplakia is a pre-malignant condition. Removal of the patches, together with avoidance of the causative factors, can prevent progression.

Tumours

Squamous carcinoma of the tongue is the most common neoplasm seen in the oral cavity. Lesions cause induration of the tongue, usually with ulceration (Fig. 30.21). Lymphatic spread occurs to the submental nodes and

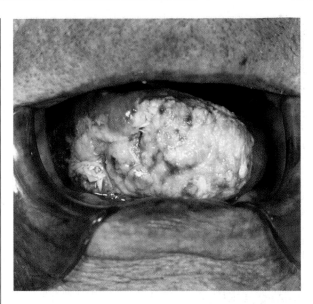

Fig. 30.21   Carcinoma of the tongue.

thence to other deep cervical nodes. Smoking and heavy spirit drinking are predisposing factors. Small lesions can be treated by local excision or radioactive implants (iridium wires), but more extensive tumours require excision with a margin of normal tissue. This often includes excision of part of the mandible.

OROPHARYNX

ANATOMY

The oropharynx lies posterior to the oral cavity between the nasopharynx superiorly and the hypopharynx and larynx inferiorly. At the junction of the mouth and oropharynx are the tonsils, which consist of lymphoid tissue. Together with the adenoids (see above) and the lingual tonsil in the base of the tongue, they form a lymphoid system known as Waldeyer's ring. This system is important in the development of immunity during early infancy, but subsequently can be removed without ill effect. The pharynx itself is surrounded by three constrictor muscles arranged one inside the other like a stack of bottomless beakers.

DISEASES OF THE OROPHARYNX

Pharyngitis

Viral infection of the pharynx is common and is often associated with coryza. Symptomatic relief can be obtained from analgesics. Sore throat with exudate over the tonsils is a common manifestation of infectious mononucleosis (glandular fever). This disease is due to the Epstein–Barr virus and also causes cervical adenopathy and hepatosplenomegaly. Irritation of the pharynx may be due to tobacco smoke and acid reflux.

Tonsillitis

This is due to bacterial infection of the tonsils, usually with *Strep. pyogenes*. Patients present with episodic sore

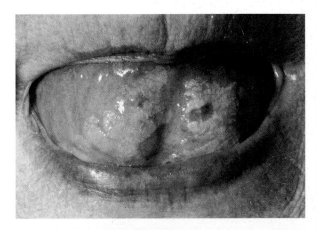

Fig. 30.20   Leucoplakia of the tongue.

30

EBM 30.2 ANTIBIOTICS FOR ACUTE SORE THROAT

'Antibiotics should not be withheld in severe cases. Penicillin V 500 mg 6-hourly for 10 days is the dosage used in the majority of studies.'

'Practitioners should be aware that infectious mononucleosis may present with severe sore throat. Ampicillin-based antibiotics should be avoided in infectious mononucleosis.'

'Sore throat should not be treated with antibiotics to prevent development of rheumatic fever or acute glomerulonephritis.'

Scottish Intercollegiate Guidelines Network. SIGN Guideline 34; 1999.
For further information: 🖳 www.sign.ac.uk

EBM 30.3 INDICATIONS FOR TONSILLECTOMY

'The following are indications for tonsillectomy: sore throats due to tonsillitis, five or more sore throats per year, symptoms for at least 1 year, or episodes of sore throat that are disabling and prevent normal functioning.'

Scottish Intercollegiate Guidelines Network. SIGN Guideline 34; 1999.
For further information: 🖳 www.sign.ac.uk

BOX 30.3 TONSILS AND ADENOIDS

- Adenoids are large in small children but become smaller with age
- They may cause nasal obstruction and be involved in the pathogenesis of otitis media with effusion and sleep apnoea in children
- Tonsils may require removal because of recurrent tonsillitis or peritonsillar abscess in adults and children. Children with sleep apnoea may also benefit from tonsillectomy
- Unilateral tonsillar enlargement may be due to squamous carcinoma or lymphoma

---

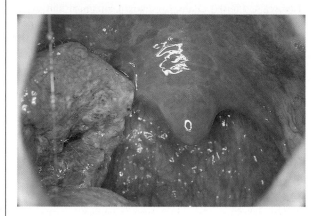

Fig. 30.22 Carcinoma of the tonsil.

throat associated with fever and malaise. Tonsillitis must be differentiated from viral sore throats, which are not usually associated with pyrexia and often form part of a more generalized upper respiratory tract infection. Infectious mononucleosis can easily be confused with tonsillitis (EBM 30.2). Tonsillitis may be complicated by the development of a peritonsillar abscess (quinsy). This may require incision and drainage. Recurrent tonsillitis can be successfully treated by tonsillectomy (EBM 30.3).

Snoring and sleep apnoea

Snoring arises because of obstruction within the pharynx during sleep or vibration of the soft palate. In some cases, it is associated with apnoeic episodes. These individuals tend to sleep poorly, wake unrefreshed and become drowsy during the day. If significant apnoea is confirmed by overnight monitoring, the use of nasal continuous positive airway pressure (CPAP) may be indicated. Simple snoring can be improved by weight loss and reduction of nocturnal alcohol intake. Sleep apnoea syndrome can also occur in children and is usually cured by adenotonsillectomy in this group.

Tumours

Lymphomas occur in the younger age group and cause enlargement of the affected tonsil, producing a smooth swelling. Squamous carcinoma occurs in older patients and usually presents with ulceration of the tonsil (Fig. 30.22). Treatment is by radiotherapy or surgery.

HYPOPHARYNX

ANATOMY

Below the oropharynx, the aerodigestive tract divides into an air passage (larynx/trachea) and an alimentary passage (oesophagus). The entrance to the air passage is protected by the epiglottis, a mobile cartilaginous structure, and by the ability of the vocal cords to close together. The entry of material into the oesophagus is controlled by a ring of muscle, the cricopharyngeus. Lateral to the larynx, the pharynx continues inferiorly on both sides into a blind-ended pit known as the pyriform fossa (Fig. 30.23).

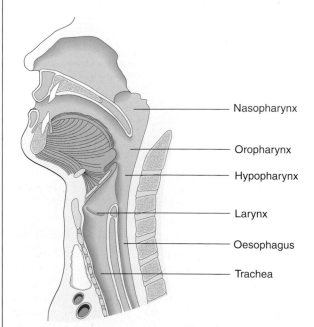

Nasopharynx

Oropharynx

Hypopharynx

Larynx

Oesophagus

Trachea

Fig. 30.23 Anatomy of the pharynx and larynx.

PHYSIOLOGY OF SWALLOWING

Swallowing is achieved by the coordinated contraction and relaxation of muscles. It is initiated by the tongue, which pushes the bolus to the back of the mouth. The pharyngeal constrictor muscles propel it towards the oesophagus, and the cricopharyngeus relaxes to receive it. A peristaltic wave then carries it on down the oesophagus to the stomach.

ASSESSMENT

Clinical features

Obstruction of the oesophagus and disorders that interfere with the muscle activity involved in swallowing cause dysphagia. Physical obstruction causes dysphagia that is worse for solids, whereas neurological disorders cause more difficulty with liquids. Hypopharyngeal pain may be felt locally or retrosternally, or may be referred to the ear (Table 30.1).

Examination

The pharynx can be assessed in the clinic using a mirror or a flexible fibreoptic rhinolaryngoscope. Under general anaesthesia, the pharynx and oesophagus can be directly inspected using rigid endoscopes. A fibreoptic oesophagoscope can be used to visualize the oesophagus after the administration of local anaesthesia and sedation.

Imaging

A barium swallow will show structural abnormalities within the pharynx and oesophagus, and also gives some information about the dynamics of swallowing. Video recording can be used to provide additional information about the details of the swallow. CT can be used to identify spread of oesophageal lesions into surrounding tissues and to demonstrate lesions causing external compression of the oesophagus.

DISEASES OF THE HYPOPHARYNX

Pharyngeal pouch

This is formed by mucosal herniation through the weakest part of the pharyngeal musculature (Killian's dehiscence). It develops when pharyngeal muscle contraction is not associated with adequate relaxation of cricopharyngeus. It causes dysphagia for solids and regurgitation of food, sometimes several days after it was swallowed. In most cases, it is possible to divide the party wall between the pouch and the oesophagus and staple the edges together with a specially designed instrument, introduced via an endoscope. This creates a segment of oesophagus that is wider than the rest. If this is not possible, the pouch can be excised via a neck incision.

Tumours

Squamous carcinoma may arise from the pharyngeal walls, the epiglottis, the pyriform fossa or the upper oesophagus (post-cricoid region). Post-cricoid carcinoma is sometimes preceded by the development of a thin membrane in the upper oesophagus, a post-cricoid web. This is associated with iron deficiency anaemia, glossitis and stomatitis (Paterson Brown–Kelly syndrome). The web itself causes some dysphagia, and treatment of the anaemia can

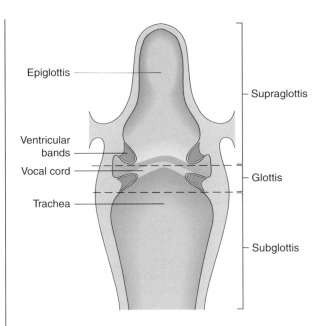

Fig. 30.24 Regions of the larynx.

prevent progression to tumour. Other pharyngeal tumours are associated with smoking. Hypopharyngeal tumours are treated by radiotherapy or surgery.

LARYNX

ANATOMY

The larynx has a cartilaginous framework. Superiorly, it is supported and protected anteriorly by the thyroid cartilage. Inferiorly lies the cricoid cartilage, which connects to the trachea (Fig. 30.24). Within the laryngeal lumen, two soft tissue folds pass from anterior to posterior. The superior of these are the ventricular bands or 'false cords'. Inferiorly lie the (true) vocal cords, which are responsible for phonation. These consist of a vocal ligament covered with a mucosa. The free edge of the mucosa is important in achieving glottic closure and voice quality.

PHYSIOLOGY OF VOICE

Voice production requires an air supply from the lungs, the presence of normally functioning vocal cords to create vibrations, and the tongue and mouth to articulate the vibrating air source into speech.

ASSESSMENT

Clinical features

Hoarseness of the voice is the cardinal symptom of laryngeal dysfunction. Patients may also complain of pain locally or referred to the ear (Table 30.1). The voice is weak and breathy in unilateral vocal cord palsy, but rough and husky in severe laryngitis and laryngeal cancer. Patients with psychogenic dysphonia often have a squeaky voice quality.

Examination

The larynx can be inspected in the clinic using a mirror, rigid telescope or flexible fibreoptic rhinolaryngoscope. Under general anaesthesia, a better view can be obtained using a rigid endoscope and operating microscope.

Imaging

CT can be used to assess the spread of laryngeal lesions to surrounding tissues.

DISEASES OF THE LARYNX

Congenital disorders

A number of congenital abnormalities of the larynx may occur, but most are rare. The most common disorder is laryngomalacia, a condition in which the laryngeal cartilages are not stiff enough to prevent collapse of the larynx during inspiration. This causes inspiratory stridor and dyspnoea, which becomes worse during upper respiratory infections. Most children grow out of the problem by the age of 2 and do not require active intervention. In severe cases, surgical division of the aryepiglottic folds can produce improvement.

Laryngitis

Inflammation of the vocal cords is the most common cause of hoarseness. Acute laryngitis frequently follows an upper respiratory tract infection. Antibiotics are of no value but steam inhalations may be helpful. The common predisposing factors for chronic laryngitis are smoking, acid reflux and excessive voice use. The vocal cords appear red or pink during the acute phase. In chronic laryngitis, they may be markedly swollen (Reinke's oedema). This pattern occurs in smokers who talk a lot. In these cases, surgical drainage of the submucosal space produces improvement. In other cases, thickened red cords or keratotic plaques (leucoplakia) may be seen.

In individuals who abuse their voices, vocal nodules that are situated at the junction of the anterior third and the posterior two-thirds of the vocal cords may develop. These can be removed, but may recur if voice abuse is not modified. In many patients, the vocal cords appear normal and the problem is functional rather than structural. Speech therapy is often helpful in these cases.

Vocal cord palsy

Unilateral cord palsy is the most commonly seen variant. Left vocal cord palsy may be caused by invasion of the recurrent laryngeal nerve by a bronchial carcinoma. The right recurrent nerve is not at risk because it does not pass down into the chest. Damage to the recurrent laryngeal nerves in the neck may occur as a result of surgery, trauma or neoplastic invasion. Unilateral palsy causes a weak breathy voice. The voice may be improved by the injection of Teflon or fat lateral to the vocal ligament. Bilateral cord palsies cause airway obstruction rather than dysphonia.

Tumours

Carcinoma of the larynx is the most common form of head and neck cancer, and is almost always a squamous carcinoma. The most important aetiological factor is smoking, but a few cases are seen in non-smokers. Patients

---

BOX 30.4 CARCINOMA OF THE LARYNX
• Persistent hoarseness in smokers should be assumed to be carcinoma of the larynx until proved otherwise
• T_1 glottic tumours can be cured by radiotherapy in up to 90% of cases
• More extensive tumours and those not cured by radiotherapy may require removal of the larynx
• Following laryngectomy, the trachea is brought out on to the surface of the neck. Speech may be regained by using swallowed air or by creating a fistula containing a one-way valve between the trachea and the pharynx

Table 30.3 CAUSES OF UPPER AIRWAY OBSTRUCTION
Children
• Inhaled foreign body
• Acute epiglottitis
• Laryngotracheobronchitis
Adults
• Inhaled foreign body
• Acute epiglottitis
• Tumour
• Laryngeal trauma
• Bilateral vocal cord palsy

complain of a hoarse voice. Uncommonly, they present with airway obstruction or haemoptysis. Tumours may arise from any of the three regions of the larynx: glottis, supraglottis or subglottis. The most common site is the vocal cord. As this area has no lymphatics, these tumours only metastasize to lymph nodes when they spread into an adjacent area. Tumours arising from the other regions do not cause hoarseness at first and therefore tend to present later.

Most laryngeal tumours are treated by radiotherapy. In T_1 lesions of the vocal cord, this modality produces cure in up to 90% of cases. Early laryngeal tumours may also be treated by excision, using a laser. The outlook is less favourable in more advanced tumours and there may be a case for primary surgery. Surgery also has a role in cases where radiotherapy fails to control the tumour. Operative treatment usually involves total removal of the larynx. In these circumstances, the trachea is brought out on to the surface of the neck as an end tracheostome. Patients can regain speech by swallowing air and using a segment of the pharynx to make it vibrate when it is expelled. Alternatively, a device with a one-way valve can be inserted between the pharynx and trachea. This allows air from the trachea to be diverted into the pharynx.

TRACHEOSTOMY

Tracheostomy may be required to relieve acute upper airway obstruction (Table 30.3). It is carried out by creating a window in the anterior tracheal wall at the level of the second and third tracheal rings and introducing a suitable tube. When short-term airway support and the causative pathology allow, the situation is better managed by passing an endotracheal tube. Cricothyrotomy (Fig. 30.25) provides

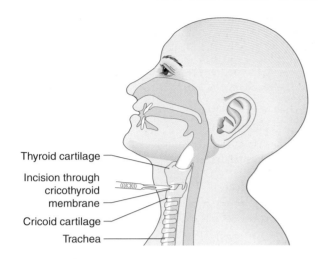

Thyroid cartilage

Incision through cricothyroid membrane

Cricoid cartilage

Trachea

Fig. 30.25 Cricothyrotomy.

a rapid short-term solution to airway obstruction and can be carried out with makeshift equipment. Foreign bodies in the upper airway can be displaced by turning a small child upside down. In a larger individual, a 'bear hug' around the chest and abdomen may expel the item (Heimlich's manoeuvre).

Tracheostomy may also be of value to reduce the dead space in patients with respiratory disease and to facilitate artificial ventilation.

NECK

ANATOMY

Knowledge of the anatomy of the neck is essential if the likely origin of neck masses is to be determined (Fig. 30.26). In the midline, lie the pharynx, larynx and trachea anteriorly. The oesophagus is deep to the trachea. The thyroid gland lies anterior and lateral to the trachea in the lower neck. Laterally, the sternomastoid muscles run from the sternum and clavicles inferiorly to the mastoid process superiorly. Between them and the midline structures is a space containing the carotid arteries and jugular veins. The vagus

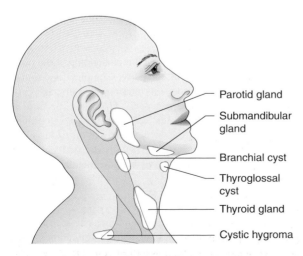

Parotid gland

Submandibular gland

Branchial cyst

Thyroglossal cyst

Thyroid gland

Cystic hygroma

Fig. 30.26 Lymph node groups in the head and neck.

nerve is closely related to the great vessels. Along the course of the jugular vein lies a chain of lymph nodes (deep cervical chain). There are also lymph nodes in other regions of the head and neck (Fig. 30.27). In the submental region lie the submandibular salivary glands, which have ducts that run in the floor of the mouth to open anterior to the tongue. The parotid salivary glands lie posterior to the angle of the mandible and anterior to the external auditory meatus (Fig. 30.28). The parotid duct opens into the mouth in the cheek close to the second upper molar tooth. The facial nerve runs through the parotid gland and emerges as a number of branches. The submandibular salivary gland is the second largest and is situated in the floor of the mouth medial to the mandible (Fig. 30.29). Its duct passes anteriorly and opens just below the tip of the tongue. The sublingual salivary gland lies in the floor of the mouth anteriorly, close to the opening of the submandibular duct. The mucosa of the mouth contains numerous small accessory salivary glands.

ASSESSMENT

Clinical features

Most neck masses are painless, but infection and malignant disease may cause pain. Rapid enlargement of a mass makes malignant disease more likely. Salivary gland swellings due to duct obstruction enlarge when the patient eats; there may also be a bad taste in the mouth.

Examination

Palpation of the neck should generally be carried out from behind. It is important to establish the size, shape, site and consistency of the swelling. Fixation to the skin or underlying structures should be established.

Imaging

CT can be used to assess most neck masses and will sometimes reveal lymph node swellings that have not been detected clinically. Cystic swellings can be differentiated from solid ones by ultrasound. Plain X-rays can be used to demonstrate salivary calculi (Fig. 30.30). Both CT and MRI are of value in assessing salivary gland swellings (Fig. 30.31). The introduction of contrast into the duct of a salivary gland (sialogram) can be used to confirm the presence of a calculus or to demonstrate inflammatory changes.

DISEASES OF THE NECK

Skin and subcutaneous swellings

Sebaceous cysts occur commonly in the head and neck region and may require removal. They are characterized by having a punctum. Furuncles or boils arise as a result of infection in hair follicles. Drainage may be required. When infection spreads to involve the dermis and subcutaneous tissue, a carbuncle is produced. It may have multiple discharging sinuses. In some cases, wide excision may be required. The possibility of underlying diabetes mellitus should be considered. Kaposi's sarcoma occurs in patients with AIDS.

Thyroglossal cyst

The thyroid gland begins its development in the base of the tongue. It descends into the neck, attached to the tongue by

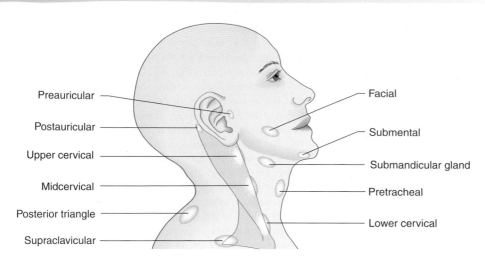

Preauricular

Postauricular

Upper cervical

Midcervical

Posterior triangle

Supraclavicular

Facial

Submental

Submandicular gland

Pretracheal

Lower cervical

Fig. 30.27   Lymph node groups in the head and neck.

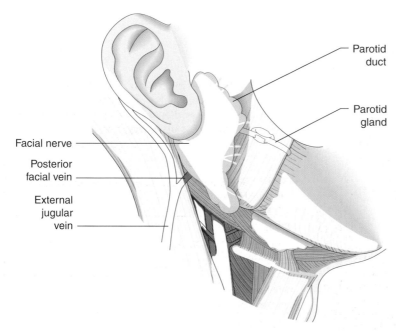

Parotid duct

Parotid gland

Facial nerve

Posterior facial vein

External jugular vein

Fig. 30.28   Anatomy of the parotid gland.

the thyroglossal duct. Under normal circumstances, this duct disappears, but if part of it is retained, a thyroglossal cyst may develop. This is a midline swelling usually situated just above the upper border of the thyroid cartilage. It moves on swallowing or tongue protrusion. These cysts can become infected. Occasionally, the descent of the thyroid gland to its normal position in the lower neck is arrested. Thyroglossal cysts must therefore be differentiated from thyroid tissue by carrying out an isotope or ultrasound scan. Treatment is by surgical excision. The centre of the hyoid bone and the persistent thyroglossal duct up to the base of the tongue should be excised with the cyst to ensure complete removal.

Branchial cyst and fistula

Swellings lying laterally in the upper neck may be branchial cysts. The aetiology of these swellings is uncertain. They are thought to be remnants of the second and third branchial arches. They more often present in adult life, which calls into question their status as congenital abnormalities. The cysts contain opaque fluid with cholesterol crystals.

Lymphoid tissue is found in their walls. They may become infected and usually require excision. Branchial fistulae may occur between the skin surface low in the neck and the tonsil. Infection often occurs and excision is usually required.

Other cystic swellings

Cystic hygroma is a rare benign lymphangioma of the neck, which usually presents in early life. Complete excision is difficult, leading to frequent recurrence. Dermoid cysts may also occur in the upper neck. They arise because of sequestration of squamous cells during development. Laryngocoeles occur as a result of herniation of laryngeal mucosa laterally into the neck. They distend with air during the Valsalva manoeuvre and may become infected. Excision is usually required.

Lymph node swellings

Lymph nodes in any of the groups present in head and neck may become enlarged in response to infection in their area of drainage. Primary neoplasms (lymphomas) and

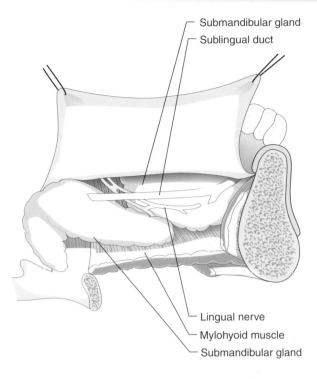

Submandibular gland
Sublingual duct

Lingual nerve
Mylohyoid muscle
Submandibular gland

Fig. 30.29   Anatomy of the submandibular salivary gland.

30

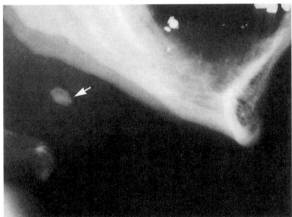

Fig. 30.30   X-ray showing a submandibular salivary calculus.

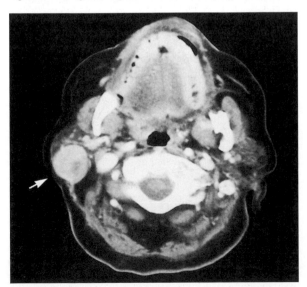

Fig. 30.31   CT scan showing parotid tumour.

Table 30.4   CAUSES OF LYMPHADENOPATHY
Infective **Bacterial** • Pyogenic infection in drainage area (e.g. streptococcal tonsillitis) • Tuberculosis • Brucellosis
Viral • Infectious mononucleosis • Cytomegalovirus • Human immunodeficiency virus (HIV)
Protozoal • Toxoplasmosis
Neoplasms • Lymphoma • Metastatic squamous carcinoma • Other metastatic tumours
Systemic disease • Collagen diseases • Sarcoidosis • Amyloidosis

secondary deposits, usually from squamous carcinomas of the head and neck region, should always be considered as a possible cause. Table 30.4 presents possible causes of cervical adenopathy.

When cervical adenopathy is noted, the upper aero-digestive tract must be carefully examined to exclude a tumour. This usually involves direct examination of the mouth, pharynx, nasopharynx, larynx and oesophagus. When inspection of these areas does not reveal an abnormality, palpation of the tonsils and tongue may reveal an occult tumour. Random biopsies from the nasopharynx may also reveal an unsuspected tumour. If no tumour can be found, there may be a need to excise the swelling for histological examination. However, small

30

BOX 30.6   SALIVARY GLAND SWELLINGS

- Swellings in the submandibular gland are more often due to calculi, but those in the parotid gland are commonly benign neoplasms
- The most common salivary gland tumours are pleomorphic adenomas and adenolymphomas (Warthin's tumour)
- Parotid swellings generally require removal with a cuff of normal salivary tissue (superficial parotidectomy)
- The facial nerve runs through the parotid gland as a series of branches and is at risk during parotid surgery

---

Table 30.5   PAROTID NEOPLASMS

Benign
- Pleomorphic adenoma
- Adenolymphoma

Intermediate
- Oncocytoma
- Mucoepidermoid tumour

Malignant
- Squamous carcinoma
- Adenoid cystic carcinoma
- Adenocarcinoma
- Lymphoma

---

mobile lymph node swellings can be observed and need only be removed if they enlarge.

Salivary gland disease

Swellings of the submandibular salivary gland are more likely to be due to obstruction of the submandibular duct by a stone or chronic inflammation. By contrast, swellings of the parotid gland are usually benign tumours.

Calculi cause salivary gland swelling by blocking of the duct. Some but not all are radio-opaque. They may pass spontaneously but are more likely to remain in situ.

Provided they are in the main duct, it is possible to remove them by opening the duct. If they are within the substance of the gland, they are usually not accessible. In these circumstances, removal of the submandibular gland may be required. In other cases, there are no calculi, but inflammatory changes can be demonstrated within the duct system of the gland by injecting contrast down its duct and taking X-rays (sialogram). Chronic sialadenitis may also be an indication for removal of the submandibular gland. Removal of the parotid gland should be avoided if possible because of the risk of damage to the facial nerve.

Salivary gland tumours

A large number of different tumour types are found in the salivary glands (Fig. 30.32). The most common are the pleomorphic adenoma (mixed salivary tumour) and the adenolymphoma (Warthin's tumour). These tumours are benign, but malignant tumours and others of variable behaviour also occur (Table 30.5). Benign parotid tumours are treated by excision with a cuff of normal tissue (superficial parotidectomy). Care must be taken to avoid damage to the facial nerve, which runs through the gland between the deep and superficial lobes. Submandibular gland tumours are treated by excision of the gland. Malignant tumours are treated by more radical surgery, with or without radiotherapy.

Carotid body tumours

Also known as chemodectomas, these are rare tumours arising from chemoreceptor tissue in the carotid body. They present as pulsatile swellings in the upper neck at the level of the carotid bifurcation. The diagnosis can be confirmed by angiography. Biopsy is hazardous because of the risk of bleeding. Surgical excision may be required

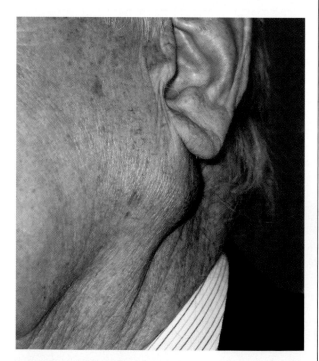

Fig. 30.32   Parotid swelling.
The mass is most likely to be a benign tumour.

31

M. GREEN

Orthopaedics

INTRODUCTION

Orthopaedic surgery involves the assessment and management of congenital, developmental (growing skeleton), traumatic and degenerative conditions of the bones and soft tissues. Assessment begins with history and examination, and is frequently followed by investigations such as plain X-rays, ultrasound, computed tomography (CT) or magnetic resonance imaging (MRI). Management may be conservative or operative, and many conditions can be treated successfully by non-surgical means.

HISTORY

Particular points in the orthopaedic history include the following.

Age
This will often help to distinguish degenerative conditions (elderly) from those related to an underlying congenital, birth-related or developmental problem (young).

Birth history
There may be a direct link between events around the time of birth and conditions such as upper limb weakness (traction injury to the brachial plexus), cerebral palsy (hypoxia) and dysplastic disease of the hip (more common in a breech delivery or first child).

Childhood
Abnormalities in the development of the growing skeleton may result in a range of conditions, some of which are associated with visible deformity. Sometimes, however, such apparent deformity is just a stage of normal development. For example, some children go through a phase of being bowlegged and anxious parents need to be reassured that this is a normal variation and not a disease.

Dominant hand
This is particularly relevant to upper limb conditions.

Occupation
Degenerative processes may be consequent upon, or at least exacerbated by, occupational use of the upper limb. The need to return a patient to employment may also affect the way and urgency with which a condition is treated.

Trauma
Many conditions follow a clearly defined episode of trauma, the nature and mechanism of which can help make the diagnosis. For example, sudden injury to the knee, with acute swelling followed by instability, is highly suggestive of anterior cruciate ligament (ACL) rupture.

Details of previous treatment
The condition may have been treated by means of physiotherapy, acupuncture, osteopathy, steroid injection and drugs over many years in primary care prior to referral to an orthopaedic surgeon. Previous operations performed on the same joint or area may affect both the current options for surgery and the chance of success. Other illnesses, such as polio, may have lifelong consequences and require a strategy for planned intervention over many years.

Past medical history
If operative intervention is planned, then general fitness for anaesthesia and surgery must be carefully assessed and the patient medically optimized. The consequences of other comorbidity must also be considered. For example, the presence of open leg ulcers in a patient about to undergo a hip replacement will increase the risk of prosthetic joint infection and the ulcers should be healed, if possible, prior to surgery.

Drug history
With regard to analgesia, changing the dose or preparation may result in significant relief of symptoms. Other drugs, such as warfarin or clopidogrel, may need to be stopped prior to surgery.

EXAMINATION

Examination should include all the other systems (cardiovascular, respiratory and neurological), as well as the specific limb and joint. Examination of the limb and joint comprises looking, feeling and then asking the patient to move.

Look
In lower limb conditions, observe gait, the use of a stick, and the ability to get out of a chair unaided and walk across the consulting room. Observe any joint or limb asymmetry or limb wasting, deformity, malalignment or shortening. Look for scars (previous operations or trauma), which may give clues to the cause of the current problem.

Feel
Palpate around the joint or limb. Establish areas of pain, and try to relate these to anatomical structures (e.g. tendons, joint lines etc.). Establish the presence of any swelling.

Move (active and passive)
Ask the patient to move the affected part (actively) through its full range of movement. Observe limitations of movement, pain, difficulty or apparent weakness. Then (passively) move the limb or joint, stopping in response to pain or stiffness. Observe limitations of movement, range, crepitus or discomfort. Test the neurovascular status of the limb (sensation to light touch and pinprick, motor power in each muscle group, pulses, colour) and compare with the other side.

This may be followed by provocative tests or tests that may examine specific functions. Examples include testing for shoulder impingement or asking the patient to stand on one leg to test the power of the abductor muscles of the hip (Trendelenburg test).

31

INVESTIGATIONS

Plain X-rays
These may be used to evaluate almost all bone pathology. Alignment (the degree of varus or valgus deformity), as well as true bone length, can be quantified. X-rays are also routinely used to confirm the correct position of bones, joints or prostheses after surgery.

Ultrasound
This is frequently used to evaluate soft tissue pathology (e.g. tendon ruptures, bleeds into soft tissues, other muscular or tendinous pathology) and to guide biopsy (e.g. tumours). As a dynamic technique, it can be used to visualise the movements of tendons and muscles under direct vision.

Nerve conduction tests and electromyography (EMG)
These are used to evaluate nerve entrapment syndromes, nerve injuries, neuropathies and abnormalities of muscular contraction.

Computed tomography (CT)
Although CT has largely been replaced by MRI, it provides excellent images of bone and soft tissues (Fig. 31.1) and will also supply three-dimensional information of help in reconstruction (Fig. 31.2). CT is also used to guide biopsy.

Magnetic resonance imaging (MRI)
MRI also provides excellent images of soft tissue, joint (Fig. 31.3) and bone pathology, but without exposure to radiation. It is widely used in virtually all branches of orthopaedics for diagnosis and pre-operative planning.

Bone scans
These can be used to assess a number of bone conditions, including infection and tumours (Fig. 31.4).

DESCRIPTION OF DEFORMITY

With patients in the anatomical position (i.e. lying on their back with their palms pointing up to the ceiling), limb deformities are described relative to the midline (away = valgus, towards = varus) and relative to the alignment of

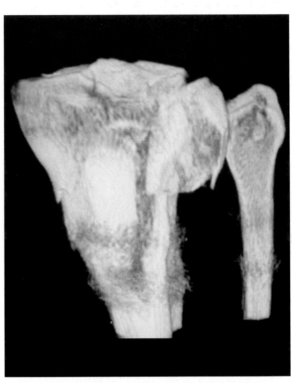

Fig. 31.2 A three-dimensional reconstruction of the tibia at the site of a tibial plateau injury, showing involvement of multiple fragments of bone.

31

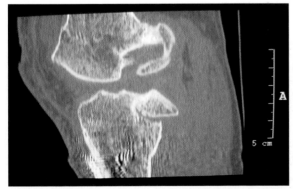

Fig. 31.1 A CT scan of the knee, showing injury to the attachment of the posterior cruciate and avulsion of a bone fragment.

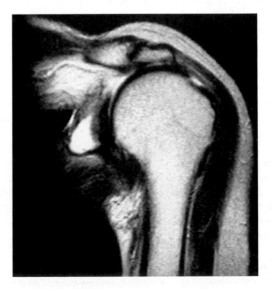

Fig. 31.3 An MRI scan of a shoulder through the level of the acromioclavicular joint and the glenohumeral joint.

31

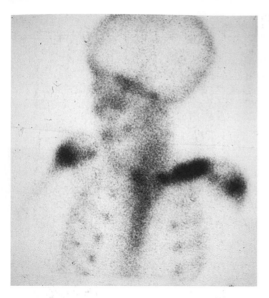

Fig. 31.4 An example of a bone scan showing increased uptake of radioactive tracer in the clavicle: in this case, indicative of infection.
There are also increased areas of uptake in the shoulders and sternum.

the limb below the joint or deformity. For example, with respect to the knees, bowleggedness is a varus deformity, while knock-knees are a valgus deformity (Fig. 31.5). With the patient viewed from the side, there is a range of descriptive terms available. For example, hyperextension

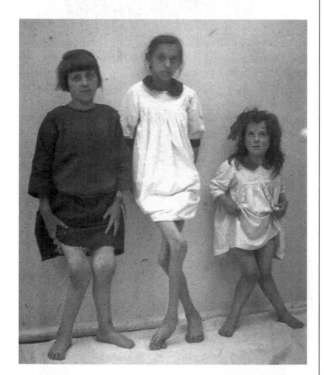

Fig. 31.5 Historical slide of children, showing deformities of the knees.
All the children show valgus knee, i.e. knock-kneed, deformities.

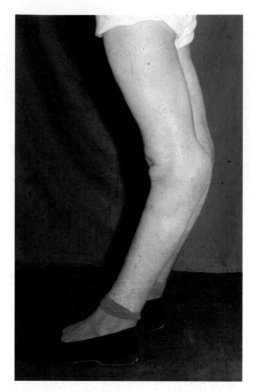

Fig. 31.6 A recurvatum deformity of the knees with hyperextension.

of the knee joint is known as recurvatum (Fig. 31.6). The three types of spinal deformity are:

- *kyphosis*: forward flexion ('the kyphotic kisses his knees').
- *lordosis*: the opposite, extension, or bent-over-backwards deformity; this represents the normal alignment of the lumbar and cervical spine.
- *scoliosis*: a sideward deformity that is normally associated with a degree of rotational deformity (Fig. 31.7).

OSTEOARTHRITIS: DEGENERATIVE DISEASE OF THE JOINTS

Osteoarthritis (OA) of a joint may occur as a primary idiopathic condition or secondary to problems such as malalignment (following, for example, intra-articular trauma) or over-stressing (obesity, overuse). In some patients, there is a strong genetic component. OA may occur in any joint (shoulder, elbow, wrist and hands) but predominantly affects those that are weight-bearing (hip and knee) (Figs 31.8 and 31.9). Idiopathic OA is generally of slow onset and affects the elderly. Secondary OA can affect the young and may develop quite rapidly where joint injury leads to malalignment. On plain X-ray, OA is associated with:

- joint space loss due to loss of articular cartilage
- sclerosis of the joint surface, with the development of increased density of the bone just under the joint space

- osteophytes
- cystic change.

In some patients, this may progress to loss of bone, leading in turn to shortening of the limb and loss of height.

Treatment of OA may be conservative or operative. The former focuses on the use of drugs and physical methods of pain and stress relief to the joint.

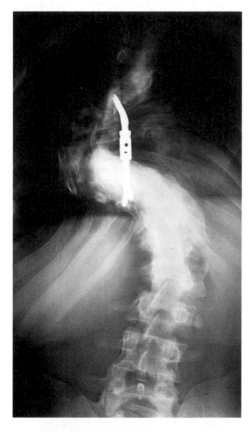

Fig. 31.7   An X-ray of the thoracic and lumbar spine, showing gross scoliosis of both.

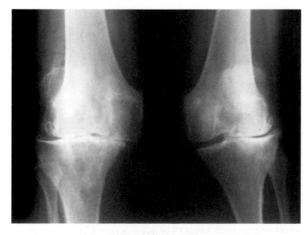

Fig. 31.8   Bilateral knee osteoarthritis.
The left knee (on the right-hand side in the illustration) shows predominantly lateral wear and has a valgus deformity. The right knee has osteoarthritis of both medial and lateral compartments.

A

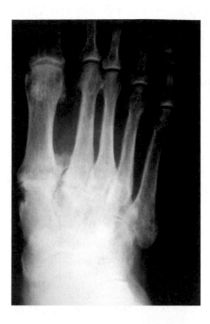

B

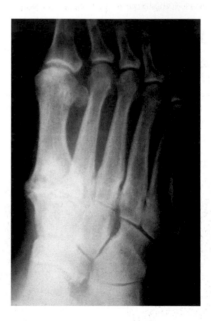

Fig. 31.9   Osteoarthritis can affect any joint.
Here, the first toe metatarsophalangeal and the tarsometatarsal joints are clearly arthritic as a result of osteoarthritic change.

MEDICAL MANAGEMENT OF OA

Drug therapy
Simple analgesics, such as paracetamol, with or without the inclusion of non-steroidal anti-inflammatory drugs (NSAIDs), are the mainstay of treatment. More powerful analgesic combinations may be introduced, if simple analgesics prove inadequate.

Off-loading
This involves the use of aids, such as a walking stick and weight loss, aimed at reducing the forces passing

through the joint. In the obese, weight loss is essential, particularly if the patient is likely to need surgery in the future, as it may reduce by 50% the risks of joint replacement surgery.

Injections

Introducing a mix of steroid and local anaesthetic into the joint may reduce inflammation and ease pain.

Compounds of hyaluronic acid

These are designed to supplement the natural joint levels of hyaluronic acid essential to normal functioning of articular cartilage and are now in common use. They work best in early OA but have little, if any, effect in late-stage disease.

Other conservative treatments

Physiotherapy and hydrotherapy both have a part to play in the control of symptoms, especially in early disease. Building up lost muscle bulk (frequently lost due to reduced activity) provides the joint with an increased degree of muscular control and may lead to considerable symptom improvement. Other treatment modalities, such as acupuncture, are recognized to have a valuable role in the conservative management of early OA.

SURGICAL MANAGEMENT OF OA

Failure of conservative methods normally leads to consideration of surgical intervention; in the patient unfit for surgery, benefit may be gained from referral to a pain therapist. The main operative interventions include osteotomy, replacement and fusion. Certain joints, particularly the knee, may benefit from a more minimal approach, such as arthroscopic debridement. This may help when a patient complains of physical symptoms indicative of underlying mechanical problems, such as locking or discomfort related to meniscal problems. Generally, just washing out the joint does not give tremendous benefit in OA.

Osteotomy

This is useful in the younger patient, in whom joint replacement may not be advisable. The aim is to change the axis of the joint, so that a portion of the joint surface that has thus far been protected from wear and tear now forms the weight-bearing area. For example, with respect to the knee, although there may be severe OA of the medial compartment in conjunction with a varus (bowlegged) deformity, the lateral compartment may have well-preserved articular cartilage. Over-correcting the varus deformity by means of osteotomy (removing wedges of bone from the tibia), so that body weight is now largely transmitted through the lateral compartment, may lead to significant improvement in symptoms, thus delaying the need for joint replacement (Fig. 31.10).

Excision arthroplasty

The joint surfaces are excised, giving a 'joint' formed of scar tissue. For example, in Keller's procedure, the metatarsal–phalangeal joint is excised to treat hallux valgus; in a Girdlestone's operation, the femoral head is excised. The hip heals in a very shortened position and patients require a significant shoe raise to equalize the

A

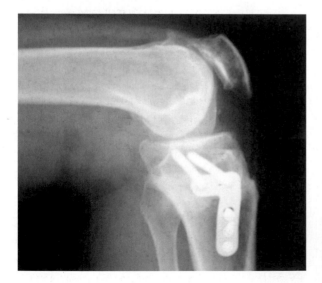

B

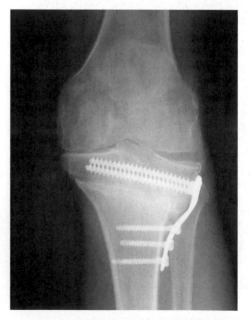

Fig. 31.10 An example of an osteotomy to the proximal tibia.
A The osteotomy site has been fixed by a plate and screws. B The cut of the osteotomy lies between the top two screws and the bottom three screws.

length of their legs, but the scar joint is relatively pain-free. Nowadays, this would be regarded as a salvage procedure of last resort after, for example, removal of an infected hip prosthesis.

Joint replacement
The hip, knee and shoulder, and indeed almost any joint, can now be partially or completely replaced in a number of different ways with varying degrees of success.

Hemi-arthroplasty
In this operation, only one-half of the joint is replaced, leaving half of the joint intact. It is normally the natural socket—for example, the acetabulum—that is left untouched. The most common example is following fracture of the femoral neck in the elderly. Such patients usually have low demand on the joint, and the hemi-arthroplasty gives adequate function without risking many of the complexities of a total hip replacement. Variations on the hemi-arthroplasty theme are used in other joints: for example, resurfacing of the humeral head.

Total joint replacement
This entails resurfacing of both sides of a joint (Fig. 31.11). The choice of materials for the weight-bearing surfaces varies, depending on the joint and prosthesis in question. Currently, metal against a high-density polyethylene is the most common, although new prostheses involving metal on metal have been developed for use in young people (Fig. 31.12). In small joints, such as those of the hand in patients with rheumatoid arthritis, silastic is often used as a buffer between the two joint surfaces.

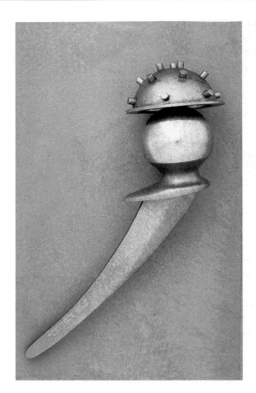

Fig. 31.12   A very early hip replacement design that used metal on metal bearing surfaces.
Although this is now obsolete, the concept of metal on metal bearing is experiencing a comeback with improvements in engineering.

Arthrodesis
Any residual cartilage is removed down to bleeding cancellous bone before the joint is rigidly fixed with complete loss of movement (Fig. 31.13). Small joint fusions of toes and fingers are the most common examples. Fusion of a large joint, such as the hip or knee, will obviously have a significant effect on mobility and will throw additional stress on the joints above and below, leading to or exacerbating OA. Thus, pre-existing OA in the joints either proximal or distal to the joint being considered for fusion is a contraindication to arthrodesis.

Interposition arthroplasty
The joint is excised and the residual space is filled with autogenous or allograft material. For example, the trapezium in the hand is excised and the space filled with a rolled-up tendon, such as palmaris longus.

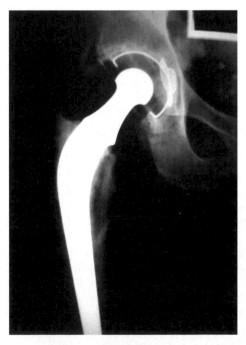

Fig. 31.11   A Charnley total hip replacement.
The acetabulum contains a high-density polyethylene socket that is radiolucent, and a wire to mark the position of the acetabulum. The femur contains a metal prosthesis. Both acetabulum and femoral components are cemented in with a polymethylmethacrylate cement.

RHEUMATOID ARTHRITIS AND INFLAMMATORY DISEASE OF JOINTS

The majority of patients with inflammatory joint disease, most commonly rheumatoid arthritis (RA), have been assessed and treated by a rheumatologist prior to orthopaedic referral. However, RA may present primarily to the orthopaedic service and, as such, must be remembered in the differential diagnosis. Orthopaedic surgeons must have a good working knowledge of the condition and its

31

31

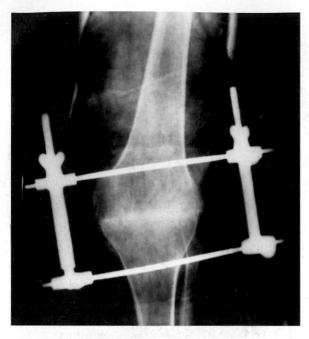

Fig. 31.13   An arthrodesis of the knee joint.
The joint has been excised and the bone surfaces have been brought together. The clamps apply pressure to enable the bone ends to be compressed, so as to increase the chances of healing.

medical treatment. Other groups of doctors must also be aware of the complications of RA. For example, anaesthetists must know the risks of endotracheal intubation in patients with RA, who may have instability of the C1/C2 spine as a result of loss of the restraining ligaments. Many of these patients are on long-term steroids and other immunosuppressants that will affect the presentation and treatment of many medical and surgical conditions.

BONE AND JOINT INFECTION

PRIMARY INFECTION

Primary infection of the bones (osteomyelitis) or joints (septic arthritis) is rare and secondary to haematogenous transmission of microorganisms. Primarily a disease of childhood, osteomyelitis presents with acute pain and loss of function (reluctance to use the limb), and often follows a bout of respiratory or skin infection. The most common sites are the long bones of the lower limb. In children, 90% of cases are due to *Staphylococcus aureus*. By contrast, adults often present with rare and unexpected organisms as a result of other comorbidity, immunosuppressant therapy, indwelling prosthetic material (e.g. renal dialysis catheters) or intravenous drug abuse. The importance of obtaining some form of positive microbiology from blood cultures or bone samples prior to starting antibiotics cannot be over-emphasized. Poorly treated acute osteomyelitis may lead to chronic osteomyelitis associated

with a life-long risk of acute exacerbations and sinus formation.

SECONDARY INFECTION

Osteomyelitis secondary to trauma (compound fracture) or operation (insertion of metalwork) is relatively more common than primary osteomyelitis. Dead bone (sequestrum) acts as a reservoir of infection and, although this may be walled off by new bone growth (involucrum), infection, once established, may lie dormant for many years before reactivating. Orthopaedic operations (without preceding trauma) are a relatively rare cause of true osteomyelitis (although any foreign prosthesis placed in bone may become infected). Osteomyelitis in the presence of a prosthesis will almost certainly necessitate removal of that prosthesis.

OVERVIEW OF JOINT REPLACEMENT SURGERY

Knee and hip replacements are by far the most common procedures, although shoulder, elbow, wrist and finger replacements may all be performed. With regard to the knee, there has also been a move away from the traditional total joint replacement towards replacing just that part of the joint affected by OA (Fig. 31.14 and 31.15). These advances permit less invasive surgery and quicker recovery. Successful joint replacement surgery is associated with a low infection and revision rate for prosthetic failure: ideally, less than 95% at 10–15 years (Figs 31.16 and 31.17). Revisional joint replacement surgery is much more complex and is associated with greater rates of complications and further device failure. Post-operative infection is broadly divided into early and late. Early infections are usually purulent, occur within the first few weeks, and may be eradicated with an early debridement and appropriate antibiotics, but may necessitate removal of the prosthesis. Late infection is usually due to more indolent organisms such as *Staph. epidermidis*, may follow a bacteraemia or colonization at the time of implantation, often presents as early loosening and frequently leads to the requirement for revisional surgery.

OVERVIEW OF ARTHROSCOPIC SURGERY

Arthroscopic techniques have been adopted in most areas of orthopaedics. The ability to stitch soft tissues, place suture anchors into bone, and drill and ream bone through the scope has permitted the development of arthroscopic-assisted:

- *repair*: menisci in the knee and the rotator cuff in the shoulder
- *stabilization of unstable joints*: the recurrently dislocating shoulder or knees with ligament ruptures
- *joint fusion*: ankle
- *ligament reconstruction*: anterior cruciate ligament.

A

B

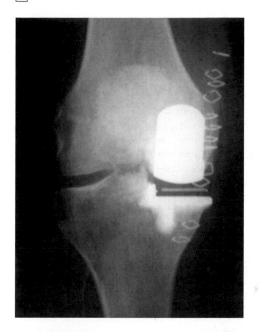

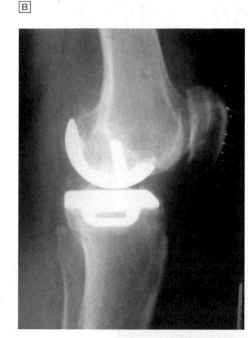

31

Fig. 31.14 A local resurfacing of the tibia and the femur for osteoarthritis of the medial compartment of the knee joint. This is a unicompartment joint replacement.

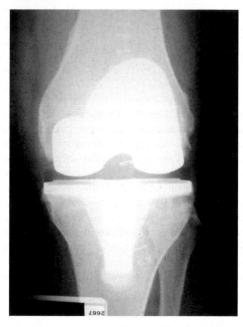

Fig. 31.15 A normal knee replacement, showing the resurfacing of the femur with a femur-shaped component. The tibial component can be seen as a metal base plate that holds the plastic bearing surface, which creates the gap between the femur and tibia.

PAEDIATRIC ORTHOPAEDIC SURGERY

The growing child presents particular challenges, and certain disease processes may only occur at certain stages of childhood. Surgery must be planned carefully so as not to interfere with the growth plates. Parents often require strong reassurance. The physician should be aware of the following conditions.

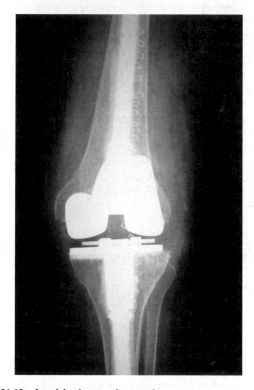

Fig. 31.16 A revision knee replacement. As can be seen when contrasted with the normal knee replacement in Figure 31.15, this is more complex and requires stems that go up the femur and down the tibia to create extra stability.

DYSPLASTIC DISEASE OF THE HIP (DDH)

This is more common in breech deliveries, the first-born and females. It is due to inadequate development of the hip joint (Fig. 31.18), and presents in a wide spectrum of

31

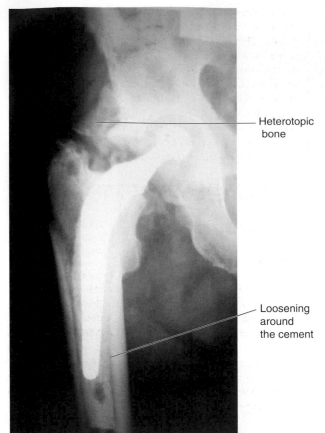

— Heterotopic bone

— Loosening around the cement

Fig. 31.17 Failure of a total hip replacement.
The hip is surrounded by heterotopic ossification and the cement mantle (surrounding the femoral prosthesis) has started to come loose.

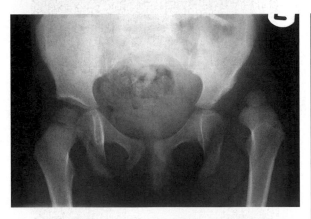

Fig. 31.18 Dysplastic disease of the hip, showing a dislocated left hip.

severity. If diagnosed in the newborn, milder forms, in which the femoral head has a tendency to sublux from the acetabulum, are best treated using a 'harness device' that allows freedom of movement while holding the femoral head in the joint. More severe forms, where there is actually fixed dislocation, may require operative reduction.

PERTHES' DISEASE

This is a self-limiting disease due to avascular necrosis of a portion of the developing femoral head. The cause is unknown but disease tends to occur between 4 and 10 years of age and is more common in males. An early stage of inflammation and synovitis is followed by a regenerative stage, in which the necrotic area is replaced by viable bone (re-ossification). Clinically, the onset is slow and the child complains of pain and limping. Treatment aims to relieve pain and prevent deformity while the femoral head is healing. Prognosis depends on the age of onset, degree of involvement of the femoral head, and adequacy of treatment; in general, the older the patient, the worse the outcome.

CEREBRAL PALSY (CP)

This is a disorder of movement and posture due to a defect in the developing brain? CP is usually caused by adverse birth events, such as hypoxia and infection, and comes in a variety of forms (spastic, athetoid, ataxic, mixed) and extents: monoplegia (one limb—rare), hemiplegia (one side of the body affected), diplegia (both lower limbs affected), tetraplegia and quadriplegia. Contractures can be treated with regular stretching, botulinum toxin, tendon release or muscle transfer. Bony abnormalities may require osteotomy.

SLIPPED UPPER FEMORAL EPIPHYSIS (SUFE)

The femoral head epiphysis weakens and the head slips, resulting in the upward and anterior displacement of the femoral neck. SUFE is of unknown aetiology. It usually develops between 10 and 16 years old, and is most common in boys at the time of their growth spurt; it is found more frequently in the short, fat, hypogonadal or hypothyroid child, suggesting a hormonal influence. It is a bilateral condition in 25% of cases. It frequently presents with referred pain to the knee and is thus commonly misdiagnosed as a knee problem. The condition may present as a chronic slip that occurs over a few months, or acutely after a seemingly minor episode of trauma. Treatment involves pinning of the slip, using a screw, together with corrective osteotomy if there is any significant residual deformity after healing.

CONGENITAL CLUB FOOT (TALIPES EQUINOVARUS OR CTEV)

This is an idiopathic fixed deformity of the foot, which is frequently bilateral. There may be a genetic component and it is twice as common in males. Simple methods of treatment include strapping and splinting for minor deformities, and surgical correction where conservative methods have failed.

SCOLIOSIS

This can be divided into structural and non-structural. 'Non-structural' scoliosis is secondary to some other problem (e.g. inequality of leg length, lumbar disc prolapse) and disappears when the underlying cause is removed. Structural scoliosis can be caused by a variety of conditions, although 90% of childhood cases are idiopathic. Unlike the non-structural form, there is an accompanying rotational deformity. The usual presentation is between 10 and 13 years of age, and the condition is more common in females. Usually, it is asymptomatic and, if there is pain, one should think of other reasons for the scoliosis (e.g. tumour). The treatment of scoliosis is complex but involves spinal bracing and surgical intervention.

ANGULAR DEFORMITIES

Genu varum (bowlegs) is often seen in very early childhood. It often corrects and tends to genu valgum (knock-knees) between 18 months and 3 years; this then corrects by 4–7 years. It is important not to forget alternative diagnoses, such as rickets and Blount's disease (idiopathic abnormality of the upper medial tibial epiphysis).

MUSCULOSKELETAL TUMOURS

Musculoskeletal tumours may arise from cartilage, skeletal muscle, synovium or bone, and may be benign or malignant. They are rare, and usually present with deep-seated pain that often continues into the night, or with a lump. There may be a history of incidental trauma, to which the symptoms are frequently attributed. High-grade tumours may have a short history (of several months), whereas the more benign lesions have a prolonged course. Clues to malignancy include rapid growth, fracture through unusual bone, destruction of the bone cortex and invasion into the soft tissues. Primary bone tumours are rare; they occur largely in the second decade of life and frequently affect the metaphysis. The most common malignant tumour is osteosarcoma, 50% of which will occur around the knee. The next most common is Ewing's sarcoma. Once a bone tumour is suspected, the patient should be referred immediately to the (supra)regional specialist treatment centre for biopsy, staging and definitive treatment. Over the last decade, advances in combination treatment (chemotherapy, radiotherapy, and excisional and reconstructive surgery) have resulted in considerable improvements in long-term prognosis.

31

THE UPPER LIMB

THE SHOULDER

Anterior dislocation

The shoulder is especially prone to dislocation, with or without fracture (Fig. 31.19). Instability with recurrent dislocation is significantly reduced if the shoulder is immobilized in a position of neutral external rotation, i.e. with the arm pointing forward. (The traditional position has always been immobilization in internal rotation, with the arm across the body in a sling.) Recurrent anterior dislocations used to be treated with open repair, but arthroscopic stabilization appears to be as effective and is growing in popularity.

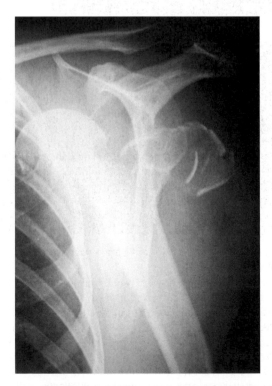

Fig. 31.19 A fracture dislocation of the humeral head, showing the humeral shaft and head as separate pieces, as well as portions of the greater tuberosity.
All are separate from the normal anatomical position of the femoral head, and the glenoid can be clearly seen in the background of the X-ray.

Impingement syndrome

Weakness through disuse, degeneration and tearing of the rotator cuff muscles (supraspinatus, infraspinatus, subscapularis) predisposes to superior subluxation of the humeral head against the acromion, leading to so-called impingement pain. Steroid injections and physiotherapy may be effective. If there is a bony spur at the front of the acromion that is contributing to the impingement, this can be removed arthroscopically (subacromial decompression).

Rotator cuff tear

Tears may be present in up to 50% of the population over 60 years of age but most are asymptomatic. They may occur spontaneously or as a result of quite minor trauma. The pain often affects the deltoid area and, like impingement pain, may be worse at night. Symptomatic tears are best repaired and, in the right hands, arthroscopic techniques are as good as, if not better than, open methods.

Osteoarthritis

OA can affect the glenohumeral or the acromioclavicular joint (ACJ). ACJ OA is treated with either injection or excision of the joint. If conservative methods fail, glenohumeral joint OA may be treated with either a shoulder replacement or a resurfacing.

THE ELBOW

Tennis and golfers' elbow

The most common pathologies to affect the elbow are inflammation of the lateral (tennis) or medial (golfers') epicondyle at the point of insertion of the muscle mass. The mainstays of treatment are bracing and strapping, injections and physiotherapy. If these fail, operative release of the tendinous insertion may be warranted.

Rheumatoid elbow

Options include a synovectomy, with debridement of the joint and excision of the radial head; interposition and covering the joint surfaces of the elbow with fascia; and total elbow replacement.

THE HAND AND WRIST

Wrist disease

The more common causes of wrist pain include scaphoid fracture (see below), severe arthritis, avascular necrosis of particular bones, and damage to the triangulo-fibrocartilage complex.

Carpal tunnel disease

The median nerve is compressed, either by the tunnel itself or by its contents: for example, by a synovial swelling. Symptoms include pins and needles or sensory loss in the territory of the median nerve (a variable area of supply normally including the palmar aspect of the thumb, index and middle fingers, with a variable amount of the ring finger involved). Treatment involves decompression of the tunnel by releasing the thick palmar fascia overlying the median nerve.

Trigger finger

Thickening of the flexor tendon causes it to jam under the pulley system that would normally allow the tendon to slide backwards and forwards. Injection around the tendon or release of the first pulley results in a cure of the condition.

Dupuytren's disease

Thickening of the palmar fascia draws the fingers (predominantly the fifth) into a flexed and deformed position, resulting in disability and loss of function. It is more common in diabetics, epileptics and those with other connective tissue contractures (e.g. Peyronie's disease of the penis). Surgery is only considered if there is significant disability. It involves dissecting and removing the thickened fascial bands, taking great care to preserve the often intimately associated nerves and blood vessels. In severe cases, amputation of the little finger may be a better option.

THE LOWER LIMB

THE HIP JOINT

As discussed above, the main problems are the late complications of young persons' diseases of the hip and OA. Treatment ranges from conservative methods through osteotomy to joint replacement surgery. Where a remnant of articular surface remains intact, osteotomies may be extremely useful to realign usable portions of cartilage against each other.

Avascular necrosis of the femoral head

This typically presents with severe pain, often at night, and initial X-rays may appear normal. MRI is usually diagnostic. If the head has not collapsed, it is usually decompressed via a channel drilled up the femoral neck (core decompression). If the head has collapsed, then total joint arthroplasty may be the treatment of choice.

Hip arthroscopy

This is a relatively new procedure and enthusiasts suggest that there are a large number of pathologies that can be treated with this technique. Certainly, debridement of the joint and removal of loose bodies can be achieved successfully. Treatment of other conditions remains to be proven.

THE KNEE JOINT

History

This is extremely important and often points to the likely diagnosis. Inability to carry on playing sport immediately after an injury hints at a ligament rupture. Rapid swelling within a few minutes or hours suggests a major injury within the knee. A large haemarthrosis occurring within the first few hours after an injury indicates a

31

major ligament tear, a peripheral tear of the meniscus or an osteochondral fracture. All of these conditions require further evaluation. Ligament injuries may present in clinic with a history of preceding injury and subsequent instability. Often, this is a feeling of an inability to trust the knee on trying to move from side to side, although the knee may feel stable when the person is running in a straight line. Regular episodes of giving way are thought to accelerate the development of OA. Patterns of injury do tend to coexist and may be related to certain mechanisms of injury.

Meniscal injuries

These are relatively common and may be crudely divided into two major groups. The younger the patient, the more likely the injury is to be purely a traumatic tear of the medial meniscus. As the patient gets older, the chances of a degenerative tear of the lateral meniscus increase. Symptoms may consist of swelling and localized pain in the knee, particularly around the joint line. If a fragment of meniscus is loose and can get into the joint space, true locking may occur, with a loss of ability to extend the knee.

Osteoarthritis

This is very common and may affect the whole of the knee (tricompartmental OA), or just particular compartments such as the medial or patellofemoral. Symptoms may be precisely localized both to precipitating events and to an anatomical site; for example, pain going up and down stairs reflects patellofemoral disease, while in isolated medial OA the pain may be well localized to the medial side of the knee. The knee lends itself to surface replacements purely of the affected parts, and isolated medial and patellofemoral joint replacements exist, as well as total knee replacements. At least some of the partial knee prostheses are as successful as a total joint replacement. Surgeons vary as to whether they replace the patella or not. When patients are asked for consent for replacement knee joints, it is customary to warn them that the prosthesis will last for 10–15 years but, in fact, many prostheses continue to function well beyond this limit and there is no sudden dramatic increase in the rate of revision once the 10 years have passed.

THE FOOT AND ANKLE

Injury to the supporting ligaments may lead to instability and recurrent giving way of the ankle. Ankle replacements for OA do exist but they have fairly restricted indications, and severe arthritis may best be treated by ankle fusion. Although fusion restricts the range of movement, it is not as debilitating as fusion of the knee or hip and effectively removes all the pain. There are multiple foot deformities, including flat feet with loss of the medial arch (pes planus) and excessive arching of the foot (pes cavus), which can lead to chronic foot pain and difficulty in walking. OA with deformity of the toes is common and may be treated by either joint excision or fusion. The most common deformity is hallux valgus (more commonly known as a bunion), in which the great toe is deviated in a valgus

direction at the metatarsophalangeal joint. Treatment includes the use of special footwear, excision of the prominent medial eminence, soft tissue realignment or osteotomy. Frequently, the other toes may be deformed either in a medial/lateral plane (where the toes cross over each other) or in a superior/inferior plane (such as in a hammer toe). As for the great toe deformity, this may be treated with either fusion or excision of the joint.

TRAUMA AND FRACTURES

GENERAL APPROACH

Management of the (multiply) injured patient requires a team approach, and often entails joint management by a number of different specialties, from the time of initial resuscitation in the accident and emergency department right through to the definitive treatment of each injury. Certain patterns of injury can be anticipated. For example, patients who fall from a height and land on their feet may be expected to have sustained injury to calcaneus, tibial plateau, hip and pelvis. At impact, patients tend to fall forward, often leading to spinal fractures.

EXAMINATION

Careful examination of each injured limb includes:

- *Skin*. Ascertain whether any skin breaks communicate with any underlying fracture.
- *Circulation*. The most common cause of absent pulses is kinking or compression of the artery by the fracture. Often, a reduction of the fracture (realigning the fracture into the anatomical position) or application of traction results in the pulses' return.
- *Nerves*. Certain injuries may have a high associated risk of neurological injury, manifest by loss of power and/or sensation. For example, the axillary nerve is at risk from shoulder fracture dislocation and its integrity should be documented prior to reduction (Fig. 31.19).

JOINT DISLOCATION

Reduction of the joint must be performed as soon as possible, either in the accident and emergency department under sedation and/or local anaesthetic blocks (e.g. anterior dislocation of the shoulder), or in the operating theatre under general anaesthesia. In the rare case where closed reduction fails, open surgical reduction may be performed.

FRACTURE MANAGEMENT

Classification
Fractures are usually classified by:

- whether they are in communication with the skin surface (open or compound) or not (closed)
- their appearance on X-ray: for example, comminuted (in multiple pieces, Fig. 31.20), spiral (where the fracture curves in a large spiral around the long axis

31

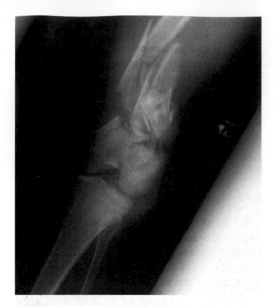

Fig. 31.20   A comminuted fracture of the distal femur involving the knee joint as well.
The femur can be seen to have broken into multiple (comminuted) fragments.

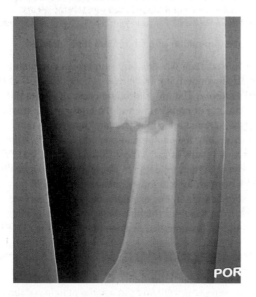

Fig. 31.21   A transverse fracture of the femoral shaft with some displacement.

of the bone) or transverse (straight across the bone, Fig. 31.21)
* anatomical site: for example, intra-articular (involving the joint surface, Fig. 31.22), metaphyseal, epiphyseal or diaphyseal.

Children

Fractures often behave differently in children. Because their bones are more pliable, children may suffer from greenstick fractures, in which the cortex of the bone does not break but bends instead. Fractures may also affect the growth plate (epiphysis) of the bone, leading to problems with slowing

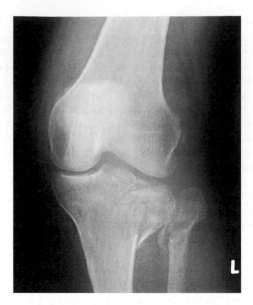

Fig. 31.22   An intra-articular fracture of the lateral tibial plateau of the knee.

of the growth of the bone (growth arrest) or deformity of the growing bone. Generally, fractures heal much more quickly in children.

Principles of fracture healing

There are many differing ways of treating fractures. However, they all have the same fundamental objectives: namely, the close approximation of uncontaminated, well-vascularized bone ends in a stable configuration that will maximize bone and soft tissue healing without deformity or loss of function.

Compound fractures

These must be treated within 6–8 hours by means of:

* removal of all the damaged and dead tissue.
* thorough cleaning of the wound, preferably by means of pulsed lavage using a powerful water jet system and many litres of fluid ('the solution to pollution is dilution').
* stabilization of the fracture to minimize further contamination. Depending on the degree of (potential) contamination, this may be by definitive or temporary fixation. Temporary external fixators are often attached by means of pins to the bones either side of the fracture site to allow access to the wound while imparting stability.

Intra-articular fractures

It is essential that the joint surface be reconstructed as accurately as possible to maximize long-term joint. In certain fractures of the humeral and femoral heads, joint replacement may be the best option.

Conservative treatment

Closed fractures with good healing potential are usually treated with external stabilization using a simple bandage, plaster of Paris (POP) or a synthetic lightweight cast. The initial cast must not encircle the whole circumference of the limb. Use of a 'back slab' of plaster allows the limb to swell and avoids the potential risk of a compartment syndrome. Once the acute swelling has settled, then the cast may be completed to become a circumferential (full) cast. Displaced fractures often require manipulation under some form of anaesthetic prior to immobilization in POP.

Compartment syndrome

This paragraph is especially important; please read it very carefully and commit it to memory. The diagnosis of compartment syndrome must be considered in any patient in POP who complains of increasing pain in the limb, with or without neurological symptoms. The presence of pulses does not exclude compartment syndrome. If compartment syndrome is suspected or cannot be excluded, the POP must be split down to skin immediately, even if the fracture position is lost such that remanipulation is required. Missed compartment syndrome has devastating consequences for the patient, cannot be rectified and is a common cause of medicolegal litigation. If splitting the POP fails to relieve the symptoms of a compartment syndrome very quickly, then further urgent, possibly surgical, decompression will be required and you must seek senior help urgently.

Operative treatment

This involves the use of devices that are broadly divided into those that remain external to the skin (see above) and those that are internal (screws, plates and nails, Fig. 31.23). The details of their use are beyond the scope of this book but depend on fracture type, site and morphology. Some devices are 'dynamic', in that they allow controlled collapse

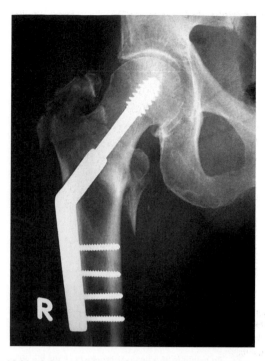

Fig. 31.24   A dynamic hip screw, a device used to secure hip fractures where the hip fracture is extracapsular as shown.
The device is dynamic, as the screw can collapse down as the fracture heals.

of the fracture, leading to compression of the bone ends and, hopefully, better healing (Fig. 31.24).

SOME SPECIFIC FRACTURES

The detailed treatment of individual fractures is beyond the scope of this book. However, you should be aware of the following.

Fractures of the femoral neck

These are generally seen in the elderly with osteoporotic bone, as a result of low-velocity falls on to the hip. They are extremely common and utilize very considerable health-service resources. Such fractures are divided into:

- *extra-capsular*, occurring outside the margins of the joint capsule, particularly the metaphysis of the femur
- *intra-capsular*, involving the femoral neck within the capsule.

This differentiation is important because blood reaches the femoral head via the capsule and runs along the femoral neck. Extra-capsular fractures are normally reduced and stabilized using a pin and plate system, commonly known as a dynamic hip screw (DHS), which allows sliding and impaction of the fracture site as the patient walks (Fig. 31.24).

Undisplaced intra-capsular fractures are commonly pinned in the hope that the blood supply to the femoral head has been preserved and avascular necrosis of the femoral head will not develop. Displaced intra-capsular fractures are frequently treated with a joint replacement. In

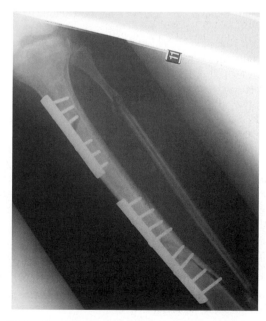

Fig. 31.23   The use of plate fixation to secure two fractures of the tibia.
Note that a fracture of the fibula has been deliberately left to heal by conservative methods.

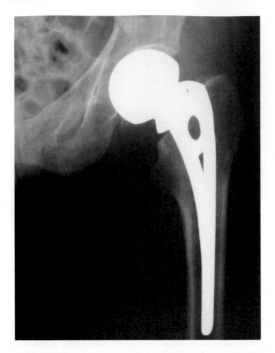

Fig. 31.25   An example of a hemi-arthroplasty of the hip, where only the femoral part of the hip joint has been replaced.
This type of procedure is commonly used after a displaced intracapsular fracture of the hip.

older patients, this is often a hemi-arthroplasty (see above and Fig. 31.25). Younger patients and those expected to rehabilitate to a higher level of activity usually receive a total hip replacement.

Colles' fractures

These are distal radial fractures, usually sustained as a result of falling forward on to an outstretched hand; they produce dorsally based (dinner fork) deformity of the distal fragment. This is most commonly seen in the osteoporotic elderly. Two well-described complications are compression of the median nerve and (usually delayed) rupture of the extensor pollicis longus tendon. A Smith's fracture is similar but has volar displacement of the distal fragment.

Forearm fractures

The principle behind all forearm fractures is that it is difficult to fracture one bone and have displacement and shortening without there being another injury to the other bone in the forearm or to the proximal or distal joint. The fracture(s) may occur at any point along the length of the radius and ulna. Although in the child it may be permissible to treat these conservatively, in the adult midshaft fractures are almost invariably fixed back into anatomical alignment using an open reduction and plate fixation. Correct anatomical alignment is essential to allow correct pronation and supination of the forearm.

Scaphoid fractures

These may present with often subtle symptoms and signs: typically, pain and tenderness in the anatomical snuffbox following a fall on the outstretched hand. Initial X-rays may fail to demonstrate the fracture and, if clinical suspicion is high, it is wise to immobilize the wrist and repeat the X-ray at 2 weeks. If suspicion is still high but the X-rays appear normal, then further imaging should take place. The scaphoid gains its blood supply for the proximal portion through blood vessels that pass from proximal to distal. Thus, a fracture of the scaphoid that crosses the bone in a transverse fashion may disrupt the blood supply and lead to non-union or necrosis of the bone and collapse with subsequent arthritic change.

Ankle fractures

These can involve any portion of the distal tibia or fibula. Technically, the fractures involving the actual articular surface of the distal tibia are known as tibial plafond fractures, whereas fractures involving either the medial or lateral malleoli (and certain combinations of fibula injury) are ankle fractures. The types and classification of ankle fracture are outside the scope of this chapter but, depending on the displacement or the threat to joint stability, will determine whether the fracture can be treated conservatively or requires internal fixation. Conservative treatment will consist of a plaster cast for around 6 weeks. The same length of time would be required for healing to take place, even if the fracture were fixed by internal fixation.

Tibial plateau fractures

These are intra-articular fractures of the knee joint involving the tibial plateau in varying forms. Treatment depends on age, the patient's functional level and the degree of displacement. A large proportion of these fractures will require internal fixation to achieve the best clinical result. Complications include knee stiffness and development of OA. Non-union is unusual, as the tibia at this point is normally well vascularized.

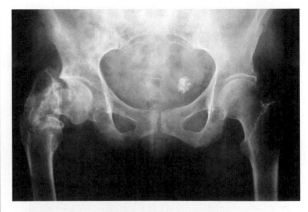

Fig. 31.26   This fracture has healed in a malunited position and would be called a malunion.

Index

Note: Page numbers in italics refer to pictures and diagrams.

B